EXPERT PRAISE FOR
*WHAT YOU NEED TO KNOW ABOUT PSYCHIATRIC DRUGS*

"Psychiatrists should 'prescribe' this book for all their patients taking psychiatric drugs. Just about every conceivable question about the benefits and risks of psychiatric drugs is answered in this book."

John Talbott, M.D.
Chairman, Department of Psychiatry
University of Maryland

"The authors, respected experts in their fields, have provided up-to-date, thorough information in language that is clearly understandable to the public. This is simply the best reference text on psychopharmacology that I have seen for use by both patients and their doctors. *Psychiatric Drugs* performs a much-needed public service in the realm of mental health."

H. Keith H. Brodie, M.D.
Duke Professor of Psychiatry and Law
and President, Duke University

"This user-friendly yet comprehensive guide, illustrated with actual case histories, will be tremendously helpful to consumers and their families."

Laurie Flynn
Executive Director
National Alliance for the Mentally Ill (NAMI)

"This crystal-clear text provides patients and their families with the up-to-date information they are seeking from us to better cope with the stresses of living with psychiatric illness. This text should be required reading for all non-medical students and professionals in mental health practice and will be a tremendous boon to the classroom teacher."

Susan Matorin, M.S., C.S.W., A.C.S.W.
Senior Lecturer, Cornell Medical School
and Director of Social Work,
Payne Whitney Clinic, New York

**Also by Stuart C. Yudofsky, M.D.**

*The Psychiatric Evaluation in Clinical Practice*
(with Roger A. MacKinnon, M.D.)

*Principles of the Psychiatric Evaluation*
(with Roger A. MacKinnon, M.D.)

**Also by Robert E. Hales, M.D.**

*The American Psychiatric Association Annual Review. Volumes 4–8*
(with Allen J. Frances, M.D.)

*Be All That You Can Be: The US Army Total Fitness Program*
(with Diane Hales)

*Textbook of Administrative Psychiatry*
(with John Talbott, M.D. and Stuart Keill, M.D.)

**Also by Stuart C. Yudofsky, M.D., and Robert E. Hales, M.D.**

*The American Psychiatric Press Textbook of Neuropsychiatry, Second Edition*

*The American Psychiatric Press Textbook of Psychiatry*
(with John Talbott, M.D.)

*The Journal of Neuropsychiatry and Clinical Neurosciences*
(editors)

**Also by Tom Ferguson, M.D.**

*Medical Self-Care: Access to Health Tools*

*The People's Book of Medical Tests*
(with David Sobel)

*The Smoker's Book of Health*

*The No-Nag, No-Guilt, Do-It-Your-Own-Way Guide to Quitting Smoking*

*Helping Smokers Get Ready to Quit: A Positive Approach to Smoking Cessation*

*Hidden Guilt: How to Stop Punishing Yourself and Enjoy the Happiness You Deserve*
(with Lewis Engel, Ph.D.)

*The Stethoscope Book & Kit*
(with Linda Allison)

# What You Need to Know About Psychiatric Drugs

**Stuart C. Yudofsky, M.D.**
Professor and Chairman, Department of Psychiatry and Behavioral Sciences
*Baylor College of Medicine*

**Robert E. Hales, M.D.**
Chairman, Department of Psychiatry
*California Pacific Medical Center*

**Tom Ferguson, M.D.**
President, Self-Care Productions
*Austin, Texas*

Ballantine Books    *New York*

Copyright © 1991 by Stuart C. Yudofsky, M.D., Robert E. Hales, M.D., and Tom Ferguson, M.D.

All rights reserved under International and Pan-American Copyright Conventions. Published in the United States by Ballantine Books, a division of Random House, Inc., New York, and distributed in Canada by Random House of Canada Limited, Toronto.

This edition published by arrangement with Grove Weidenfeld, a division of Grove Press, Inc.

Grateful acknowledgment is made for permission to reprint from *An Invitation to Health* (fourth edition) by Diane Hales, copyright © 1989 by Benjamin/Cummings Publishing Company, and for permission to reprint from *American Psychiatric Glossary*, edited by Evelyn M. Stone, copyright © 1988 by American Psychiatric Press.

Library of Congress Catalog Card Number: 91-58327

ISBN: 0-345-37334-0

Cover design by Kristine V. Mills

Manufactured in the United States of America

First Ballantine Books Edition: June 1992

10  9  8  7  6  5  4  3

*No longer silent about our illnesses,*
   *no longer passive in our care.*
*To those among us—and our families—who suffer*
   *from psychiatric disorders.*

# Acknowledgments

IN writing this book we have drawn upon the work of thousands of researchers, teachers, and clinicians. We are well aware of our debt and can only express our sincere gratitude to everyone who has contributed, directly or indirectly, to the extraordinary body of knowledge that comprises contemporary psychopharmacology.

We have been very lucky to have the help of four outstanding colleagues in preparing this manuscript:

• Kevin Sloan, M.D., wrote our chapter on antidepressant drugs while working in close collaboration with the authors as a senior resident in psychiatry at the University of Chicago. He is currently a staff psychiatrist on the faculty of the Albert Einstein Medical Center in Philadelphia.

• Viktoria Erhardt, M.D., wrote our chapter on antipsychotic drugs while working in close collaboration with the authors while a senior resident in psychiatry at the University of Chicago. She is currently a staff psychiatrist on the faculty of Chicago Medical College.

• Terry Hugg, M.D., wrote our chapter on drugs for attention-deficit hyperactivity disorder while working in close collaboration with the authors. Terry, a child psychiatrist, was Director of Education at the Department of Psychiatry, University of Texas School of Medicine, Houston, at the time he wrote the chapter.

• Jonathan Silver, M.D., wrote our chapter on psychiatric drugs of the future while working in close collaboration with the authors. Jon is currently Assistant Professor of Clinical Psychiatry at Columbia University College of Physicians and Surgeons and Director of Neuropsychiatry at Columbia Presbyterian Medical Center.

These four physicians showed extraordinary patience, good humor, and flexibility as they worked with us through countless revisions of their manuscripts.

We thank Ira, Stanley, and Marcia Gumberg—dear friends, bibliophiles, and visionaries in the support for and the development of hospital-based medical services—for their advice, direction, and encouragement in the earliest stages of this project.

We thank particularly Susan Meenan, Executive Director of the National Depressive and Manic Depressive Association; Laura Guilfoyle, Executive Director of the Alliance for Mentally Ill of Greater Chicago; Helen Lockwood, volunteer and long-time member of the Alliance for Mentally Ill of Greater Chicago; and Gwill Newman, who has served as president of the National Alliance for Research on Schizophrenia and Depressive Disorders and as president of the Brain Research Foundation, for their line-by-line review of the text and innumerable corrections and constructive suggestions. As both leaders and representatives of those humanitarian advocates for better care and increased funding for research into mental illnesses, these individuals brought perspectives, information, and experience that we found invaluable.

We also thank Ruth and Dan Edelman, philanthropists and pioneers in mental health advocacy through public relations and political activism. Through their ideas and support, much of this book took shape.

We thank Joy Yudofsky Behr and Dr. Janice Koster, for giving up their summer vacations to proofread the "galley sheets" and for their editorial suggestions throughout each phase of the book's development.

We wish to thank the many academic psychiatrists who have been our teachers and colleagues and our students, who have imparted to us much of the information that is found in this book.

We owe a double thanks to Lewis Engel, Ph.D., who not only offered valuable suggestions on the manuscript but also graciously allowed us to adapt some of the guidelines for finding a therapist he and Tom Ferguson originally developed for the book *Imaginary Crimes* (Boston: Houghton Mifflin, 1989).

We would like to thank Dan Green and Tom Bryan for their special enthusiasm and support for the book.

We are grateful to our gifted, capable, and enthusiastic literary agent, Charlotte Sheedy of the Charlotte Sheedy Literary Agency, who guided us from the initial stages of planning the book and finding a publisher to the final stages of production and publication of the text.

We owe a very special thanks to Bill Strachan and Walt Bode, our editors at Grove Weidenfeld. Bill served as our advocate, collaborator, and chief support person from the very beginning of this project, providing enthusiasm, constructive criticism, and a quiet confidence. His unstinting efforts made this a much better book. Walt joined us later in the project and helped shape the final phases of the book's production.

Our spouses, Beth Yudofsky, Diane Hales, and Meredith Dreiss, have supported this project in a thousand ways, from reading and commenting on the manuscript, to taking on an extra portion of household and parenting tasks, keeping our spirits high, and, when necessary, reminding us that there were other things in life than "the book." None of us could have taken on a work of this magnitude were it not for the solid primary bond we each feel for our respective life partner.

But above all, we would like to express our appreciation and thanks to the thousands of patients—and to the families of patients—we have had the privilege to know and work with. They have gently pointed out our blind spots, and have helped us understand the benefits, hazards, and limitations of drug treatment. Even more important, they have helped us to appreciate the importance of family and group support, self-care, and other nondrug approaches.

# Contents

# Caution to Patients

This book is not designed to replace the interaction between you and your physician. Rather, it is crafted so that you may be an informed and active participant in a constructive and beneficial doctor-patient relationship. Do not take any medications or change the way in which you are taking your medications without the full involvement of your physician.

# Introduction: How to Use This Book

YOU are probably reading this book because you—or a family member or friend—are taking or are considering taking one of the more than a hundred psychiatric prescription drugs now available. Or you may work in a medically related field or be a mental health professional looking for a concise, up-to-date review on the current uses of psychiatric drugs.

This book is *not* designed to replace the interaction between a patient and his or her physician, psychiatrist, or other mental health professional. A person taking a psychiatric drug needs a great deal of information in order to be an active participant in this essential doctor-patient partnership. Indeed, we would hope it would help improve the usefulness of these essential doctor-patient dialogues.

We decided to write this book because we often found it difficult to cover these topics adequately within the limited scope of an office visit: Despite our best attempts to answer the questions asked by our patients and their families, they would frequently have new questions once they had left our offices. Indeed, many questions did not even occur to the patient until he or she had been taking a drug for several days or weeks. It seemed to us that there was a great need for a concise, up-to-date summary of the key points of psychiatric drug use in a form our patients and their families could discuss and review at home. This book is our attempt to provide that information.

## Special Issues Associated with the Use of Psychiatric Drugs

Many people taking psychiatric drugs experience periods of intense psychological turmoil. Some are struggling to combat biological depression. Others are battling one of the schizophrenias. Still others suffer disturbing and disruptive mood swings characteristic of manic-depressive illness. Such psychiatric disorders frequently affect an individual's ability to concentrate, think logically, or trust the recommendations of mental health professionals. It is especially important for people taking psychiatric drugs to have continual access to clear, precise information about any proposed or current medications. We hope that this book will provide people who are currently taking psychiatric drugs with ready access to the information they seek—in a form they can consult during times of reduced stress, decreased anxiety, and heightened attention and concentration.

Psychiatric drugs produce side effects. These can affect every aspect of a person's mental and physical functioning—alertness, attention, coordination, energy level, interpersonal relationships, judgment, mood, sleep patterns, and more. Many people taking these drugs overlook uncomfortable or disabling side effects because they consider them either a part of the original disorder or a necessary part of the treatment. We hope that this book will help patients and their families recognize, manage, and avoid the many side effects these drugs can produce.

In any given year, only about one-fourth of those who suffer from mental illness seek the help of a mental health professional. Many people do not even realize that they have a *treatable* mental illness. We hope that this book will help convince more people that they too could benefit from psychiatric help.

Many of those taking psychiatric drugs become addicted because they did not understand how habit-forming these drugs can be. We hope that this book will help prevent drug addictions. We also hope it will help those who have already become addicted to understand the addictive process and try to overcome their addiction in the safest and most effective ways.

Many individuals hesitate to take a psychiatric drug even though their physicians try to convince them that they would benefit greatly from taking it. Some refuse because they overestimate the risks or underestimate the benefits of the drug. Others have been subjected to injurious, ineffective, or inadequate treatment in the past and are understandably afraid that their unpleasant experiences will be repeated. Still others decline treatment because of the stigma attached to taking a psychiatric medication. In this book, we hope to provide those considering a psychiatric drug with a balanced, realistic view of the benefits and hazards of these medications.

Psychiatric treatments are often more controversial than other medical treatments. Different physicians frequently suggest totally different solutions to the same psychiatric problem. We hope this book will provide an objective second opinion.

Some psychiatric drugs don't begin working right away; others continue to affect us long after we have stopped taking them. We hope this book will help explain the many ways in which persons taking these drugs will benefit from following the recommended dosage regimens.

Many psychiatric drugs are effective only at certain blood levels, and many people taking these drugs don't experience the desired effects because their doses are too high or too low. Lab tests can determine whether a person is getting the right dose. Other tests can detect early signs of harmful side effects. This book will help patients understand the importance of drug monitoring and other laboratory testing for those taking these drugs.

Some psychiatric treatments are either still in the experimental stage or are so new or specialized that most physicians know little about them. This book will provide consumers with guidelines for finding and working with physicians who specialize in the drug treatment of such emotional and behavioral problems as panic disorder, substance abuse, and aggression.

Older people are frequent users of psychiatric drugs, and those over sixtyfive are also particularly vulnerable to their side effects. This book will help older people understand the special benefits and hazards they may encounter in taking these drugs—and the strategies they and their physicians may use to achieve the optimal effects with the lowest risks.

Any licensed physician—or any dentist—can prscribe psychiatric drugs. Although many psychiatrists, family practitioners, internists, and other specialists are highly knowledgeable and skilled in utilizing psychiatric drugs, it is also a fact that many professionals who commonly prescribe psychiatric drugs have little or no special training or up-to-date knowledge base in this area. Some are prescribed inappropriately, while many other useful, safe, and proven psychiatric drugs—especially the antidepressants—are commonly ignored or misused. This book will provide to intelligent consumers and interested mental health professionals alike a balanced, state-of-the-art review of psychiatric drugs.

## Questions to Ask Before Taking Any Psychiatric Drug

- Exactly what *is* the psychological problem that you (or your family member or friend) are facing? Is your problem a sign or a symptom of a medical illness or a primary psychiatric disorder? If it is a psychiatric disorder, what is the official American Psychiatric Association diagnosis of your condition?
- What are the most effective nondrug therapies for this condition?
- Can a psychiatric prescription drug help to alleviate, manage, or solve this problem?
- Can nondrug therapies be used instead of drug therapy? Can they be used as a supplement to drug therapy?
- What are the positive (therapeutic) effects this drug may provide?
- How likely is it that this drug actually *will* provide these effects?
- How does this drug work? Exactly where in my body does it achieve its therapeutic effects?
- Which side effects can this drug produce? Which are rare and which are common? Which are harmless and which can be truly dangerous? Which are reversible and which can be permanent?
- Does my age, my physical condition, or any preexisting medical illness present special problems or require any special precautions?
- Can this drug interact with any other food, drug, or other substance? Can it interact with any other drugs I am taking?
- Which medical examinations or tests will be necessary before I begin taking this drug? Will I need to have any regular physical examinations and laboratory tests while I am taking this medication?
- Under which conditions should I check back with the mental health professional who prescribed this drug?
- How do I know that this drug is working? How long does it take to achieve its effects?
- How long should I continue to take this drug?
- Are there particular times (e.g., with meals, before sleeping) when I should take this drug?
- How should I take and store this drug? Do I need to take special precautions to keep others from using or abusing this drug?
- Can this drug lose its effect while I am taking it?
- What will I do if the drug does not work? Are there other drugs that can be added to the first one to make it work better? Are there other classes of drugs that might also be helpful if this drug doesn't work?

• How long should I stay on this drug after my psychiatric symptoms go away?

• Is it likely that I will become addicted to this drug?

• Are there any special precautions that must be taken while discontinuing this drug? Can I discontinue the drug suddenly or is it necessary to reduce my dosage gradually? Is there any chance that I will experience withdrawal effects when I stop taking this drug?

• If my psychiatric symptoms recur after I stop taking this drug, will the same drug at the same dose be effective in the future?

• How can I find out if any new, safer, more specific, or more effective drug approaches have been discovered to treat my psychiatric disorder?

• Under which conditions should I stop taking this drug?

• How much does this drug cost? Is it available in a less expensive form? Is there a less expensive drug that can provide the same or similar benefits?

• Is there anything else I should know before I fill my prescription for this drug?

The answers to these questions can be found in the chapters that follow, but we hope that you will consider your reading of this book as the beginning, not the end, of your efforts to familiarize yourself with your problem and the remedies available.

The aim of *What You Need to Know About Psychiatric Drugs* is to provide relevant and easy-to-understand information for those people and their families who are now taking or considering the use of psychiatric drugs. We also have endeavored to craft a book that is easy to use. As physicians and psychiatrists, we are aware that different people learn and access information in different ways; we have tried to take these differences into account in devising the book's format.

People who are *visual learners* prefer terse summaries in which the most important information is highlighted in charts and special type. Others understand best from real-life examples or stories such as the case histories in this book. Others like the logical, systematic presentation of information that characterizes most well-wrought textbooks. We have used all of these formats and several more to accommodate most readers—especially those of us who like a combination of learning formats. The examples below can serve as representative guidelines about the many ways in which *What You Need to Know About Psychiatric Drugs* may be used.

**Q.** *My son has just been diagnosed as having schizophrenia. His doctor has prescribed Thorazine. How do I know that he is on the right drug and what the risks and side effects of this drug are?*

**A.** First, look up schizophrenia in the index, which will refer you to p. 167, where the characteristics of this disorder are reviewed. We have endeavored to provide clear descriptions of each major psychiatric illness for which medications are used. If the signs and symptoms that your son exhibits match the description and diagnostic features of schizophrenia, you may also wish to read the representative case history of a person suffering from schizophrenia on p. 170. Usually, by this point, you will recognize clearly the diagnosis and characteristic features. If the descriptions of schizophrenia in the book do not match the clinical picture of your son, we recommend you discuss this discrepancy with his psychiatrist.

Second, look up Thorazine in the index of the book. The index will refer you to p. 197 in Chapter 7 on antipsychotics, where you will learn that this is the trade name for chlorpromazine, as well as to its listing on p. 409 in the Individual Drug Listings. You will learn that it is one of many medications used to treat schizophrenia and other illnesses that involve psychosis. The benefits, risks, side effects, and many other important clinical features of Thorazine will be described in both Chapter 7 and the Individual Drug Listings.

**Q.** *Two weeks ago, my family practitioner placed me on the antidepressant Elavil. My vision has become blurred—especially when I read the newspaper. My ophthalmologist checked my eyes and said they're okay. Can this problem possibly be due to the drug?*

**A.** Look up Elavil in the index of the book. You will be referred to Chapter 3 on antidepressants, where you will learn that this is the trade name for the drug amitriptyline—to p. 43, where side effects are discussed, as well as to p. 381 of the Individual Drug Listings, where side effects of this medication also are listed. Both sections will indicate that blurred vision is an early-onset side effect of most heterocyclic antidepressants—including Elavil. You will be advised of the implications of this side effect, whether the side effect is permanent or reversible, whether or not to inform your doctor, and how to deal with the problem.

**Q.** *I am a recovering alcoholic who attends Alcoholics Anonymous. Although I have been successful for three years in not drinking alcohol, I still feel sad much of the time. I have problems falling asleep and staying asleep, and I have lost fifteen pounds over the past year without dieting. I think I may be depressed. I would like to know more about* *depression—particularly if antidepressants really work and if there is a danger that I will become addicted to them.*

A. Although this book is designed to be used in collaboration with your physician and mental health professional and although one must be warned against making diagnoses for oneself (even mental health professionals themselves must avoid this dangerous pitfall), this book contains a wealth of information about mental illness and its treatment. It is intended to be a good resource about how to approach seeking professional help and how to evaluate the quality of that help once you get it.

First, look up depression in the index, which will refer you to Chapter 3 on antidepressants. The characteristic signs and symptoms of depression are listed on p. 21. You will also find the case study of Carl in Chapter 3 and you will likely find that your symptoms are consistent with his.

Next, read in Chapter 3 about antidepressants to learn whether or not you feel you should discuss this option with a psychiatrist.

The addictive potentials of all psychiatric drugs are discussed in the respective chapters (in this case, Chapter 3, p. 42), as well as in the Individual Drug Listings.

Q. *My pediatrician has prescribed the drug Ritalin for my nine-year-old son. I would like a second opinion from a psychiatrist. How do I find a qualified psychiatrist, and what questions should I ask him or her about the drug?*

A. First, look up the drug Ritalin in the index. You will be referred to Chapter 10, where you will find that this is the trade name for methylphenidate, as well as to p. 502 of the Individual Drug Listings, where the uses, risks, and benefits of this drug are described in detail.

Next, read in Chapter 10 about the characteristic features of attention-deficit hyperactivity disorder (ADHD)—the most common condition for which this drug is prescribed. There is extensive information about the appropriate use of Ritalin in children in the context of a comprehensive treatment plan.

Finally, beginning on pp. xvi and xviii read thoroughly *all* the points raised under Special Issues Associated with the Use of Psychiatric Drugs and Questions to Ask Before Taking Any Psychiatric Drug.

Q. *I am a psychiatric social worker, and I wish to learn more about the use and misuse of psychiatric drugs. Can this book be of help?*

**A.** This book is an up-to-date data-based resource. Much of the relevant information found in the chapter on psychopharmacology in our textbook *The American Psychiatric Press Textbook of Psychiatry* is covered in this book. We endeavored to keep the format and content both clear and interesting, so that the book could be read cover to cover and remain stimulating and nonrepetitive. You may, however, wish to read a chapter that pertains to a specific patient with particular symptoms (e.g., panic attacks) to gauge whether psychiatric medications may be indicated or should be considered as a component of a comprehensive treatment plan.

First, look up panic in the index. There, you will be referred to Chapter 5 on antipanic and antiphobic drugs. You may wish to read this chapter for an update on biological perspectives of panic.

You will note in Chapter 5 that antidepressants are often used, and that alcohol and antianxiety drugs are often misused in the treatment of panic. You may also wish to refer to Chapter 3 on antidepressant drugs and Chapter 9 on antiaddiction drugs as you consider your treatment plan.

Finally, you may wish to consider sharing this information with your client by suggesting that he or she read specific sections of this book, which has been devised to be safe and useful for patients and their families. Thereafter, you may consider reviewing, together in the treatment setting, the ideas and options presented in the book.

We hope that you will discuss your conclusions, concerns, and further questions with your physician. Repeat this process as appropriate, consulting both this book and your doctor. You may also wish to consult some of the books or groups mentioned in the following chapters.

You will be able to develop a more sophisticated understanding of your condition and will be much better prepared to play an active role in managing it. More important than the most effective drug are caring, responsible, motivated, well-informed networks of patients, family, health-care professionals, and friends playing active roles in managing their own problems.

Those who suffer from psychiatric illnesses have many opportunities for improvement and recovery, and it is our hope that this book will become yet another useful resource.

Stuart C. Yudofsky, M.D.
Robert E. Hales, M.D.
Tom Ferguson, M.D.

# PART I

# Basic Information

# Chapter 1

# The Age of Psychiatric Drugs

APPROXIMATELY one of every three people will suffer from a mental illness at some point in life. Over the last forty years, we have seen a revolution in psychiatry's effectiveness as many mental illnesses have been treated with drugs.

A few decades ago, people with severe psychiatric illnesses were routinely relegated to a lifetime of emotional torment, social stigma, and lengthy incarceration in state mental institutions. The use of new psychiatric drugs and other innovative treatments have reduced the number of mentally ill in institutions by more than 50 percent. Psychiatric medications have brought new hope for individuals with depression, manic depression, schizophrenia, and many other types of mental illness. Psychiatric drugs are now among the most commonly prescribed of all medications. Within the last few years, researchers have developed new drug treatments for anxiety attacks, attention-deficit hyperactivity disorders, alcoholism and other chemical dependencies, aggressive disorders, dementias, eating disorders, pain syndromes, panic disorders, phobias, sleep disorders, and many other mental and emotional problems. And researchers are working to discover more specific and effective psychiatric drugs for the future.

3

## The Humane Treatment of Mental Illness

For most of human history, people with mental problems were subject to ostracism, stigmatization, and physical persecution. It was not uncommon for people with auditory or visual hallucinations to be labeled witches or demons and put to death. By the 1850s, physicians began to consider mental problems as types of illnesses. They joined together with family members of the mentally ill to wrest the "treatment" of the emotionally disabled away from the religious and legal authorities. Up to that time, there was only one legal classification of mental illness: idiocy.

By the turn of the century, the early psychiatrists had described more than a dozen different mental illnesses. This enabled clinicians to offer more specific treatments and more accurately predict likely outcomes. But there was little agreement as to the criteria for establishing a diagnosis. Until very recently, the same patient might be diagnosed by one physician as having manic-depressive illness and by another as having schizophrenia. It was not until 1980 that psychiatrists, with the publication of the American Psychiatric Association's *Diagnostic and Statistical Manual III* (DSM III), agreed on a unified system for classifying mental illnesses.

## The Understanding of Brain Chemistry

Over the past two decades, we have begun to learn a sufficient amount about the brain—and about what happens in mental illness—to provide the basis for such a unified system of diagnosis. The human brain is the most complex entity in the observable universe. Hundreds of billions of small nerve cells called neurons communicate with each other by releasing tiny quantities of chemicals, called neurotransmitters. Among the most important known neurotransmitters are norepinephrine, epinephrine, dopamine, serotonin, gamma-aminobutyric acid (GABA), and acetylcholine.

Our most critical physical and mental capacities depend on an orderly system of chemical communication among the neurons of our brain. However, these communications can be disrupted by many factors including physical injury, poisons, abused substances like drugs and alcohol, infections, cancer, neurologic disorders, or psychological stress. These and a variety of other stressors produce changes in our brain chemistry and physiology. Often changes that result in mental illness occur only in the brains of those with genetic predispositions to a particular mental illness. In some cases, psychiatric drugs can help restore mental health by affecting the number or activity of these neurotransmitters and/or the brain receptors on which they act.

## The Classification of Mental Illness

Ironically, one of the most important advances in the age of psychiatric drugs was not a discovery or a drug. It was a book—the result of hundreds of thousands of hours of labor by hundreds of different researchers, clinicians, and other mental health professionals; it is the ultimate expression of the long-awaited unified system for the classification of mental illness. This book, published by the American Psychiatric Association under the title *Diagnostic and Statistical Manual*, has revolutionized the practice of psychiatric diagnosis and treatment. The most recent edition, published in 1987 and titled *Diagnostic and Statistical Manual, Third Edition-Revised*, is universally and fondly referred to by practitioners and researchers as the DSM-III-R.

In the DSM-III-R, mental disorders are described as psychological patterns that cause distress or disability in one or more important areas of functioning: on the job, in school, or in social or family life. The manual defines the specific clusters of signs, symptoms, and history that experts currently use to diagnose each specific mental illness. It emphasizes the importance of using specific signs and symptoms, as opposed to older diagnostic methods, which were based on speculation and theories as to the possible causes of the disorder.

The DSM-III-R and its predecessors have provided mental health professionals with much more precise guidelines for making a psychiatric diagnosis. The standards it has set have led to enhanced communication between research scientists, clinicians, patients, and family members. And it provides a mechanism by which our diagnostic and classification systems can be revised and improved as our knowledge increases. Currently, teams of psychiatrists and scientists are working on the next update of this diagnostic system, the DSM-IV, to be published in 1992.

Thus, the conditions discussed in this book adhere closely to the classification system used in the DSM-III-R. For each mental illness, we provide and discuss the specific DSM-III-R criteria used to diagnose it. A listing of all conditions described in the DSM-III-R appears in the Appendix.

The DSM-III-R also makes it clear that certain conditions should *not* be labeled as mental disease. These include:

• The expected, reasonable, and self-limiting reactions to unfortunate life events, such as intense feelings of grief or sadness associated with the death of a loved one, the fear associated with exposure to dangerous situations, or the psychological trauma that may follow an assault, illness, or injury.

• The usual variances that are found in human expressions, reactions, and political or religious choices. It is thus important to remember that persons who have political, religious, or attitudinal disagreements with their mental health professionals, their community, or with their government do not necessarily have a mental illness.

It will never be an easy task for anyone, whether mental health professional, layperson, lawyer, or judge, to decide what behaviors are the true signs of a mental disorder and which are simply a normal and expected response to external stimuli or an expression of individual style, preference, or belief. But, thanks to the DSM-III-R, we now enjoy the highest degree of professional and lay agreement ever about what a mental disorder is.

# Chapter 2

# Frequently Asked Questions About Psychiatric Drugs

**Q.** *Is mental illness hereditary?*

**A.** While not every mental disorder is genetically transmitted, many of our most common and disabling mental illnesses have hereditary features. A predisposition for a variety of mental illnesses can be genetically transmitted from generation to generation. This means that if you have certain kinds of mental illnesses—mood disorder, panic disorder, phobia, manic-depressive illness, schizophrenia, obsessive-compulsive personality disorder, and perhaps even alcoholism—your children and grandchildren will be at greater risk of developing the same mental illness you have than the children and grandchildren of a person who does not have a family history of that mental illness.

However, this does not mean that the disease itself is inevitable. For example, Mary Blake may inherit a predisposition to depression, which will appear only as the result of severe psychological stress. Thus a given level of stress may trigger depression in Mary but not in her sister Joan, who did not inherit that characteristic. In other cases, an inherited condition may express itself regardless of circumstance. Thus, a good family history is always an important part of any psychiatric interview.

We routinely take a detailed family history of psychiatric and other medical disorders for every patient whom we see. This often proves extremely helpful in understanding and diagnosing an individual's psychiatric conditions, and it frequently helps us to identify other family members who may also benefit from treatment. If Mike Schultz, who is suffering from depression, tells us that his mother also experienced periods of depression and was treated effectively with a particular antidepressant drug, it may well be a good idea for Mike to take the same drug.

Even though some mental illnesses have an inheritable component, you should not necessarily assume that your children or grandchildren will inherit it. It is possible, for example, for people with manic-depressive illness *not* to transmit the illness or even the predisposition to the illness to any of their offspring. On the other hand, it is entirely possible for people to pass on a genetic predisposition for a mental illness even though they themselves never experienced any symptoms of that mental illness.

In each chapter of this book we have included information about the hereditary aspects of the mental disorders that are discussed. Many of our patients do worry that they might pass their mental disorder on to their children. If you or a member of your family has an emotional or mental illness and has questions about the implications of this illness for the children, grandchildren, or other relatives, we suggest you consult a psychiatrist familiar with the biologic aspects of mental disorders. By obtaining accurate information about the chances of transmitting your illness to your children, you will be able to make informed decisions about family planning. If there is a chance that a condition might be passed on in this way, you may want to ask your doctor how to detect and treat the early signs of these conditions. Our patients are usually reassured by the statistical data we provide, and they are comforted by the good news that, even if the illness is transmitted to their children, there are almost always safe and effective treatments available.

**Q.** *What are psychiatric drugs? How are they usually taken?*

**A.** A psychiatric drug is any drug that has been proved safe and effective in the treatment of a mental disorder as defined by the DSM-III-R. We have also included information about drugs that are useful in treating disabling symptoms associated with such mental disorders as agitation, irritability, anxiety, and insomnia.

The vast majority of psychiatric drugs are taken orally in tablet, capsule, or liquid form. A few drugs may, on occasion, be given by injection—either into a muscle or directly into the bloodstream. It may well be that in the future, some drugs will be introduced directly into the brain.

**Q.** *Who can prescribe psychiatric drugs?*

**A.** Any physician (M.D. or D.O.) or dentist who is licensed to prescribe drugs can legally prescribe psychiatric drugs. Psychiatric drugs are commonly prescribed by many different kinds of physicians: general practitioners, family physicians, pediatricians, specialists in internal medicine, and physicians from other specialties. In most cases, the physicians who have the most training and experience in prescribing psychiatric drugs are psychiatrists, family practitioners, and specialists in internal medicine.

Psychiatrists are physicians who specialize in the assessment and treatment of people with mental illnesses. For the past decade, most psychiatric training has included extensive emphasis on the appropriate, safe, and effective use of psychiatric drugs. Psychiatrists who have completed three years of approved postgraduate psychiatric residency training and have passed an extensive battery of rigorous tests of their skills and knowledge in psychiatry receive a special certificate certifying them as *board certified* in psychiatry.

Many capable and experienced therapists—psychologists, social workers, and other mental health professionals who do not have medical degrees and who therefore cannot prescribe drugs—work in close collaboration with psychiatrists when one of their clients requires a medication. In many such cases, the client continues to see his or her regular therapist, but, in addition, occasionally sees the psychiatrist to make sure that the drug he or she is taking is working effectively, that no dangerous side effects are emerging, and that other medical illnesses do not complicate the condition.

As we will see in the chapters that follow, it sometimes requires great expertise to choose the right dose of the right drug for a given individual. This expertise can only be gained through extensive experience. Although two of us (Yudofsky and Hales) specialize in the use of drugs in the treatment of psychiatric illness, we regularly seek the advice of other professionals who have greater expertise in specialized areas. Such consultations can be especially useful when a patient's illness has not responded to the usual treatment or when a side effect becomes particularly bothersome.

**Q.** *How can I find a psychiatrist who is experienced in prescribing psychiatric drugs?*

**A.** One of the best ways is to ask your family practitioner for a referral to such a psychiatrist. You should feel free to ask the psychiatrist how frequently he or she uses drugs to treat patients with similar problems. But you should not automatically assume that the psychiatrist will determine that drugs are the answer for your particular problem. He or she may well suggest individual or group psychotherapy or some specialized type of counseling instead of or in addition to drug treatment.

The psychiatrist you seek may be identified as a biologically oriented psychiatrist, a psychopharmacologist, or simply as a psychiatrist with a great deal of experience and competence in the use of psychiatric drugs.

Other ways to obtain a referral:

• Ask your local mental health society or mental health association.

• Call your local medical school or your local hospital or medical center's department of psychiatry and ask to be referred to an expert or subspecialist in the use of psychiatric drugs.

• Call the nearest office of the American Psychiatric Association to ask for a referral. For the address and phone number of the nearest office, contact the national office:

**American Psychiatric Association**
1400 K Street, N.W.
Washington, D.C. 20005
(202) 682-6000

• There are special benefits in seeking a referral to a recommended psychiatrist through one of the many self-help advocacy groups for the mentally ill. For information on finding the right self-help group, please refer to the next question.

**Q.** *I would love to get some advice from other people who have successfully dealt with a similar problem. Is there any way I can do this?*

**A.** Yes, and we strongly suggest that you do so. There are an estimated 500,000 active self-help groups in the United States alone. Many of these specialize in the same mental health problems we cover in this book. These groups can help you find a psychiatrist who is an expert in your particular area of concern. They can also provide other vital information, literature, and support.

Ask your mental health professional to refer you to the appropriate advocacy group in your area.

**Q.** *How do I find the right mental health professional?*

**A.** Finding the right mental health professional is like finding a good pair of running shoes: (1) You shouldn't necessarily accept the first pair you are offered. (2) Just because they are expensive doesn't mean they are the best. (3) If they don't feel comfortable, they are definitely not for you.

Once you obtain your list of recommended experts, it is important that you make your own final decision about choosing a mental health professional. We suggest that you ask yourself the following questions about your present—or your prospective—professional therapist:

• Do I feel safe? Do I feel that I can tell this person my deepest thoughts, fantasies, and fears? Or does he or she seem somehow disrespectful, unreliable, distant, harsh, critical, or judgmental? (Your therapist should make you feel safe and hopeful, not tense and frightened.)

• Do I feel understood? Does the professional really listen to the details of my predicament? Does he or she really seem interested in understanding and helping me? Or does he or she seem more interested in retaining control, demonstrating expertise, or plugging me into some set psychological theory? Do I feel my professional understands what I am going through? (A professional who can't understand your predicament is unlikely to be of much help.)

• As a result of my initial meeting or meetings with my professional, do I feel at least a bit better about myself? Do I feel a bit less anxious, less guilty, less depressed, more hopeful, or more clear?

• After discussing my problem with my professional, do I feel that I understand the nature of my psychiatric problem—and the pain and limitations it is causing—somewhat better?

• Do I fully agree with and support the treatment plan my professional has proposed? Do I fully understand and support the therapies he or she has chosen?

• Do I feel some sense of excitement about my progress? Do I feel that I have been making reasonable progress and have a reasonable chance of making steady and rapid progress in the future?

• Does my mental health professional have my full confidence and trust?

If your answer to any of these questions is *no* or even *maybe*, we would strongly suggest seeking a second opinion from another qualified mental health professional. All too frequently we are consulted by people who have spent many years seeing a mental health professional who has made them feel uncomfortable (or in the case of unethical therapists, "too comfortable" in the early stages of treatment). In many such cases, the treatment has gone on and on with no clear treatment plan and no progress. When we ask those people why they waited so long before seeking a second opinion, they usually tell us they blamed themselves or didn't trust their own feelings. You should *always* pay attention to your feelings and instincts—and those of your friends and family—in choosing a mental health professional.

If, when you raise the topic of getting a second opinion, you experience any resistance at all from your current mental health professional, this is often a good indication that you are with the wrong person. A competent mental health practitioner never feels threatened and will almost always benefit from the advice and counsel of a competent professional colleague.

**Q.** *Has it ever been scientifically proved that psychiatric drugs really work?*

**A.** The answer to this question is a resounding yes. All the major classes of drugs discussed in this book—antidepressant agents, antianxiety agents, antipsychotic agents, lithium, and many others—have been found safe and effective by a variety of well-controlled scientific studies. In these studies, the drugs were compared with placebos (pills containing no active ingredients) in situations in which neither the patient, the physician, nor the researcher knew which subjects were receiving the drug and which were receiving a placebo—a so-called double-blind trial. As a result, psychiatric drugs—when used appropriately—are among the safest and most effective drugs currently in use.

**Q.** *Do psychiatric drugs just cover up an emotional problem, or can they really treat the underlying condition?*

**A.** It is important to distinguish between controlling a symptom, reversing the underlying condition temporarily, and reversing that underlying condition permanently. Some psychiatric drugs help control symptoms, while others reverse the underlying disorder as long as the person continues to take the drug. Many drugs do both.

Few, if any, drugs can permanently reverse an underlying condition. However, by relieving a problem temporarily, a drug may make it easier for the body's own natural processes to restore permanently normal functioning.

The antidepressants provide a good example: in addition to treating the specific symptoms of depression (e.g., sadness, fatigue, guilt, suicidal thoughts, inability to experience pleasure), antidepressants can also reverse the altered brain chemistry that produces these signs and symptoms. Antidepressants cannot change the genes that make a person susceptible to depression. Treatment with an antidepressant will usually result in long periods (i.e., many years) when a patient is free from depression—even though the medication has been discontinued.

**Q.** *Are psychiatric drugs addictive?*

**A.** Many psychiatric drugs are *not* habit-forming. Others can be powerfully addictive. The following drugs are unlikely to be addictive: antidepressants, antimanic agents, and antipsychotic agents. The following drugs can be addictive: antianxiety agents (including the benzodiazepines), most sedative agents (particularly barbiturates), and many analgesics (particularly the opiates). Stimulants may be addictive in people who are *not* being treated for attention-deficit hyperactivity disorder.

We provide information on the addictive potential of each category of drug discussed in this book. For those agents that can lead to dependency, we provide precise instructions about how to avoid or reduce dependency.

**Q.** *Are antidepressant drugs similar to such "uppers" as amphetamines, alcohol, and cocaine? Do they produce highs or euphoria?*

**A.** More than 99 percent of the antidepressants currently prescribed by psychiatrists are not stimulants or uppers. These antidepressants elevate the mood only in those people who are suffering from depression. They would have little or no mood-elevating effect in a nondepressed individual. People do not request or crave higher doses of antidepressants as they do with most addictive drugs. Antidepressants are not addictive and are rarely abused—even by those individuals who are highly prone to substance abuse.

Other drugs, such as amphetamines, alcohol, and cocaine (which are not antidepressants), may temporarily elevate mood, but are also likely to produce addiction. The mood-elevating effects of these drugs typically occur only the first few times a person takes the drug. Larger or more regular doses are then required to reproduce the initial high. After sustained use of these agents, no mood-elevating effect occurs, and the person must take large amounts of the drug in order not to feel the pain and anxiety associated with drug withdrawal.

**Q.** *Isn't taking a psychiatric drug like using a crutch?*

**A.** We are often asked whether psychiatric drugs prevent people from dealing directly with their problems. Some patients say they believe that taking a psychiatric drug constitutes "giving up" or "not fighting the problem directly." We disagree.

Overcoming any problem, particularly a psychiatric illness, requires enormous will and fight on the part of the individual—whether a drug is used or not. Sometimes people with a severe emotional illness (e.g., biochemical depression) will *not* be able to deal with their life problems effectively until the biological components of their illness are treated with psychiatric drugs.

We must emphasize again that psychiatric drugs alone are rarely sufficient to overcome the many dimensions of emotional illnesses. They should be considered as just one of many parts in a multiple-strategy treatment plan in which the final goal is to work through the emotional disorder.

We thus encourage our patients to think of psychiatric drugs as tools rather than as crutches. Refusing to use an effective psychiatric drug to treat an emotional or mental problem is like refusing to use a hammer to build a house. Psychiatric drugs can enable you now and again to use your own initiative, ability, and effort to overcome your illness.


**Q.** *Do some psychiatric drugs have dangerous side effects?*

**A.** All drugs prescribed by physicians produce results other than those for which they are prescribed. Such actions are called side effects. Some disturbing and bothersome side effects (e.g., dry mouth, dizziness, constipation) frequently occur with the use of psychiatric drugs—particularly during the first few days or weeks of treatment. Some side effects can actually be beneficial. Others are harmless but mildly distracting. Some can be dangerous. A few can be life-threatening.

When people first begin taking antidepressants, they will typically experience the sedative side effects of the drug for several days before they first notice the antidepressant effects. This may well help them overcome their insomnia and may alleviate the feelings of anxiety that are often associated with depression. Once the depression has been effectively treated, the associated symptoms of anxiety and insomnia are reversed by mechanisms entirely distinct from sedation.

A conscientious physician never recommends a psychiatric drug without first considering the potential side effects it may produce in that particular patient. Physician and patient should discuss these matters frankly before they agree on a treatment. The physician must clearly explain both the potential benefits *and the risks* of any recommended drug. The patient and the patient's family may then make an informed decision about whether or not to accept the recommendation.

By meticulous physical evaluation, precise selection of the drug, careful adjusting of the dose, and comprehensive follow-up, your physician should almost always be able to prevent the occurrence of dangerous side effects.

In the chapters that follow, we have attempted to describe the most common side effects for each category of psychiatric drugs. We have also explained how to recognize these side effects and how to treat them if they should occur.

**Q.** *Will I still feel like myself if I take a psychiatric drug?*

**A.** It is mental illness, not psychiatric drugs, that causes people to feel different, unusual, or unlike themselves. The purpose of a psychiatric drug is to help an individual to return to his or her normal state of feeling, functioning, self-esteem, and self-expression. Thus, if a psychiatric drug is working correctly, it should make you feel much *more* like yourself.

If you find that you do *not* feel like yourself after taking a psychiatric drug, you should contact your psychiatrist or prescribing physician immediately. Explain exactly what you are experiencing and ask your doctor whether you should (1) reduce your dose or (2) discontinue the drug.

**Q.** *Are psychiatric drugs expensive?*

**A.** Psychiatric drugs range from inexpensive to very expensive, but if a drug is really needed, it is usually worth the cost. Most studies show that psychiatric drugs are the single most important factor in reducing the overall cost of mental illness—to the individual, the family, and society. Deciding *not* to use a particular psychiatric drug when it is truly needed may be the most expensive and pain-producing decision that you can make.

Prices of drugs may vary substantially from place to place and in the years to come. In many cases, you and your physician will face a choice between some drugs that are less expensive and others that are more expensive. In some cases, the drug you need may be available in a less expensive generic form. Do not hesitate to ask your doctor if there is an equally effective but less expensive alternative.

**Q.** *Why don't I believe you when you say a psychiatric drug will help me?*

**A.** Feelings of hopelessness, self-doubt, lowered self-esteem, pessimism, and difficulty in trusting others are common symptoms of many psychiatric illnesses. Effective physicians are usually able to combine their scientific knowledge with their interpersonal skills to create a level of confidence sufficient to encourage a patient to try a potentially helpful drug. Family members, support groups, and client advocates can also reverse the doubts and distrust that are components of many mental illnesses. We encourage you to acknowledge and discuss all your feelings—including your fears and your doubts—with your family, your friends, your self-help group, your mental health professional, and your whole treatment team. We would also encourage you to read widely about your condition and the various treatments available. With the possible exception of life-threatening conditions, a responsible professional will propose alternatives, answer your questions, and support your own choices as to treatment. The more you know about your condition, the greater the contribution you can make to your own care.

**Q.** *Should I tell my employer that I am taking a psychiatric drug?*

**A.** Greater numbers of enlightened employers are realizing that psychiatric disorders are no different from other medical illnesses and should not be associated with stigma, shame, or embarrassment. Nonetheless, we all live in the real world, and each situation must be judged individually.

Some psychiatric drugs can affect an individual's ability to handle hazardous equipment, and this must be considered in a decision about whether or not to inform your employer. Most psychiatrists and other mental health professionals are experienced in counseling individuals about such decisions. Such discussions should be an integral part of your relationship with your mental health professional.

It may occasionally be necessary to seek the counsel of an attorney or other appropriate counselor in the job setting to make sure that your rights are not violated. Employers must recognize that it is, for the most part, people with *untreated* psychiatric illnesses, not those receiving effective, medically supervised treatment, who should be of most concern.

**Q.** *What do I do if the psychiatric drug doesn't work?*

**A.** If an initial treatment with a psychiatric drug is not effective, there are almost always other effective drugs to try. Two of us (Yudofsky and Hales) spend a great deal of time providing second opinions and professional consultations for patients who have not responded to the usual treatments with psychiatric drugs. In most of these cases, these treatments were appropriately conceived and carried out, but the patient did not improve. Nonetheless, we are almost always able to suggest alternative approaches and, if these also prove ineffective, alternatives to our alternatives.

We are able, in the end, to recommend effective drugs to nearly all patients whose prior treatment with drugs was unsuccessful. A useful rule of thumb is that if you have a psychiatric illness that is known to respond to psychiatric drugs, do not become discouraged if the first, second, or even the third drug regimen does not prove effective.

The fact that a drug does not produce the desired results does not necessarily mean that the physician who prescribed the drugs is at fault. The inherent complexity of the human brain is such that one cannot always predict which of the many available drugs may prove effective for a given individual. With each unsuccessful trial of a new drug, your physician will learn more and more about the way your illness responds to treatment. The next drug should have an even greater likelihood of working.

You should not be discouraged if your initial trial of drug therapy is unsuccessful. However, if you lose confidence in your physician, do not hesitate to seek out a second opinion from a competent psychiatrist experienced in the use of psychiatric drugs.

**Q.** *What can be done about the stigma associated with mental illness?*

**A.** The more we have come to understand the biological processes that contribute to mental illness, the less stigma our society has attached to these conditions. Both epilepsy and Parkinson's disease were originally considered the results of moral depravity. We now accept them as straightforward neurological disorders. Thus the stigma, embarrassment, and guilt in patients with seizure disorders and Parkinson's disease have been dramatically reduced.

The same thing is now happening with mental disease. As we have learned more and more about the biological bases of these conditions, there has been less and less social stigma attached to them. In addition, the growing number of support groups and advocacy groups for the mentally ill (patients, family members, and mental health professionals) has become our strongest and most hopeful weapon against the fear, prejudices, and misinformation that are the foundations of these outmoded attitudes.

**Q.** *Why do I feel so alone in dealing with my mental illness?*

**A.** You may feel alone, but the fact is that you are *not* alone. Feeling alone is a common symptom of many emotional illnesses. In the past, the social stigma and the accompanying embarrassment and guilt about emotional illnesses drove many people to conceal these difficulties. Today, self-help and advocacy groups provide a powerful network of information and support for the mentally ill and their families. We have repeatedly found that patients who involve themselves with these groups benefit greatly and experience a speedier and more successful recovery.

Two of the largest and most effective of these groups are the National Alliance of the Mentally Ill and the National Depressive and Manic Depressive Association. Founded in 1979 by 254 people, the National Alliance of the Mentally Ill (NAMI) currently has more than 150,000 members, 11,000 affiliate groups, and coalitions operating in all fifty states. Members of NAMI are the relatives and friends of people with serious mental illnesses, people who suffer from mental disorders, and many concerned professionals. NAMI operates a toll free HELPLINE where people can get answers to questions about mental illness and information about affiliate groups and other services. They offer self help including ongoing meetings for people with mental illnesses and their families where they can share concerns, learn more about psychiatric disorders and receive practical advice on insurance, medical treatment, housing, employment, and community services. Also offered is public education which can help reduce the stigma that so typically surrounds mental illness as well as advocacy at federal, state, and local levels to help bring about improved services and increased funding through research related to mental illness. NAMI can be reached by dialing 1-800-950-NAMI. The National Depressive and Manic Depressive Association (NDMDA) also began in the 1970s, and today has 250 chapters worldwide and more than 35,000 active members.

New alliances between advocacy groups and mental health professionals are among the most important and encouraging of all current developments in the entire mental health field. Such alliances are becoming stronger with each passing day and are already exercising significant political clout at national and local levels. It is our hope that through the combined efforts of advocacy groups and professional societies such as the American Psychiatric Association, the American Psychological Association, the National Association of Social Workers, the National Institute of Mental Health, and many others, we will be able to ensure increased funding for clinical services and for research related to the problems and needs of the emotionally ill. Working together, we can make great strides toward the day when the loneliness and isolation experienced by those with mental problems— like the shame and secrecy once associated with neurological illness— will be considered an unfortunate historical aspect of our distant past.

# PART II

# Categories of Psychiatric Drugs

# Chapter 3

# Antidepressant Drugs

WE all know what some aspects of depression feel like. Everybody feels sadness and discouragement after a death, a divorce, a serious illness, or a major disappointment. We feel exhausted, empty, incapable of dealing with one more thing and, often, more than one thing. This is a natural, healthy, and understandable response.

However, we may sometimes experience these same hopeless, discouraged feelings when we have had no recent trauma, no sudden loss. Or we may be plagued by relentless sadness and pervasive gloom that seem out of all proportion to the events that may have triggered such. At last, after all our efforts to ignore or deny these feelings, we must finally admit it: We are feeling depressed.

Depression is the state of feeling despondent, cheerless, gloomy, glum, low-down, blue, unhappy, out of sorts, discouraged, lifeless, or vaguely sad for no apparent reason. We feel empty, defeated, spent. We seem to have lost all our old energy, all our old faith in ourselves. Even if we tell ourselves that things will feel better tomorrow, the next day things seem even worse.

Our despondency may grow deeper and deeper until it is an inescapable bottomless pit: The whole world seems barren and empty. We toss and turn all night. We often awaken hours before daylight and cannot fall back to sleep. Our minds are filled with worries, fears, and negative thoughts. We blame ourselves for misfortunes of the past, feel guilty and overcome with pessimism and self-doubt. Often we are preoccupied with issues or concerns that we feel we have no power to alter—such as how we may have mistreated a loved one who has died or how we will "survive" financially if our business goes bad. When morning comes, we can barely summon the energy to drag ourselves out of bed.

These gloomy feelings may continue for weeks or months at a time. We may despair of finding help and may even become convinced that death offers the only possible way out. In extreme cases, we may think of ways to kill ourselves and may even make an attempt on our own lives.

People who are depressed often complain of having little interest in activities they previously found pleasurable. They may feel tired most of the time, yet may find it impossible to get a good night's sleep. They frequently find themselves crying for no apparent reason. Although they feel bad the whole day, early mornings are the worst time.

Seriously depressed people usually have difficulty concentrating. Many have a hard time carrying out their usual daily responsibilities at home or at work. They often lose their appetite. Even when they force themselves to eat, food just doesn't taste good. They frequently lose weight. Depressed people sometimes appear to move, talk, and think very slowly. Other common symptoms of depression include restless agitation, pacing, hand-wringing, and high levels of anxiety. Often people with depression take antianxiety pills to feel less "nervous," or they take sleeping pills, or they take both. These make depression much worse. Often they turn to alcohol, and this is like throwing gasoline on a fire. In such cases, depression almost always deepens dramatically.

## How Common Is Depression?

Depression is among the most widespread of mental disorders. Most of us feel depressed from time to time, but we frequently hide our depressed feelings from others. When we do let down our defenses and share these experiences, we are almost always surprised to find that many—perhaps most—of our friends and associates have grappled with similar problems.

Even that upbeat friend of the sunniest imaginable disposition may turn out to be intimately familiar with the dark, silent corners of depression. When word got around that we were writing this book, we were besieged by requests for draft copies of this chapter. Most of those requests came from friends we would never have identified as feeling the least bit depressed.

It is helpful indeed to remember that if you are feeling depressed, you are not alone. Many of the great figures of our time have experienced severe episodes of depression. Winston Churchill referred to his own depression as a "black dog" that could turn up at the most unexpected moments. Poet May Sarton found that pulling the weeds out of her garden was an excellent therapy for her own negative moods. Indeed, psychiatrists, psychologists, and other therapists see so many cases of this disorder that they often refer to depression as the common cold of their profession.

Anyone can experience depression: old or young; rich or poor; black, white, Hispanic, or Asian; male or female. About 3 percent of adults in the United States will experience severe depression in any given six-month period. About 5 percent will experience a major depression at some time during their lives.

Women are three to four times as likely to experience a major depression as are men. The blood relatives of a person who has experienced severe depression are more likely to become depressed. A first episode of a major depression is more common between the ages of twenty-five and thirty than in any other five-year period.

Two groups are at highest risk of depression: those who abuse alcohol, cocaine, or other drugs, and those who have experienced a previous episode of severe depression.

## Normal Depressed Mood

In most cases, a depressed mood is part of a normal reaction to change or loss. The death of a close relative will make most of us feel severely depressed. But smaller losses may also produce moderately or profoundly depressed feelings: a move, a divorce, a separation from a loved one, the death of a pet, an illness, the loss of a body part or body function. The loss of a cherished goal (e.g., realizing that we will never attend a certain college, will never marry a certain person, will never have children, or will never become the president of our company) can also trigger feelings of depression.

In all these cases, the depressed mood is part of your normal reaction to a specific situation. These depressed feelings may actually provide you with the energy and direction you need to make the changes that will make your new situation tolerable.

# Normal Grief

Grief after the death of a loved one is probably the most common cause of severe depression. If the deceased was our spouse or a close friend or family member, we will usually begin to experience intense grief within two or three days after the death. These feelings may continue for six to twelve months.

During this period of intense grief, we may experience feelings of depression, anger, poor appetite, and insomnia. We may become preoccupied with thoughts of the lost person and guilt about things done or left undone.

Grief is a normal process, and most people gradually work through it with a combination of self-care and the help and support of their closest friends and family members. But sometimes a grief reaction continues much longer or becomes much more severe. In such cases, professional treatment may help the person complete the grieving process and return to a normal, undepressed mood.

### Margaret Allen: Normal, Uncomplicated Bereavement

Margaret Allen never experienced depression until Larry, her husband of forty years, died of a sudden heart attack. For the first few days after her husband's death, Margaret was kept busy with the funeral arrangements, the reading of the will, and a hundred other administrative details. But over the next six weeks, she began to feel sadder and sadder. She lost interest in all her usual activities. She lost her appetite. It was unpleasant for her to be at home: Everything reminded her of Larry. She felt too listless and exhausted to go elsewhere.

She kept thinking of things she and Larry had always hoped to do together: the Hawaiian cruise; that trip to France and Germany; the purchase of a vacation home. She tortured herself by recounting all the cruel things she had ever said to him. During these six weeks, she spent much of her time crying.

Margaret was lucky to have a number of supportive friends who came to see her every day. Her son also stopped by frequently. Her three other children lived farther away, but they all came to stay with her briefly and called her several times a week.

Gradually, over the next six months, Margaret's mood improved and she began to socialize again. She found that she was able to enjoy herself once more. Although there were still times when she missed Larry terribly, the loss gradually became more bearable. She also began to remember the good times. On the first anniversary of Larry's death, Margaret was sad for most of the day, but by the following day she had returned to her normal more cheerful mood.

Margaret was able to work through her grief with the help of her supportive family and her extensive social network. Although she had a serious grief reaction, she was able to overcome her painful feelings without medications or formal counseling. Other people in similar circumstances might have benefited from talking with a member of the clergy or with a mental health professional.

## Adjustment Disorder with Depressed Mood

Sometimes a loss will trigger a period of depression that goes well beyond a normal grief reaction. Psychiatrists call this an adjustment disorder—a maladaptive reaction (to a change or loss) that occurs within three months of the original event. In contrast to the depressed mood experienced after a loss, this kind of reaction does *not* serve an adaptive purpose. It is longer, more severe, or otherwise out of proportion to the loss that triggered it. Antidepressant medications are rarely needed, but psychotherapy and other forms of counseling can be extremely useful in helping you sort out the causes of your problem and the possible solutions.

### CHERYL PATRICK: ADJUSTMENT DISORDER WITH DEPRESSED MOOD

Cheryl, an accountant, took time off to be with her three children when they were small. When the youngest was two, Cheryl went back to work at a tax-advisory firm.

She soon found that she hated her new job. The office was a madhouse, her new colleagues were not so well trained, and her supervisor emphasized volume at the expense of quality. Unfortunately, Cheryl and her husband, Brad, had made some large installment purchases, so Cheryl couldn't quit.

Although Brad promised to help with the cleaning and cooking, he never followed through. Cheryl became progressively overwhelmed with her multiple responsibilities. She frequently lay awake at night trying to figure out how she could handle it all. She felt depressed and drained most of the time. It just didn't seem that she could possibly handle everything she had to, especially feeling the way she did.

Cheryl began to snap at her children and husband over petty issues. She became impatient with the secretaries at work and, on occasion, with clients and colleagues. After three months on her new job, she was constantly angry.

At last, Cheryl decided to see a therapist. After meeting with Cheryl for two preliminary sessions, her psychologist, Susan Richards, suggested that she appeared to be suffering from an adjustment disorder with depressed mood. Dr. Richards recommended a fourteen-week course of short-term psychotherapy. Cheryl agreed to meet with her twice a week for seven weeks, then once a week for another seven weeks.

In treatment, Cheryl began to see that her current situation was just another example of a pattern she had been repeating since junior high: She would overschedule herself and would then find herself both unable to cope with her commitments and unable to ask for help. She remembered that her own parents had rarely been available to her, telling her that they were "too busy" to spend time with her. Cheryl soon learned that she could get their attention by creating emergencies. She had, for instance, once waited until the weekend before her seventh grade science fair project was due to start on it. As a result, she received both parents' total attention for the hectic weekend.

At her therapist's suggestion, Cheryl began negotiating with her husband for a more equitable distribution of household chores. Through the support and insight gained in her treatment and through key changes that she made in her behavior, Cheryl was gradually able to regain control of her life. Her mood improved gradually—in tandem with the progress that she made in understanding herself better, changing self-defeating patterns, and improving the ways she related to and dealt with other people.

## Mild Depression

Mild depression (dysthymia) is simply a less severe form of depression. According to the DSM-III-R criteria, a diagnosis of mild depression is made when the person exhibits a depressed mood and has at least two of the following symptoms: appetite problems, sleep problems, low energy, poor self-esteem, poor concentration, and feelings of hopelessness.

These symptoms must have been present for at least two years with no break for longer than two months at a time.

### JOHN BEALE: MILD DEPRESSION

At age forty-five, John was a moderately successful salesman in the men's clothing department of a local department store. Although he had hoped to move into management, he had received no promotion in the past six years. His supervisor observed that John knew the merchandise and had talent at fitting a style to the customer, but he lacked zest, vitality, and initiative. As a result, John was continually passed over for promotion. He regularly saw younger and less experienced salesmen sell more clothes and be promoted above him.

John's social relationships were also a problem. Although he had dated a variety of women over the years, these women would typically complain that they found him boring and "a downer." When asked for specifics, they explained that John complained constantly, and was emotionally draining to be around. When a woman would begin to pull away from the relationship, John would rarely pursue her. "It wouldn't make a difference," he lamented. "I guess I'm just a born loser."

John had slept poorly and had complained of a lack of energy for many years. He had come to consider a day when he felt anything other than "depressed" a good day. John had a hard time remembering when he really felt good. "Maybe when I was in the ninth grade, but I'm not sure." After a salesman he had trained was promoted to be his supervisor, John stated: "I hit an all-time low in self-disgust."

For a detailed account of John's treatment and recovery, see p. 39.

## Major Depression

Major depression is one of the most painful of human conditions. People suffering from a major depression will typically exhibit intensely anxious and severely depressed moods. In many cases, they may exhibit a complete loss of interest in all their usual activities or pastimes.

To meet the DSM-III-R criteria for major depression, a person must have experienced strong feelings of depression for two weeks or more in the absence of any loss or change that might have triggered feelings of depression. In addition, at least four of the following additional symptoms must be present: sleep problems, appetite problems, lack of energy, physical agitation, physical slowing, difficulty concentrating, excessive guilt, and suicidal thoughts.

If four or more of these symptoms have been present for at least two weeks, and have been present for the greater part of each day, then the person is suffering from a major depression.

A major depression is a very serious psychiatric condition. Without treatment it may become worse. Severe depression is an extremely painful state. Most people with major depression say that the experience is worse than other medical conditions they have suffered, including broken bones, appendicitis, or pneumonia. A depressed person usually experiences profound feelings of despair and hopelessness, and intense guilt. Thus, anyone who is experiencing a major depression is at considerable risk of suicide.

---

**WARNING:**

**If you believe that you (or a friend or family member) may be suffering from a major depression, we very strongly advise you to seek help from a mental health professional at once. If you are feeling an urge to kill yourself right now, please call your local 911 or other emergency number immediately. Tell the operator that you are afraid you may attempt to kill yourself. Ask them to send a police officer or a paramedic team to make sure you do not hurt yourself and to help you get immediate psychiatric care. Or ask a family member or neighbor to drive you to the nearest hospital emergency room immediately. Tell the emergency room personnel that you are (or your friend is) having powerful suicidal urges. Crisis intervention will protect you from harming yourself and begin a process of understanding, assessment, and treatment that almost always reverses self-destructive intentions and leads to recovery from depression.**

---

Even if you are sure that there is no chance you might kill yourself, if you are experiencing a major depression, we strongly suggest that you arrange an emergency session with a qualified mental health professional.

Suicide is a very real threat for those with major depression. An estimated 10 to 25 percent of people with a major depression try to kill themselves within five years of the onset of their depression. Unfortunately, a high number succeed. As highly effective therapies for this disorder are available, this is a tragic waste of life and a source of great stress for family members and others.

In some cases, people who are experiencing a severe depression may also be experiencing psychotic symptoms, e.g., hearing voices (auditory hallucinations) or believing ideas that have no basis in reality (delusions). Those who are experiencing such symptoms are especially likely to commit suicide and must be taken at once to the nearest emergency room. For a more extensive discussion of hallucinations, delusions, and other psychotic symptoms, see Chapter 7.

## CARL ZELAND: MAJOR DEPRESSION

Carl, a thirty-two-year-old construction worker, was recently promoted to foreman. His new responsibilities turned out to be much more demanding than he had thought. The other foremen, his former bosses, were cold and difficult to work with. His old work buddies became distant and suspicious.

He began to feel unmotivated. He felt as if he had lost all his energy. He felt sad, was irritable, and thought that he was a "bad person" for no specific reasons. He no longer enjoyed his weekly bowling evenings or spending time with his children. He became obsessed with the details of his work but, nonetheless, performed poorly on the job. It seemed to Carl that he had lost all his old enthusiasm. His family noticed that he was more and more withdrawn.

Carl had never previously had a problem with drinking, but he now began to stop off at a neighborhood tavern to have several beers on his way home from work. He explained that he needed to drink in order to relax and get his mind off his work. Over a period of several weeks, his drinking increased. Soon he drank six to eight beers every evening, and began to drink during the day on the weekends. The drinking helped Carl fall asleep, but he would wake up at three or four in the morning and would lie awake tossing and turning until it was time to get up at 6:30 A.M. As a result, he would be even more exhausted the next day.

As the weeks went by, Carl's drinking increased. He began calling in to work sick. He felt he lacked both the energy and self-confidence to deal with the problems his job entailed. When he stayed home from work, he would often lie in bed with the covers pulled over his head. Usually, he would take "a drink or two" in the morning "to settle my nerves."

Carl also lost all interest in sex. He would become angry with his wife when she showed any sexual initiative. Formerly a heavy and appreciative eater, he lost all pleasure in eating and lost fifteen pounds in four weeks.

One morning, Carl told his wife that he had been thinking quite seriously of suicide. She insisted that they go together to see a family practitioner. Carl reluctantly agreed, even though he doubted that there was anything the doctor could do. In his first meeting with the family physician, Carl attributed his problems to "my total incompetence as a breadwinner, as a father, as a husband, and as a man."

A detailed account of Carl's treatment and recovery is included later in this chapter.

## Manic-Depressive Illness

For a person with manic-depressive illness, episodes of depression alternate with episodes of intense excitement and enthusiasm. During the depressed phase, the person feels all the symptoms of severe depression that have been described earlier in this chapter. During the excited or manic phase, the person may experience an elevated or irritable mood, increased energy, decreased need for sleep, and increased self-esteem all far in excess of a normal mood. The treatment for a bipolar depression is somewhat different from that of severe depression without mania. The diagnosis and treatment of manic-depressive illness is described in Chapter 6.

### RICHARD MUNGER: MANIC-DEPRESSIVE ILLNESS

By age twenty-eight, Richard had had manic-depressive illness for ten years. He experienced his first manic symptoms at age eighteen: a decreased need for sleep, elevated mood, and increased energy. Richard had to be hospitalized after he was found running up and down the local interstate in bare feet. When the state police interviewed Richard, he told them that he was training for the Olympic marathon by trying to keep pace with the cars.

During his first psychiatric hospitalization, Richard was treated with chlorpromazine and lithium, and he continued taking lithium after discharge from the hospital. Since that time, his manic symptoms had never reappeared.

Several months after discharge, Richard began to experience feelings that were completely new to him: loss of self-esteem, tiredness during the day, loss of appetite, poor concentration, and profound feelings of sadness. Both Richard and his psychiatrist recognized what was happening: He was entering the depressed phase of his illness.

After discussing the risks, benefits, and potential side effects involved, Richard and his psychiatrist chose to begin treatment with the serotonin specific antidepressant fluoxetine (Prozac). Richard also saw his therapist regularly to monitor his progress and to examine the stressful events that might have contributed to this episode. Four weeks later, Richard was feeling fine and functioning in his usual fashion. Had Richard and his psychiatrist not recognized the early onset of depression and begun treatment quickly, his depression would likely have become much more severe.

For more on the diagnosis and the treatment of manic-depressive illness, see Chapter 6.

## Atypical Depression

*Atypical depression* is a term that mental health professionals apply to a set of symptoms that meet the criteria for a major depression but are unlike the usual picture. A typical depression might include such symptoms as depressed mood, lack of energy, insomnia, reduced appetite with weight loss, poor concentration, and thoughts and feelings of inappropriate guilt. Somebody with an atypical depression may not feel sad but, rather, anxious or irritable. The person may sleep practically all the time and may have a voracious appetite, leading to a substantial weight gain. Some individuals with atypical depression may become especially sensitive to the perceived rejection of others. They may feel deeply depressed for several days, then feel fine for several days, then become depressed again. One class of antidepressants, the monoamine oxidase inhibitors, appears to be especially effective in treating atypical depression.

### MARILYN ARCHER: ATYPICAL DEPRESSION

Marilyn had always wanted to have a large family, so she was overjoyed after each of her first two children was born. However, after the birth of her twins (her third and fourth children), things never seemed quite the same. Marilyn was having increasing difficulty taking care of the children at home. She seemed to have lost all her old energy and she could not seem to get enough sleep, even though she was sleeping ten hours every night and napping for another two hours during the day. Her mood kept getting worse and her cravings for sweets became so intense that she soon gained thirty pounds, mostly from chocolates. She eventually had to wear her maternity clothes again, because her other clothes no longer fit.

Through all these symptoms, Marilyn never felt sad, just less and less interested in life. When her mother visited, she was astonished to find Marilyn's home in disorder, her children dirty and poorly dressed.

Marilyn's husband, Jim, had tried to persuade Marilyn to see a doctor for a checkup, but she insisted that she felt fine physically. She stated that she was only tired. One day he came home to find Marilyn lying listlessly on the living room floor, the babies unchanged and hungry and the house in a state of absolute chaos. He called Marilyn's obstetrician for help. The obstetrician referred Marilyn to a psychiatrist.

Marilyn did acknowledge feeling sad, and did not fit the usual picture of depression. Nevertheless, she did have a major depression of the atypical variety. Her treatment included psychotherapy, treatment with a monoamine oxidase inhibitor, and more support at home. Three months later, she was back to her usual efficient self: Her house was shipshape and she was enjoying her new twins.

## Psychotic Depression

A very severe depression may sometimes include psychotic symptoms, such as hearing voices (auditory hallucinations), or delusions (believing in things that are not true). When people hear voices, these voices are usually highly critical. They tell the people how bad they are or call them vulgar, hurtful names. A typical delusion might include the notion that the person committed some unforgivable sins and, therefore, deserves severe punishment or retribution.

People suffering from psychotic depression may require treatment with both antidepressant *and* antipsychotic medications. Electroconvulsive therapy (ECT) may also be indicated. If left untreated, a patient with delusional or psychotic depression is very likely to attempt suicide. For more on psychosis and antipsychotic medications, see Chapter 7.

## What Causes Depression?

We don't really know what causes depression, but researchers have proposed a number of possible explanations.

### PSYCHOLOGICAL THEORIES

Some experts think of depression as an ineffective reaction to a real, threatened, or perceived loss. An important loss early in life may leave a person with a special vulnerability to later losses. Mistreatment or lack of proper nurturing behavior by parents or caregivers is also perceived as a kind of loss. If people who experienced a loss in childhood are subjected to another loss later in life, they may react by becoming depressed.

Other experts believe that depression is the result of low self-esteem and a lack of the social skills necessary to obtain positive reinforcement from others (e.g., "You did a really fine job on the Jacobson project, Carl. Good work"). If a person is unable to evoke these responses from others because he or she lacks the necessary skills, then it may be difficult for him or her to maintain a positive self-image. But at the same time, if a person suffers from low self-esteem, he or she may be unable to accept such positive reinforcement even if he or she does receive it.

Low self-esteem may also lead to "cognitive distortions," i.e., incorrect attitudes and reasoning processes leading to faulty conclusions about the world and one's own self-worth. For example, a person who forgot to let the cat out for the night might mistakenly conclude that he or she is an animal abuser and, therefore, should not be allowed to have pets.

## BIOLOGICAL THEORIES

Other experts consider depression the result of imbalance of certain chemicals in the brain. These chemicals, called neurotransmitters, include norepinephrine, epinephrine, dopamine, serotonin, and probably many others. Some antidepressant medications work by acting directly on these neurotransmitters. Neurotransmitters carry their messages to special parts of the brain neuron cell called the neuroceptors. These are also believed to malfunction during depression.

Another theory holds that depression is the result of disruptions in the sleep-wake cycle. Sleep studies of depressed people show characteristic changes in sleep patterns, and one suggested treatment for depression is to shift the times for waking and sleeping and thereby "reset the biologic clock." This approach does show some benefits in the treatment of mild depression, but the benefits are not always permanent. We believe that the symptoms and signs of depression are end results of complex biological, experiential, psychological, and social factors. Thus, all these perspectives—and more—must be addressed in the treatment of depression.

## MEDICAL CONDITIONS THAT CAN CAUSE DEPRESSION

Before seeking psychological help for depression, it is important to be sure that your depression is not the result of a physical problem. The medical conditions that most commonly produce depression include thyroid deficiency, infections, neurologic disorders, and cancers (including some undiagnosed cancers). The conditions below can also sometimes produce depression:

Addison's disease
Alzheimer's disease
brain tumors
cerebral ischemia
Cushing's disease
gastrointestinal diseases
heart failure

Huntington's disease
hyperthyroidism
hypothyroidism
infectious diseases (especially
    viral diseases)
malnutrition
multiple sclerosis

myocardial infarction (heart attack)
pancreatic disease
Parkinson's disease
rheumatoid arthritis
stroke
systemic lupus erythematosus
traumatic brain injury
various cancers
vitamin deficiencies (some)
other neurologic, collagen, vascular, and endocrine disorders

## DRUGS THAT CAN CAUSE DEPRESSION

A number of drugs (both prescription and nonprescription) can cause depression. To complicate matters, discontinuing certain medications—especially narcotic analgesics, steroids, and stimulants—can also produce depressed feelings. Some of the drugs that most commonly cause depression are listed below. In addition, many individuals have special or unusual reactions; these are called idiosyncratic side effects. Thus, if depression occurs while you are taking or discontinuing *any* medication, you should consult your physician.

alcohol (see below)
amantadine (Symmetrel)
amphetamines and similar stimulants (on withdrawal)
barbiturates
benzodiazepines
carbidopa
clonidine (Catapres)
cocaine
cycloserine (Seromycin)
estrogens
levodopa (Dopar and others)
methyldopa (Aldomet)
narcotic analgesics
oral contraceptives
propranolol (Inderal)
reserpine (Serpasil)
steroids (prednisone, cortisone, and others)
vinblastine (Velban)
vincristine (Oncovin)

**Source:** "Drugs That Can Cause Psychiatric Symptoms." *Medical Letter* 26 (August 17, 1984): 75–78.

## ALCOHOL AND DEPRESSION

Alcohol is often used to enhance social interactions and to help people relax. Unfortunately, when used on a regular basis it can increase a person's feelings of depression. Indeed, alcohol abuse is all too frequently associated with depression. People who drink heavily are at higher risk for depression, and many people drink more heavily when they are depressed.

Although we may temporarily feel stimulated or uninhibited when we drink alcoholic beverages, alcohol is actually a powerful nervous system *depressant*: It actually suppresses many important activities of the brain, such as alertness, balance, and motor coordination. This makes the brain susceptible to the development of greater depression. Most experts advise people who suffer from depression to drink little or no alcohol. Recovery from a moderate or severe depression is far more difficult (some would say virtually impossible) if the depressed person continues to use alcohol. Depressed people are sometimes tempted to use alcohol to help them fall asleep, but this is ultimately self-defeating. As soon as the alcohol has worn off, it becomes even more difficult to fall asleep. Alcohol disrupts the usual and healthy electrical rhythms of the brain that are associated with restful sleep—both in those who are depressed and those who are not.

## DO RECREATIONAL DRUGS CAUSE DEPRESSION?

Yes. Such stimulants as cocaine and amphetamines can briefly elevate the user's mood. However, the drugs leave a depressed mood behind when the effects have worn off. You may be tempted to increase the dose of these drugs to escape the withdrawal feelings. To alleviate a depression caused by recreational drugs, treat the drug abuse itself first. If, after you are off drugs, you are still depressed, then it may be necessary to treat your depression with one of the methods described in this chapter.

## IS DEPRESSION HEREDITARY?

Most biologically oriented psychiatrists believe (and we agree) that a person can inherit a vulnerability to depression. About 20 percent of those with serious depression have one or more relatives who suffer from the same disorder. In addition, intense life stresses may increase a vulnerable individual's risk of developing depression. For example, a person with a strong genetic vulnerability to manic-depressive illness may not require a great deal of stress to go into a severe depression, whereas a person with less genetic vulnerability to depression may not develop the disorder at all except under extremely high stress.

Infants and children are particularly vulnerable to stress. They require an atmosphere of love, respect, enlightened support, and direction. When children are not protected and supported—or, worse, when they are abused—their vulnerability to depression later on may be markedly increased.

## CAN STRESS CONTRIBUTE TO DEPRESSION?

It is common for people who are depressed to have experienced a major stressful event, especially a loss, shortly before the onset of their depression. But many other people become depressed without similar stresses. Stress, even chronic stress, does not in and of itself cause major depression. However, for people who are genetically predisposed to depression, stressful events can indeed bring on an episode of major depression. An important task of psychotherapy is to help identify the stresses that can contribute to depression and to develop specific ways to cope with them.

## CAN ALLERGIES CAUSE DEPRESSION?

Although sensitivities to certain foods can cause a wide variety of psychological symptoms, there is little evidence except in a few rare cases that allergies are a common cause of depression beyond being a source of discomfort and general life stress.

# How Long Does an Episode of Depression Usually Last?

Without treatment, most episodes of major depression last two to four years. They may last even longer. Depression can recur after months—or years—of normal mood. We now have so many different treatments for depression that the outlook is much brighter than it once was. Once a person is on a therapeutic dose of the appropriate medication, improvement will usually begin in as little as two to three weeks.

But even after the symptoms of depression have disappeared, a person is still at risk for recurrence. The risk is highest in the first six months after the episode begins. Thus, it is common practice to continue the drug treatment for depression for at least six months after the symptoms have disappeared.

# Why Do I Need a Medical Examination If I Have Been Feeling Depressed?

It is essential that any individual with depression have a thorough medical evaluation by a physician who is knowledgeable in the full range of medical conditions that can give rise to depression. Two of the authors of this book (Yudofsky and Hales) have evaluated hundreds of patients who have received extensive, expensive, and unsuccessful treatments of depression—only to learn that the problem was due to an undiagnosed medical condition. Because the first and most important principle of the treatment of depression is the attempt to understand its underlying cause or source, this must include a thorough and knowledgeable medical assessment.

# Nondrug Treatments for Depression

The nondrug treatments listed below can be extremely valuable in reversing depression. In some cases, they will be sufficient to control the problem altogether. And they can be a valuable supplement to drug treatment.

Although friends, counselors, and professionals may be able to suggest useful strategies, this is an area in which you yourself are the final authority. There is no standard treatment that works for everyone. We recommend that you explore all possible options, then choose the self-help methods that strike you as most promising.

## EXERCISE

One option that deserves special attention is exercise. As physical activity during the day can improve sleep and appetite (two processes that are greatly disturbed in depression), exercising regularly can often alleviate mild depressive symptoms. Exercise also may reduce irritability and anger. Feelings of accomplishment and mastery associated with exercise are helpful in combating low self-esteem.

For some patients, exercise ends up being the most important part of their treatment plans. Evelyn, a thirty-six-year-old depressed schoolteacher, began exercise walking at her therapist's suggestion. She soon went on to jogging, then to competitive running. Eventually, much to her surprise and delight, she entered and performed well in local ten-kilometer races.

"I always thought I was a terrible athlete," she told her therapist. "Now I have a wall full of ribbons."

Researchers now believe that strenuous exercise may actually promote chemical changes in the body that, like antidepressants, work to treat the associated chemical imbalances of depression. Although the data in this area are still limited, most experts believe that when performed under medical supervision, regular, judicious exercise can be an important adjunct to the treatment of depression. We believe that exercise may well turn out to be an important part of treatment for depression.

## NUTRITIONAL TREATMENTS

Nutritional approaches to the treatment of depression are still highly controversial. There is widespread agreement that nutrition is critical in maintaining good mental health and must be an essential component of any treatment of a mental disorder. It is clear that certain elements of diet (e.g., alcohol) can cause depression. Thus it is not unreasonable to think that nutritional measures may be important in the treatment of depression as well. While this is an area of great interest and much research, at the present time, researchers have identified only one nutritional approach beyond the general recommendation to eat a well-balanced diet.

The exception is based on the finding that foods containing the amino acid tryptophan appear to increase brain serotonin levels. Reduced serotonin levels have been found in certain people with depression and the mechanisms of action of certain powerful antidepressants (e.g., amitriptyline, fluoxetine, trazodone) are thought to involve increases in brain serotonin levels. Increasing serotonin through diet might be helpful for some people experiencing depression and insomnia. Milk is a good source of tryptophan, as is turkey. Recently, however, some store-bought supplements containing tryptophan have been found to cause dangerous blood-related problems. Check with your psychiatrist or general physician before taking this food supplement.

## SELF-HELP OR ADVOCACY GROUPS

People experiencing depression and having difficulty coping may find it extremely helpful to discuss their problem with a sympathetic friend or a member of the clergy. Self-help or advocacy groups, such as the National Depressive and Manic-Depressive Association, can be helpful in dealing with depression. If there is a specific problem associated with your depression (e.g., alcoholism, loss of a loved one, child abuse), a group that focuses on this particualr problem can be especially useful. Self-help groups (especially those, such as Alcoholics Anonymous, that are directed specifically toward problems that may cause or prolong depression) can be highly therapeutic.

### PROFESSIONAL THERAPY

If you decide to consider psychotherapy with a mental health professional, you will have a variety of choices: one-to-one sessions with a therapist, sessions with a therapist and your whole family, and/or group therapy.

In individual psychotherapy, the therapist will first ask you about many aspects of your present situation and past experience, and will also discuss your feelings about these events in a supportive, reassuring manner. These discussions will help you understand yourself more fully and gain insights into all the possible causes for your depressive feelings. Family and group therapy most often begin in a similar manner, but because several people are participating, there you will also have the opportunity to examine your behaviors from varied points of view. In group therapy, you will have a chance to benefit from the experience of others facing similar problems.

## JOHN BEALE: PSYCHOTHERAPY FOR DEPRESSION

(The first part of John's history is given on p. 26.)

When John went to his family physician to request a "sleeping pill," his doctor referred him for psychotherapy to Dr. Carl Burke, a clinical psychologist. Dr. Burke began twice-a-week insight-oriented psychotherapy that was geared to helping John understand the psychological origins of his low self-esteem, his lack of motivation and enthusiasm, and his problems with interpersonal relationships. Many of these problems were traced to John's relationship with his father, who was critical, emotionally distant, and competitive with John. After many months of treatment, John began to understand how his anger toward his father was "internalized" (literally, John turned this anger on himself), with the overall result that John "punished" himself by not meeting his full potential academically or vocationally. He also did not allow himself to experience pleasure. With Dr. Burke's support, John reappraised his self-worth, applied himself more at work, and assumed more initiative in dating as well as making new male friends. Simultaneously, his symptoms of depression (low energy, insomnia, sadness) improved significantly. Over time, his "mild" depressive symptoms were relieved without the use of medication.

## KAREN TOWNSAND: PSYCHOTHERAPY FOR DEPRESSION

Karen, a twenty-eight-year-old nurse, decided to see a therapist because she had been feeling depressed for nearly a year. She became aware of self-hate and low self-esteem. Her recognition of these feelings frightened her so severely that she decided to seek professional help. She was referred by a friend to a psychoanalytically oriented psychotherapist. At the time she entered therapy, Karen was listless, depressed, overweight, and unkempt. Her hair was stringy and unwashed. She told her therapist that on those rare occasions when she was asked out on dates, she declined because she was so embarrassed about the way she looked.

After several sessions of therapy and discussion of her history with her therapist, Karen recalled that when she was eleven years old she had experienced many episodes of psychological, physical, and sexual abuse from the man who later became her stepfather. Karen realized that she had "forgotten" these episodes altogether. They had been completely banished from her conscious thoughts for a decade—a psychological process called repression. She began to see the connection between these banished feelings and her deep-seated feelings of worthlessness and self-hate.

After many discussions with her therapist, Karen came to realize that she had blamed herself for her sexual feelings—which she associated with shame—and the feelings of murderous rage toward her stepfather that these experiences had triggered in her as a child. It was very helpful for Karen to be able to understand that no child should be held accountable for sexual abuse that was initiated by an adult. To her great relief, she realized that she was not "the bad person"—in fact, she deserved to feel good about herself and to experience pleasure in life as much as any other individual. These insights had a major impact on relieving her feelings of depression and low self-esteem.

Once Karen felt that she had gotten a handle on her depressed feelings and feelings of low self-worth, she was ready to turn her attention to getting her act together. She joined a health club, began working out regularly, and lost thirty pounds. Even better, she made new friends—men and women at the club. To her delight, she found that she was liked and was frequently invited to social events. This raised Karen's sense of self-worth and made her feel that she really deserved pleasure and good treatment.

## Who Should Consider Using an Antidepressant Drug?

If your depressed feelings are fairly mild and seem manageable, or if they are clearly the result of a major loss or change in your life, you may well wish to work through them on your own, by talking with a sympathetic counselor, friend, or spiritual adviser, or by reading a self-help book on depression. Indeed, it can sometimes be useful to realize that these changes in mood are part of a normal, natural, healthy process, and that it is a healthful process to experience and express, and accept these feelings. In some cases, however, your feelings may be so severe, so inexplicable, and so baffling that you may wish to seek a consultation with a psychologist, psychiatrist, or other mental health professional. (For guidelines on finding a good therapist, see p. 11.)

After discussing your feelings and concerns with your professional, you may wish to ask whether he or she thinks that you might benefit from antidepressant medication. This choice is an individual one, but as a general rule, antidepressant medication may be useful if (1) your symptoms are severe enough to interfere with your daily functioning; (2) your symptoms have continued without interruption for two weeks or more; (3) you cannot identify a triggering episode for your depression; (4) you feel that you have become incapable of enjoying life as fully as you once could; (5) your depressive symptoms do not respond to nondrug treatments.

# The DSM-III-R Criteria for Depression

You should not take an antidepressant medication for depression unless you and your physician agree that your condition meets the specifications for *major depression* or *bipolar illness, depressed* as specified by criteria in DSM-III-R. These specifications are listed in Table 1.

TABLE 1

**DSM-III-R Criteria for Major Depression**

At least five of the following symptoms have been present during the same two-week period and represent a change from previous functioning; at least one of the symptoms is either (1) depressed mood or (2) loss of interest or pleasure (do not include symptoms that are clearly due to a physical condition, mood-incongruent delusions or hallucinations, incoherence, or marked loosening of associations):

(1) depressed mood (or can be irritable mood in children and adolescents) most of the day, nearly every day, as indicated either by subjective account or observation by others

(2) markedly diminished interest or pleasure in all, or almost all, activities most of the day, nearly every day (as indicated either by subjective account or observation by others of apathy most of the time)

(3) significant weight loss or weight gain when not dieting (e.g., more than 5 percent of body weight in a month), or decrease or increase in appetite nearly every day (in children, consider failure to make expected weight gains)

(4) insomnia or hypersomnia nearly every day

(5) psychomotor agitation or retardation nearly every day (observable by others, not merely subjective feelings of restlessness or being slowed down)

(6) fatigue or loss of energy nearly every day

(7) feelings of worthlessness or excessive or inappropriate guilt (which may be delusional) nearly every day (not merely self-reproach or guilt about being sick)

(8) diminished ability to think or concentrate, or indecisiveness, nearly every day (either by subjective account or as observed by others)

(9) recurrent thoughts of death (not just fear of dying), recurrent suicidal ideation without a specific plan, or a suicide attempt or a specific plan for committing suicide

**Source:** Reproduced with permission of the American Psychiatric Association.

In most cases, you can work through these feelings using a combination of self-care, group support, and the sympathetic understanding of family members and friends. However, in some cases the depressive reaction triggered by such events may be so severe, so prolonged, and so out of proportion to the event itself that the depression itself becomes a problem. In such cases, you may well benefit from professional therapy, antidepressant medication, or both.

## Drugs Used to Treat Depression

Antidepressant agents are medications that specifically treat depression. These agents are not *mood elevators* nor do they make one high. If a person who was *not* feeling depressed took one of these medications, they would not notice any effect on their mood (although they might notice some of the side effects, e.g., dry mouth, blurred vision, and constipation). Unlike the stimulants, antidepressants have virtually no potential for abuse, habituation, or addiction. A frequent question from patients is "Will I get hooked or become dependent on antidepressants?" Our answer is an emphatic "No!"

There are four general classes of antidepressants: heterocyclics (formerly called the tricyclics), monoamine oxidase inhibitors, serotonin-specific agents, and alprazolam (Xanax).

To understand how these drugs work, we must briefly review the role of neurotransmitters in depression.

### How Do Antidepressants Work?

Neurotransmitters are chemicals that carry messages from one nerve cell to another. The first nerve cell releases a small amount of the chemical, which is then sensed by the second nerve cell. The neurotransmitters are then quickly cleared away.

They may be cleared away in either of two ways: The neurotransmitter can be recaptured by the first nerve cell and repackaged for future use; or the neurotransmitter may be broken down by enzymes in the space between the two cells.

Researchers believe that depression is, in part, the result of abnormally low levels of certain neurotransmitters (norepinephrine, epinephrine, and/ or serotonin). Antidepressant drugs can increase the levels of these chemicals by interfering with the mechanisms by which the brain rids itself of these biological compounds. The heterocyclic antidepressants and the serotonin-specific agents block the recapture of neurotransmitters, with the serotonin-specific agents blocking the recapture of serotonin. The monoamine oxidase inhibitors interrupt the enzyme monoamine oxidase, which breaks down norepinephrine, epinephrine, and serotonin in the space between the two nerve cells.

All three of these drugs act within the brain. Why does it take three to four weeks for the symptoms of a major depression to respond to these medications? This remains a mystery even to the most knowledgeable researchers and clinicians in the field. We believe that the answers to the mystery lie in part in the complex interrelationship of neurotransmitters and the receptors on the nerve cells to which the transmitters carry their message. By changing the levels of neurotransmitters at the receptor site, we change the sensitivities of the receptors, which we know are altered during the state of depression.

## EXACTLY WHAT CAN ANTIDEPRESSANTS DO?

The antidepressants can be used to treat either a single episode or recurrent episodes of depression. They can be used either while experiencing symptoms, or when a person is well but wishes to decrease the chance of a relapse. Some antidepressant medications are also used in the treatment of other disorders, including panic attacks, chronic pain, anorexia and bulimia, obsessive-compulsive disorder, cravings associated with narcotic and cocaine withdrawal, migraine headaches, and even bed-wetting.

## HETEROCYCLIC ANTIDEPRESSANTS

*Drug names*: amitriptyline (Elavil, Endep), amoxapine (Asendin), desipramine (Norpramin, Pertofrane), doxepin (Adapin, Sinequan), imipramine (Tofranil), maprotiline (Ludiomil), nortriptyline (Pamelor), protriptyline (Vivactil), trimipramine (Surmontil).

*Actions*. These medications inhibit the nerve cells' ability to reabsorb two neurotransmitters, principally norepinephrine and serotonin.

*Advantages*. The heterocyclic antidepressants are usually the drugs of first choice in the drug treatment of depression. They have been proven safe and effective for depression by many scientific studies. Seventy to 80 percent of people with major depression respond to the first heterocyclic antidepressant tried.

*Drawbacks and limitations*. Despite their enormous efficacy in the treatment of depression, the heterocyclic antidepressants pose two potential problems: their side effects, and the possibility that they could be used in a suicide attempt.

*Side effects*. Unfortunately, in addition to affecting the neurotransmitters norepinephrine and serotonin, these drugs also affect a third neurotransmitter, acetylcholine. Because heterocyclics can interfere with the effects of acetylcholine, these drugs can produce a variety of side effects: blurry vision, constipation, orthostatic hypotension (feeling light-headed when standing or sitting up suddenly), dry mouth, urinary retention, and confusion. These side effects can be quite annoying for anyone; for older people, they can be particularly disabling.

Fortunately, these side effects (researchers call them anticholinergic side effects) will generally get better or go away on their own. Sometimes, however, they may require special treatment (as in eating bran cereal for breakfast daily to prevent constipation). In some cases, these side effects are so disabling that the current medication must be discontinued and another medication substituted.

*Other possible side effects of the heterocyclics*: flushing, sweating, tachycardia, hypotension, racing heartbeat, low blood pressure, aggravation of narrow-angle glaucoma, and adynamic ileus. Also, allergic skin reactions and photosensitivity (or rashes and painful sunburns with modest exposure to the sun), blood-related problems (including changes in the white blood cells and platelets), sex-related problems (including delayed, inhibited, or retrograde ejaculation in males), tremor, speech blockage, and an increase in insomnia and/or anxiety. In addition, increased appetite with overeating, seizures in susceptible individuals, occasional parkinsonism, especially when abruptly withdrawing the drug.

*Risk of overdose*. A major drawback of the heterocyclic antidepressants is the risk of suicide or unintentional overdose. (If you take a large quantity of one of these drugs, it can kill you.) This is a particularly worrisome problem when a person has a condition—major depression—in which he or she is already at relatively high risk of attempting suicide.

The decision to prescribe heterocyclic antidepressants for a depressed person who may be at risk of suicide is very difficult. On the one hand, heterocyclics are among the most effective and easily tolerated medications for the treatment of major depression. In many cases, there may not be another drug that is both nearly so good and a great deal safer. Thus, a psychiatrist may try to minimize the risk of overdose by prescribing only a few days' supply of the medication at one time. In this way, the total amount of medication dispensed at any one time is less than the lethal amount. In addition to preventing overdose, this may encourage the depressed person to see a physician more frequently for support and assessment of suicidal risk.

Overall, if risks of overdose are minimized and the side effects are tolerable to the individual patient, these medications are among the most effective and useful drugs we have for the treatment of major depression. More people with depression have been safely and successfully treated by heterocyclic medications than by all other classes of drugs combined.

*Treatment of overdose*. A single dose of 1 g imipramine equivalent leads to severe toxic reaction. Doses greater than 2 g imipramine equivalent are sometimes fatal. The first adverse symptoms usually are not evident until one to four hours after ingestion. They are: reduced breathing, serious heart changes including dangerous changes in the heart rhythm, agitation, lowering of blood pressure, garbled speech, high fever, confusion, disorientation, and coma.

Emergency interventions in the hospital usually can prevent a person who has taken an overdose of antidepressants from dying or suffering permanent physical damage—*if the person gets medical help in time!*

### MONOAMINE OXIDASE INHIBITORS (MAOIs)

*Drug names*: isocarboxazid (Marplan), phenelzine (Nardil), tranylcypromine (Parnate).

*Actions*. Monoamine oxidase inhibitors prevent an enzyme called monoamine oxidase from breaking down the neurotransmitters norepinephrine and serotonin.

*Advantages*. These drugs are as effective as the heterocyclics in the treatment of major depression, and sometimes they may be even more useful. Monoamine oxidase inhibitors may be used as a drug of second choice to treat people whose symptoms have not improved significantly after treatment with a heterocyclic or serotonin-specific antidepressant. They may be the drug of first choice to treat "atypical" depressions, and anxious depressions.

*Disadvantages*. The major problem associated with monoamine oxidase inhibitors is the high risk of an adverse reaction, called a monoamine oxidation inhibitor reaction. This is actually a food-drug interaction in which certain foods interact with the drug to produce potentially toxic effects. The solution is simple but not always easy: avoid all foods containing tyramine, an amino acid found in many foods in the average American diet. Tyramine can interact with monoamine oxidase inhibitors to cause severe and life-threatening increases in blood pressure.

You should not take this drug unless you, or the family member you are concerned with, are absolutely sure that you will be able to keep your diet free of foods containing tyramine. If you would have a difficult time excluding cheese or beans from your diet, you should not take these drugs.

People with memory problems, and also people who would be liable for any reason to make mistakes while taking a monoamine oxidase inhibitor, should not take these drugs. There are also a number of prescription and over-the-counter medications that should be avoided if you are using one of these drugs. See Table 2. You must never take any medication without first notifying your psychiatrist for an assessment of its safety when used together with a monoamine oxidase inhibitor.

TABLE 2

### Some of the Foods and Drugs to Avoid
### When Taking a Monoamine Oxidase Inhibitor

**Foods**
High tyramine content
    Cheeses: Boursin, Camembert, cheddar, Gruyère, Stilton
    Other foods: lox, pickled herring
    Beverages: Chianti (You should not drink alcohol while being treated for depression, anyway)
Moderate tyramine content
    Cheeses: Gouda, Parmesan
    Other foods: salted herring, chicken liver, figs, raisins, broad (fava) beans, yeast products, pickles, sauerkraut, coffee, chocolate, cocoa, soy sauce, sour cream, snails, avocado, banana peels, licorice
    Beverages: sherry, beer
Low tyramine content
    Cheeses: American
    Beverages: champagne, Italian red wine, Riesling, santeone, hard liquor
**Drugs**
Medications
    amphetamines (Benzedrine), decongestants (contain phenylpropanolamine, ephedrine, or pseudoephedrine), dexatroamphetamine (Dexedrine), methamphetamine (Desoxyn), methylphenidate (Ritalin), procaine (Novocain and others)
Illicit drugs
    All substances of abuse (recreational drugs) should be avoided by people with depression and may be *highly dangerous* when combined with a monoamine oxidase inhibitor.

## THE SEROTONIN-SPECIFIC AGENTS

*Drug names*: fluoxetine (Prozac), trazodone (Desyrel).

*Actions*. Serotonin-specific antidepressant drugs inhibit the recapture of the neurotransmitter serotonin by the nerve cells.

*Advantages*. These drugs frequently produce fewer side effects (e.g., dry mouth, constipation, urinary retention, blurry vision) than the heterocyclic antidepressants. They are also often better tolerated by people with heart disease, dementia, Alzheimer's, and those who have had a stroke. In addition, some of these drugs, e.g., trazodone, have a sedating effect. That can sometimes help the person with depression fall asleep even before the antidepressant actions occur.

Fluoxetine does not usually cause sedation; it may also be the only antidepressant not associated with a weight gain. Both trazodone and fluoxetine have relatively high margins of safety when ingested in higher doses than recommended for therapeutic purposes—as in suicide attempts by overdose. Initially, these agents were used as another class of drugs for the treatment of patients whose depression did not respond to the heterocyclic antidepressants or for those people who tolerated other antidepressant medications poorly. They are increasingly being used as *first-line* treatment for depression. Fluoxetine is useful in the treatment of obsessive-compulsive disorder (see Chapter 4), and may also have antipanic and antiphobic effects.

*Disadvantages*. With trazodone, a small percentage of men develop painful erections requiring surgical treatment. In some cases, this has led to permanent impairment in erectile function. For disadvantages of fluoxetine use, see below.

## ABOUT FLUOXETINE (PROZAC)

No doubt many of you may have purchased this book because either you or a member of your family has been prescribed the medication fluoxetine (Prozac). At the time of our writing this chapter, fluoxetine has been available for only three years; yet it is currently the nation's most prescribed antidepressant medication. Over 650,000 new or renewed prescriptions for fluoxetine are being written every month. According to *Newsweek* magazine, which featured this medication on the cover of its March 26, 1990, issue, sales of the medication reached $125 million in 1988, and increased to $350 million in 1989 (more than was spent on all antidepressants two years previously), and expectations are that the drug will earn $1 billion by

1995. Not availabe as a generic drug, fluoxetine cost between $1 and $3 per capsule, which can be up to ten times the cost of the other brand name antidepressants and/or generics.

## ADVANTAGES OF FLUOXETINE

As stated elsewhere in this chapter, heterocyclic antidepressants and mono-amine oxidase inhibitors are highly effective in the treatment of depression. In addition, when used as prescribed, these medications have a high degree of safety backed by over thirty years of extensive experience. Nonetheless, fluoxetine is enjoying a level of success surpassing other antidepressants by virtue of its efficacy, convenience, side effect profile, and safety.

### Efficacy

Scientific studies have shown that fluoxetine is a powerful antidepressant medication. The drug works almost exclusively on the neurotransmitter serotonin, which is known to be an important brain chemical in the regula-tion of mood. In fact, fluoxetine is the first antidepressant marketed that blocks the reuptake of serotonin in the presynaptic nerve ending, a process that leads to dramatic increases in the availability of serotonin at postsynap-tic receptor sites in the brain. Although limitations of research strategies make it difficult to compare the degree of efficacy of one antidepressant versus another, it appears that fluoxetine may, for many patients, be more effective than certain other types of antidepressants that work in different ways on different brain messenger systems. Some scientists have gone so far as to postulate there are different types of depression based on the underlying chemical disorders. At the present time, it is clear that fluox-etine is highly effective for treating many types of depression afflicting many people, and that there are many people who respond to fluoxetine who have not responded to other types of antidepressants. However, we must add that we have also evaluated many patients who have not re-sponded to fluoxetine alone, but who have shown responses to fluoxetine only in combination with other medications (such as lithium). We have also treated patients who did not respond to or tolerate fluoxetine at all but who recovered from depression upon treatment with heterocyclic antidepres-sants or monoamine oxidase inhibitors. The take-home lesson is that fluoxetine is an important addition to our therapeutic regimen that currently is benefiting hundreds of thousands of people with depression. Nonethe-less, for those people with depression that fluoxetine cannot help, other types of antidepressants and electroconvulsive therapy (ECT) continue to hold great promise.

*Convenience—How to Take Fluoxetine*

Fluoxetine is availabe in 20 mg capsules and in liquid concentrate. The half-life of fluoxetine is long, which enables the drug to be prescribed in a once-per day dose. Although the Eli Lilly Company, which manufactures Prozac, states that most people require only one capsule per day to receive maximum antidepressant benefit, we are finding dosage requirements to be highly variable and specific to the individual patient. In the healthy young adult, we usually begin with one 20 mg capsule per day, which we recommend taking in the morning with water or with juice. If, after the first several doses, a patient has difficulty tolerating this dose, we recommend that he or she open the capsule and place a fractional dose (e.g., 50 percent) into the water or juice. Gradually, we raise the medication to the dose that shows significant antidepressant efficacy. Like other antidepressants, fluoxetine usually requires at least three weeks before depression is significantly reduced. Some patients may respond sooner than that, but a significant percentage of our patients show their maximal response after six to eight weeks of treatment. If our patients do not show a response after two or three weeks, we raise the dose of the medication. Many of our patients require 80 mg of fluoxetine before maximal antidepressant efficacy is realized; and these patients usually have no problem taking all of their medication at one time. In our experience and that of others, people with obsessive-compulsive symptoms (with or without depression) routinely require higher doses, with 80 mg being an average dose for this condition. Many of our patients have required much higher doses.

*Side Effects*

*Comparison with other antidepressants.* Like all other antidepressants, fluoxetine has many side effects—some quite serious and others just inconvenient. In general, however, fluoxetine has fewer disabling side effects than other classes of antidepressants. Fluoxetine has almost no anticholinergic side effects that lead to blurred vision, dry mouth, sluggishness, confusion, urinary problems, and constipation. In addition, it is the safest antidepressant to use in people who have severe cardiovascular disorders. It does not cause heart block or dangerously raise or lower the blood pressure in most patients. With the aging of our population and the increased incidence both of depression and heart disease in patients who are elderly, the absence of heart-related side effects is an important advantage. Fluoxetine is not associated with the increases in weight that commonly occur in patients who are being treated with heterocyclics or monoamine oxidase inhibitors. For most of those patients, the weight gain is an annoying side effect. Some patients even experience a five- to ten-pound loss of weight upon the initiation of treatment. However, in our experience, the drug is not the long-awaited safe "diet pill." After several months, our patients return to their baseline weights. Fluoxetine is not beneficial in elevating the mood of people who do not have clinical depression; nor does it seem to be effective in treating obesity—either of people who do or do not have depression.

*Troublesome side effects.* Insomnia, anxiety, and nervousness—especially during initiation of treatment—are the most troublesome side effects associated with fluoxetine. Unfortunately, more often these side effects occur early in treatment (i.e., the first several days), and many patients wish to discontinue their treatment with fluoxetine then and there. We, however, encourage our patients to try to endure these "early" side effects, as they frequently go away after the first several weeks of treatment. Occasionally, it is necessary for us to add low doses of a benzodiazepine medication (usually alprazolam [Xanax]) to enable the patient to remain on fluoxetine. We must add that this practice is somewhat controversial in that benzodiazepines may aggravate symptoms of depression and, in some people, lead to dependency. Once a patient experiences the antidepressant effects of fluoxetine, we generally taper the antianxiety agent without recurrence of the side effect. Other side effects of fluoxetine include stomach cramps, headache, diarrhea, nausea, skin rash, and, rarely, sedation. The most serious side effect associated with fluoxetine is seizures; but this is highly rare and is more common with most other types of antidepressants. Because the medication is relatively new, there is a possibility that there are other rare side effects about which we are currently unaware. There have been several case reports of patients with depression who, prior to treatment with fluoxetine, did not experience suicidal ideation or attempts; however, after the initiation of the treatment, they had intense suicidal preoccupations. The implications of this and other potential side effects of fluoxetine will require several more years of careful monitoring of patients taking the medication.

### Safety

In contrast to most heterocyclic antidepressants and monoamine oxidase inhibitors, fluoxetine is remarkably safe in situations of overdose. With most other types of antidepressants, taking several days' dose of the drug can result in significant risks to health and survival. At the present time, despite many attempts, fatalities subsequent to overdose with fluoxetine are virtually nonexistent. There have been cases of individuals taking up to fifty times their normal daily dose without fatal outcomes. Because so many patients with severe depression have thoughts of and desire to take their own lives, this added margin of safety is a great advantage (see Note, page 454). We must add, however, that little is known about the danger of combining high doses of fluoxetine (Prozac) with other medications or substances of abuse. In the absence of data, we must assume this practice is highly dangerous and potentially lethal.

## NOTE OF CAUTION

Unrealistic expectations and potentially dangerous oversimplifications often occur with important advances in medicine. In the case of fluoxetine, which now has helped hundreds of thousands of people overcome depression, a patient may become uncommonly discouraged if he or she does not respond or receives only a partial response to the medication. The experienced clinician, however, is aware of the multifaceted complexity and great variability in the symptomatology and response to treatment of depression. People with depression that is only partially treated may, paradoxically, have increased risk of suicide or other self-destructive behavior. Close clinical monitoring of all patients recovering from depression is essential— particularly to help patients understand and deal with the damage and disruptions in their personal and professional lives caused by the illness. Experienced clinical monitoring and intervention are required to assess carefully and to intervene with risk factors that may retard recovery or contribute to a future recurrence of depression. We are currently seeing an ever-increasing number of patients who have experienced some degree of improvement with medications, but who have not fully recovered from their depression. For these individuals who have not responded fully to antidepressant treatment, there are many safe and effective strategies. First, the individual must work closely with his or her physician to make "doubly sure" that there are no underlying medical disorders that are contributing to the depression. Second, possible interactions of the antidepressant with other medications and substances of abuse (including alcohol) also must be considered and appropriately dealt with. Third, the dose of the antidepressant and, where appropriate, the blood level of this medication should be considered. A great number of patients who are referred to us because of poor response to antidepressants require and will respond to higher doses of the medication. Fourth, consideration should be made of the strategy to augment the activity of the antidepressant agent by combining it with another drug. ("Augmentation therapy" is discussed more fully below, see p. 53.) Fifth, when the above considerations have not been beneficial, changing from one class of antidepressant to another class is indicated. In making a decision as to what antidepressant to choose after the first choice has not proved effective, the sophisiticated psychopharmacologist utilizes information from multiple sources—especially a patient's reaction to the side effects of the antidepressant first tried. In addition, such choices as the class of antidepressant that has proved effective in the treatment of close family members, or an antidepressant that affects a different class of neurotransmitters (e.g., from one that affects primarily the serotonin system to one that effects the catecholamine system), may be considered. Finally, as for every patient with depression, it is imperative that nondrug interventions such as exercise, stress, reduction, psychotherapy, family treatments, social support, self-help or advocacy groups, and/or dietary changes be evaluated and implemented where appropriate.

## ALPRAZOLAM (XANAX)

Alprazolam is a benzodiazepine; it has much in common with the other benzodiazepines frequently used as antianxiety agents, sedatives, and anticonvulsants (see Chapter 4). In addition, alprazolam has antidepressant properties and may be considered for a person suffering from both anxiety and depression. We, however, advise the use of antidepressants as the first line of treatment for people with both depression and anxiety.

*Advantages.* One advantage of alprazolam is that its therapeutic actions begin very quickly as compared to the heterocyclic antidepressants, whose positive effects take two to three weeks to appear. With alprazolam, the antianxiety effects begin almost at once even though the antidepressant effects usually take longer (two to three weeks).

*Disadvantages.* Among people treated with this drug for depression, a smaller proportion respond favorably than among those who are treated with a heterocyclic antidepressant. Also, unlike other antidepressants, alprazolam poses a significant risk of addiction. It is more difficult to withdraw from this drug than from most antidepressants. In fact, it is often the case that a person discontinuing alprazolam will find that anxiety returns just as strong or even stronger than it was before. As a result, many people become dependent on this drug.

## BUPROPION (WELLBUTRIN)

Bupropion is an antidepressant unrelated to all the other antidepressant medications mentioned thus far. It was originally introduced in 1986 for the treatment of depression in patients who did not tolerate or benefit from usual antidepressant therapy. A short time later, the manufacturer withdrew the drug because of reports of seizures in some patients with bulimia. Extensive research into this particular risk was undertaken, and in 1989 the drug was reintroduced with a cautionary statement that seizures occur in approximately 4 out of every 1,000 patients. (Of note is that seizures occur in about 1 out of every 1,000 patients on no medication.) Research to date indicates that bupropion may be as effective as other antidepressant medications, but more will be learned as its use becomes more common.

*Actions.* It is not known how bupropion causes its antidepressant effect. Is is clear that it does not inhibit the enzyme monoamine oxidase (as do the monoamine oxidase inhibitor antidepressants), nor does it inhibit the reuptake of norepinephrine or serotonin (as do the heterocyclic and serotonin-specific antidepressants).

*Advantages.* Bupropion causes few of the side effects usually encountered with the heterocyclic and monoamine oxidase antidepressants. It produces little or no drowsiness, does not interfere with the heart, and does not significantly reduce blood pressure. It has few anticholinergic side effects (e.g., dry mouth, blurry vision, confusion). Also, it is not associated with weight gain.

*Disadvantages.* The major problem associated with bupropion is the increased risk of seizures in bulimics. This is minimized by taking the medication in smaller doses, two or three times a day, which may be inconvenient for some people.

## Drugs That Enhance the Activities of Antidepressants— "Augmentation Therapy"

In some cases, certain drugs are used in combination with the antidepressants listed above to make receptors in the brain more receptive to the antidepressant. Such combinations should only be used under the guidance of a psychiatrist or other physician experienced with these drugs. For those individuals whose depression responds partially to antidepressant treatment and for those who do not achieve an appreciable response to antidepressant treatment at all, their psychiatrists may consider augmenting the activity of the antidepressant that they are currently taking by adding another drug of the type listed below.

### TRIIODOTHYRONINE ($T_3$, CYTOMEL, THYROLAR)

$T_3$ is a hormone naturally produced by the thyroid gland. It is now available in commercially manufactured form. Adding triiodothyronine to a heterocyclic may lead to a faster or better response, especially for those who have not experienced substantial benefit from a heterocyclic antidepressant alone. Please note that $T_3$ not only helps those individuals whose depression is associated with low thyroid function (hypothyroidism), but is useful in the treatment of people with uncomplicated depression as well.

## ANTIMANIC DRUGS (LITHIUM, CARBAMAZEPINE)

These medications may have both antimanic and moderate antidepressant actions and may be helpful for people who have not responded to standard therapy—usually used as an adjunct to heterocyclic antidepressants. These drugs may also be used when a person cannot tolerate the side effects of the standard medications.

## STIMULANTS

Although stimulants are not usually effective as antidepressants, they may sometimes be highly effective when combined with heterocyclic antidepressants. Because of the highly addictive nature of most stimulants, the clinician must exercise caution before prescribing a stimulant to patients with personal or family histories of addictive disorders. If an individual begins to increase his dose of stimulants beyond the usually low doses required for augmentation treatment, this is usually a warning sign that dependency and habituation are developing. In a very low percentage of patients, depression returns when stimulants are tapered. Closely monitored by a psychiatrist highly experienced in psychopharmacology, these patients can be maintained for years on very low doses of stimulants. Such patients do not experience the euphoric effects of stimulants and do not develop the pattern of increasing their dose. See Chapter 10 for more on stimulants.

## SEROTONIN-SPECIFIC ANTIDEPRESSANTS

On an experimental basis, we are now combining fluoxetine with heterocyclic antidepressants. The preliminary experience has been positive; but it is as yet too early to provide definitive recommendations about the safety and efficacy of this practice.

## COMBINING A HETEROCYCLIC WITH A MONOAMINE OXIDASE INHIBITOR

If you should experience little or no response to heterocyclic antidepressant treatment, your physician may suggest adding monoamine oxidase inhibitors. But as the combination of these two drugs may put you at significant risk of high blood pressure, this combination should only be considered after other treatments have failed—and then only under close supervision of a psychiatrist highly experienced in psychopharmacologic treatments. Careful monitoring of an individual's blood pressure, pulse rate, and other vital signs and symptoms is an essential component of this pharmacologic approach, which is, in almost every case, adopted only after other pharmacologic treatments have not proved sufficiently effective.

## What It Feels Like to Be On an Antidepressant

We often tell our patients that antidepressants are just the opposite of alcohol. With alcohol, you get the good effects right away. The worst side effect—the hangover—usually doesn't appear until the next morning. With the antidepressants, it's just the reverse. You will probably experience the unpleasant effects first, while the benefits may take days or weeks to appear.

### AT FIRST

The first noticeable effects of these drugs are, typically, dry mouth, blurry vision, constipation, and a feeling of light-headedness when you stand up. Although somewhat annoying, they are a positive sign: They are telling you that the drug is beginning to work. These side effects are usually quite tolerable, they often go away on their own, and they are rarely severe enough to make you discontinue the drug. The problem: their timing. The last thing a seriously depressed person needs is an additional source of stress and frustration, as minor as it may be. It can thus be especially important for the person's supportive and involved family members to encourage the depressed individual to keep his or her spirits up and to do his or her best to withstand these initial side effects—and to maintain the hope and confidence that the antidepressant effects of the agents will soon be at hand.

We usually advise physicians to start their patients on relatively low doses of antidepressants and to increase these doses gradually, constantly evaluating the patient's ability to tolerate the initial side effects, and using the patient's reaction to the side effects as a guide when increasing the dose of the medication.

Drinking water and sucking on hard candy can help one cope with dry mouth. Eating foods high in fiber (e.g., bran cereal) and taking a daily dose of a natural bulk laxative (e.g., Metamucil, Citrucel) can help prevent constipation. Stand up slowly to prevent light-headedness. Another side effect, blurred vision, usually affects only the reading of small print and goes away after several weeks.

Many people find that they become more, rather than *less*, nervous during the first couple of weeks after taking antidepressants, especially if nervousness and anxiety were prominent symptoms prior to beginning treatment. Although common in the initial phase of therapy, the nervousness should be greatly diminished as these medications begin to treat the depression. If the increase in anxiety is intolerable, it can also be treated by a brief course of the appropriate antianxiety medication (see Chapter 4). The sedative side effects of some of these drugs may prove particularly welcome to depressed people who are anxious or unable to sleep at night.

## AFTER TWO TO FOUR WEEKS AT FULL DOSE

It typically takes a long time for benefits to begin. To the depressed person, it often seems like an eternity.

It usually takes two to four weeks (and occasionally even longer) at a full therapeutic dose for the antidepressant agent to produce a positive response. And since it may take two or three weeks to get to the point where you are taking a full therapeutic dose, five or six weeks may elapse from the time you take the first pill until you feel that your symptoms have been substantially relieved. By the third week of treatment, many of the initial side effects—such as dry mouth, blurred vision, and constipation—will usually improve. Many patients at this time no longer experience these side effects. Orthostatic hypotension, or the decrease in blood pressure while sitting or standing up, may last longer. Research shows that injuries secondary to falling as a result of orthostatic hypotension are the most dangerous and debilitating early side effects of antidepressant use. This is particularly important for those with osteoporosis or others especially susceptible to bone fractures.

*It is extremely important to continue (1) taking the drug and (2) increasing the dose until a therapeutic response occurs.* The most common cause of failure in antidepressant therapy is not taking high-enough doses of the drug for a sufficient period of time. You may need to increase the dose of this drug gradually over a long period of time before you begin to feel its benefits.

Once the medication has had an opportunity to work, you should notice a gradual lessening of all your symptoms of depression: insomnia, lethargy, low self-esteem, depressed feelings, hopeless mood, anxiety, and poor sleep. It is often a friend or family member who first notices the initial signs of improvement.

In summary, then, you will know that the antidepressant is working when your self-esteem improves, feelings of hopefulness prevail, and you can return to your former—healthy—level of psychological functioning.

## How Do We Know That Antidepressants Work?

These drugs have all been proved effective in studies in which neither the patients receiving the drug, the physicians prescribing the drug, nor the researchers evaluating the results were aware which subjects were receiving the drug and which were receiving a placebo. This type of research, called a double-blind study, is the most objective kind of research, since the study design eliminates the possibility of bias on the part of the researchers. Many double-blind studies, performed worldwide, have proved that these drugs can provide substantial benefits in approximately 70 percent of those with major depression. About 20 percent experienced some symptom reduction when given the placebo.

Thus, you should have at least a 70 percent chance of benefit from the first drug you take. If the first drug does not produce the desired effect, try another drug. There are many other choices. With the great variety of treatments currently available, a skilled clinician can offer some level of relief for virtually everyone with severe depression.

## Drugs That Should *Not* Be Used to Treat Depression

Sometimes, especially when a depression is at an early stage and is mainly causing insomnia or anxiety, other medications are prescribed to try to treat the outward symptoms of depression. Sleeping pills for the insomnia, tranquilizers for anxiety, and stimulants for the depressed mood are, at times, prescribed. Unfortunately, these do not treat the underlying biologic process of depression and, usually, make depressive symptoms worse.

Although the drugs described below are sometimes used to treat depression, in our opinion this is a mistake. These drugs have not been proven safe and effective in the treatment of an uncomplicated major depression. In fact, studies have shown them to be no more effective than treatment with a placebo. Most have potentially hazardous side effects, and can make symptoms worse. Not infrequently, when the person's depression worsens and when he or she becomes exasperated by medical treatment, these drugs are used in serious suicide attempts. Thus, with the exception of a few rare situations, we recommend that *only members of the heterocyclic, mono-amine oxidase inhibitor, and serotonin-specific families of antidepressants and alprazolam be used to treat uncomplicated major depression.*

If you are suffering from an uncomplicated major depression and your physician suggests one of the drugs listed below, we suggest that you and your physician jointly review the material in this chapter and choose a more appropriate alternative.

## AMPHETAMINES AND OTHER STIMULANTS

Although amphetamines were used at one time for the treatment of depression, they are neither safe nor effective as the sole form of therapy. These drugs are used at times for treatment-resistant depressions, and there are data to suggest that they may be useful for this purpose. However, stimulants may cause or worsen psychosis, high blood pressure, agitation, and other symptoms. They also have a high potential for abuse. We believe that amphetamines and other stimulants should be prescribed only by psychiatrists for the treatment of depression. They should be used for such limited and specific purposes and their potential for abuse—both through prescriptions and illegal sources—is so great that we advise you to seek a second opinion from a psychiatrist qualified in psychopharmacology if your doctor attempts to prescribe any of the following drugs for uncomplicated depression.

*Amphetamines and other stimulants not recommended for the treatment of depression:* amphetamine, Cylert, Desoxyn, Dexedrine, dextroamphetamine, methamphetamine, methylphenidate, pemoline, and Ritalin.

## SLEEPING MEDICATIONS, ANTIANXIETY AGENTS, SEDATIVES, AND TRANQUILIZERS

These medications are often used to treat insomnia and anxiety, two symptoms commonly associated with depression. These medications are not effective in the treatment of the entire depressive syndrome. In fact, these drugs can make a depression worse through side effects and delay of efficacious treatment (see Chapters 4 and 8); we do not recommend them as the sole treatment for depression. If your doctor prescribes one of these medications alone for a major depression, we suggest you seek a second opinion from a psychiatrist qualified in psychopharmacology.

*Sleeping medications, antianxiety agents, sedatives, and tranquilizers*

*not recommended for the treatment of depression without specific consulta-
tion with your psychiatrist:*

1. Antianxiety agents—Ativan, BuSpar, buspirone, Centrax, clorazepate, chlordiazepoxide, clonazepam, Dalmane, diazepam, flurazepam,
halazepam, Halcion, Klonopin, Libritabs, Librium, lorazepam, oxazepam, Paxipam, prazepam, Restoril, Serax, temazepam, Tranxene, Valium, Valrelease;

2. Sedatives—Atarax, Benadryl, chloral hydrate, diphenhydramine,
Doriden, Equanil, glutethimide, hydroxyzine, Mepargan, meprobamate,
Meprospan, Mequin, methaqualone, methyprylon, Miltown, Moctec,
Noludar, Orgatrax, Paral, paraldehyde, Parest, Phenergan, Placidyl, pro-
methazine, Qaalude, Unisom, Valmid, Vistaril; and

3. Barbiturates—Alurate, amobarbital, Amytal, aprobarbital, butabarbital, Butisol, Luminal, Mebaral, mephobarbital, Nembutal, pentobarbital, phenobarbital, secobarbital, Seconal, Sedadrops, and Solfoton.

## ANTIPSYCHOTIC AGENTS

At times, antipsychotic medications are prescribed to treat symptoms of
anxiety or insomnia, which can accompany a depression. These medications should be used to treat psychotic symptoms (hallucinations and
delusions) or mania and are not generally effective in the treatment
of depression. Although a severe depression can include psychotic symptoms, which may respond to an appropriate antipsychotic medication, the
depressive component requires separate treatment. The potential side effects of these medications are so serious (see Chapter 7) and the potential
benefit so marginal that we do not recommend the use of these agents in an
uncomplicated nonpsychotic depression. If your doctor attempts to prescribe any of the following drugs for an uncomplicated depression, we
advise you to seek a second opinion from a psychiatrist qualified in psychopharmacology.

*Antipsychotic agents not recommended for the treatment of depression:*
acetophenazine, carphenazine, chlorpromazine, chlorprothixene, Compazine, Etrafon, fluphenazine, Haldol, haloperidol, loxapine, Loxitane,
Mellaril, mesoridazine, Moban, molindone, Navane, Orap, penfluridol,
Permitil, perphazine, pimozide, piperacetazine, prochlorperazine, Proket-
azine, Prolixin, Quide, Sempa, Serentil, Stelazine, Taractan, thioridazine, thiothixene, Thorazine, Tindal, trifluoperazine, triflupromazine,
Trilafon, and Vesprin.

**COMBINATION MEDICATIONS**

In general, especially in the initial treatment of uncomplicated depression, we do not advocate the use of combination products for treating any mental disorder. This is because one component is usually unnecessary. In the unusual case in which both are needed, the precise dose of each is restricted by the combination product's predetermined ratios; and combination products are usually more expensive than using two individual products.

At least four medications are currently marketed in the United States for the treatment of depression that also contain other drugs that are not antidepressants. If your doctor prescribes one of these combination medications, we suggest you seek a second opinion from a psychiatrist qualified in combination psychopharmacology.

*Combination medications not recommended for the treatment of depression without specific consultation with your psychiatrist:*

- Deprol (meprobamate and benactyzine)
- Etrafon (perphenazine and amitriptyline)
- Limbitrol (chlordiazepoxide and amitriptyline)
- Triavil (perphenazine and amitriptyline).

# Antidepressant Drugs: User Guidelines

**ARE ANTIDEPRESSANTS ADDICTIVE?**

Antidepressants are not addictive. Taking them will not make you dependent on them to feel well. The moods of people who are not depressed do not become elevated when taking these drugs. And stopping them, if done gradually, does not produce withdrawal symptoms. You should not discontinue these drugs abruptly, as doing so may produce a variety of flulike symptoms.

If you are being treated for severe depression, stopping these medications may result in the return of your depressed feelings.

**HOW LONG WILL I NEED TO TAKE THESE DRUGS?**

This varies considerably from person to person, but most severely depressed people will need to take these drugs for at least six months.

A very few people may find that they need to take these drugs for a year or longer, because their depression continues to recur if they attempt to discontinue the drug; but there is no evidence that these drugs have any lasting side effects after discontinuation. The clinical judgment of your psychiatrist working closely with you is usually the best guide for when to stop taking the drug.

## CAN I OVERDOSE ON ANTIDEPRESSANTS?

Yes, you can. The heterocyclics in particular can be lethal when an overdose is taken. In some cases, death can occur with overdoses as low as two to three times a person's normal daily dose.

The best way to guard against overdose is to take the medications exactly as prescribed, and to report any new symptoms or side effects to your physician immediately. There is much less danger from overdose with the serotonin-specific antidepressants.

## WHAT SHOULD BE DONE IN CASE OF OVERDOSE?

Anyone who has taken an overdose of these drugs needs prompt medical attention. If a drug overdose is suspected, go to the nearest emergency room immediately. Monitoring in the intensive care unit of a general hospital may be required.

Since overdose with these drugs is possible, and since people who are depressed are more likely to attempt suicide than people with many other kinds of mental disorder, it is very important to have a physician closely following a person who is depressed. Friends and family members should also be alert for signs that the person's depression may be worsening or that he or she may be considering or planning suicide.

## WHO SHOULD TAKE ANTIDEPRESSANTS?

Most people with severe depression can benefit from antidepressants, but as some types of depression are the result of other medical problems, you should not begin taking these drugs until you undergo a complete medical history and physical examination to rule out other medical conditions. This medical evaluation can also help to determine which antidepressants would be most appropriate.

## WHO SHOULD *NOT* TAKE ANTIDEPRESSANTS?

• If you have previously had negative reactions to a particular class of antidepressants, you should not take other drugs of that class.

• If you drive a car, fly aircraft, operate heavy machinery, or engage in other potentially dangerous activities, you should avoid antidepressants with marked sedative effects such as amitriptyline or trazodone, or you should take them only at bedtime when their sedating side effects will not interfere with your activities.

• If you cannot strictly follow the diet required when taking a monoamine oxidase inhibitor, you should avoid drugs of this class.

• If you are pregnant or are breast-feeding, you should, if possible, use nondrug alternatives for treating your depression.

• Persons with certain medical conditions should not take some of these drugs. Consult your physician for advice in your own case.

## TESTS REQUIRED PRIOR TO TAKING ANTIDEPRESSANTS

We recommend the following: (1) history and physical—a medical and psychiatric history profile, a mental status exam, a complete physical exam, and a neurologic assessment; (2) urine tests—a urinalysis and a toxicology screen for abused substances and environmental poisons; (3) blood tests— a complete blood count, electrolytes, blood urea nitrogen, serum creatinine, glucose, liver function tests, and thyroid function tests; (4) heart tests—an electrocardiogram.

## RECOMMENDED PERIODIC MEDICAL EXAMINATIONS WHILE TAKING ANTIDEPRESSANTS

If you are taking a monoamine oxidase inhibitor, frequent monitoring of blood pressure is necessary. You may wish to participate in this process by learning to take your own blood pressure at home.

For those with no medical illness (other than depression) who are taking heterocyclic or serotonin-specific antidepressants, no special lab tests or examinations are required unless you have been taking an antidepressant for over a year (as may be the case in someone with severe recurrent depression). After a year, the medical evaluation and laboratory tests should be repeated.

If you are over forty or have serious heart disease, a periodic electrocardiogram may be indicated. Check with your physician.

In some specific cases, other testing may be required. You should discuss your need for periodic medical examinations with your physician and/or your psychiatrist.

## POSSIBLE SIDE EFFECTS OF ANTIDEPRESSANTS

*Expected and Usually Manageable or Tolerable, and Occurring Early in Treatment*

Blurred vision, constipation, orthostatic hypotension (i.e., light-headedness upon standing), impaired concentration and sleepiness, dry mouth, initial increase in nervousness.

*More Rarely Occurring Side Effects*

Nausea and vomiting, increase in sweating, sensitivity to the sun, difficulty in ejaculation.

*Side Effects Specific to the Antidepressant Amoxapine*

Excessive or spontaneous flow of breast milk, irregular menstruation, sudden muscle stiffness and contractions.

## POSSIBLE ADVERSE REACTIONS

*All Antidepressants*

Depressed production of white blood cells, liver damage, irregularities of the heartbeat, muscle weakness, agitation, dizziness, tremors, loss of muscular coordination, seizures, difficulty in passing urine, loss of appetite, insomnia, worsening of glaucoma. During the first few days of treatment, some people may feel excessive restlessness and anxiety. This is an upsetting but not dangerous adverse reaction.

*Monoamine Oxidase Inhibitors*

Hypertensive crisis (dangerously increased blood pressure) when taken with tyramine-containing foods or incompatible drugs.

## CAN ANTIDEPRESSANTS INTERACT WITH FOOD?

The monoamine oxidase inhibitors (e.g., Parnate, Nardil) may interact dangerously with foods having a high tyramine content (see p. 46). None of the other classes of antidepressants interacts dangerously with foods.

## CAN ANTIDEPRESSANTS INTERACT WITH ALCOHOL?

Yes. Heavy alcohol use commonly produces depression. Such depression cannot be effectively treated unless the depressed person severely limits his or her alcohol intake. In addition, alcohol magnifies a number of the unpleasant side effects of the antidepressants. We strongly advise people who are depressed to stop drinking. It is especially important that you not drink alcohol while taking antidepressants.

## CAN ANTIDEPRESSANTS INTERACT WITH OTHER DRUGS?

Yes, particularly other antidepressants (monoamine oxidase inhibitors), alcohol, and abused substances such as cocaine, amphetamines, and depressants.

## DIFFERENCES AMONG THE ANTIDEPRESSANTS

### Heterocyclic Antidepressants

Most sedating: amitriptyline, trimipramine, and doxepin.
Least sedating: desipramine and protriptyline.
Most anticholinergic: amitriptyline, imipramine, trimipramine, doxepin, fluoxetine, and hazodone.
Least anticholinergic: desipramine, nortriptyline, and protriptyline.

## OTHER CONSIDERATIONS

### Antidepressants and Panic Attacks

Antidepressants can be very useful in the treatment of panic attacks. For more on the diagnosis and treatment of panic and phobias, see Chapter 5.

### Antidepressants and Chronic Pain

Antidepressants can be useful in the treatment of chronic pain—but first have a comprehensive medical evaluation. Although many antidepressants are used in the treatment of pain, the drug amitriptyline (Elavil) appears to be among the most effective.

### Antidepressants and Migraine Headaches

Heterocyclic and serotonin-specific antidepressants (e.g., amitriptyline, fluoxetine) are sometimes used to help prevent and treat migraines.

### Antidepressants and Bed-Wetting (Enuresis)

Imipramine and some other heterocyclic antidepressants are occasionally used to treat chronic bed-wetting in children (in cases in which no physical cause for the lack of bladder control can be found). The use of psychoactive medications for this purpose is extremely controversial, however. When used in such cases, the drug usually stops the bed-wetting; but the problem often recurs as soon as the child stops taking the medication.

### Use During Pregnancy and Breast-Feeding

These drugs have not been demonstrated to be safe during pregnancy. Antidepressant use during pregnancy should be limited to those cases in which the patient is at high risk for harming herself or others if not treated. As these medications can be secreted in the breast milk, nursing mothers should also either use nondrug alternatives or should bottle-feed the infant.

### Precautions for Those over Sixty

People over sixty may be unable to tolerate high doses of antidepressants, since they are more susceptible to the side effects of these drugs (especially blackouts or dizziness after standing up suddenly, confusion, and memory impairment). Initiating the medication at very low doses and increasing the daily dose very slowly can help reduce the occurrence of these side-effects. Serotonin-specific antidepressants are often indicated because of their reduced side-effect profile.

## WHO SHOULD PRESCRIBE ANTIDEPRESSANT DRUGS?

Only physicians who are familiar with the therapeutic and side effects of these medications should prescribe them; and then only if they are prepared to do the necessary preliminary evaluation and follow-up monitoring required. Choosing the right dose of the right antidepressant for a given patient often requires considerable clinical experience.

## HOW CAN THESE DRUGS BE MISUSED?

### In General

These drugs should not be used unless (1) you have had a complete medical history and physical examination taken by a qualified physician and the predrug laboratory tests recommended for the drug you will be taking, (2) you understand and accept the fact that you are taking this drug on a trial basis, and that there is a chance that it will not turn out to be the right drug for you, and if this is the case, you will be willing to try other therapies; (3) you have arranged to see your doctor for periodic follow-up visits.

If you achieve a good therapeutic response, you will be able to stop taking these drugs in about six months (exception: if you are suffering from severe or recurrent depression). Your original treatment plan should include a schedule for discontinuing the medication at a certain date.

## Abuse

Since antidepressants do not produce a high, they are not commonly used for recreational purposes. Patients rarely increase their doses of these drugs spontaneously. Therefore, antidepressants are rarely, if ever, abused.

## SUSAN EAMES: UNSUCCESSFUL USE OF ANTIDEPRESSANTS

Before her youngest daughter left for college, Susan spent most of her time caring for her home and four children; afterwards, things went rapidly downhill. The house seemed far too empty. Susan toyed with this project and that, but found nothing that really excited her. She found herself easily distracted. She realized that she was having a hard time simply getting through the day.

A little brandy always seemed to make things better. By the time her daughter came home for Christmas vacation, Susan was taking four to five large drinks a day. Her husband began suspecting something was wrong when he called her at home in the middle of the day and heard her slurred speech.

At the urging of her husband and her brother, Susan went to see her family physician, Dr. Pearson. After taking a complete history and giving Susan a full physical examination, the doctor delivered his verdict: Susan had become depressed. When her doctor asked her about her use of alcohol, Susan was too embarrassed to tell the truth; she maintained that she drank only occasionally.

Dr. Pearson prescribed an antidepressant. Unfortunately, no family consultation or psychotherapy was included in the treatment plan. In fact the daily dose prescribed by Dr. Pearson (100 mg per day of amitriptyline) was not sufficient to achieve a therapeutic level, although Susan had the side effects of sedation and mental confusion.

One evening, her husband came home to find Susan comatose with two empty bottles of scotch and several empty medicine containers on her bed. Susan was pronounced dead on arrival at the general hospital emergency room. The failure of the physician to communicate more closely with Susan's husband and family, the failure to treat her alcoholism, the improper use of antidepressants, and the failure to refer Susan for counseling all contributed to the tragic outcome.

## CARL ZELAND: SUCCESSFUL USE OF ANTIDEPRESSANTS

The first part of Carl's history is given on p. 29.

The family physician who saw Carl recognized that in order to recover from his depression, Carl would need to take three important steps: stop drinking, take an antidepressant medication, and have individual counseling (psychotherapy). At first, Carl protested that he couldn't possibly give up alcohol. It was the only way he could get to sleep. Dr. Higgins gently explained that the alcohol was also one of the principal causes of Carl's sleeplessness. Dr. Higgins gave Carl a comprehensive physical exam and laboratory testing including blood tests, liver function tests, and an EKG. He also referred to Carl to Alcoholics Anonymous.

When Carl finally agreed, Dr. Higgins prescribed an antidepressant medication, trazodone—at an initial dose of 50 mg at bedtime—with instructions to increase the dose to 50 mg per day as long as there were no significant side effects. Because Carl said he had been thinking about suicide a great deal, Dr. Higgins gave him only a two-day supply.

After three days of this regimen, Carl reported he was sleeping a bit better and that he had stopped drinking. The doctor told Carl that this dry mouth meant that the medication was getting into his system and beginning to work. He also said that the result of all laboratory tests were negative; no thyroid, liver, or other physical problems were found; there was no reason to suspect any other physical causes of depression.

Dr. Higgins also met with Carl's wife and with other family members, weekly on four occasions, to help them monitor Carl's progress and to pick up any warning signals that Carl might be getting more rather than less suicidal. For the first four weeks, he saw Carl four times per week. During this time, he gave Carl a great deal of encouragement and support for not drinking and for staying with the treatment plan.

After a month, Carl was feeling somewhat better. He was sleeping better, had more self-confidence, and derived more pleasure from his work and home life. Carl now saw a psychotherapist three times a week for three weeks. They began to discuss the feelings and events that had led to Carl's depression. Over the next several weeks, Carl began to feel much better. His wife noticed it first. A week later, Carl himself noticed that he was sleeping much better, and that he felt more refreshed and energetic during the day.

As his psychotherapy continued, Carl began to take a good look at his negative self-concepts. He began to see that his feelings of "total incompetence as a breadwinner, as a father, as a husband, and as a man" were the result of his depression and not an accurate self-appraisal.

After seven weeks, Carl felt completely normal again. His appetite had returned and he was his usual energetic, robust self. His pharmocatherapy did not end at this point, however. Dr. Higgins explained how depression might recur if he stopped the medication, and he advised Carl to continue taking the antidepressant for at least six months. During this time, Carl continued his psychotherapy once a week to discuss his feelings of anxiety and despair whenever he perceived that his collegues were not supportive, and to review all of his problems in adjusting to his new job as foreman. With his therapist's advice, Carl made some new resolutions such as not expressing anger and becoming defensive when his authority was questioned at work, and communicating more openly about work problems with his superior. By attending meetings of Alcoholics Anonymous, Carl came to understand how he had misued alcohol in an unsuccessful effort to manage anxiety and to sleep. He continued to attend A.A.

Two years later, Carl is doing well. He has been off medication for more than a year, and has had no further depressed feelings. He looks back on the depression as one of the worst times of his life, but he acknowledges that he learned a great deal from it.

He now feels more in control of his life than he ever felt before. "I've also realized just how much I really mean to my family, and how much they mean to me. Also, I now find I can do my job without constantly worrying how other people will judge me or whether they will get angry with me when I have to make an unpopular decision. It's just too bad I had to wait so long or suffer so much to learn some of these lessons."

## Electroconvulsive Therapy and Depression

A combination of individual self-help, individual and group psychotherapy, self-help groups, addiction treatment (for example, for alcohol addiction), and supportive friends, plus the antidepressant medications described in this chapter, can help control most cases of depression. However, if after all these treatments your depression continues unabated, your physician may raise the possibility of using electroconvulsive (shock) therapy, ECT.

Some of us remember hearing horrible stories of patients who were harmed by ECT treatment. While we deplore the mistakes of the past, we can assure you that modern ECT offers hope to many depressed people who have not responded to other treatments. While it may not be the treatment of first choice in most situations, if you or your family member has tried drugs and therapies without success, ECT may well be a useful treatment for depression. For an overview of ECT treatment, see Chapter 13.

## Recommended Reading on Depression and Manic-Depressive Disorder

There are many useful self-help books on depression and manic depression. Following is a list of several of the more recent books that can be ordered through the National Alliance for the Mentally Ill (NAMI), 2101 Wilson Blvd. Suite 302, Arlington, VA 22201, (703) 524-7600:

Gold, Mark S., M.D. *The Good News About Depression: Cures and Treatments in the New Age of Psychiatry.* New York: Villard Books, 1987.

Goodwin, Frederick K., M.D. *Depression and Manic-Depressive Illness*, "Medicine for the Layman." Bethesda, MD: U.S. Department of Health and Human Services, 1982.

Greist, John, and James Jefferson. *Depression and Its Treatment: Help for the Nation's Number 1 Mental Problem.* Washington, D.C.: American Psychiatric Press, 1984.

Klein, Donald, and Paul H. Wender. *Do You Have a Depressive Illness?* New York: New American Library, 1988.

Lobel, Brana, and Robert M. A. Hirschfield. *Depression: What We Know.* Rockville, MD: U.S. Department of Health and Human Services and NIMH, 1985.

Papolos, Demitri, and Janice Papolos. *Overcoming Depression.* New York: Harper and Row, 1987.

## Chapter 4

# Antianxiety Drugs

ANXIETY has both mental and physical components. It is a state of uneasiness of mind, a vague sense of undefined danger. Anxiety resembles fear; but for the person who is afraid, the danger has an obvious source. In the case of the anxious person, there is usually no identifiable danger. Nevertheless, the person is plagued by constant worry, which, if intense and prolonged, can produce considerable mental suffering. The anxious person may also experience pain and apprehension, and may amplify concerns about relatively minor issues that have arisen or might arise in the future.

People suffering from high levels of anxiety frequently speak of feeling agitated, restless, *keyed up* or *on edge*. They sometimes describe themselves as *apprehensive, concerned, distressed, nervous, irritable, panicked, troubled, uneasy,* or *upset*. They frequently complain of confused thinking or difficulty in concentrating. They are fearful of "losing control."

The anxious person usually experiences physical distress including nausea, diarrhea, or abdominal symptoms; rapid, intense heartbeat; night terrors; muscle tension, aches, or soreness; easy fatigability; sweating; cold or clammy hands; dizziness or light-headedness; dry mouth; frequent urination; hot flashes or chills; trouble swallowing; or a lump in the throat.

70

Anxiety is the most widespread of all psychological problems. A recent study found that 8 percent of adults living in U.S. cities had experienced one or more periods of severe anxiety during the preceding six months. Another recent study found that about 2 percent of British children at any given time experience severe anxiety. Women are twice as likely to be severely anxious as are men. Rates are roughly the same for all socioeconomic groups in the United States.

Some people suffer a higher than average level of anxiety all their lives, while others experience repeated relatively brief episodes of severe anxiety. These recurring anxiety attacks may start at any age, but most frequently begin between the ages of fifteen and thirty-five, and may persist through old age.

## Types of Anxiety

Physicians sometimes speak of a person who is intensely anxious as suffering from an *anxiety disorder*. This is simply a medical term to describe a person feeling intense, prolonged anxiety (i.e., for more than two weeks). It does *not* necessarily mean that you have a permanent or incurable condition.

Sometimes an anxiety disorder falls into one of these clearly defined categories:

1. phobia
2. agoraphobia
3. panic attacks
4. obsessive-compulsive behavior
5. posttraumatic stress disorder
6. performance anxiety

### SUZANNE MILLER: PHOBIA

It was not until a promotion took her to New York that Suzanne's fear of dogs became a serious problem. As long as she lived in Dallas, she had been able to keep her environment dog-free. She'd had her suburban home enclosed by a high fence. She never went out except by car, and she drove directly to her office building's parking garage.

New York was another matter. She bought a co-op apartment in a building that prohibited pets, but she was shocked to find that people walked their dogs all hours of the day and night. It was simply not possible to walk anywhere without encountering dogs.

For a while, Suzanne did fairly well. She had her doorman hail a cab each morning after making sure there were no dogs in sight. She sprinted from the cab to her office building, and had her evening cab pick her up at the loading dock, where dogs were not allowed. She avoided going to theaters and restaurants, since there was always the risk of encountering a dog. She also avoided going to the grocery store. She lived on food deliveries from nearby restaurants and became a virtual prisoner in her own apartment.

As she was going to work one morning—eight months after she moved to New York—the elevator doors opened on a lower floor, and two lively wire-haired terriers bounded in. Suzanne screamed and fainted. The next day she consulted a psychiatrist who specialized in the drug treatment of phobias.

A phobia is a persistent irrational fear of a specific object, activity, or situation—in Suzanne's case, it was dogs—that is so strong that it results in an overwhelming urge to avoid the object, activity, or situation that produces it. People with such phobic fears usually realize that their feelings are irrational, but find themselves going to seemingly absurd lengths to avoid the intense feelings that are triggered by the object of their phobia. Fear of flying and fear of heights are two common phobias. Another common phobia, agoraphobia (see below), is the fear of being in a place or situation from which escape might be difficult, embarrassing, or impossible in the event of a sudden catastrophe.

For a more extensive discussion of phobias, see Chapter 5.

## AGORAPHOBIA

People with agoraphobia (literally: *fear of gathering places,* or *of open spaces*) are terrified of being in situations in which sudden harm may come upon them, but help will not be available. They therefore do all they can to avoid crowds, bridges, tunnels, and public transportation. Steve was an accountant who suffered from an intense fear of crossing bridges. He drove twenty-five miles out of his way each day to avoid crossing a bridge on his way to work. He refused to travel out of his small town for fear of having to cross a bridge.

People with agoraphobia may restrict their normal activities, sometimes to the point where they will not leave home unless accompanied by a person they trust. People with agoraphobia sometimes come to depend heavily upon one specific person, who is sometimes called the person's phobic partner.

For additional information on agoraphobia, see Chapter 5.

### EMILY ENGLANDER: PANIC ATTACKS

Emily experienced her first panic attack on a Saturday afternoon while driving to a nearby shopping center to have lunch with a friend. "I was stopping at a red light, and suddenly I couldn't catch my breath," she remembers. "It seemed as if somebody had sucked all the oxygen out of the car. At the same time my arms, my legs, and my mouth all went numb. I was possessed by a horrible feeling of terror and dread. I was sure I was dying of a heart attack.

"Bystanders called an ambulance, and I was rushed to the hospital. The doctors found nothing wrong. When I returned home, I experienced another panic attack. Again I went by ambulance to the hospital. This time my doctor told me he thought I'd had a panic attack. I reluctantly agreed to see a psychiatrist."

A panic attack is a period of intense anxiety and fear that occurs unexpectedly in the absence of any situation (e.g., an auto accident, the death of a loved one) that might normally produce such feelings. Without any apparent reason, the person experiences a sudden sense of overwhelming apprehension, fear, terror, and a sense of impending doom. People experiencing panic attacks may fear that they are in great danger of dying or that they may lose control of themselves and go crazy. These feelings may be accompanied by a racing heartbeat, dry mouth, sweating, or cold, clammy hands; dizziness, nausea, a sensation of being unable to breathe, or other physical symptoms.

People who experience panic attacks typically do so while engaged in a routine activity such as washing the dishes, driving their car, or walking in the park. Most panic attacks last between five and twenty minutes. They can occur as frequently as several times a day or as rarely as once or twice a year. Some people who have experienced panic attacks experience great anxiety about the possibility of future attacks. A somewhat similar kind of experience may occur at night while a person is asleep. These are called night terrors.

For more on panic attacks, see Chapter 5.

### JOHN EVANS: OBSESSIVE-COMPULSIVE BEHAVIOR

Shortly after he started his sophomore year of college, John Evans, aged eighteen, began worrying that his father might develop a brain tumor. In spite of continued reassurances by his family and his father's physicians, John was persistently haunted by these obsessive thoughts—to the point where he began staying home from class so that he could come to his father's aid in case of a life-threatening medical emergency. He awakened his father several times a night to make sure he was all right. Despite all reassurances and all evidence to the contrary, John continued to be plagued by these irrational fears. When the family finally consulted a psychiatrist, John was diagnosed as having severe anxiety accompanied by obsessive-compulsive behavior.

For a detailed account of John's treatment and recovery, see p. 101.

Obsessions are recurring irrational ideas, thoughts, impulses, or images. People experiencing obsessive thoughts recognize that these ideas don't make sense, but are simply unable to stop the flow of irrational ideas or images. Obsessions frequently involve dirt, contamination, diseases, real or imagined trauma, or other frightening or unpleasant themes.

These obsessive thoughts frequently lead to compulsive behaviors—repeated activities or rituals performed in response to an obsessive thought. Through these compulsive behaviors, a person seeks to prevent, neutralize, or undo some dreaded event. John's compulsive behavior involved his continuing expressions of concern for his father's health. John would wash his hands every ten or fifteen minutes because he was fearful that his germs would contaminate his father and make him deathly ill. After washing, he would touch articles of his father's clothing in an attempt to use "magic" to protect his father from the dreaded brain tumor.

Many of us engage in obsessive-compulsive activities from time to time. It may be as benign as checking several times to be sure that the oven is turned off or that we locked the front door of our house. However, an estimated 2 to 3 percent of adults experience marked obsessive-compulsive behavior. The symptoms span a wide range—from almost adaptive to so disruptive that a person cannot function. In certain situations, obsessive traits may provide distinct benefits. For example, many career athletes, lawyers, and physicians tend to obsess about the details of their professions. Not many of us would complain if we learned that the brain surgeon who would be operating on us tended to obsess about the cleanliness of the operating rooms and the minute details of our illness. (His or her family might complain about the time away from home and the distraction that this behavior entailed.) However, as obsessive-compulsive behaviors become more extreme, they can interfere with functioning in all realms. If a neurosurgeon were so obsessed with germs that he or she was distracted while operating, this would be a serious problem.

A tendency to obsessive-compulsive behavior may be partly hereditary. Such behavior may be linked to a decreased level of the chemical messenger serotonin in the brain. New drugs that increase serotonin may therefore prove effective in the treatment of obsessive-compulsive behavior (see Chapter 3).

Antianxiety agents have only limited value in the treatment of obsessive-compulsive conditions. Because this is usually a long-term personality pattern, the use of antianxiety drugs may lead to dependency. Among the most useful approaches to obsessive-compulsive conditions are supportive psychotherapy, behavioral treatments, and such self-help measures as exercise and relaxation techniques. If symptoms are severe, treatment with serotonin-stimulating antidepressants should be considered. For more on such treatments, see Chapters 3 and 14.

## JAKE NICHOLS: ANXIETY FOLLOWING A TRAUMATIC EXPERIENCE (POSTTRAUMATIC STRESS DISORDER)

Jake Nichols was a marine field commander in Vietnam. He experienced a long succession of horrors and tragedies during his year of service there. On one occasion, 75 percent of his platoon was killed in an intense enemy attack.

After he returned to civilian life, Jake found himself endlessly reliving his painful experiences overseas. He lost all interest in work, friends, and family; he sat around all day drinking beer and discussing the war with other Vietnam vets. Every time he saw a Vietnamese-American or heard the sound of helicopters, he would be overwhelmed by disabling feelings of anxiety and impending doom.

Many people who have lived through a deeply troubling life event find themselves having recurring recollections or dreams about the traumatic incident. The original events that trigger such a reaction may include a serious threat to one's life or the lives of one's family, the destruction of home or property, serious auto or plane crashes, rape, murder, suicide of a loved one, or wartime experiences. Psychiatrists call this condition a *posttraumatic stress disorder.*

Persons afflicted with this condition may find themselves endlessly replaying the disturbing occurrence. They may make heroic efforts to avoid people, places, objects, or situations that remind them of their upsetting ordeal. Some individuals completely suppress the memory of painful experiences. Psychiatrists call this *psychogenic amnesia*.

Although antianxiety drugs may help a person get through a particularly difficult few days, they are not recommended for long-term use in this condition. There is currently no accepted long-term pharmacological treatment for posttraumatic stress disorder. Researchers are currently studying the effects of beta blockers, the antihypertensive drug clonidine, antidepressants, and other experimental drugs for posttraumatic stress disorder.

Most individuals who suffer from posttraumatic stress disorder do best with a combination of self-help, support groups, and supportive sessions with a counselor or therapist. Support groups composed of others who have experienced similar trauma (e.g., those who have experienced rape, suicide in the family, family alcoholism, the death of a child, or those who are Vietnam veterans, or belong to families of people with serious head injuries) can be especially helpful.

## PERFORMANCE ANXIETY

Performance anxiety, also known as social phobia, stage fright, or exam nerves, is a special type of anxiety that develops only under certain situations—typically during public speaking or other public performances. People who suffer from performance anxiety are usually afraid of acting in a way that will make them feel humiliated or embarrassed. A young man who suffers from performance anxiety described his symptoms as follows: "My mind goes completely blank. My mouth becomes dry, and I have such a lump in my throat it feels impossible to speak. I'm paralyzed by fear and am terrified I might faint and humiliate myself even further." There is now good evidence that many people who suffer from performance anxiety can be treated by beta blockers along with psychological and behavioral therapies.

# What Causes Anxiety?

## MEDICAL CONDITIONS THAT CAN PRODUCE ANXIETY

Some physical conditions can produce all the symptoms associated with intense, prolonged anxiety. These include anemia, asthma, emphysema, low blood pressure, heart disease, an overactive thyroid gland (hyperthyroidism), and low blood sugar (hypoglycemia), as well as a number of other conditions (see Sidebar 1). If you are troubled by continuing

## Sidebar 1: Medical Conditions That Can Produce Anxiety (Panic Disorder)

*Cardiovascular/respiratory*
  asthma
  cardiac arrhythmias
  chronic obstructive pulmonary
    disease
  congestive heart failure
  coronary insufficiency
  hyperdynamic beta adrenergic
    state
  hypertension
  hyperventilation syndrome
  hypoxia, embolus, infections
  mitral valve prolapse
*Endocrine*
  carcinoid
  Cushing's syndrome
  hyperthyroidism
  hypoglycemia
  hypoparathyroidism
  hypothyroidism
  menopause
  pheochromocytoma
  premenstrual syndrome
*Neurologic*
  collagen vascular disease
  epilepsy

  Huntington's disease
  multiple sclerosis
  organic brain syndrome—
    delirium, dementia
  vestibular dysfunction
  Wilson's disease
*Substance-related*
  Intoxications
    anticholinergic drugs
    aspirin
    caffeine
    cocaine
    hallucinogens, including
      phencyclidine (angel dust)
    steroids
    sympathomimetics
    THC
  Withdrawal symptoms
    alcohol
    narcotics
    sedative hypnotics

anxiety of an unknown cause, we suggest that you have a thorough medical examination by a good internist (a physician who specializes in internal medicine) to determine whether a medical condition may be responsible. If no physical cause is found, you may wish to consider self-help measures, professional counseling, and/or drug treatment.

## SOME MEDICATIONS CAN PRODUCE ANXIETY

A wide variety of prescription and over-the-counter medications—cold medicines, diet pills, thyroid supplements, stimulants, antidepressants, sleeping pills, blood pressure medications, caffeine-containing medications, and many other drugs—can produce the symptoms of anxiety. To complicate matters even further, discontinuing certain drugs—especially antianxiety drugs—can produce a marked increase in anxiety symptoms. Discontinuing some other drugs—especially sleeping pills, pain pills, and blood pressure medications—can also produce anxiety symptoms.

## CAFFEINE AND ANXIETY

High doses of caffeine can produce symptoms that are indistinguishable from those of an anxiety attack. High caffeine intake is one of the most common—and most overlooked—causes of anxiety. Many of the most troublesome cases of prolonged, unexplained anxiety disappear rapidly when the formerly anxious individual simply eliminates or reduces his or her caffeine consumption.

The pharmacological effects of caffeine can include nervousness, irritability, agitation, headache, rapid breathing, muscle twitching, and a tremor in the hands. People who ingest high doses of caffeine also frequently complain of insomnia and other sleep disturbances. Other symptoms of excessive caffeine intake can include sensitivity to touch, ringing in the ears, and visual flashes of light. Withdrawal from caffeine can produce irritability, anxiety, nervousness, inability to work effectively, lethargy, restlessness, and headache. This self-scoring quiz (see Sidebar 2) will help you calculate your daily intake of caffeine.

Symptoms of caffeinism are most common in those who take in more than 250 to 300 mg of caffeine per day—the equivalent of two to four cups of strong coffee. Caffeine's potential as a source of anxiety symptoms is often overlooked by health professionals. A surprising number of people who seek medical treatment for anxiety are never asked about their caffeine intake. Thus, if you drink coffee, tea, or colas, or are taking pain medications that contain caffeine (e.g., Excedrin), and are experiencing anxiety, you should decrease or eliminate your caffeine intake. If you seek professional advice for anxiety-related symptoms, be sure to let your counselor or health professional know how much caffeine you consume each day.

---

## Sidebar 2:  What's Your Daily Caffeine Consumption?

Coffee        ___ cups   @ ___ mg = ___ mg
 (fill in dose from Table 1)

Tea         ___ cups   @ ___ mg = ___ mg
 (fill in dose from Table 1)

Cola drinks      ___ cups   @ ___ mg = ___ mg
 (fill in dose from Table 2)

OTC drugs      ___ cups   @ ___ mg = ___ mg
 (fill in dose from Table 3)

Other sources             ___ mg
 (chocolate 25 mg per bar, cocoa 13 mg per cup)

            Daily total   ___ mg

    I would prefer my daily total to be about   ___ mg

---

## ALCOHOL AND ANXIETY

Under certain conditions, alcoholic beverages may help reduce anxiety and increase social comfort for certain individuals. It is thus easy to see how some people who suffer from persistent, severe anxiety may grow dependent on alcohol. Unfortunately, alcohol can also produce a wide variety of side effects and toxic effects—including increased anxiety levels. It can severely disrupt social interactions, and it has a powerful potential for addiction and abuse. Thus alcohol itself can quickly become a much more serious problem than the original anxiety it was used to supposedly treat.

Although the occasional use of alcoholic beverages may be harmless in the psychologically healthy individual, people with persistent, severe anxiety should not attempt to use alcohol as an antianxiety agent. When used regularly for this purpose, the hazards of alcohol far outweigh its benefits.

## IS ANXIETY HEREDITARY?

A tendency to anxiety seems to run in certain families. Studies show that about 55 percent of the close relatives of people with persistent anxiety problems will also have high anxiety levels. Only about 2 percent of the close relatives of people with normal anxiety levels have high anxiety levels.

TABLE 1

**Caffeine Content of Coffee, Tea, and Cocoa**
**(mg per serving—average values)**

| | |
|---|---|
| Coffee, instant | 66 |
| Coffee, percolated | 110 |
| Coffee, drip | 146 |
| Teabag, 5-minute brew | 46 |
| Teabag, 1-minute brew | 28 |
| Loose tea, 5-minute brew | 40 |
| Cocoa | 13 |

TABLE 2

**Caffeine Content of Cola Beverages (mg per 12-ounce can)**

| | |
|---|---|
| Coca-Cola | 65 |
| Dr. Pepper | 61 |
| Mountain Dew | 55 |
| Diet Dr. Pepper | 54 |
| TAB | 49 |
| Pepsi Cola | 43 |
| Diet RC | 33 |
| Diet-Rite | 32 |

TABLE 3

**Caffeine Content of Over-the-Counter Drugs (mg per tablet)**

| | |
|---|---|
| Anacin | 32 |
| Aqua-ban | 100 |
| Bivarin | 200 |
| Caffedrine | 200 |
| Dristan | 16 |
| Empirin | 32 |
| Excedrin | 64 |
| Midol | 32 |
| No Doz | 100 |
| Pre-mens Forte | 100 |
| Vanquish | 33 |

**Source:** Bunker, M. L., and McWilliams, M. "Caffeine Content of Common Beverages." *Journal of the American Dietetic Association*, 74 (January 1979): 28–32.

## CAN ALLERGIES CAUSE ANXIETY?

Although sensitivities to certain foods can cause a wide variety of psychological symptoms, including anxiety, except for a few rare cases there is little evidence that allergies are a common cause of anxiety symptoms.

## CAN LOW BLOOD SUGAR (HYPOGLYCEMIA) CAUSE ANXIETY?

Low blood sugar does, indeed, produce anxiety. However, this is a relatively rare cause of anxiety, and your internist can establish whether you suffer from this condition by laboratory blood tests such as fasting glucose levels.

# Nondrug Treatments for Anxiety

Once possible physical causes have been ruled out, nondrug treatments for anxiety should be considered. Such treatments seek to improve your overall health status, reduce the external sources of stress, and help you learn new patterns of processing information so that a given stimulus is experienced as less stressful. Self-help measures can also help increase your ability to relax, and to engage in enjoyable and fulfilling activities.

Although friends, counselors, and professionals may be able to suggest some useful strategies, this is an area in which you yourself are the final authority. There is no standard treatment that works for everyone. We recommend that you explore all possible options, then choose the treatments that strike you as most promising.

### PSYCHOLOGICAL TREATMENT FOR ANXIETY

People with feelings of severe anxiety may find it helpful to discuss the problem with a sympathetic friend or with a member of the clergy. Self-help groups can also be a good source of support, advice, and help. You may wish to discuss setting up a series of regular therapy sessions with a psychologist, psychiatrist, social worker, psychiatric nurse, or other health professional.

Professional psychotherapy may take place either one-to-one with a therapist, or in a group session. In individual psychotherapy, a professional counselor will usually ask questions about many aspects of your past experience and present situation in order to understand you more fully and to gain insights into the possible causes of your anxiety. Most counselors also provide support, reassurance, and encouragement. The goal of psychotherapy is to increase your understanding of the causes of your anxiety, and to decrease these feelings through understanding, support, and reduction in life stresses. Psychoanalysis is an intensive form of individual treatment in which an individual meets frequently (e.g., four times per week) with a psychoanalyst over a protracted time period (several years). The focus is less on supportive and directive counseling and more on uncovering and treating unconscious conflicts that may be the source of your anxiety. If you or your physician believe that psychological treatment may be helpful, you may wish to seek several opinions covering the different options before deciding which approach seems most promising and compatible.

## EXERCISE

One option that deserves special consideration is exercise. While exercise is not everyone's cup of tea, if you already have some interest in exercise, it may prove an extremely useful tool in the management of anxiety.

One of us (Yudofsky) is an avid swimmer. He works out with a masters swim team and swims several miles at least five times per week. Immediately after his swimming workout, he experiences a profound feeling of relaxation and well-being. He sometimes begins a swimming session tense and overly concerned about some minor or major problem at work or at home, but, by the time he gets out of the water, his excessive worries have usually vanished.

But swimming is not the answer for everyone. One of us (Ferguson) becomes extremely tense in the water but loves to put on his running shoes and set off at a slow, steady jog down a quiet country road—or on a treadmill at his health club. He experiences the same feeling of comfortable, worry-free well-being after a long run. The third author (Hales) is also a regular jogger and has written a book with his wife on exercise and fitness. We all experience varying levels of anxiety in our daily lives, and we have found relief and, perhaps, prevention in regular exercise.

Many researchers believe that vigorous exercise produces important chemical changes in the body. These biochemical changes reduce anxiety and increase our ability to tolerate stress and discomfort. It may well be that these substances are also triggered by other commonly used stress-reduction methods such as meditation, laughter, and interactions with close friends and family members. Among the benefits of these natural approaches to mental health is that there are few risks of side effects.

## NUTRITIONAL APPROACHES TO ANXIETY

As there are undoubtedly a number of well-established nutritional *causes* of anxiety (e.g., caffeine, alcohol), it is not unreasonable to think that there may be nutritional measures that may relieve anxiety as well. This is currently an area of great interest and research. Although there is so far no definitive proof for the following conclusions, some researchers now believe the following: (1) Foods containing the amino acid tryptophan may increase brain serotonin levels. If so, this might be helpful for people experiencing insomnia and depression. Milk is a good source of tryptophan. The time-honored home remedy "a hot glass of milk at bedtime" may thus turn out to have a scientific basis. Turkey is also a good source of tryptophan. This may explain why some people feel unusually sleepy after a big Thanksgiving dinner. (2) Foods containing the amino acid tyrosine may increase brain levels of dopamine and norepinephrine, which appear to buffer the effects of stress. Good sources of tyrosine include meat and fish. (3) A high-carbohydrate diet may have some antianxiety effects.

None of these nutritional effects has been confirmed by double-blind studies. Please note that at the time of the writing of this book, L-tryptophan is not available for purchase as a dietary supplement because of a possible life-threatening, blood-related side effect. See Chapter 8 (p. 224) for more on this problem.

# Who Should Consider Using an Antianxiety Drug?

You may wish to consider using an antianxiety drug if:

1. Symptoms of anxiety are prolonged.
2. There is no reasonable cause for anxiety.
3. Anxiety symptoms are so severe that they interfere with your daily functioning or keep you from enjoying the ordinary pleasures of life.
4. Your anxiety symptoms do not respond to nondrug treatments (see Nondrug Treatments for Anxiety on p. 81.)

# What Is an Antianxiety Agent?

Although the old-fashioned term *tranquilizer* is still sometimes used, most experts now prefer the term *antianxiety agent* to describe the drugs that have proven effective in the treatment of anxiety. Unfortunately, a number of other medications, both prescribed and over-the-counter, are also sometimes prescribed or recommended in an attempt to treat anxiety. All of the FDA-approved drugs have been proven safe and effective when used correctly. The nonapproved drugs have not.

In our opinion, the *Physician's Desk Reference* (PDR) has contributed to confusion among both physicians and layfolk about the distinction between tranquilizers and antianxiety agents. Consumers should realize that one function of the PDR is the presentation and promotion of the products of the pharmaceutical industry. It therefore should not be considered an unbiased source of consumer drug information. It is not subject to the same impartial editorial review as a scientific journal. We believe that the continuing use in the PDR of the outdated term *tranquilizer* as the title for its section that includes the antianxiety agents leaves many physicians, mental health professionals, and patients unaware that many of the drugs listed in this section have never been approved for the treatment of anxiety, and do not, in fact, safely reduce anxiety for most people. We are not being purists in emphasizing this point; many people are needlessly exposed to serious side effects as the result of this confusion.

## Drugs That Should *Not* Be Used to Treat Anxiety

Although the following drugs are sometimes used to treat anxiety, in our opinion this is a mistake. These drugs have not, to date, been proved safe and effective in the treatment of uncomplicated anxiety. Some have potentially hazardous side effects. With the exception of a few rare situations, we recommend that only members of the benzodiazepine family and three other types of drugs—BuSpar (buspirone), antihistamines, and beta blockers—be used to treat anxiety. These drugs are described below.

If you are suffering from uncomplicated anxiety and your physician suggests one of the following drugs, we suggest that you and your physician jointly review the material in this chapter and choose a more appropriate alternative. A second opinion from a psychiatrist experienced in psychopharmacology may also be required.

### ANTIPSYCHOTIC AGENTS

The drugs listed below are normally used to treat psychotic conditions. These drugs are not recommended for the treatment of uncomplicated anxiety. They were formerly called the *major tranquilizers*. This is extremely misleading since the sedation produced by the antipsychotic agents is actually a side effect. We recommend the use of antipsychotic agents only in those cases in which anxiety is directly related to well-documented examples of psychotic thinking, e.g., hallucinations or delusions.

If your doctor attempts to prescribe any of the following drugs for uncomplicated anxiety, we suggest you seek a second opinion.
*Brand names:* Compazine, Etrafon, Haldol, Lidone, Loxitane, Mellaril, Moban, Navane, Orap, Permitil, Prolixin, Quide, Serentil, Stelazine, Taractan, Thorazine, Tindal, Trilafon, and Vesprin.
*Generic names:* acetophenazine, chlorpromazine, chlorprothixene, clozapine, fluphenazine, haloperidol, loxapine, mesoridazine, molindone, perphenazine, pimozide, piperacetazine, trifluoperazine, triflupromazine, thioridazine, and thiothixene.

## TRIAVIL

This drug is a combination of the antipsychotic drug Trilafon (see p. 196) and the antidepressant drug amitriptyline (see p. 44). It has never been proved effective in the treatment of anxiety. This combination of drugs can needlessly expose a patient to serious and potentially dangerous side effects, including tardive dyskinesia (see p. 186). If your doctor attempts to prescribe this drug for uncomplicated anxiety, we suggest you seek a second opinion.

## MEPROBAMATE

Although the drug meprobamate (brand names: Miltown, Equanil, Meprospam, SK-Bamate) was widely prescribed for anxiety in the 1950s and 1960s, it has now been replaced by the safer and more effective benzodiazepine antianxiety agents and other antianxiety medications described elsewhere in this chapter. If your doctor attempts to prescribe meprobamate for uncomplicated anxiety, we suggest you inquire further about this choice or seek a second opinion. Meprobamate is also marketed as a component of several combination products: i.e., Deprol, PMB-200, and PMB-400.

# The Benzodiazepines

The benzodiazepines are now the most widely used psychiatric drugs, but before 1960, the most frequently used antianxiety drugs were the barbiturates. Barbiturates are highly sedating, impair coordination, are addictive, trigger anger and depression in some people, and may be lethal when combined with alcohol or taken in overdose. The newer benzodiazepines are much more effective in the treatment of anxiety, have fewer side effects, and are less dangerous in overdose. When chlordiazepoxide (Librium), the first benzodiazepine antianxiety drug, became available in 1960, it started a revolution in the drug treatment of anxiety that has continued to the present day. Diazepam (Valium) was introduced in 1962 and soon became even more popular. By 1977, Americans were receiving fifty-four million prescriptions per year for diazepam and thirteen million per year for chlordiazepoxide.

Today, six of the top twenty-five best-selling prescription drugs are benzodiazepines. American physicians write one benzodiazepine prescription per year for every two U.S. adults. An estimated 10 percent of Americans took a benzodiazepine in 1987. Of those currently taking these drugs, 31 percent have been taking them for a year or more.

For many years, diazepam was the most commonly prescribed psychiatric drug. It has recently been dislodged from the number-one spot by its newer cousin alprazolam (Xanax). More than 25 percent of all new benzodiazepine prescriptions are now written for alprazolam.

A 1982 study found that 14 to 15 percent of high school seniors had used antianxiety drugs for recreational purposes. These drugs are also frequently used by adults who are addicted to alcohol, barbiturates, and opiates. One study found that 65 to 70 percent of patients in two methadone centers tested positive for benzodiazepines.

The most frequently prescribed benzodiazepines are as follows (approximately ranked according to frequency of use):

1. alprazolam (Xanax)
2. diazepam (Valium)
3. clorazepate (Tranxene)
4. lorazepam (Ativan)
5. oxazepam (Serax)
6. prazepam (Centrax)
7. chlordiazepoxide (Librium)
8. halazepam (Paxipam)

## WHAT IT FEELS LIKE TO BE ON BENZODIAZEPINES

Benzodiazepines make most anxious people feel calmer, more relaxed, and less apprehensive. These drugs frequently produce a feeling of pleasant well-being. Their effects are experienced usually very shortly (minutes to hours) after the drug is first taken. But like alcohol and many other drugs, the benzodiazepines affect different people in different ways. Because people respond differently, and because some benzodiazepines make some people feel sleepy, we suggest that a person taking a benzodiazepine for the first time should take a single, small dose in a protected situation in which there is no need to perform occupational duties, drive, operate machinery, or prepare for important tasks or examinations. For certain people who are highly anxious, it may require that the dose of the benzodiazepines be built up over several days or even longer before the antianxiety effects are experienced.

## HOW DO WE KNOW THAT THE BENZODIAZEPINES WORK?

Medical researchers frequently use double-blind studies to measure a drug's effectiveness. In such studies, neither the patient receiving the drug, the physician prescribing the drug, nor the researcher measuring the patient's responses knows whether the patient is receiving the drug being tested or a placebo.

Several dozen such double-blind studies have proved that the benzodiazepines are effective in treating anxiety. However, improvement is observed in only about 65 to 70 percent of people with anxiety, and there is no way of knowing, in advance, who will benefit. This means that approximately 30 to 35 percent of anxious persons taking these drugs may not experience significant benefits. People who have responded positively in the past are likely to do so again at a later date. Those who do benefit will usually experience a positive response to treatment within the first week.

## THERAPEUTIC EFFECTS OF THE BENZODIAZEPINES

The benzodiazepines can relieve mild to moderate anxiety. They can be used to treat either short- or long-term anxiety, but long-term use (i.e., for more than four weeks) can lead to dependence and increase the risk of side effects.

Benzodiazepines are also sometimes prescribed to treat insomnia, agitation, epilepsy, and alcohol withdrawal. They are sometimes used as muscle relaxants in the treatment of muscle spasm. They are also frequently given to patients about to undergo surgery to help them relax or as a method of brief anesthesia.

## EXACTLY WHAT DO THE BENZODIAZEPINES DO?

The mechanisms by which the benzodiazepines produce their antianxiety effects are still not completely understood. It is known that the brains of both humans and laboratory animals contain benzodiazepine receptors. Animal studies show that the stronger a drug's affinity to those binding sites, the greater its therapeutic effect. The neurotransmitter gamma-aminobutyric acid (GABA) can stimulate benzodiazepine binding sites. GABA is known to exert a calming effect on laboratory animals.

## HOW LONG CAN I TAKE BENZODIAZEPINES SAFELY?

You can become both physically and psychologically dependent on these drugs within two to four weeks. If you have a special problem with chemical dependency or alcoholism, the time required for benzodiazepine dependence may be even briefer—one or two doses. Thus long-term use of benzodiazepines (more than four weeks) is usually not recommended. For most people, taking moderate doses of benzodiazepines for two weeks or less carries little risk of addiction. But if you take these drugs for three or four weeks or more, and then stop abruptly (i.e., without tapering down), you may experience both psychological and physical withdrawal symptoms.

Psychological symptoms of withdrawal may include anxiety (sometimes called *rebound anxiety*), irritability, restlessness, insomnia, impaired memory and concentration, or panic attacks—some of the same symptoms that led you to take these drugs in the first place. Common physical side effects of withdrawal may include upset stomach; shaking of the hands; muscle twitching; sensitivity to light, sound, and touch. Other possible physical effects include rapid heartbeat, increased blood pressure, and muscle cramps.

For persons taking doses greater than the normally recommended therapeutic dose, even more severe withdrawal symptoms may occur; the most severe are confusion, seizures, and delirium (an excited, confused, near-psychotic state).

The drugs in the benzodiazepine family that are eliminated from the body most rapidly (e.g., lorazepam, alprazolam, triazolam) can cause withdrawal symptoms within one to two days after the drug is discontinued. The benzodiazepines that are cleared from the body more slowly (e.g.,

Valium) typically produce withdrawal symptoms that begin on the fifth to tenth day following the last dose.

Withdrawal effects are more likely to occur if the drug is stopped abruptly. Thus, one should withdraw from these drugs gradually, not all at once. For example, a person who has been taking 10 mg of Valium per day for a week may be advised to take 6 mg per day for two days, then 3 mg per day for two days, then 1 mg per day for two days before stopping the drug— rather than stopping abruptly. Withdrawal from the more rapidly eliminated benzodiazepines must proceed more slowly. For a person who has been on a total of 3 mg alprazolam (Xanax) per day for more than three weeks, we recommend reducing the dose by 0.25 mg each week until the drug is stopped altogether. This withdrawal procedure may take several months. In general, the higher the dose and the longer you have been taking it, the greater the chance that you will experience withdrawal symptoms. But the kind and severity of withdrawal symptoms vary a great deal from person to person.

The take-home lesson is that these drugs are effective in the treatment of anxiety, *but* they should be taken for the shortest possible time. Some people use the medications episodically and briefly during anxiety peaks or times of high stress—such as a single tablet one or two times a month. In these cases, care must be taken that the dose frequency does not gradually increase and that the prescribing physician is aware of the regimen and any changes in it.

## CAN I OVERDOSE ON A BENZODIAZEPINE DRUG?

Although it is possible to overdose on benzodiazepines, it is not easy to do so. While as few as ten to twenty capsules of amibarbital (a barbiturate) may prove fatal, the fatal dose of diazepam (Valium), a benzodiazepine, is fifty to one hundred tablets (if not combined with alcohol). Although the benzodiazepines are frequently used in suicide attempts, attempts made with benzodiazepines alone rarely result in death. One recent study found that benzodiazepines were responsible for only 2 of 1,239 drug overdose deaths. We must emphasize, however, that the combination of a benzodiazepine with other drugs—especially alcohol or barbiturates—can be highly lethal and has resulted in large numbers of deaths.

## BENZODIAZEPINE OVERDOSE

Signs of benzodiazepine toxicity include sedation, reduced coordination, slurred speech, poor concentration, decreased breathing rate, confusion, and problems with memory. If these symptoms are present, the person should be taken to the nearest emergency room; blood studies and life-supporting measures may be required. The medical treatment of benzodiazepine overdose may include intravenous fluids, a respirator to assist breathing, and keeping the person away from driving and other potentially dangerous situations until he or she is fully recovered.

## WHO SHOULD TAKE BENZODIAZEPINES?

Benzodiazepines should be used only after consultation with and under the direction of a knowledgeable physician. A complete physical examination and testing are usually advised to rule out medical conditions that can produce anxiety. If it is determined that the anxiety is not the result of an underlying medical condition, then you and your doctor should discuss the pros and cons of using a benzodiazepine drug.

These drugs are best used for short periods, and as one of several measures to deal with anxiety. For example, a benzodiazepine might be used to help calm a man who had witnessed the death of his daughter in an auto accident. In such a situation, the drug might be prescribed for a period of one week, to be accompanied by supportive psychotherapy and an opportunity for the individual to spend time with other family members and clergy, to discuss his feelings and to receive sympathy and encouragement.

If you receive a prescription for a benzodiazepine, it is important that you understand the possible side effects and interactions with drugs and foods. You and your physician should jointly agree on a treatment plan and arrange for a predetermined time and method for discontinuing the drug.

Except under special circumstances (e.g., as an adjunct to chemotherapy in the treatment of cancer), a physician who provides anxious people with re-peated refills of prescriptions for these drugs is doing them a great disservice because there is such a high risk of addiction. *Certainly,* a physician should not regularly refill prescriptions for benzodiazepines without close and regular monitoring of a patient's physical and emotional status.

## WHO SHOULD *NOT* TAKE BENZODIAZEPINES?

- People who have previously had negative reactions or serious side effects with benzodiazepines
- People who must fly aircraft, drive, or operate heavy machinery
- People with a history of drug dependence
- People with Alzheimer's disease, stroke, multiple sclerosis, or other brain disorders

- People with anxiety that recurs after benzodiazepines are discontinued
- People with serious depression
- Women who are pregnant
- Women who are breast-feeding

## TESTS REQUIRED PRIOR TO TAKING BENZODIAZEPINES

We recommend the following (many of the tests listed below are described in the Glossary):

*Patient's History and Physical Examination*

   medical history
   mental status examination
   physical examination
   neurologic assessment

*Urine Tests*

   urinalysis
   urine drug screening

*Blood Tests*

   complete blood count
   serum electrolytes
   urea
   calcium
   uric acid
   alkaline phosphotase
   total bilirubin
   SGOT
   SGPT
   T3
   T4
   TSH

*If Warranted by Other Findings*

   chest X ray
   serum catecholamines
   24-hour urine catecholamines
   thyroid scan

## RECOMMENDED PERIODIC EXAMINATIONS WHILE TAKING BENZODIAZEPINES

Because benzodiazepines do not generally have harmful effects on body organs and because we do not recommend taking benzodiazepines on a long-term basis, periodic laboratory tests or medical examinations are usually not needed.

## POSSIBLE SIDE EFFECTS OF BENZODIAZEPINES

### Drowsiness

These drugs may make you feel sleepy or drowsy. Clinicians refer to this as a *sedative effect*. Feelings of drowsiness are often most severe within the first few days of treatment. The sedative effects of these drugs usually diminish with continued use.

If sleepiness becomes a significant problem, you may wish to ask your doctor to switch you from a benzodiazepine with a slow elimination rate, e.g., prazepam (Centrax), chlordiazepoxide (Librium), halazepam (Paxipam), chlorazepam (Tranxene), or diazepam (Valium), to one with an intermediate elimination rate, e.g., lorazepam (Ativan), oxazepam (Serax), or fast elimination rate, e.g., alprazolam (Xanax). Reducing the dose during the day will also minimize sleepiness. A larger dose an hour before bedtime will often help you fall asleep, and may help reduce daytime sleepiness.

### Impaired Coordination

This side effect, technically called psychomotor impairment, is among the most dangerous of all the benzodiazepine side effects, as it can impair coordination while driving or operating potentially hazardous machinery. Drivers taking these drugs are at five times the risk of being involved in traffic accidents. Reducing the dose or switching from a benzodiazepine with a slow elimination rate to one with an intermediate or fast elimination rate can help minimize, but not eliminate, this side effect. Even so, you should not drive or operate potentially hazardous heavy machinery while you are taking these drugs.

### Impaired Memory and Concentration

Judy first began taking diazepam (Valium) (20 mg per day) for her premenstrual anxiety. Because it made her feel so relaxed, she soon began taking it throughout the month. After several months, she began to experience troublesome lapses in memory. She forgot people's names and had so much trouble studying for exams that she was forced to drop out of her MBA program. Although she was only thirty-three, Judy became convinced that she was suffering from Alzheimer's disease. Once she stopped taking diazepam, her memory returned to normal.

Benzodiazepines may affect your ability to remember what you read, heard, or saw while you were taking these drugs. These drugs appear to affect the process by which information is transferred from short-term memory to long-term memory. Some people taking these drugs may experience so-called *benzodiazepine amnesia* in which they lose all memory of their actions during certain periods. Memory impairment may be most severe with certain types of benzodiazepines, e.g., lorazepam (Ativan) and triazolam (Halcion), and is even more severe when benzodiazepines are taken intravenously.

Like the other side effects described above, benzodiazepine amnesia can be minimized by reducing the dose and by switching from a benzodiazepine with a slow elimination rate to one with an intermediate or fast elimination rate.

## Muscular Weakness

Some people taking these drugs may find their legs growing heavy as they climb stairs or walk up hills. Others experience a reduced ability to lift heavy objects or to engage in other sustained physical activities. Like most of the other benzodiazepine side effects, muscle weakness is most pronounced in those taking benzodiazepines with a slow elimination rate. Effects are less pronounced with those family members with intermediate or fast elimination rates. The muscular weakness disappears altogether when you stop taking the drug.

## If Side Effects Are Unacceptable

If, despite all attempts at switching to a different benzodiazepine or reducing your dose, it is not possible to reduce these side effects to an acceptable level, you may wish to discuss with your physician the possibility of switching to buspirone (BuSpar), a new antianxiety agent. Buspirone appears to be as effective as the benzodiazepines for many kinds of anxiety, but it has a different set of possible side effects. If switching from a benzodiazepine to buspirone, you must first taper down and discontinue the old drug. But please note: Buspirone does not prevent the withdrawal effects of benzodiazepines.

For more on buspirone, see p. 97.

## POSSIBLE ADVERSE REACTIONS TO THE BENZODIAZEPINES

A few people have unusual, individual reactions to these drugs. Contact your doctor immediately if you experience any of the following:

- unusual feelings of intense anger
- outbursts of unaccustomed rage, hostility, or violence
- intense feelings of depression
- intense anxiety or irritability
- severe insomnia

## CAN BENZODIAZEPINES INTERACT WITH FOODS?

Benzodiazepines do not interact dangerously with foods.

## CAN BENZODIAZEPINES INTERACT WITH ALCOHOL?

Drinking alcoholic beverages will increase all the side effects of benzodiazepines, especially the sedative effects and their tendency to slow your breathing. This is a major public health problem with the widespread use of both benzodiazepines and alcohol in our society. If you suffer from prolonged or recurring anxiety, don't drink any alcoholic beverages at all.

Alcohol also increases the memory lapses associated with the benzodiazepines. This can result in a dangerous situation in which a person, forgetting how much medication has been taken, takes repeat doses while drinking alcohol. High doses of benzodiazepines plus alcohol can impair a person's ability to breathe and can lower blood pressure. This can result in coma and death. Thus it is extremely important that you not drink alcoholic beverages if you are taking benzodiazepines.

## CAN BENZODIAZEPINES INTERACT WITH OTHER DRUGS?

A number of other drugs can interact with benzodiazepines. You should not take any other drug—either prescription or nonprescription—unless you assure yourself through consultation with your physician that there is no possibility of such interactions. The drugs listed below should not be combined with benzodiazepines except under carefully monitored conditions in the hospital:

*Narcotics* (e.g., Demerol, Percodan, codeine, morphine, Talwin)

These drugs increase the sedative effects of the benzodiazepines. This combination can seriously reduce your breathing rate and can be deadly. Do not use narcotics if you are taking benzodiazepines.

*Barbiturates and Other Sedatives* (e.g., phenobarbitol, pentobarbital, Seconal, Tuinal)

These drugs also increase sedation and may depress breathing to dangerous levels if combined with benzodiazepine or other antianxiety drugs.

*Other Benzodiazepines*

It is unnecessary and may be unsafe to take more than one benzodiazepine at a time.

*Sleeping Pills*

It is unnecessary and may be unsafe to take a sleeping pill while taking a benzodiazepine. If you need help in sleeping, talk with your doctor about a treatment plan that calls for a larger dose of your benzodiazepine shortly before bedtime.

*Antidepressants and Other Medications*

The anxiety associated with depression should be treated with antidepressants (Chapter 3). In most cases, benzodiazepines make depression worse!

*Drugs that reduce the liver's ability to remove benzodiazepines from the body increase all the actions and side effects of these drugs*: ulcer drugs, e.g., cimetidine (Tagamet); birth control pills; propranolol, used to treat hypertension, heart disorders, migraines, etc.; disulfuram (Antabuse), used in the treatment of alcoholism.

### DIFFERENCES AMONG THE BENZODIAZEPINES

All members of the benzodiazepine family are equally effective in treating anxiety. Psychiatrists select a benzodiazepine based on its side effect profile.

Lorazepam (Ativan) has less effect on the liver. This drug may be better suited for those taking ulcer medications, birth control pills, propranolol, disulfuram, or other drugs that may affect liver function.

Three of the benzodiazepines—alprazolam (Xanax), lorazepam (Ativan), and oxazepam (Serax)—are cleared from the body more quickly. They are thus more likely to produce withdrawal symptoms when discontinued. These drugs are also less likely to produce such side effects as sedation; impairment of coordination, concentration, and memory; and muscular weakness.

One member of the benzodiazepine family, alprazolam, is somewhat less sedating.

Alprazolam and the anticonvulsant benzodiazepine clonazepam (Klonopin) may have antipanic effects (see Chapter 5). Alprazolam may have antidepressant effects as well.

## BENZODIAZEPINES AND DEPRESSION

Under most circumstances, benzodiazepines are not a suitable treatment for depression or for anxiety associated with depression. Many people suffering from depression find that their depression grows even worse after they take benzodiazepines. Also, depressed people often use benzodiazepines in suicide attempts. The best drugs for treating combined anxiety and depression are currently the antidepressants. Unfortunately, benzodiazepines are prescribed for many people with depression. Not only do their symptoms of depression become worse, but they often remain unaware of the powerful therapeutic benefits of the antidepressants. One reason we wrote this book is that on numerous occasions we have provided consultation to people who have suffered from prolonged bouts of painful depression. They tell us, "I tried medications and they didn't help." When we inquire which medication, the response is often "Valium," a drug that makes depression worse.

For more on antidepressant drugs, see Chapter 3.

## BENZODIAZEPINES AND OLDER PEOPLE

Many elderly people and some younger people with brain disorders such as Alzheimer's disease may be especially sensitive to the side effects of the benzodiazepines. If these drugs are used with such patients, they should be used in very low doses and monitored very closely. Oversedation, memory impairment, confusion, disorientation, and poor coordination resulting in serious falls are the most common problems.

## BENZODIAZEPINES AS SLEEPING PILLS

If you are taking a benzodiazepine for anxiety and need help in sleeping, talk with your doctor about taking a larger dose of the drug shortly before bedtime.

# Other Effective Drugs for Anxiety

### BUSPIRONE (BUSPAR)

Although this new antianxiety agent has a different chemical structure from the benzodiazepines, recent studies suggest that it is just as effective in the treatment of most kinds of anxiety. The good news is that buspirone lacks many of the troublesome side effects that make it difficult for some people to take the benzodiazepines. Buspirone is much less sedating than the benzodiazepines. It does not cause memory loss. Because it does not impair coordination, those who need to drive can take this drug without increasing their risk of traffic accidents. BuSpar does not interact dangerously with alcohol. While it appears that there is little risk of overdose from buspirone, since the drug is still relatively new, more data are needed to confirm this observation. This drug has little potential for addiction, and thus may be used for periods longer than four weeks.

However, buspirone has some problems of its own. People taking a benzodiazepine can't switch directly to buspirone but must taper off their present drug before starting the new one. Buspirone must be taken at least three times per day, while some of the benzodiazepines can be taken only once a day. Because there may be a lag period of one to three weeks between the time a person begins taking buspirone and the time antianxiety effects appear, this drug cannot be used in emergency situations in which a quick response is desired. People with anxiety are understandably impatient for the quick results that are possible with benzodiazepines but not buspirone. Buspirone may produce the following side effects: nervousness, insomnia, dizziness, light-headedness, gastric upset, nausea, diarrhea, and headaches.

In summary, buspirone appears to have as much to offer as an antianxiety agent. This drug, or other related antianxiety drugs, may in time become the treatment of choice for anxiety. However, because buspirone is a relatively new drug, further studies are needed before a final appraisal of effectiveness and long-term safety can be made.

### ANTIHISTAMINES

Antihistamines, which have some sedative properties, may have some mild effects on anxiety. These drugs are relatively safe, as they are not habit-forming. In general, however, they are far less effective than benzodiazepines in the treatment of anxiety. Many individuals find these drugs so highly sedating that they interfere with the normal activities of daily life.

If your doctor suggests an antihistamine for the treatment of anxiety, feel free to ask about the reasoning behind this choice. If there is some reason that you cannot take a benzodiazepine or buspirone, if the sedative effects would be of benefit, or if you need an antihistamine for other medical conditions, this could be a reasonable choice.

## BETA BLOCKERS

Epinephrine and norepinephrine are two neurotransmitters involved in the brain's coordination of our reactions to danger or stress—the so-called fight-or-flight reactions. These neurotransmitters can act on specific receptors in the neurons, called beta receptors. Researchers believe that the beta receptors in our brain and nervous system are responsible for modifying our reactions to stressful situations. Drugs that block these beta receptors can help diminish the physical manifestations of danger, stress, or anxiety (e.g., racing heartbeat, sweating, and "butterflies in the stomach"), and perhaps reduce mental manifestations of anxiety as well.

While the use of beta blockers for general anxiety and aggressive behavior is still under study, these drugs have proved especially effective in the prevention and treatment of performance anxiety. People who experience performance anxiety on certain occasions—e.g., an actress who must perform at an audition, a student who must defend his master's thesis before a panel of professors, or a businesswoman who must give a speech to her company's board of directors—may benefit by taking a predetermined and pretested dose of beta blockers one hour in advance. These drugs do *not* appear to impair performance and may do just the opposite. In a study of musicians who suffered from performance anxiety, a panel of musical experts rated their performances on the drug as superior to their performances without it.

The beta blocker propranolol is most frequently used for this purpose. Effective doses vary from person to person, but the usual range is 40 to 320 mg per day in divided doses. These drugs have few side effects and are not addictive.

If you suffer from performance anxiety and are interested in learning more about using a beta blocker for performance anxiety, we suggest that you consult a psychiatrist who specializes in the drug treatment of psychological problems.

For more on beta blockers, see p. 122.

# Clomipramine (Anafranil) in the Treatment of Obsessive-Compulsive Disorder

Obsessive-compulsive disorder is officially categorized by the American Psychiatric Association as a form of anxiety. The clinical aspects of this disorder are, therefore, described earlier in this chapter (p. 74). Nonetheless, the medications that have been shown to be successful in treating the symptoms of severe obsessive-compulsive disorder are in the antidepressant class. At the present time, there is only one medication that has approval from the Food and Drug Administration (FDA) to be marketed as a specific treatment for obsessive-compulsive disorder: clomipramine (Anafranil). Another medication that does not have FDA approval but shows great promise in the treatment of obsessive-compulsive disorder is fluoxetine (Prozac).

## ABOUT CLOMIPRAMINE (ANAFRANIL)

Clomipramine is in the tricyclic antidepressant category of medications, and it is chemically closely related to the antidepressant imipramine (Tofranil). Clomipramine has been used on an international basis for over twenty years in the successful treatment of depression. One important pharmacologic property of clomipramine is its powerful effect on the neurotransmitter serotonin. Specifically, clomipramine inhibits the reuptake of serotonin in presynaptic neurons, and this chemical property is believed to be responsible for its strong effects in the treatment of obsessive-compulsive disorder. These effects have been documented by several well-controlled double-blind studies that have been conducted both in the United States and in Europe, where clomipramine has been proved to be clearly more effective than placebo or other antidepressant agents. It is interesting that its close chemical relative imipramine (Tofranil) has not been shown to have any antiobsessive or anticompulsive properties. Clomipramine became available for the first time for nonexperimental or restricted use in the United States in February 1990.

## BEGINNING TREATMENT WITH CLOMIPRAMINE

Once your psychiatrist has diagnosed you to have obsessive-compulsive disorder with symptoms sufficiently severe to require treatment with clomipramine, the medical and laboratory testing that has already been described for other heterocyclics should be performed. Clomipramine is supplied in capsules of 25 mg, 50 mg, and 75 mg strengths. As with other heterocyclic antidepressants, we initiate treatment with very low doses (25 mg daily) and increase the dose gradually as tolerated. Usually the dose is raised to approximately 100 mg per day over the first two weeks of treatment. For children and adolescents, we raise the dose more slowly. As with the use of heterocyclic antidepressants in the treatment of depression, most patients do not show significant response to the drug until two or three weeks *after* they have been on a treatment level (150 mg to 250 mg per day). The usual maximum dose for adults is 250 mg per day, and for adolescents, 200 mg per day or 3 mg per kg, whichever is lower.

## SIDE EFFECTS OF CLOMIPRAMINE

Side effects of clomipramine are nearly identical to those that have been described for other heterocyclic antidepressants (see pp. 44). Among the most common side effects are sedation, hand tremor, dry mouth, dizziness, constipation, headache, insomnia, decreased sexual drive, sweating, weight gain, blurred vision, and problems with ejaculation. Anxiety and nervousness also may occur, but less frequently. Less common side effects include memory impairment, muscle twitching, rash, diarrhea, loss of appetite, flushing, sore throat, runny nose, problems urinating, menstrual changes, impotence, muscle pain, and problems tasting food. As with other heterocyclics this medication is highly toxic in high doses and is of significant danger when used in a suicide attempt.

## SPECIAL ISSUES ASSOCIATED WITH USE OF CLOMIPRAMINE

Clomipramine is present in the milk of nursing mothers, and, therefore, it cannot be used if a mother continues to nurse her baby. Many children and adolescents have used this medication for both the treatment of depression and obsessive-compulsive personality disorder. However, at the present time, it is uncertain whether or not the long-term treatment with clomipramine may alter the growth and development of children. Clomipramine's safety and efficacy in children below the age of ten have not been established.

## About Fluoxetine (Prozac) in the Treatment of Obsessive-Compulsive Disorder

Because it is a relatively new drug, there are fewer controlled scientific studies testing the effects of fluoxetine for the treatment of obsessive-compulsive disorder as compared with clomipramine. Nonetheless, like clomipramine, fluoxetine has potent effects on brain serotonin; so fluoxetine is currently being used by both research scientists and clinicians to treat patients with obsessive-compulsive symptoms. Our initial experience with fluoxetine for the treatment of obsessive-compulsive disorder has been highly rewarding—with results that approximate those of clomipramine: substantial reduction in symptoms (by at least 50 percent) in a high percentage of patients treated. Because fluoxetine has a more mild side effect profile than clomipramine, we anticipate an increased use of fluoxetine for the treatment of this disorder.

### THE TREATMENT OF JOHN EVANS

John Evans's obsessions and compulsions as they relate to his fears that his father would develop a fatal brain tumor are described briefly on p. 74. His psychiatrist, Dr. Norman Miller, first focused on what he believed to be the hostile and competitive relationship between John and his father. Dr. Miller met twice a week with John, and reviewed his early life history. Dr. Miller also met once a week with John in the company of both parents. After three months of this treatment, John's symptoms became far worse—to the point that he was no longer able to attend college classes or enjoy any recreational activity. Dr. Miller's psychological treatment emphasized "uncovering deep-seated hostilities" that John had for both parents. The result was that not only did John become overtly enraged with his parents, but his obsession that his father would die from cancer intensified to the point that it plagued his mind virtually every minute of the day. Although Dr. Miller opposed this approach, John's father pursued a second opinion from another psychiatrist. Dr. Miller told Mr. Evans, "You are sabotaging the treatment of your son. The only reason that you wish to have a second opinion is to avoid facing your son's hostility and the fact that you have been a less than perfect parent."

It was only after Mr. Evans's first visit with Dr. Elizabeth Kostner that he acknowledged to himself just how dissatisfied and frustrated he had been with Dr. Miller's treatment and approach: "From the first minute, I did not feel comfortable with or have confidence in Dr. Miller. He seemed aloof; he never answered any of my questions directly; he used psychological jargon (such as displacement, anal retentive, loculated aggression, etc.) that I never really understood. He tended to blame me and my wife for causing John's illness, but he never would give us a clear treatment plan about how to make things better. Worse than feeling ashamed and blamed by Dr. Miller, John didn't seem to get any better under his care. He got only worse." Although distrustful of all psychiatrists after his experience with Dr. Miller, Mr. Evans liked Dr. Kostner almost immediately. Unlike Dr. Miller, Dr. Kostner did not mind being asked about her academic credentials or about her philosophic approach to treating psychiatric illness. Dr. Kostner appeared to both Mr. and Mrs. Evans a "real human being." Although she did not spend a great deal of time talking about herself, she also did not keep her own life a total mystery. For example, Mr. and Mrs. Evans were greatly relieved when Dr. Kostner said, "I can assure you from my experience of being a mother of three children that all of us are 'less than perfect parents.' It is not my opinion that your treatment of John fully explains the nature and severity of his symptoms. There are important recent scientific data to suggest that there are biologic and, perhaps, genetic predispositions to severe obsessive-compulsive personality disorder. More important, we now know with confidence that certain medications in combination with psychosocial approaches are highly effective in treating the symptoms of most individuals with this disorder."

Before finding Dr. Kostner, Mr. and Mrs. Evans and John had been greatly opposed to the use of psychiatric drugs. Their pediatrician had given John the drug thioridazine (Mellaril) for anxiety when John was in high school, and this medication made John lethargic and, later, stiff. I did nothing to help his anxiety. However, Mr. and Mrs. Evans quickly developed a high degree of confidence in Dr. Kostner, and they encouraged John, who was understandably discouraged and reluctant, to try the medication clomipramine (Anafranil) that Dr. Koster recommended. To everyone's surprise and delight, within less than a month, John's painful obsessional thoughts were markedly reduced. The treatment also included individual therapy and family therapy, which served to bring the family closer together rather than placing them at odds with one another. By the third month of treatment with medication, John's obsessive thoughts and compulsive acts had virtually disappeared. He was now able to return to college, concentrate on his studies, and resume long-abandoned friendships with his peers.

The case of John Evans illustrates at least five important points:

1. Patients and families should trust their own instincts and feelings regarding the choice of physicians and therapists. It can be highly confusing if "a blaming therapist" holds responsible a patient or a family member when improvement does not occur. Skilled clinicians are able to deal with the sensitive and embarrassing issues without patients or families feeling accused or demeaned.

2. A clear and acceptable treatment plan should be proposed within the first several meetings with the clinician. If, after discussion with the clinician, this treatment plan does not make sense to the family, a second opinion from a consulting psychiatrist should be pursued.

3. Dr. Miller's discouragement of a second opinion should have set off a "warning bell." As we have stated previously in this book, as clinicians we have uniformly found that second opinions do not "muddy the water" for us or our patients. Rather, they consistently provide important new information, or help to substantiate, support, and lend confidence to a treatment plan that is already in place.

4. In general, the most severe and disabling psychiatric illnesses (such as severe obsessive-compulsive disorder, manic depressive illness, schizophrenia, etc.) require multifaceted approaches that often, although not always, include individual treatments, family treatments, support groups, and medications.

5. People who have been plagued and discouraged by years of tormenting psychiatric symptomatologies and ineffective treatments should retain hope. The breakthrough in the use of medications to treat obsessive-compulsive disorder is relatively recent. This is a symbol for the real hope and promise of novel, safe, and effective pharmacologic interventions for other intractable psychiatric illnesses or symptoms.

## Nondrug Treatments of Obsessive-Compulsive Disorder

Behavioral treatments and psychological treatments also have varying degrees of benefit in treatment of patients with obsessive-compulsive personality disorder. We recommend that all patients receiving clomipramine also receive regular psychotherapy and behavioral treatments simultaneously to optimize these specific benefits. We must emphasize, however, that obsessive-compulsive personality disorder is one of the most disabling and painful conditions in all medicine. We have evaluated and treated many patients who have failed to benefit from many years of psychological and behavioral treatments, but who, following treatment with clomipramine or fluoxetine, have shown extraordinary improvement. Upon treatment with medication, they were able to make greater strides in their psychosocial treatments.

## Who Should Prescribe Antianxiety Drugs?

Benzodiazepines are the most frequently prescribed psychiatric drugs. Prescriptions for benzodiazepines may be written by physicians and dentists—who may have little or no training in the use of these complex drugs or in understanding the conditions for which they are being prescribed. As with other types of medication, the proper use of antianxiety agents and nondrug measures for anxiety frequently requires a specially trained professional. Thus, if you are prescribed any psychiatric drug—including benzodiazepines—you should be especially careful to review the indications, side effects, and potential problems of these drugs on your own, as well as in consultation with a *competent* professional. If you develop any problems with these drugs (e.g., bothersome side effects, unmanageable emotional problems, memory impairment, confusion, poor coordination), if you are confused about your diagnosis or the indications for the drug, if you find that your anxiety symptoms are not reduced after taking a benzodiazepine, if you find that you must use the drug for more than three or four weeks, or if you find you are becoming dependent on the drug, we recommend that you seek a consultation with a knowledgeable physician.

## How Do I Find a Psychiatrist with an Up -to-Date Knowledge of the Antianxiety Drugs?

Another good approach is to contact the department of psychiatry at the nearest medical school or teaching hospital. Most will have a special clinic for treating anxiety and related problems. Such a clinic may be called Anxiety Clinic, Anxiety Disorder Clinic, Phobia and Panic Clinic, Obsessive-Compulsive Disorder Clinic, the Psychopharmacology Clinic, or other similar names. The psychiatrists who work in these clinics are experts in the drug management of anxiety-related disorders. Such specialists may be able to provide the services you need, or they may be able to suggest a local practitioner who is an expert in your particular area of concern. Your family physician may also be able to refer you to a psychiatrist with an up-to-date knowledge of these drugs.

## ROBERTA BAKER: UNSUCCESSFUL USE OF ANTIANXIETY DRUGS

Roberta Baker, aged forty-eight, is recently widowed New Jersey letter carrier. She first received diazepam (Valium) from a cardiologist, Dr. Perkins, after she hurt her back while helping a co-worker move a heavy locker. The drug made her feel both relaxed and pleasantly high. For Roberta, the feeling was quite similar to the effect of drinking two or three glasses of wine.

It was a difficult time in Roberta's life. Six months before, Jonathan, her husband of twenty-eight years, had died of congestive heart failure. They had loved each other very much, and Roberta now felt lost without him. She kept torturing herself with guilty feelings—if only she had cooked more nutritious meals and encouraged him to exercise and stop smoking, he might still be here with her.

The insurance money had lasted only a few months. After that she had to sell the house. She hated her job, resented the cramped duplex she lived in, and resented having to pinch pennies. The effect of wine was a feeling Roberta knew well. She had consumed four or five glasses of white wine almost every evening since Jonathan had died. It was the only way she knew to dull the emotional pain. Her drinking and her depression had grown so bad that Chris, her twenty-five-year-old son who lived in California, had asked her not to visit her grandchildren over the holidays. This made her even *more* depressed. Roberta was now drinking to the point of intoxication once or twice a week. She soon discovered that combining white wine and diazepam made her feel even more relaxed. Even better, she found that taking diazepam the day after a drinking binge helped to steady her hands, calm her nerves, and make her less irritable.

Roberta saw only one problem with the arrangement: she kept running out of diazepam. As Dr. Perkins had originally prescribed diazepam as a muscle relaxant, Roberta found that she was forced to pretend her back was still bothering her, even though the pain had gone away long ago. She felt guilty about this deception, but saw no other solution. She was afraid that she would simply not be able to cope if her supply of diazepam were cut off. After her third office visit for back pain, her doctor increased her dose from 2 mg to Valium three times per day to 5 mg five times per day. After her fifth visit, he referred her to an orthopedic physician.

The orthopedist did a series of tests, which all, naturally enough, proved negative. He referred Roberta to a rehabilitation counselor, who prescribed a regimen of exercise and weight loss. When the rehabilitation specialist asked her about alcohol intake and benzodiazepine use, Roberta, embarrassed, claimed that she averaged only a glass of wine at night and an "occasional" diazepam use. The rehabilitation expert didn't check with Roberta's original doctor or with her supervisor at work, both of whom, at this point, were quite aware of Roberta's problems with alcohol and diazepam.

Roberta tried one more reconciliation with her son. When he informed her that he wanted nothing more to do with her, Roberta grew terribly angry and depressed. She increased her intake of diazepam to 10 mg five times per day, and increased her wine consumption to two bottles per night. She refused to attend the recommended exercise, nutrition, and weight control sessions. When her doctor refused to increase her prescription, she obtained a prescription from another physician who asked few questions and didn't even perform a physical examination. Occasionally, she even purchased diazepam illegally from a drug dealer she knew.

As her alcohol and drug intake increased, Roberta began to miss more and more work. When she did report to work, she was frequently abusive to supervisors and co-workers. She was involved in several accidents while on the job and received three police summonses for driving while intoxicated. After a series of warnings, she was finally fired from her job. Two weeks later, Roberta locked herself in her duplex, got into a hot bath, took one hundred 10 mg Valium tablets and drank a fifth of bourbon. Her suicide note read as follows: "I am taking my own life because I feel that the whole world is against me. No one knows how much I suffer. All I ever wanted was to be a good wife and a good mother and now I find it impossible to be either. All I want now is a chance to rest and to be free of this suffering and this pain. I love you all. Love, Roberta."

Luckily a concerned friend happened to stop by and found Roberta unconscious on the floor. By the time the paramedics arrived, she was in a deep coma. They got her to the hospital just in time to save her life.

Roberta's experience with diazepam is entirely too common. Thousands—perhaps hundreds of thousands—of benzodiazepine users are knowingly or unknowingly abusing these drugs with the unwitting (and, rarely, witting) complicity of their physicians. So what went wrong? Here are some of the wrong turns on the road to Roberta's suicide attempt:

1. *Failure to take a complete history and perform a physical exam.* Dr. Perkins should never have prescribed diazepam without a complete history and physical. A careful history would have revealed Roberta's shaky psychological situation and her increasing alcohol intake. It would have also turned up a strong family history of alcoholism. The appropriate laboratory tests would have drawn attention to early liver damage and other signs of Roberta's heavy drinking.

2. *Lack of a jointly negotiated treatment plan*. The use of a benzodiazepine to treat muscle pain or tension is sometimes appropriate, but these drugs should never be used without a treatment plan that includes a firm discontinuation plan and date.

3. *Lack of personal communication and self-responsibility*. Roberta failed to recognize the signs of deepening depression and to take effective measures—such as discussing her problems with friends, seeking advice from a clerical counselor, joining a support or mutual aid group for widows, reading books and articles on grief and depression, or seeking professional psychotherapy.

4. *Lack of professional communication and involvement*. The four health professionals involved—Dr. Perkins, the orthopedist, the rehabilitation expert, and the other physician who gave Roberta a diazepam prescription—failed to communicate with one another. Thus none was able to see the whole picture: death of a spouse, and other family problems; deepening depression; alcohol abuse; diazepam abuse; and deterioration of occupational and social functioning.

5. *Lack of involvement and communication among family and friends*. Although they were all aware of the problem, none of Roberta's family, friends, or co-workers took an active role in trying to bring a positive resolution to the problem. They did not communicate with one another, and they did not talk with any of the professionals involved in Roberta's care. Most of all, they didn't talk to Roberta herself. Although her son, Chris, would angrily confront her with being "a goddamn drunk" each time she called him, he did not suggest any positive solutions to her problems: that she might benefit from attending a meeting of Alcoholics Anonymous or one of the local self-help groups for depression. Roberta's co-workers and supervisors never brought Roberta's drug and alcohol problems to the attention of the Post Office's employee assistance program.

## SUZANNE TRIPITT: SUCCESSFUL USE OF ANTIANXIETY DRUGS

Suzanne, aged thirty-six, is a high school mathematics teacher. She is married to Harry Tripitt, a successful Omaha real estate developer. The Tripitts have two teenaged daughters, Pamela and Rebecca. On March 1, 1989, while taking her morning shower, Suzanne found a small, hard lump in her left breast. Her grandmother had died of breast cancer years before. Ever since, Suzanne had been terrified by the thought that she, too, might one day develop breast cancer. She had yearly checkups and examined her breasts on the first day of every month. She was sure that the lump had not been there the month before.

After dinner that evening, she mentioned the lump to her husband. They decided that she should consult her gynecologist, Dr. Doris Meyers, at once. Harry insisted on accompanying Suzanne. The next morning, after performing a physical examination and a mammogram, Dr. Meyers sat down with the Tripitts and told them that the mammogram indicated that there was a good chance the lump *was* malignant, and that Suzanne had breast cancer. She praised Suzanne for her careful self-exam and for coming in to see her so quickly. A breast cancer specialist recommended breast surgery. Since the lump was discovered when it was still very small, there was an excellent chance for a complete cure.

At this point, Suzanne became so anxious that she was no longer able to discuss her condition with her husband, her daughters, or Dr. Meyers. "The mere thought of having some surgeon cut into my breast reduced me to a state of trembling jelly," she remembers. "My hands were shaking, my heart was pounding. I was crying all the time. I couldn't eat. I couldn't stand to see anyone. I paced the floor constantly. I tossed and turned all night. And if I did drop off to sleep I was immediately awakened by horrible nightmares of dying or being disfigured."

After several days of this severe anxiety, Suzanne finally agreed with her doctor's suggestion that she should consult a psychiatrist, Dr. Eileen Goldman, who had been a great help to some of Dr. Meyers's other patients. Suzanne agreed. "But it was only because I hoped she could give me something to calm me down."

Suzanne told Dr. Goldman that she had experienced similar feelings of anxiety and panic on three other occasions—all times of extreme stress. Dr. Goldman also learned that Suzanne's mother, grandmother, brother, and two maternal aunts had also experienced periodic bouts of severe anxiety. Laboratory tests confirmed that Suzanne had no other physical problems. Dr. Goldman also made sure that Suzanne had never had previous problems with drugs or alcohol.

After a great deal of discussion, Suzanne Tripitt and Dr. Goldman agreed on the following treatment plan:

Suzanne would take a 5 mg diazepam (Valium) tablet upon waking, and another after lunch. She would take one 5 mg tablet one hour before bedtime. She would continue on this regimen until the day of her surgery—which was ten days away—and for a week thereafter. Following this she would first taper down, then stop the drug over a period of one week.

Dr. Goldman and Suzanne would have two one-hour sessions per week over the next two months to discuss Suzanne's feelings and what to expect before, during, and after surgery. They both decided that it would be especially important for Suzanne to discuss the feelings she experienced at the age of seven, watching her grandmother die of breast cancer. Also, before surgery, Suzanne and Dr. Goldman would meet with her husband and their two teenaged daughters for two hour-long appointments to discuss ways they could be supportive to Suzanne in the weeks and months to come. Suzanne would meet with members of the surgical team to discuss preparations for surgery and what to expect afterward. She would attend regular meetings of Reach for Recovery, a support group for women who have had breast cancer surgery.

Suzanne had a very favorable response to her first dose of diazepam. "I could feel my mind and body relaxing for the first time in days. It was as if a big propeller inside my chest had suddenly stopped whirling." The medication made her feel slightly sleepy, a sensation she liked. The dose shortly before bedtime made it easier for her to fall asleep.

After taking diazepam for two days, Suzanne was able to return to work. Because of the sedative effects and possible loss of coordination from the drug, she agreed not to drive.

The surgeons were able to remove the lump with only a small bit of surrounding tissue. Suzanne recovered quickly and experienced so little anxiety during her recovery that she decided she no longer needed the diazepam. She tapered down and quit during her six-day stay in the hospital. After her release, Suzanne decided to continue weekly therapy with Dr. Goldman to help her understand her feelings of vulnerability to illness and to help her work to improve her relationship with her husband.

Suzanne's experience provides a fine example of an appropriate, enlightened, and successful use of an antianxiety drug. Suzanne, her family, and her two physicians did everything right:

Suzanne took the initiative and responsibility for her own health care by examining her own breasts and bringing the lump to her doctor's attention. She may well have saved her own life.

Suzanne's family provided support during each stage of her care and recovery. They did not tease or ridicule her for her dramatic psychological response to the diagnosis. They were understanding and supportive and communicated frequently and clearly with Suzanne's physicians.

Suzanne's physicians also communicated clearly—with Suzanne, her family, *and one another*.

Dr. Goldman, the psychiatrist, did not rely on the drug alone to solve the problem. Instead, she recommended a combination of psychotherapy, family therapy, and judicious drug use. She did not limit the focus of treatment to one problem, but dealt with a full range of Suzanne's psychological needs. The focus was not only on Suzanne's response to having breast cancer but on other issues that emerged as the result of the precipitating stress.

Dr. Goldman chose a drug regimen that would ease Suzanne's anxiety quickly and help her get to sleep, and she chose a drug that was easy to discontinue.

Because diazepam has high potential for abuse, Dr. Goldman first gave Suzanne a schedule for tapering down and stopping the drug. Then Suzanne received the first dose.

## Living with Anxiety

Although anxiety may sometimes be a symptom of hidden psychological conflict, an inherited biochemical trait, a learned habit, a response to stress, or a combination of any or all of these, in its milder forms anxiety may also be a healthful and helpful emotion. Anxiety can alert us to be wary of subtle dangers, such as a stranger with bad intentions. Some forms of anxiety (e.g., before a game or before a test) can spur us on to higher achievement. Most of us experience mild anxiety symptoms from time to time, and many of us have learned to benefit from them. You may wish to consider consulting a psychologist, psychiatrist, or other counselor for help with your feelings of anxiety if they interfere with your school or work performance, your personal relationships, or your enjoyment of normally pleasurable activities.

While antianxiety drugs can be of some use in specific instances, we strongly advise against "turning to the pill bottle" each time you experience mild or moderate anxiety. In the long run, you will be much better off taking steps to understand the sources of your anxiety, modifying the factors that give rise to it, and learning to turn your anxiety to your own benefit.

The following books may supplement certain topics discussed in the chapter:

## Recommended Reading on Anxiety

Gold, Mark S. *The Good News About Panic, Anxiety, & Phobias.* New York: Villard Books, 1989.

Rapoport, Judith L. *The Boy Who Couldn't Stop Washing.* New York: E.P. Dutton, 1988.

Salzman, Leon, *Treatment of the Obsessive Personality.* New York: Jason Aronson, Inc., 1980.

# Chapter 5

# Antipanic and Antiphobic Drugs

LIKE anxiety, panic has both mental and physical components. Panic is a feeling of sudden, intense apprehension and fearfulness. People experiencing a panic attack feel as if they are in a life-threatening situation. They may believe that they are experiencing a heart attack or having a nervous breakdown. Panic is almost always associated with the sense of a loss of control, and feelings of confusion and extreme dread.

People experiencing a panic attack may feel that they are somehow outside their body, looking down at themselves. (Psychiatrists call this *depersonalization*.) Occasionally, a person will experience the frightening sensation that his or her body has turned into wood or into some other inanimate substance, or that they are somehow no longer themselves. (Psychiatrists call this *derealization*.)

## Panic

### PHYSICAL SYMPTOMS

Physical symptoms accompanying a panic attack may include light-headedness, dizziness, and tightness or pain in the chest. People experiencing a panic attack may be painfully aware of a rapid, powerful heartbeat. In the midst of a panic attack, people will typically feel that they cannot catch their breath even though they are breathing rapidly. Some panic attack victims experience shortness of breath (such as one might feel after vigorous exercise), others feel as if they are being smothered. To compensate for these feelings, they often take rapid and shallow breaths, which psychiatrists call *hyperventilation*. There may be numbness or tingling in the lips, around the mouth, or in the fingers or toes. Some other symptoms: sweating, flushing, choking sensations, nausea, abdominal distress, chills, and trembling.

Panic attacks usually develop with little or no warning. Although they mimic the normal response to danger, they take place in the absence of any stimuli that would normally produce such a reaction.

### How Long Does a Panic Attack Usually Last?

Panic attacks can appear with dramatic suddenness and may disappear as abruptly as they began. Most panic attacks will stop of their own accord without any special treatment. The length of a panic attack can vary greatly from individual to individual. Most panic attacks last only a few minutes; some pass in seconds; in rare cases, they may continue for several hours.

### Anticipating a Panic Attack

Many people who have had previous panic attacks develop a condition psychiatrists call *anticipatory anxiety*. This is a prolonged state of anxious anticipation of another panic attack. In extreme cases, anticipatory anxiety may be present during most of their waking hours.

### Does a Panic Attack Mean You Have a Physical Disorder?

People who have recently experienced a panic attack may fear that they are suffering from a serious, undiagnosed medical condition—generally some type of heart disorder. They may quite understandably feel confused when they receive a clean bill of health from their physicians. If such people do not receive proper counseling, they may continue to seek a second, third, or fourth opinion from various medical specialists, even though they are repeatedly told that no medical problem can be detected.

Such behavior reveals how terrifying and upsetting a panic attack can be. A person who has experienced one or more of them may feel desperate to regain some sense of control. They would actually be relieved to learn that they had a disabling disease. As one patient with frequent panic attacks recently told us: "The worst thing about my symptoms is that no one seems to know what is causing them. Any condition this rare certainly must be very dangerous and very hard to treat."

It can be immensely satisfying for the psychiatrist seeing an individual with a previously undiagnosed panic disorder to be able to say: "You *do* have a medical disorder, and I know *exactly* what it is. It is called panic disorder, and all the symptoms that you have described to me are common and characteristic of this condition. The good news is that, in almost all cases of panic disorder, we are able to treat successfully the symptoms. And in most cases we can also help you to identify and solve the problems that are giving rise to these frightening reactions."

## About Phobias

Phobias are persistent, irrational fears or apprehensions that are associated with certain objects or situations. People experiencing phobias will become extremely anxious when they encounter the objects or situations that give rise to their phobias. They will also feel a strong urge to avoid the objects or situations that produce these anxious feelings.

### SIMPLE PHOBIAS

In simple phobia, the individual's irrational fear is of a specific object, activity, or situation. This fear may be so strong and compelling that it results in an overwhelming urge for that individual to avoid the object, activity, or situation altogether. Individuals who experience phobias usually recognize that their feelings are irrational, but they find themselves unable to cope with their fears and anxieties in any way other than attempting to avoid completely the objects, situations, or activities that seem to trigger their fears.

The hallmark of a simple phobia is that the individual symptoms are usually elicited by and certainly are the most intense when confronted by the feared object such as the snake or dog, or situation such as a closed elevator. In most cases, the person experiencing the phobia does not fear the object or situation itself. What is feared is some dire outcome from being in a specific situation—being bitten, suffocating, falling, etc. Common simple phobias include fear of heights, fear of closed spaces, fear of flying, fear of certain animals such as dogs, fear of germs, fear of thunder and lightning, fear of blood, fear of crowds, and fear of various illnesses. Virtually any object or situation may become the focus of a simple phobia.

Although unsettling and upsetting, the anxieties and fears associated with simple phobias are usually not so intense as those associated with panic disorder. The avoidance behavior of simple phobias often gives the individual some measure of relief. Nonetheless, avoidance behaviors often can and usually do become severely disruptive to social and occupational functioning.

## PERFORMANCE ANXIETY AND OTHER SOCIAL PHOBIAS

Individuals with a social phobia have a fear of specific social situations—usually one in which they are performing. When they must give a talk or participate in some other kind of public performance (especially those in which they feel they will be evaluated, scrutinized, or criticized by others) they may experience intense feelings of shyness, shame, embarrassment, and apprehension. When these individuals must actually perform, they will typically experience bodily symptoms that resemble those of panic: tremor, hyperventilation, racing heartbeat, sweating, and dry mouth.

Speaking before an audience is the most common type of performance anxiety. This condition may be highly disabling to students at all levels of their education and for many individuals who are expected to make verbal presentations as part of their work. People with performance anxiety and other social phobias will go to almost any length to avoid speaking or performing in public. This can result in great cost: they may lose their jobs, suffer in their student evaluations, suffer in their professional lives, and experience severe blows to their self-esteem.

## AGORAPHOBIA

People with agoraphobia are fearful of being trapped in places where escape may be difficult or embarrassing or wherein they may be helpless in the face of a known or unknown danger. Common places or situations that evoke terror and avoidance are large public places such as theaters, shopping centers, or athletic stadiums; crowds; public transportation such as airplanes and trains; bridges; and parks.

People with agoraphobia restrict their daily activities to avoid these places. Some do so to the point of becoming virtual prisoners in their own homes. Because they fear that they may become helpless in the face of either known or unknown harm, a person with agoraphobia may develop a highly dependent relationship on a specific person without whose company he or she will not leave home. This individual is called the *phobic partner* of the person with agoraphobia. Sometimes the phobic partners may help a person with agoraphobia cope with the limitations imposed by the disorder. But sometimes the phobic partner may promote this dependency by reinforcing the agoraphobic person's fears.

There is an important association between panic attacks and agoraphobia. Agoraphobia often appears shortly after a panic attack. The situation or place that the person with agoraphobia avoids somehow becomes associated with the panic attack. The helplessness and dread that the individual fears may constitute a memory—conscious or unconscious—of the panic experience. The phobias, panic, and depression frequently occur in the same individuals or the same families. Some researchers believe that all of these symptoms are part of a single underlying biologic disorder that is genetically transmitted. There thus seems to be a significant relationship between depression, manic depression, and anxiety disorders.

## NORMAN STEIN: PANIC ATTACK AND AGORAPHOBIA

Norman Stein, a forty-eight-year-old accountant, was enjoying an evening at the symphony with his wife, Evelyn, when he suddenly felt he was having a heart attack. His chest felt tight, his heart raced and pounded, he felt he couldn't catch his breath, and the room began to spin around him. An aching pain moved down his left shoulder and into his forearm. He felt so weak that he was barely able to attract his wife's attention. She nearly jumped out of her chair when he whispered, "Evelyn, I think I'm dying."

She helped him stagger to the lobby. Someone called an ambulance. Norman's symptoms did not diminish during the ride to the hospital. Despite his panting, he felt as if he were suffocating. In the emergency room, the pain in his chest increased, and he was transferred immediately to the cardiac intensive care unit.

Over the next several days, Norman underwent intensive laboratory testing and continuous monitoring of his vital signs; but no abnormality was ever found. His cardiologist assured him that he could find no evidence of a previous heart attack or any present cardiac disorder.

Rather than being relieved by this optimistic report, Norman became infuriated with his medical team for not finding a definitive cause for what he was now calling "my heart attack." Dr. Mark Meyer, Norman's cardiologist, stated that there were many possible causes for his experience—from (1) a transient viral infection to (2) something Norman had eaten that "didn't agree with him," to (3) an emotional reaction.

When Dr. Meyer mentioned this latter possibility, Norman flew into a rage. "Are you trying to tell me that I'm some kind of lunatic, or that I made this up, or that it's somehow all in my mind?" he demanded. "No," replied Dr. Meyer, "all I am saying is that whatever caused your condition cannot be found at the present time using batteries of tests. At present, we cannot find any evidence that your cardiovascular system or any other system is impaired."

Norman replied, "What I hear you saying is that you weren't able to find out what is wrong with me, so you're blaming it on my nerves. How do I know that I won't have another attack?"

After his discharge from the hospital, Norman discussed his health concerns with several of his friends and with his senior partner at his accounting firm. He decided to take a medical leave of absence until he could arrive at some "definitive conclusions" about his "medical problems." On the recommendation of several of his friends, Norman contacted a variety of specialists, all of whom did their best to assure him that they could find no evidence of any illness. Nonetheless, Norman was not reassured.

Terrified that "an attack" might occur at any time, Norman severely restricted his activities. "I might not survive if my next attack happens in a place where I can't get help," he reasoned. He therefore spent most of his time in his home, where he had installed sophisticated equipment for monitoring his pulse, blood pressure, and heart rhythm as well as a system for calling emergency medical help.

After reading newspaper accounts of a famous athlete who, despite regular exercise and having routine physicals, died from a cardiac arrhythmia, Norman became convinced that his "attacks" stemmed from a rare and hard-to-diagnose electrical abnormality of his heart. On the rare occasions that Norman left home, Evelyn always accompanied him. And he was careful not to go too far from hospitals with cardiac intensive care units.

Four and a half months after his first attack, Norman experienced a second attack with symptoms almost identical to the first. Again he was taken by ambulance to the hospital and admitted under Dr. Meyer's care. Again, no physical source of his symptoms was detected by physical examination and laboratory testing. This time, Dr. Meyer had a long talk with Evelyn in which he communicated to her his strong suspicion that there was "an emotional factor" underlying Norman's problems. He urged Evelyn to try to persuade Norman to see Dr. Beverly Young, a consulting psychiatrist who specialized in caring for the psychiatric problems of patients on the medical and surgical services.

Dr. Young reviewed carefully the symptoms Norman had experienced during his panic attack. She also learned that Norman's maternal grand-mother began to have what were then called *fits* when she was in her early thirties. She had almost never left home during the last forty years of her life. Norman's mother and sister both suffered from recurrent depression. Although neither had been hospitalized, both had taken antidepressants on several occasions.

Dr. Young told Norman that she was quite sure that he was suffering from panic attacks with agoraphobia. When Norman responded by saying, "What you're telling me, Dr. Young, is that it is all in my head, and that I am not really sick," Dr. Young responded, "That is not at all what I am saying. I view your illness as a medical illness that has both biological and psychological features. I am going to give you several scientific articles to read as well as chapters from psychiatric textbooks on various aspects of panic attacks and agoraphobia. In this way you can come to understand that you have a well-defined and treatable medical illness, about which you have no reason to be ashamed."

Norman read and reread the articles given to him by Dr. Young and was astonished to learn that other people had endured almost the exact same symptoms that he had experienced. He agreed to work with Dr. Young on a treatment plan that involved psychological interventions, behavioral inter-actions, and medications. Because he had experienced "only" two episodes of panic, both he and Dr. Young concluded that it was not necessary at this time to place him on a heterocyclic antidepressant—which might prevent future panic attacks.

Norman learned relaxation skills and other behavioral techniques that he could employ if he felt a panic attack beginning. Dr. Young also gave Norman a prescription for alprazolam (Xanax), a benzodiazepine antianx-iety agent. She instructed him to keep several tablets with him at all times, and to take one if he had any sense that a panic attack might be starting.

Dr. Young advised Norman that his return to work should be an important part of his treatment. Norman, his wife, and Dr. Young all spoke openly with Norman's business associates regarding Norman's condition. His co-workers, thus informed, provided Norman with a great deal of support and encouragement. In the weeks that followed, Norman was able to return to work, where he gradually assumed all his former activities.

After a third episode of panic occurred at work, Norman, Evelyn, and Dr. Young met again. With Dr. Young's encouragement, Norman decided to begin taking imipramine (Tofranil), a heterocyclic antidepressant. The dose of the drug was built up gradually to 250 mg per day, and Norman remained on a full dose of this drug for one year. At the end of a year, he gradually reduced his dose, then stopped the drug altogether. It has now been six years since he went off the drug. During that time, Norman has not experienced another panic attack.

Norman's experience demonstrates several important principles about panic attacks, agoraphobia, and their treatment:

• Panic attacks are terrifying to the person affected.
• Both patients and their physicians may at first believe their symptoms are due to a physical problem, usually a heart problem.
• Agoraphobia, when it develops, often occurs after a panic attack.
• People who have had a panic attack may initially be reluctant to admit that such experiences might be a result of a psychological disorder.
• Like Norman, some people who have experienced panic attacks may attempt to discourage their medical team from seeking psychiatric intervention.
• A careful history will often uncover both panic disorder and depression in other family members.

The successful treatment of Norman's panic disorder and agoraphobia also illustrates several important points about recovery from these conditions:

• The understanding, encouragement, and support of the affected person's spouse, family, friends, and working associates are all extremely important.
• The person with the problem must be fully informed on all aspects of panic disorder and agoraphobia. Dr. Young acted very wisely when she provided Norman with copies of recent review articles from psychiatric journals.
• A successful treatment plan will usually involve several elements: psychological counseling; discussions with family, friends, and co-workers; learning new relaxation and stress management skills; and, in some cases, taking one or more prescription drugs.
• By making it clear that it was Norman who would make the major decisions about treatment, Dr. Young helped him overcome the fear of losing control—his principal fear.
• The treatment plan should be a flexible one. All parties should realize that if the first plan does not control the problem, they can always try other techniques.

*Medical Workup*

As with other psychiatric disorders, we recommend a thorough medical evaluation to make sure that the panic disorder has no medical ("organic") cause. See Sidebar 1 in Chapter 4 for medical conditions that can produce panic disorder. Even if a panic disorder is diagnosed, this does not rule out the possibility that another psychiatric or medical illness is also causing panic and affecting the patient. It is therefore important for people who experience a panic disorder to consult with both a mental health professional and a medically oriented physician.

### Treatment Plan

Even though many panic disorders can now be treated with drugs, drug treatments do not succeed alone. They should be considered as one part of a four-stage plan.

Stage One: Psychiatric drugs (usually monoamine oxidase inhibitors or heterocyclic antidepressants) are used to block the panic attacks. These medications appear to block both the physical expressions of panic—such as racing of the heart—and the psychological aspects—such as anxiety and apprehension.

Stage Two: The person should be helped to understand the exact nature of the panic and phobias in his or her life. This will help to alleviate fears (e,g., that the patient is suffering from an undiagnosed cardiac disease) or incorrect implications (e.g., that the patient is "crazy," infantile, lazy, etc.).

Stage Three: The person who has experienced panic attacks should receive encouragement and support from his or her psychiatrist, spouse, family, friends, and work associates—and in some cases from self-help groups for people with panic disorders.

Stage Four: The person should learn new stress management and relaxation techniques and social skills to help reverse the patterns that may have emerged as a result of the panic disorder, e.g., social withdrawal, alcohol dependence, low self-esteem.

## Suggested Treatments

### TREATMENT OF PANIC WITH HETEROCYCLIC ANTIDEPRESSANTS

The heterocyclic antidepressant imipramine (Tofranil) is the most commonly utilized antidepressant to treat panic attacks. Imipramine has been shown effective in treating panic disorder in 50 to 90 percent (depending on the particular scientific outcome study) of all patients treated. Combining imipramine with psychological and behavioral treatments increases the percentage of patients who benefit.

One commonly recommended regimen is to start a patient on 10 mg of imipramine at bedtime, and then to increase the dose by 10 mg every other night until a dose of 50 mg is reached. Thereafter, the dose is raised by 25 mg increments every three days, or by 50 mg weekly, to as high as 300 mg per day—or until the panic is fully blocked. For most people with panic attacks, this will require at least 150 mg of imipramine per day. For some, doses higher than 300 mg per day may be necessary. If a person's symptoms of panic do not respond to high oral doses of imipramine or other hetero- cyclics, blood levels should be measured and doses adjusted accordingly. If symptoms do not respond at adequate blood levels, changing the drug to a monoamine oxidase inhibitor or to a serotonin-specific antidepressant is indicated.

Once all symptoms of panic have disappeared, the person should be maintained on the heterocyclic antidepressant for six months or more to prevent relapse. Thereafter, the antidepressant should be tapered slowly and eventually discontinued.

Approximately two-thirds of the patients will not experience reemer- gence of their panic attacks after discontinuation of their medications. We recommend continuing heterocyclics for at least an additional year for those patients whose panic symptoms emerge upon a first tapering of their medication.

The side effects of heterocyclic antidepressants and of the newer serotonin-specific antidepressants (which increasingly show evidence of antipanic effects) and other medical aspects of the use of these classes of medications are discussed in Chapter 3.

### TREATMENT OF PANIC WITH MONOAMINE OXIDASE INHIBITORS

Monoamine oxidase inhibitors are as effective as heterocyclic antidepres- sants in the treatment of panic attacks. But because of the dietary restric- tions necessary for their safe use (see Chapter 3), these drugs are used less frequently than heterocyclics. For those patients who cannot tolerate cer- tain side effects of heterocyclic antidepressants, or for those patients whose panic has not responded to heterocyclic antidepressants, monoamine oxi- dase inhibitors can be an excellent alternative.

Monoamine oxidase inhibitors are used in the same fashion and in the same doses to treat panic disorder as they are to treat depression. Occa- sionally, 90 mg phenelzine (Nardil) is required for the effective treatment of panic. Phenelzine treatment is usually begun at 15 mg per day in the mornings for three days. This is followed by 30 mg in the morning for four days, and thereafter followed by 45 mg daily each morning for one week. If a patient's symptoms of panic remain after he or she has been on a dose of

45 mg for one week, the dose should be raised to 60 mg and held there for at least fourteen days. Thereafter, the dose may be gradually raised, if necessary, to 90 mg per day or until a patient's symptoms of panic are no longer present. One monoamine oxidase inhibitor, tranylcypromine (Parnate), is usually begun at 10 mg taken in the morning and increased, if necessary, by approximately 10 mg per week until the symptoms are removed or until the upper limit of 80 mg per day is reached.

## TREATMENT OF PANIC WITH SEROTONIN-SPECIFIC ANTIDEPRESSANTS

As we write this book, the results of scientific studies are emerging on the use of serotonin-specific antidepressants in the treatment of panic. Fluoxetine (Prozac) is the medication that has been evaluated in most of the studies, and this drug appears to be as effective as the heterocyclic antidepressants and the monoamine oxidase inhibitors in blocking panic. In our own practices, we have had excellent results in using fluoxetine to treat panic, and we follow the same dosage regimens and clinical practices that we do when treating depression with this drug. We predict that, as with depression, the use of fluoxetine and other serotonin-specific antidepressants will become the drug most frequently chosen for treating panic.

## TREATMENT OF PANIC ATTACKS WITH BENZODIAZEPINES

With the exception of alprazolam (Xanax), high-potency benzodiazepines are rarely used for the treatment of panic attacks. This is because their usefulness for panic and phobia is questionable and their potential for dependence is high. In addition, it is much more difficult for a patient to withdraw from a benzodiazepine than from an antidepressant drug. *Rebound* panic and anxiety upon withdrawal from benzodiazepines is more common with these drugs.

Nonetheless, several studies show that alprazolam is an effective antipanic drug that works faster and has fewer side effects than heterocyclic antidepressants. Our practice is to limit the use of benzodiazepines in the treatment of panic to those patients who have either severe anticipatory anxiety accompanying their panic disorder or to those whose panic symptoms intensify during the initial phases of antidepressant treatment. We never use benzodiazepines for patients who have a history of drug dependency.

For many patients, we use relatively low doses of alprazolam (e.g., 0.25 mg four times per day) at the same time that we initiate treatment with and increase the doses of the heterocyclic antidepressant. Once we are relatively certain that the panic symptoms are blocked by the heterocyclic antidepressant, we *slowly* taper the alprazolam until it is discontinued.

When used by itself to treat panic, higher doses of alprazolam are required than for the treatment of general anxiety disorder. We recommend beginning with 0.25 mg four times a day and raising the dose by 0.25 mg every three days. We continue to raise the dose until the patient's panic symptoms are no longer present. Some patients may require doses of up to 10 mg per day in divided doses for as long as eight months.

Most patients respond within two to three weeks after the initiation of treatment. The same alprazolam side effects we described in Chapter 4 occur when alprazolam is used to treat panic disorder. Because of the relatively high doses of alprazolam that are necessary to treat panic, certain patients may become so sedated that a treatment dose cannot be achieved.

## PSYCHOPHARMACOLOGIC TREATMENT OF AGORAPHOBIA

The treatment of agoraphobia usually includes:

Stage One: Treating the underlying panic disorder with an antidepressant.

Stage Two: Treating the person's anticipatory anxiety with psychotherapy and/or an antianxiety agent.

Stage Three: Treating the avoidant behavior with behavioral treatments, self-help groups, or other nonpharmacologic interventions.

Social phobias and simple phobias are, for the most part, best treated with nondrug methods. Treatment usually involves systematic exposure to the feared object or situation under carefully controlled and professionally guided conditions. For example, a patient may first imagine coming in contact with the feared object, then look at pictures of the feared object, and gradually, with encouragement and support, build up to entering the presence of the feared object and even touching or holding the object. These same principles and techniques are frequently effective in the treatment of certain social phobias.

## THE USE OF BETA BLOCKERS IN THE TREATMENT OF PERFORMANCE ANXIETY

A person experiencing performance anxiety will typically experience both psychological symptoms (e.g., fear, tension, difficulty in concentration) and physical symptoms (e.g., rapid heartbeat, tremors, heartburn, nausea, vomiting, diarrhea). Many of these functions are regulated by the part of the brain influenced by a family of drugs called the beta blockers (or, more formally, the beta adrenergic receptor antagonizing agents).

Beta blockers are drugs that can block the beta receptors in your nervous system. Beta receptors are divided into two classes: beta-1 receptors, which have stimulatory effects on heart muscle, and beta-2 receptors, with a dilating effect on the small air channels (bronchioles) in the lungs and the blood vessels throughout your body. Some beta blockers (e.g., atenolol and metroprolol) block only the beta-1 receptors. Other so-called nonselective beta blockers (e.g., propranolol, nadolol, timolol, and pindolol) block both beta-1 and beta-2 receptors.

Beta blockers can also be classified by their specific activities in the body. One important quality of a beta blocker is its ability to dissolve in a lipid solution. Researchers often speak of the lipid solubility of a particular beta blocker. The more lipid soluble the medication, the more quickly it will enter the brain. Propranolol, by far the most widely used beta blocker, is highly lipid soluble. The drug atenolol, on the other hand, has a low lipid solubility and thus is very slow to enter the brain and central nervous system.

Another important quality of any beta blocker is its half-life. This reflects how long the drug survives in the body in its active form. Oral propranolol has a half-life of approximately twelve hours. It must therefore usually be taken twice per day. Another drug, nadolol, has a longer half-life, approximately sixteen to twenty hours. It can thus usually be taken only once per day.

Beta blockers are more likely to produce side effects in persons with preexisting asthma and other pulmonary disorders, congestive heart failure, insulin-dependent diabetes mellitus, significant vascular disease, hyperthyroidism, angina pectoris, and several other medical conditions. When taken by people with a prior history of depression, beta blockers may also increase the risk of developing a depressive episode. It is therefore important for a person to undergo a complete medical history and an evaluation before taking these drugs.

While the treatment of performance anxiety with beta blockers is still controversial, some of the research in this area is among the most interesting and creative in all of medicine. Most studies compare the effect of a single dose of a beta blocker with that of a placebo on subjective distress or objective performance when volunteers are engaging in a broad range of performance, stressful, or competitive situations. Approximately twenty controlled studies have been conducted in this area. Most have used a single administration of a relatively low dose of the beta blocker (e.g., 40 mg propranolol, 5 mg pindolol, or 100 mg atenolol).

Some studies have examined the effects of beta blockers on the performances of musicians—with both the performing individuals and a musically knowledgeable panel assessing the quality of the performances. Most of these studies have concluded that the beta blocker improved the quality of the performance.

Researchers have also studied the effects of beta blockers on students taking examinations, surgeons performing operations, pilots flying helicopters, public speakers giving talks before large audiences, and sporting performances ranging from bowling to riflery. In more than half of these studies, anxiety was relieved. In approximately half of the studies, there was objective evidence of improved performance.

For this reason, although treatment of performance anxiety has not yet been listed by the FDA as an officially approved use of the beta blockers, many physicians have already begun to prescribe low doses of these drugs to help people deal with the symptoms of performance anxiety. While we agree that the present medical literature is inconclusive about the efficacy of beta blockers for this use, we believe that future research involving the use of higher doses of beta blockers for prolonged periods of time may demonstrate that this category of medications is, indeed, helpful for many individuals. Our current advice for using beta blockers in the treatment of this condition can be summarized as follows:

• Consult your family physician and, perhaps, a competent mental health professional to be certain of the diagnosis of performance anxiety and to identify clearly the source of your anxiety. It is particularly important to be sure that you have no underlying medical illnesses that may be contributing to your feelings of anxiety. Please consult Chapter 4 for an overview of the medical examination and testing recommended before any drug treatment for anxiety. In addition to the tests listed there, your physician should rule out bronchospastic pulmonary disorders, congestive heart failure, insulin-dependent diabetes mellitus, significant vascular disesase, persistent angina, and hyperthyroidism.

• Once your physician has determined that it is medically safe for you to take a beta blocking drug for performance anxiety, we advise a trial dose of 40 mg propranolol, to be taken about two hours before a routine performance situation—when you might expect some mild anxiety. Since you may be somewhat nervous about using a drug for the first time and because there is a small chance of unexpected side effects, you should take your initial dose in a safe, secure situation—ideally, a rehearsal or practice session. You should not use this drug for the first time in any situation that involves any risk of physical danger (e.g., mountain climbing, piloting an aircraft) or in situations that might have far-reaching implications in your life (e.g., a college entrance interview or specialty medical boards). Following these precautions, any unexpected side effects from the beta blocker will not result in serious consequences.

• Once it has been established that you can tolerate a single dose of 40 mg propranolol without disabling side effects, *under your doctor's guidance* you should take a low dose (20 to 40 mg) approximately two hours prior to a situation in which you expect significant performance anxiety. Note that the half-life of a beta blocker extends approximately eight hours following a single dose, so that if the performance extends for a prolonged period of time, the medication should be administered at the same dose every eight hours.

• If this regimen proves effective, the same procedure should be repeated under your doctor's guidance as required for treatment of any future performance anxiety. If you receive only partial relief from anxiety, the dose should be gradually increased by 20 mg during successive performances until you receive adequate relief.

• If you find that you receive little or no benefit from the dose described above, you and your physician must decide whether your anxiety is sufficiently severe or the nature of the performance is sufficiently important to consider long-term treatment with a beta blocker. In your discussion of the possible risks and benefits of such treatment, you should be sure you understand and accept the fact that beta blockers are not FDA-approved for the treatment of any anxiety disorder, and the scientific knowledge on the prevention of performance anxiety is at present quite limited.

• If you and your physician agree on long-term preventive treatment, we recommend your taking propranolol at 20 mg three times a day, and increasing the dose by 20 mg, as tolerated, every four days to a total dose of 40 mg three times per day. If you receive only a partial relief from performance anxiety at this dose, we suggest taking an additional single dose of 80 mg of propranolol prior to the performance. You and/or your doctor should monitor your blood pressure and heart rate on a regular basis. If you have no cardiovascular illnesses, we advise skipping the dose of medication if your systolic blood pressure drops below 90 mg of mercury or if your heart rate drops below fifty beats per minute. If you experience severe dizziness, loss of coordination, or wheezing, you should reduce your dose or stop taking the drug and immediately inform your physician.

We advise physicians to maintain their patients on 240 mg propranolol per day for at least six weeks before concluding that their performance anxiety is not responding to this approach. Serum levels of all the other antipsychotic or anticonvulsant medications you may be taking must be monitored when you are taking a beta blocker.

When discontinuing propranolol after taking the drug for an extended period of time, the dose must be reduced a little at a time. We suggest reducing the dose by 20 mg a day until you are on a total of 40 mgs per day. You should then reduce your dose by 20 mgs every other day (and more slowly than that if you have hypertension or any other cardiovascular disorder).

Let us emphasize once again that beta blockers are powerful and potentially hazardous medications and should be used only under the direct care of a knowledgeable physician.

## NONDRUG TREATMENT OF PANIC ATTACKS AND PHOBIAS

There are many effective nondrug treatments for both panic disorders and phobias. These include self-help groups, psychotherapy, behavioral treatments, cognitive retraining, relaxation techniques, and many other helpful approaches. Because a full discussion of these approaches is beyond the focus of this book, we recommend reading an overview of psychological and behavioral treatments in a standard textbook of psychiatry such as *The American Psychiatric Press Textbook of Psychiatry*, edited by Talbott, Hales, and Yudofsky (Washington, D.C.: American Psychiatric Press, 1988), pp. 855–907; or Dr. Michelle G. Craske's excellent review, "Cognitive-Behavioral Treatment of Panic," *Review of Psychiatry*, Vol. 7 (Washington, D.C.: American Psychiatric Press, 1988), pp. 121–137. Excellent bibliographies can be found in both references.

# Frequent Questions About Panic and Phobias

**Q.** *Can chemicals and other substances produce panic attacks?*

**A.** In susceptible individuals, a broad range of chemicals, drugs, and other substances can produce panic. Approximately one-half to two-thirds of people with a prior history of panic will experience a panic attack if they are given an intravenous infusion of sodium lactate. Important is that this response does not usually occur in people with psychiatric conditions other than panic disorder. Intravenous sodium lactate does not produce panic in people whose panic disorders have been successfully pretreated with imipramine or alprazolam. This induction of panic under experimental conditions tells scientists that there is probably a biochemical component to panic disorder (i.e., it is not a "purely" psychological problem), and it also helps confirm the efficacy of drugs for panic. Panic is also induced when people prone to panic disorders inhale carbon dioxide; but this does not occur in those without a history of panic disorder. Several studies have shown that caffeine can induce panic attacks in people with histories of panic disorder, but not in patients who do not have panic disorder. Please note that in all experimental inductions of panic, neither the patient nor the doctor knows whether the patient is receiving lactate, caffeine, carbon dioxide, or a different, nonactive (placebo) substance. Finally, panic may also be induced in susceptible individuals by certain substances of abuse— particularly tetrahydrocannabinol (the active ingredient in marijuana) and cocaine. Alcohol does not usually produce panic. In fact, certain people with panic disorder attempt to treat their condition with alcohol. Unfortunately, this approach can lead to alcohol dependence and the many disabling psychological and medical problems associated with this devastating condition.

**Q.** *Are panic disorders hereditary?*

**A.** Several carefully designed studies have shown that panic disorder occurs in much higher rates in relatives of individuals with panic disorder than it does in the relatives of other people without panic disorder. One study showed that the risk of panic disorder is approximately 25 percent among relatives of a person with panic disorder. This percentage compares with only approximately 2 to 3 percent among the relatives of any selected individual without panic disorder. In genetic studies involving twins, anxiety disorders with panic attacks were five times as common among monozygotic, or identical, twins than they were among dizygotic, or fraternal, twins. This finding is interpreted by scientists as an indication that panic disorder is hereditary and transmitted genetically, since monozygotic, or identical, twins have the same genetic makeup.

**Q.** *Can allergies cause panic disorder?*

**A.** Although sensitivities to certain foods can cause a wide variety of psychological symptoms, including panic and anxiety, except for a few rare cases there is little evidence that allergies are a common cause of anxiety symptoms.

**Q.** *Can hypoglycemia or low blood sugar cause panic?*

**A.** Although anxiety may be associated with low blood sugar, there is little, if any, evidence that indicates that a panic attack or panic disorder is associated with low blood sugar. Attempts to produce panic attacks by lowering blood sugar do not produce panic—even in panic-prone individuals. Glucose-tolerance tests, which indicate tendencies toward hypoglycemia, are within the normal ranges in patients with panic disorder. Finally, lactate-induced attacks are not accompanied by hypoglycemia. All this evidence suggests that low blood sugar is *not* associated with panic attacks or panic disorder.

**Q.** *How common is panic disorder? How common are phobias?*

**A.** Several investigators have found that approximately 10 percent of the population report a history of at least one panic attack. However, a far smaller percentage of people meet the American Psychiatric Association's strict diagnostic requirements for panic disorder. Approximately 1 percent of the population at any given time carries this diagnosis, and between 1 and 2 percent of the population will develop this disorder in their lifetimes. Phobic disorders, on the other hand, are much more common, with approximately 5 percent of the population having one type of phobic disorder at any given time. Simple phobias are about twice as common as agoraphobia or social phobia.

**Q.** *What drugs should* not *be used to treat panic or phobias?*

**A.** Although many drugs—including antipsychotics, barbiturates, other sedatives, and even lithium—are sometimes used to treat panic, in our opinion this is a mistake. These drugs have not, to date, been proved safe or effective in the treatment of panic attacks or phobic disorders. Many have potentially hazardous side effects. With the exception of a few rare situations, we therefore recommend that only members of the antidepressant families, selected benzodiazepines, and beta blockers be used to treat panic or phobic disorders. It is particularly important not to take antipsychotic agents or combination drugs that include an antipsychotic agent to treat panic or phobic conditions. If you are suffering from panic disorder or phobia and your physician suggests the use of an antipsychotic agent, we request that you and your physician jointly review the material in this chapter and choose a more appropriate alternative.

**Q.** *How long does a panic disorder last?*

**A.** Untreated, panic disorder may begin quite early in life and persist literally for a lifetime. Before the advent of modern psychopharmacologic and other treatments of panic and phobic disorders, large numbers of people were severely disabled by their symptoms. In taking family histories of our patients with panic disorders, we commonly hear of parents, grandparents, and great-grandparents who remained imprisoned in their homes for much of their adult lives. Although panic and phobic disorders recur in certain individuals (i.e., they return later—even after successful treatment), this is unusual. In general, we prescribe antidepressants for six months to one year after the medications have removed the symptoms. Thereafter, most patients may discontinue their medications—without the recurrence of panic or phobic symptoms. Concomitant psychological, behavioral, group, and/or other treatments also help to prevent recurrence.

**Q.** *Is there any association between alcohol and panic disorder?*

**A.** There is a strong association between alcohol and panic disorder. Almost every study that has investigated the issue has shown that panic disorder is highly prevalent in hospitalized patients who were being treated for alcoholism. It is not yet known whether or not alcohol, ingested at high doses over prolonged periods of time, induces panic, or whether panic-prone individuals are drawn to alcohol in an attempt to obtain relief from their panic attacks. For certain individuals with panic disorder, alcohol, in very low amounts, can have some calming effects on the apprehension and fears associated with panic. Unfortunately, continued or prolonged use of alcohol for this purpose brings a rebound phenomenon in which the panic becomes more pronounced and more frequent as the effects of alcohol wear off. One can easily understand how panic- or phobic-prone individuals may tend to increase their consumption of alcohol by using more and more alcohol to treat the very emotional reactions elicited by alcohol withdrawal. The overall result is that the panic and phobic symptoms become progressively worse, while the degree of dependence on alcohol becomes greater. The important lesson is that alcohol and panic disorder are a very dangerous combination.

**Q.** *Can withdrawal from medication or drugs cause panic disorder?*

**A.** Yes, withdrawal from a wide range of prescribed medications, over-the-counter drugs, and so-called recreational drugs can give rise to symptoms identical to those that occur during panic attacks. The most common substances that produce such symptoms upon their withdrawal are alcohol, opiates and other analgesics, barbiturates and other sedatives, and psychiatric medications (including heterocyclic antidepressants and benzodiazepines). Short-acting benzodiazepines such as alprazolam (Xanax) pose a particular problem. Although this drug has been proved to be an excellent antipanic medication, the fact that it is short-acting causes its antipanic actions to disappear quickly. In addition, alprazolam may be associated with a condition called *rebound anxiety*, which, in fact, may be panic and anxiety resulting from drug withdrawal. It is sometimes difficult for psychiatrists to determine whether their patients' symptoms are the results of (1) incompletely treated panic or (2) withdrawal from benzodiazepine. For this reason, we advocate the use of antidepressants as the pharmacologic treatment of first choice for panic attacks and agoraphobia. We do not prescribe benzodiazepines to people with panic disorders and a history of substance abuse or dependence.

**Q.** *Can poisons in our environment result in panic attacks?*

**A.** There is good evidence that certain toxic chemicals in our environment can produce symptoms similar to panic attacks. Included in this list are certain substances such as arsenic, mercury, bismuth, and other elements that can produce severe anxiety as well as irritability and mood swings. Recently, mercury has been traced not only to industrial pollution, but also to marijuana grown in regions of Hawaii with high mercury content. Volatile chemicals can also give rise to symptoms of profound anxiety and panic. Workers in industries associated with volatile gases (e.g., refineries, chemical plants, paint factories, aircraft refueling settings, anesthetic-producing factories) are at particularly high risk for chemical toxicities that may lead to panic symptoms. Additionally, insecticides and fertilizers containing substances called organophosphates may cause changes in brain chemistry that also give rise to profound anxiety, panic, and other serious psychological changes. As with the carcinogenic effects of environmental poisons, the psychological effects of these poisons often go unrecognized, their effects unproved, for many years before they are detected as the source of panic and other medical problems.

# Recommended Reading on Panic and Phobias

Gold, Mark S. *The Good News About Panic Anxiety and Phobias*. New York: Villard Books, 1989.

# Chapter 6

# Antimanic Drugs

Mania is a state of excessive excitement or enthusiasm. A person in a manic mood feels euphoric, excited, expansive, and may experience wild flights of fancy. People in the grip of mania can appear tremendously energetic. They may report feeling excited or high all the time.

During a manic period, people who are normally cooperative may become hyperactive or aggressive. They may commit themselves to unrealistically ambitious projects. A person in a manic state may come to believe that certain fantasies are actually true. For example, they may astonish family members and friends by announcing that they are about to dance for the Bolshoi Ballet, join the New York Yankees, or address the United Nations—even though they have no training or experience in these areas. Clinicians call such mistaken beliefs *delusions of grandeur*.

People in the midst of manic episodes typically speak in loud, rapid voices. They may become irritable if you attempt to interrupt them. They may act in ways that seem excessively dramatic and theatrical—almost as if they were playing the part of a character in a play. They may become angry at those who try to help them and may hold forth against others who have supposedly wronged them.

People experiencing a manic episode often find themselves unable to sleep or even to sit still. Such individuals are often brought to the hospital emergency room by baffled family members, who complain that the patient had been keeping the whole family awake by talking or singing all night.

People in the grip of mania often make unnecessary or extravagant expenditures. John, a thirty-year-old lawyer with a modest income, agreed to buy three new Mercedes automobiles—at a cost of $120,000—during a two-month manic episode. Others may invest their money in foolish business enterprises or may simply give it away. Judy, a twenty-nine-year-old account manager, invested $20,000 in a high-risk movie production company after she stopped taking her antimanic medication. She subsequently lost all her savings.

Individuals suffering from mania frequently appear to have little need for sleep and may express the opinion that sleep is a complete waste of time. Joan, a nineteen-year-old college student, went for four nights without sleeping while writing several long term papers. She considered these papers so exceptional that she expected to receive a Pulitzer Prize. Her professor found them wildly incoherent and gave her a failing grade for the course.

A person in a manic state may also experience an unusual degree of distractibility, rapid flow of disjointed thoughts, and periods of sexual hyperactivity or promiscuity.

# Mania

### FRIENDS AND FAMILY

Mania can be a particularly difficult mental disorder for friends and family to understand. People experiencing mania often appear to enjoy their manic episodes. They frequently deny that they are ill and may resist treatment. In some cases, the symptoms of mania can be mistaken for signs of real genius. Indeed, it often seems that people suffering from mania produce more problems for others than they do for themselves.

### MANIC STAGES

• Mild mania (sometimes called hypomania): The person will exhibit an unusually cheerful or elevated mood during which he or she may appear overly confident and grandiose. You will be able to understand the manic person, but his or her thinking may seem muddled and may not lead to any clear conclusions. In psychiatric terms, such thinking is called *tangential* or *non–goal-directed*. Jim, a forty-year-old insurance agent, called the president of a multinational oil company to give him advice about a projected takeover of another company while in a state of mild mania. Mild mania is sometimes the earliest stage of a manic episode, however some people may maintain a mild manic state for long periods without progressing to more severe forms of mania. When these hypomanic episodes alternate with periods of mild to moderate depressions, the term *cyclothymia* is used. If the manic symptoms are so severe as to disrupt a person's social, work, or school functioning, *bipolar illness* is the term used to describe this emotional state.

• *Moderate mania.* This is a more advanced stage of mania. The individual may become extremely irritable—or openly angry, hostile, or argumentative. The person may begin to exhibit grandiose or paranoid delusions. Bob, a thirty-two-year-old hospital attendant, came to believe that he was a famous thoracic surgeon. He stormed into an operating room without mask or gown and attempted to operate on a patient.

• *Severe mania.* In the most severe form of mania, thoughts and ideas flow through the individual's mind at an uncontrollable pace. Severely manic individuals may become very physically active. Hospitalized manic patients can frequently be found racing up and down the hallways of the psychiatric ward, making emphatic gestures and talking incessantly.

## WHEN MANIA USUALLY DEVELOPS

A person's first episode of mania usually occurs in the late teens or early twenties. Some people may have their first severe episode—one that requires hospitalization—in their twenties or thirties. A few people do not experience their first manic episode until their forties or fifties. Mild mania sometimes begins in the late teens, with as many as 35 percent of these teenagers later developing a full-blown bipolar disorder or major depression.

## MANIA AND DEPRESSION

About 90 percent of people who experience manic episodes also experience severe episodes of depression. In most cases, mania is just one phase of a more complex disorder in which periods of mania alternate with periods of depression. Psychiatrists call this combination *manic-depressive illness* or *bipolar disorder*.

Mania without depression is relatively rare. For every ten people with manic-depressive illness, there is only one who experiences mania without depression. Three-fourths of those with bipolar disorder will experience one or more periods of mania before they experience their first episodes of depression.

Roughly 1 percent of North Americans will exhibit manic-depressive illness at some time in their lives. Of these, about half will have one parent with a history of either depression or bipolar illness. In contrast, individuals who experience depression without mania rarely have a manic-depressive parent.

Treatments for the depressive episodes of manic-depression are the same as the treatment of depression without mania. These treatments are discussed in Chapter 3.

## DRUGS THAT CAN PRODUCE MANIA

• *Medically prescribed steroids.* Steroids are a common cause of drug-induced mania. John, a nineteen-year-old asthmatic, was given prednisone, a steroid, to help control his asthma. Within two days he began to exhibit agitated behavior, restlessness, and inability to sleep. He complained of racing thoughts. He talked incessantly and was unable to sit still. When the prednisone was discontinued, his symptoms disappeared.

• *Steroids used by bodybuilders and athletes.*

• *Antidepressants.*

• *Other drugs:* Isoniazid (an antituberculosis medication); L-dopa (a medication used to treat Parkinson's disease); marijuana, LSD, cocaine, PCP, and mescaline; and medications that are prescribed to treat hyperactivity in children can also cause drug-induced mania. Medications prescribed to treat hyperactivity in children that may also produce maniclike symptoms are: dextroamphetamine (Dexedrine), methylphenidate (Ritalin) and pemoline (Cylert).

## DISEASES THAT CAN PRODUCE MANIA

• epilepsy
• multiple sclerosis
• hyperparathyroidism
• hyperthyroidism

## SELF-HELP GROUPS FOR MOOD DISORDERS

**Depressives Anonymous**
329 East 62nd Street
New York, NY 10021
(212) 689-2600

Depressives Anonymous helps anxious and depressed people change troublesome behavior patterns and attitudes. Professional counselors are part of the program. The group publishes a newsletter and will help interested persons set up new chapters in localities where one does not already exist.

**National Depressive and Manic-Depressive Association**
53 West Jackson Boulevard
Suite 505
Chicago, IL 60604
(312) 939-2442

The National Depressive and Manic-Depressive Association provides mutual support for patients with manic-depressive or depressive illness, and their families—and education to help overcome the stigma of manic-depressive disorder. They can put callers in touch with existing groups, or provide a how-to kit for those who would like to join with others in their area to form new chapters. They also provide phone help, doctor referrals, a newsletter, and other literature on manic-depressive illness.

**Helping Hands**
109 Chestnut Street
Andover, MA 01810
(617) 475-6888

Helping Hands provides support for people with manic-depressive and obsessive-compulsive disorders. This group sponsors a nationwide network of support groups for these conditions. They can provide a wide range of information and offer advice on finding specialized treatment for these conditions. Helping Hands also sponsors informal correspondence and telephone support networks.

## PSYCHOTHERAPY FOR MANIA

Psychotherapy can be extremely helpful for patients with mania or bipolar disorders. During manic episodes, a great amount of emotional turmoil affects both the individual and his or her relationships with a spouse and other family members. A good relationship with a mental health professional is of great benefit during these difficult periods. Psychotherapy can also help the person suffering from mania:

• Learn to recognize when his or her mood is becoming too high. This can be the tip-off of increased risk for such self-damaging acts as buying sprees, sexual indiscretions, unwise commitments, etc.

• Separate the positive from the negative aspects of manic depression.

• Learn to manage the emotional roller coaster as he or she passes from a period of mania into a period of depression.

## Drugs Used to Treat Mania

In most cases, lithium carbonate is the drug of choice for people experiencing mania. It is available either in regular or in time-release preparations. For children with mania, a flavored lithium preparation is available.

Some patients with severe mania, especially those who pose a possible threat to themselves or others, may also benefit from antipsychotic medications prior to beginning lithium. These treatments are discussed in Chapter 7. Such treatment can help the person calm down until lithium has a chance to become effective.

A second frequently used drug for manic disorders is carbamazepine (Tegretol), an anticonvulsant medication that has recently been found to be effective in treating mania. Lithium and carbamazepine are currently the most widely used drugs for this condition. Several of the newer and experimental drugs for the treatment of mania are described in a later section.

### How Do These Drugs Work?

*Lithium*

Nobody really knows how lithium works. Some researchers think it acts through regulating the movement of calcium in and out of nerve cells. Others believe that lithium regulates the central nervous system by controlling the sensitivity of receptors on the nerve cells. Lithium is effective in treating both the manic and depressive phases of manic-depressive disorder.

*Carbamazepine*

Researchers believe that carbamazepine may control mania because of its ability to control *kindling*. In kindling, repeated psychological stresses may produce seizurelike activity in the pathways within the nervous system that transmit the impulses that produce manic behavior. While lithium can be used to treat both the manic and the depressive phases of bipolar illness, carbamazepine is used only to treat mania. In patients with manic-depressive illness, other treatments may be needed when the person becomes depressed.

## WHO SHOULD TAKE THESE DRUGS?

### Lithium

This is the drug of first choice for most people who are experiencing a manic episode. Manic behavior usually diminishes after seven to ten days of lithium treatment. As we have previously mentioned, lithium will usually prevent both manic and depressive episodes in patients with bipolar illness. Patients with milder forms of mania, such as cyclothymia, may also benefit from lithium.

Lithium is sometimes used in combination with carbamazepine. It is also sometimes used in combination with heterocyclic antidepressants to treat patients who do not respond to antidepressants alone. Lithium is sometimes given to patients following electroconvulsive therapy to keep them from again becoming depressed.

### Carbamazepine

Carbamazepine is usually the drug of second choice for mania. It is usually used to treat manic-depressive disease in patients who have not responded to lithium. In some such cases, a person may take both carbamazepine and lithium. It is also used with patients who experience unpleasant side effects when taking lithium. Carbamazepine can help control manic episodes. It can also be taken to prevent future episodes. This drug is best for individuals who experience frequent episodes of mania. Such episodes, which psychiatrists call *rapid cycling*, frequently respond more favorably to carbamazepine than to lithium.

## TESTS REQUIRED PRIOR TO TAKING LITHIUM

For a list of lab tests required for those taking lithium, see Table 1, p. 140.

### Medical History

• If you have a medical record from another doctor or hospital, your present doctor should obtain it and read it.
• Have any of your blood relatives (i.e., parents, brothers, sisters, grandparents, aunts, uncles) had kidney disease?
• Have any of your blood relatives had thyroid disease?
• Have you ever had any kind of heart disease?

*Physical Examination*

• Your physician should examine your heart, your kidneys, and the thyroid gland in your neck.

*Urine Tests*

- complete urinalysis
- twenty-four-hour urine volume
- urine specific gravity (You should drink no fluids for twelve hours before this test.)
- creatinine clearance

*Blood Tests*

- blood urea nitrogen (BUN)
- blood creatinine
- serum electrolytes
- $T_3$ radioactive iodine uptake (T3RIA)
- $T_4$ radioactive iodine uptake (T4RIA)
- thyroid stimulating hormone (TSH)
- antithyroid antibody test
- blood calcium level
- fasting blood glucose
- complete blood count (CBC) with differential

*Other Tests*

- electrocardiogram (EKG) (strongly recommended if the person has a history of heart disease or is over forty)
- weight

## TESTS REQUIRED PRIOR TO TAKING CARBAMAZEPINE

For a list of lab tests required for those taking carbamazepine, see Table 2, p. 141.

*Medical History*

• If you have a medical record from another doctor or hospital, your present doctor should obtain it and read it.

• Have you ever had a low red blood cell count, low white blood cell count, or any bleeding problems?

• Have you ever had any form of liver disease?

*Physical Examination*
- Your physician should perform a complete physical with special emphasis on the examination of the liver and on any signs of bleeding.

*Blood Tests*
- complete blood count (CBC) with platelet count
- serum glutamic oxalacetic transaminase (SGOT)
- serum glutamic pyruvic transaminase (SGPT)
- lactic dehydrogenase (LDH)
- alkaline phosphatase

## How Can These Drugs Be Misused?

Neither lithium nor carbamazepine is commonly abused. In contrast to the benzodiazepines that are used to treat anxiety, neither lithium nor carbamazepine is addictive. And neither lithium nor carbamazepine produces cross-tolerance when combined with other drugs, such as alcohol or benzodiazepines.

## Precautions to Observe While Taking These Drugs

*Lithium*
- Do not allow yourself to become dehydrated.
- Let your primary care physician know that you are taking lithium, since there are some drugs that you should not take with lithium.
- If you miss a dose, don't take extra pills the next time.

*Carbamazepine*
- Call your doctor if you suddenly develop a high fever or bleeding problems.

## Periodic Laboratory Evaluations Required While Taking These Drugs

*Lithium Blood Levels*

It is vitally important that persons taking lithium measure the levels of these drugs in their blood at regular intervals. When you first begin taking lithium, your doctor will check your blood lithium level twice a week until you reach the desired therapeutic level. You will then have this test once a month for the first six months you are taking the drug. Once you have maintained a therapeutic blood level for six months, the test is usually repeated every three months for as long as you take the drug.

Therapeutic lithium blood levels may range from 0.5 to 1.5 milliliters equivalents per liter (mEq/liter). After six months, blood levels may range between 0.5 and 0.8 mEq/liter.

## Carbamazepine Blood Levels

Those taking carbamazepine should be sure that their carbamazepine blood levels are measured every week until a therapeutic level, usually approximately 4 to 12 micrograms per milliliter, is obtained. Serum blood levels should then be monitored every month for the first three months and every three months thereafter.

TABLE I

**Laboratory Tests Required for Those Taking Lithium**

| TESTS | FREQUENCY |
|---|---|
| *Urine* | |
| creatinine clearance | every six months |
| twenty four-hour urine volume | only if indicated |
| urine specific gravity | only if indicated |
| *Blood* | |
| TSH | every six months |
| calcium | after one month, then at yearly intervals |
| fasting blood glucose | yearly |
| CBC with differential | yearly |
| *Other* | |
| EKG | one month after stable lithium level, then yearly |
| weight | every three months |

TABLE 2

**Laboratory Tests Required for Those Taking Carbamazepine**

| BLOOD TESTS | FREQUENCY |
|---|---|
| complete blood count (CBC) with platelet count | every two weeks for the first two months, then every three months |
| SGOT | every month for the first two months, then every three months |
| SGPT | every month for the first two months, then every three months |
| LDH | every month for the first two months, then every three months |
| alkaline phosphatase | every month for the first two months, then every three months |

## POSSIBLE SIDE EFFECTS

Side effects are effects other than the desired therapeutic effects of the drug. In most cases, these are manageable and tolerable and do not require you to discontinue the drug. Side effects that pose such significant risk or discomfort that the drug must be discontinued are called adverse reactions (see below).

### Lithium

The most common side effects of lithium include tremor, weight gain, nausea, diarrhea, and skin rashes. These side effects are quite common and are often mild and tolerable. (If you find them intolerable, discuss a different treatment with your doctor.)

• Effects on the kidneys. About 60 percent of people taking lithium experience frequent urination. This problem can usually be managed by (1) drinking lots of fluids (i.e., ten to twelve glasses of water per day), and (2) asking your doctor to keep the daily lithium dose as low as possible. You may be able to manage this problem by taking a single daily dose of lithium—discuss this with your doctor.

• Effects on the thyroid gland. About 20 percent of people taking lithium may experience a depressed function of the thyroid gland (hypothyroidism). This occurs more frequently in women and in people with certain thyroid abnormalities (e.g., thyroid antibodies). Thyroid function tests are usually obtained both before and after starting lithium treatment. Symptoms of hypothyroidism may include heat and cold intolerance, a coarsening of the hair, lethargy, and muscle weakness. If you do develop hypothyroidism, your physician or psychiatrist should consult with an endocrinologist to decide the best way to deal with the problem. Possible alternatives include taking thyroid hormone replacement or discontinuing lithium.

• Effects on the parathyroid glands. Fifty percent of those taking lithium experience an increase in both their serum calcium and their parathyroid hormone levels within the first four weeks of starting the drug. Of these, about 10 percent (5 percent of all patients on lithium) develop symptoms of hyperparathyroidism. These symptoms may include mood changes, anxiety, delirium, aggressiveness, sleep disturbances, apathy, or confusion. If there is only a mild elevation of calcium, symptoms will be nonexistent or mild and lithium can usually be continued. If your serum calcium remains above normal limits and your symptoms are severe, you should stop taking the drug.

• Effects on the nervous system. About half of all patients taking lithium experience a resting tremor—a tremor when not moving the hand. After you have been taking lithium for several weeks, the tremor will frequently become less noticeable. If it does not, the beta-adrenergic blocking drug propranolol (Inderal) can be used to treat it. Some people who take lithium experience memory and concentration problems. This side effect is more common in people with neurologic disorders, such as stroke or epilepsy, and may also be more frequent in the elderly. If you become forgetful or confused after starting lithium, notify your psychiatrist, who may wish to prescribe a different type of antimanic medication.

• Effects on the heart. Lithium may cause changes in your electrocardiogram (EKG), but in most cases these changes are completely harmless. Your doctor should take an EKG before you start taking this drug. (This is called a baseline EKG.) This can then be compared with later EKG readings to see whether the drug has caused any changes. If you have severe cardiac disease or develop irregular heartbeats after starting lithium, your psychiatrist should arrange a consultation with a cardiologist.

• Weight gain. People on lithium frequently complain of gaining weight. Since lithium causes patients to produce more urine, they must drink a large amount of liquid to replace the fluids lost. Choosing high-calorie fluids (e.g., soft drinks) will increase weight gain.

• Skin reactions. Five to ten percent of those taking lithium experience a skin rash. Others report hair loss, hair thinning, and a straightening of the hair. Lithium may also produce acne and may make psoriasis worse. If you develop a bothersome skin problem after starting lithium, you should arrange a consultation with a dermatologist.

• Effects on the gastrointestinal system. Many people taking lithium report some nausea and diarrhea. Although these symptoms usually occur with toxic blood levels of lithium, they may sometimes occur even when lithium is within the desired therapeutic range. Such side effects may result from a rapid increase in blood levels rather than from the absolute level itself. Taking smaller doses or using a slow-release formula (e.g., Lithobid or Eskalith CR) may help minimize these side effects. Taking your lithium with meals may also help.

• Effects on the blood cells. Lithium sometimes produces an increase in the number of white blood cells. This change is usually benign and carries no risk. In fact, lithium is sometimes used to raise white blood counts in those with low white counts. A baseline white blood cell count should be recorded and this test should be repeated at regular intervals so that an infection unrelated to lithium treatment may be more readily recognized.

## Carbamazepine

The most serious toxic side effect of carbamazepine treatment is aplastic anemia, a very rare condition, occurring less than once in 50,000 cases, in which the bone marrow stops making all three major types of blood cells: red blood cells, white blood cells, and platelets. Aplastic anemia can be fatal. Thus it is important for your psychiatrist or physician to check closely for any sign of decreased blood cell production, fever, or abnormal bleeding.

About 10 percent of people taking carbamazepine have depressed white blood cell counts. Less than 5 percent experience some decrease in the blood's clotting ability (as measured by the platelet count) or a mild anemia (lowering of the red blood cell count).

You should obtain red and white blood cell counts and a platelet count before starting this drug. These tests should be repeated every two weeks during the first two months you take carbamazepine. If any of these tests shows moderate decreases during the initial phases of carbamazepine treatment, more frequent blood counts will be obtained. If any of these tests shows a dramatic drop, it may be necessary to discontinue the drug. Ask your doctor about your test results.

If you develop a fever, infection, or weakness, or notice signs of bleeding under the skin, in your nailbeds, or in the whites of your eyes while you are taking carbamazepine, you should stop the drug and contact your physician immediately.

Carbamazepine may also affect your liver, producing an allergic-type response within several weeks of beginning treatment. This is why various liver function tests (SGOT, SGPT, LDH) are conducted.

Carbamazepine can also produce blurred vision, constipation, and dry mouth. Other side effects include dizziness, drowsiness, and difficulty waking. All these symptoms are the result of carbamazepine's effects on the central nervous system. They are much more prevalent during the early phases of treatment. As treatment progresses, the intensity or frequency of these side effects usually diminishes.

## POSSIBLE ADVERSE REACTIONS

Adverse reactions are side effects that pose such significant risks or discomfort that the drug must be discontinued.

### Lithium

Adverse reactions to lithium are most common in patients with high lithium blood levels, that is, in excess of 1.5 mEq/liter. Ordinary therapeutic levels in the range of 0.5 to 1.5 mEq/liter rarely produce lithium toxicity. When lithium blood levels reach between 1.5 and 2.0 mEq/liter, a person may experience vomiting, abdominal pain, dizziness, slurred speech, difficulty walking, lethargy, and muscle weakness. At levels between 2.0 and 2.5 mEq/liter, nausea and vomiting become more intense. The person may experience convulsions, delirium, stupor, coma, and blurred vision. If lithium blood levels exceed 2.5 mEq/liter, the patient may experience convulsions, renal failure, and death. Thus, it is very important to have your blood lithium levels tested regularly. This is especially important during exercise in hot weather. You should avoid dehydration and should be sure to drink plenty of fluids while taking lithium.

Lithium can also damage the kidneys. Regular blood and urine tests can help detect the early signs of kidney damage.

Lithium may also affect the thyroid and parathyroid glands. Regular thyroid function tests (for the thyroid) and blood calcium levels (for the parathyroid) can help detect any signs of problems in these vital organs.

Lithium should be used with special caution in people who have had previous heart attacks, irregularities of the heartbeat, or other cardiovascular problems.

### Carbamazepine

The most serious adverse reaction to the use of carbamazepine is aplastic anemia. This condition is relatively rare, and frequent blood counts are necessary to detect it. Also, bleeding may occasionally occur because of a lowered platelet count. People taking carbamazepine may be at higher risk for infection because of the lower white blood cell count. The most serious side effect on the liver is a *hypersensitivity hepatitis*—in which the liver's ability to cleanse the blood of waste products is reduced. If hypersensitivity hepatitis occurs, carbamazepine must be stopped.

## POSSIBLE DRUG INTERACTIONS

### Lithium

Lithium is excreted unchanged by the kidneys into the urine. Consequently, drugs that may alter the kidney's ability to remove lithium from the blood will affect lithium blood levels. If the serum plasma levels of lithium are increased, a person may experience some of the side effects described earlier: in particular, gastrointestinal complaints (abdominal cramps, nausea), and/or tremors.

- Diuretics, e.g., chlorothiazide (Maxzide), Diupres, Hydropres, Diuril. Hydrochlorothiazide diuretics, frequently used to treat high blood pressure, decrease the kidney's ability to remove lithium from the bloodstream. This results in *increased* blood lithium levels. Thus patients taking these drugs will generally require *lower* doses of lithium.
- Tetracycline, e.g., Sumycin, Achromycin. This antibiotic, frequently used to treat infections and acne, may *increase* lithium levels. Persons taking both lithium and tetracycline will thus generally need *lower* doses of lithium.
- Theophylline, e.g., Bronkaid, Constant-T, Marax, Mudrane, Primatene, Quibron, Respbid, Slo-phyllin, Sustaire, Theo-dur, Theospan SR. Theophylline and theophylline-containing compounds *decrease* serum lithium levels. Thus, persons taking these drugs with lithium may require *higher* doses of lithium.
- Nonsteroidal anti-inflammatory drugs, e.g., indomethacin (Indocin), ibuprofen (Advil, Midol, Motrin, Nuprin). These agents may increase lithium levels. Persons taking these drugs may require *lower* lithium doses.
- Antipsychotic medications. Antipsychotic agents are frequently used in conjunction with lithium and/or carbamazepine during the early phase of treatment of mania. Even though there may be some increased risk of toxicity (and even, in rare cases, death), the benefit of treating a manic episode that is unresponsive to lithium or carbamazepine alone may be considerable, and must be balanced against the risk of possible adverse side effects. See Chapter 7 for more information.

### Carbamazepine

While drug interactions involving lithium are quite common, interactions with carbamazepine are much less frequent:

• Cimetidine (Tagamet), a medication used to treat ulcers, may increase blood carbamazepine levels by decreasing the rate at which the liver breaks down the drug.

• Erythromycin, an antibiotic, can increase plasma carbamazepine levels.

• Isoniazid (INH), a drug used to treat tuberculosis, can increase plasma carbamazepine levels.

• Darvon, a pain medication, can increase plasma carbamazepine levels.

• Barbiturates, e.g., phenobarbital, amobarbital (Amytal), pentobarbital (Nembutal), secobarbital (Seconal), may *decrease* blood carbamazepine levels by speeding up its breakdown in the liver. Thus, patients who are taking phenobarbital may require higher doses of carbamazepine.

## How These Drugs Make You Feel

### Lithium

Lithium can even out the intense ups and downs a manic or manic depressive may experience when not taking medication. When lithium is taken for the treatment of mania, irritability, euphoria, increased motor activity, restlessness, agitation, racing thoughts, and other related symptoms usually diminish. These and other symptoms associated with the manic *high* are usually markedly reduced by lithium. The patient should begin to feel reasonably normal after several weeks of treatment.

At the same time, the patient may experience such side effects as dry mouth, a frequent need to urinate, a slight tremor of the hand, a bloating sensation, or stomach cramps. These side effects usually peak about one to two hours after taking lithium. Some people find that by taking a single bedtime dose of lithium, unpleasant side effects can be kept to a minimum—and they occur while the person is asleep.

### Carbamazepine

Patients taking carbamazepine may experience most frequently blurred vision, constipation, or dry mouth. Others may occasionally feel drowsy during the day or get dizzy, especially when they suddenly get up from sitting or lying down. Usually these symptoms decrease the longer the patient is on the treatment.

## How to Take These Medications

Lithium is usually begun at a daily dose of 600 to 900 milligrams (mg). The medication is taken in 300 mg tablets two or three times a day with meals to reduce such gastrointestinal side effects as nausea, diarrhea, and stomach cramps. After four to five days, and depending upon blood levels, lithium is increased slowly in 300 mg increments every four to five days until therapeutic blood levels (0.5 to 1.5 mEq/liter) are achieved and the patient shows reduced euphoria and irritability, less motor hyperactivity, and slowed thoughts. For the treatment of acute manic symptoms, blood levels of 1 to 1.5 mEq/liter are desirable. During maintenance treatment, levels of 0.5 to 1.0 mEq/liter are usually adequate to control symptoms.

Some patients with more severe manic-depressive illness in which symptoms reappear if lithium blood levels drop slightly (if they forget to take their medication) may require relatively sustained and high levels of lithium without a wide variation in blood levels. They should use lithium in time-release capsules. In contrast to regular lithium tablets, which come in 300 mg doses, the sustained-release tablets come in both 300 mg and 450 mg strengths.

Time-release capsules usually produce fewer gastrointestinal side effects. Since they are usually taken twice a day instead of three or four times a day, lithium blood levels are more consistent and you are less likely to forget to take your medication.

## Carbamazepine

Carbamazepine is usually begun at a daily dose of 400 mg: 200 mg twice a day. The dose is usually increased by 200 mg every five to seven days until therapeutic levels are obtained (usually between 4 and 12 mEq/ml). Blood levels are usually obtained weekly. A complete blood count, including a platelet count, should be obtained every two weeks for the first two months of treatment. Liver function tests (SGOT, SGPT, LDH, alkaline phosphotase) should be obtained once a month for the first two months of treatment.

The most common side effects of carbamazepine are blurred vision, constipation, and dry mouth. Some patients also complain of dizziness, drowsiness, and loss of coordination. These symptoms usually occur during the early phases of treatment and diminish as treatment continues. In contrast to lithium, weight gain does not appear to be a problem.

## OTHER DRUGS USED TO TREAT MANIA

For people who do not respond to either lithium carbonate or carbamazepine alone, some clinicians may use a combination of the two. This combination can be an effective one for many patients. The side effects associated with these combinations are similar to those experienced if each medication were taken alone. As you may expect, you need to be especially careful to follow your doctor's treatment recommendations.

Several other drugs are being used to treat mania on an experimental basis:

• The antiseizure medication valproic acid (Depakene). Dose: 30 to 60 mg per kg of body weight per day with plasma levels of approximately 50 to 100 micrograms per ml.

• The benzodiazepine anticonvulsant clonazepam (Klonopin). The recommended dose has ranged dramatically from 1.5 to 20 mg per day. Since Klonopin can be addictive, it should not be taken by people who have drug-abuse or drug-dependence problems. Like many addictive drugs, clonazepam may produce tolerance and withdrawal symptoms.

• The high blood pressure drug clonidine (Catapres) has also been used to treat mania.

• The heart drug propranolol (Inderal) has been used to treat acute manic episodes. Dosages as high as 3 g a day have been used.

• Verapamil (Isoptin, Calan), a drug used in the treatment of irregular heartbeats and high blood pressure, has also been found effective in the treatment of mania.

# Case Studies

### JOHN WRIGHT: SUCCESSFUL USE OF ANTIMANIC MEDICATION

This twenty-four-year-old medical student was brought to the emergency room by his roommate, who reported that John had become increasingly irritable, talkative, and distracted over the past month. Over the previous week, these symptoms became so intense that John found himself completely unable to prepare for an important anatomy exam. Instead of studying, he had been spending his time buying clothes he couldn't afford—and charging them. He ran up huge bills he was incapable of paying.

John had stopped studying and had stopped going to class. He had apparently stopped sleeping, and spent the nights pacing around the apartment. When asked about his strange behavior, he explained that he was busy designing a new artificial heart and did not want to go to class because he was afraid someone would read his thoughts and steal his idea. He repeatedly referred to himself as an outstanding surgeon. This struck his roommate as bizarre, since John was a first-year medical student and had had no prior engineering or surgical experience.

John was unable to sit still during the psychiatric interview. He paced up and down the room, interrupted the psychiatrist, and made irrelevant comments about the psychiatrist's clothes, the stock market, baseball scores, and other unrelated matters. When the psychiatrist asked John to show him his plans for his new artificial heart, he took out a bundle of hastily scribbled notes that, as far as the psychiatrist could tell, made no sense at all.

John's suit, shirt, and tie were dirty and wrinkled. He had neither shaved nor combed his hair for several days. He explained that he expected to win the Nobel Prize and had been sleeping in his clothes so that he would be appropriately dressed when the press arrived.

John had never had a manic episode before. However, he had been severely depressed for a few weeks during his junior year in college. At that time he had complained of chronic fatigue and lethargy, and had experienced a fifteen-pound weight loss. A university physician had prescribed an antidepressant. The medication produced a marked improvement in John's mood and he had not felt depressed since.

A month before coming to the emergency room, John had begun to feel that medical school was "getting to him." He began taking diet pills to increase his energy and to lose weight. After he began taking the pills, his thoughts began to race and he felt little need for sleep. He grew irritable and began to distance himself from his friends.

John's grandfather had required frequent hospitalizations for what John described as *crazy behavior*: "He would go around preaching to people in the middle of the night about the end of the world and the need to repent." John's grandfather eventually committed suicide.

John was hospitalized on the inpatient psychiatry service. He received two 5 mg tablets of haloperidol (Haldol) per day for the first week. His psychiatrist took a careful history and performed a comprehensive physical examination. John also received a battery of laboratory tests, including an electrocardiogram (EKG).

John was also treated with lithium carbonate. For the first few days, he took a 300 mg pill three times per day. At first he experienced some mild stomach cramps—a side effect—but these diminished once he began taking his medication with meals.

Over the following two weeks, John gradually increased his dose until he was taking a total of 1,500 mg of lithium per day: three 300 mg tablets at bedtime and two at breakfast. With this dose, he experienced three mild side effects from the medication: a slight tremor of his hands, an increased frequency in urination, and a slight weight gain.

Two months after his visit to the emergency room, John's manic symptoms were well under control and he was able to return to medical school. During his weekly follow-up visits with his psychiatrist, John reported that when he forgot to take his lithium he would again experience increased irritability and agitation and a decreased need for sleep. But as long as he took his medicine regularly, he maintained a normal, nonmanic mood.

After taking lithium for several months, John found that he could maintain his normal mood on a lower lithium dose, 900 mg a day, taken at bedtime.

John successfully completed medical school and is now a dermatologist living in southern California. He continues to take lithium, is happily married, and has experienced no further episodes of mania or depression.

John's case illustrates the positive outcome often achieved with lithium therapy. The drug effectively combats the irritable mood and confusing thoughts associated with bipolar disorder. By taking this medication, John was able to achieve his professional goal of becoming a physician and to establish a normal personal life. And because he took most of his medication at night, John experienced only minimal side effects from the drug.

John's case also illustrates several other important points about mania:

• Like John, many people with bipolar illness have a blood relative with a similar condition.

• Many first-time manic patients have experienced a prior depressive episode.

• Certain medications, such as the stimulant diet pills John took, may precipitate a manic episode in vulnerable individuals.

• John's case also illustrates that medication alone is not the whole answer. John also saw a psychiatrist once a week for several months. These sessions helped John gain important insights into his symptoms and helped him understand why he needed to take lithium.

## EMILY MANNERS: UNSUCCESSFUL USE OF ANTIMANIC DRUGS

This forty-nine-year-old divorced, unemployed woman was brought to the emergency room by police after she had physically attacked several male patrons in a neighborhood bar. When the police arrested her, they noted that she appeared intoxicated. She shouted rather than spoke. Her words seemed to rush out at a rapid rate. It was almost impossible to interrupt her. When the police were able to talk with her, they noted that she was easily distracted by passing cars or people passing on the sidewalk. She could not respond to simple questions, and, in the words of the officer at the scene, "her thinking was not quite right."

Emily had been hospitalized six months earlier for similar disruptive behavior. Her medical record revealed six hospital admissions over the last ten years for treatment of bipolar illness and alcohol abuse. She would take lithium for a few days or weeks and would then discontinue the drug. After stopping her medication, she would begin drinking heavily—becoming manic and abusive—and would once again end up in the hospital.

Emily was first hospitalized at age twenty-seven with severe symptoms of mania. Her thoughts would race, her need for sleep was greatly decreased, and she became increasingly irritable and argumentative. She began going to bars after work, drinking, and going to bed with men she had picked up in these bars.

When her symptoms of mania began, Emily was a secretary at a law firm. Her fellow secretaries became increasingly resentful of her disruptive behavior. She was subsequently fired from her job after a screaming episode with her boss. Her husband eventually divorced her because of her promiscuous behavior.

As time went on, Emily's manic episodes became more and more frequent. At first, she would experience a manic episode about every two to three years. At the time of her latest hospital admission, she was experiencing episodes every nine to twelve months. Emily repeatedly refused to take her medication for more than a month at a time, saying, "It slows me down too much."

Between her manic episodes, Emily has experienced periods of depression so severe that she has been unable to get out of bed or dress for days at a time. During these periods, she will typically lose weight and lie in bed feeling that life is not worth living. As she loses weight, her sex drive disappears. These periods usually come in the fall, and she can almost anticipate that they will last about three to four months. She describes these periods as recurrent "low" periods and explains that she has become accustomed to them.

Emily currently lives alone in a small, shabby apartment, supported by her monthly welfare check. She is unable to hold a job. She has no friends, and spends her days aimlessly wandering the streets or watching TV in her apartment. She becomes sexually hyperactive and drinks heavily during her manic episodes—and remains in bed when she is feeling depressed. She is currently two months behind in her rent, and has been threatened with eviction.

Emily's alcoholism makes her bipolar disorder even more difficult to manage. During those times when she is neither depressed nor manic, her alcohol abuse impairs her thinking and makes goal-directed behavior almost impossible. This unfortunate combination has thus led to her gradually deteriorating social and economic situation.

Emily has refused individual psychotherapy, group psychotherapy, Alcoholics Anonymous, and treatment at both an alcoholism program and medication clinic. She has never gained the insight necessary to recognize that she has two severe psychiatric illnesses—bipolar illness and alcoholism—both of which would benefit from treatment. Her continuing resistance to treatment makes her long-term prognosis quite bleak.

# Lithium Carbonate

Brand names: Eskalith, Lithane, Lithotabs, Eskalith CR (sustained release), Lithobid (sustained release), Cibalith-S (liquid form)

Common street name: lithium

Drug family: antimanic agents, mood stabilizers

Availability: by prescription only

Tablets: Available in 300 mg and 450 mg tablets (only Eskalith CR is available in a 450 mg tablet)

Capsules: Available in 150, 300, 450, and 600 mg capsules (Eskalith)

Liquid: Cibalith-S is available in a dose of 8 millequivalents (mEq) per 5 ml of liquid in a 450 ml bottle. One teaspoon, 8 mEq, is equivalent to approximately 300 mg of the carbonate preparation.

Other routes of administration: This drug is given only by mouth.

## Is This Drug Available in Generic Form?

Yes. The generic name of this drug is lithium carbonate. The carbonate capsules are available from Roxane Pharmaceutical Company.

## How to Store and Take This Drug

Because of the toxic side effects associated with high dosages, this drug should be stored in a dry, tightly closed, tamperproof container. It should be kept away from children. Most clinicians recommend that you begin with a low, divided dose of lithium carbonate at either 300 mg twice a day or 300 mg three times a day. For treatment of acute mania, this dose is increased up or down to achieve a serum blood level of approximately 1 to 1.5 mEq/liter. In older patients or in those with kidney impairment, a lower dose should be used. Lithium usually takes approximately seven to ten days before therapeutic benefits are achieved. For acute mania, an antipsychotic agent is usually also prescribed for the first week to ten days.

Once the acute manic episode has been treated, lithium doses are reduced to achieve serum blood levels of approximately 0.5 to 1.0 mEq/liter. Additionally, the whole dose may be taken at night to decrease the likelihood of gastrointestinal and other side effects. Taking several doses throughout the day with meals also has been reported to decrease gastric side effects. People will usually remember to take their medication once or twice a day.

## DO NOT TAKE THIS DRUG IF:

- You have preexisting kidney disease or are on kidney dialysis.
- You have sick sinus syndrome of your heart.
- You are pregnant or attempting to get pregnant.
- You are breast-feeding.

## INFORM YOUR PHYSICIAN BEFORE TAKING THIS DRUG IF:

- You are taking thiazide diuretics for hypertension.
- You have a history of hyperthyroidism or are taking thyroid medication.
- You have a family history of kidney disease.
- You have a family history of thyroid disease.
- You have a history of cardiac disease (previous heart attack, arrhythmias, etc.).

## POSSIBLE SIDE EFFECTS OF ANTIMANIC DRUGS

These are the expected and tolerable effects that can occur in addition to the desired therapeutic effects:

- resting tremor of the hands
- weight gain
- rash (red, flat, broad, diffuse rash that frequently will appear on chest or back but could appear anywhere)
- increased urination
- nausea immediately after taking medication (decreased by taking medication immediately after meals)
- mild diarrhea

## POSSIBLE ADVERSE REACTIONS

These are unusual, potentially hazardous reactions. Stop taking the drug and notify your physician if these develop:

- development of a goiter or mass in the neck
- confusion
- sleep disturbances
- difficulty in walking
- dizziness
- slurred speech
- extreme tiredness or excitement
- muscle weakness

## WARNINGS AND CAUTIONS

- If you lose a significant amount of fluids through exercise or heat, be sure that you drink plenty of liquids.
- When operating a vehicle or machinery, be careful while taking this medication; it may impair your alertness.

## INTERACTIONS WITH FOODS AND BEVERAGES

- rarely a problem with lithium

## INTERACTION WITH OTHER DRUGS

See Individual Drug Listings.

## HOW MUCH WILL IT COST?

Lithium is a simple saltlike compound, and the usual price is quite inexpensive (less than five cents per tablet).

## HOW TO AVOID ADDICTION

- Lithium is not associated with tolerance, dependence, or abuse.

## EFFECTS OF OVERDOSE

See Individual Drug Listings.

## LABORATORY EXAMINATIONS REQUIRED WHILE TAKING THIS DRUG

- thyroid function tests
- blood urea nitrogen (BUN)
- serum creatinine
- urine creatinine clearance
- serum calcium
- fasting blood glucose
- serum white blood cell count
- EKG
- monitor weight

# Carbamazepine (Tegretol)

Brand name: Tegretol.
Common street names: None.
Drug family: Antiseizure medications.
Availability: By prescription only.
Tablets: Available in 200 mg tablets or 100 mg chewable tablets. Tegretol is also available in 100 mg per 5 cc suspension.
Other routes of administration: None.

## IS THIS DRUG AVAILABLE IN GENERIC FORM?

Yes. The generic name of this drug is carbamazepine. Tegretol is the trade name for the carbamazepine tablets. The suspension, in generic form, is manufactured by CIBA-Geigy Pharmaceutical Company. Carbamazepine is currently available under its generic name from three other companies: Lederle, Martec, and Warner Chilcott.

## HOW TO STORE AND TAKE THIS DRUG

Keep it in a tightly closed, tamper-resistant container. Carbamazepine should be begun in a dosage of approximately 200 mg twice a day (for a healthy adult male, two 100 mg tablets at twelve-hour intervals during the day). The dose should be gradually increased by approximately 200 mg a day every five to seven days until a serum plasma level of from 4 to 12 micrograms per milliliter is obtained. If the dose is increased too rapidly, you may experience dizziness, difficulty walking, and other adverse effects. This drug is not approved by the FDA for the treatment of mania. However, its use in treating mania represents a potentially beneficial application. Many psychiatrists use carbamazepine to treat patients who do not respond to lithium. If you have questions concerning the use of this drug, you should consult your physician. If you have difficulty swallowing the medication, you can take the chewable form.

## Do Not Take This Drug If:

- You have a history of liver disease.
- You have experienced an allergic, aplastic anemia (i.e., failure of your bone marrow to produce essential blood components) due to medication.
- You have a history of a low white count or low platelet count.
- You had a previous hypersensitivity reaction to this medication.
- You have had bone marrow depression or known sensitivity to any of the heterocyclic antidepressants.
- You are taking monoamine oxidase inhibitors.
- You have a history of narrow-angle glaucoma.
- You are breast-feeding.
- You are pregnant or planning a pregnancy.
- The patient is less than six years of age.

## Inform Your Physician Before Taking This Drug If:

- You have ever had an allergic reaction to any drug.
- You have narrow-angle glaucoma.
- You have had a sensitivity reaction (rash, difficulty breathing, etc.) to any heterocyclic compounds.
- You stopped taking monoamine oxidase inhibitors within the last fourteen days.
- You have had an adverse hematologic reaction to any drug.
- You have had severe dermatologic reactions to medications in the past.

## Possible Side Effects

These are expected and tolerable effects that can occur in addition to the desired therapeutic effects:

- drowsiness
- nausea
- vomiting
- problems walking (ataxia)
- dizziness

## WARNINGS AND CAUTIONS

You should be aware of early signs or symptoms of a potential bleeding problem or low white count: fever, sore throat, easy bruising, ulcers in the mouth, or bleeding under the fingernails.

## INTERACTIONS WITH FOODS AND BEVERAGES

Because the most common side effects are sedation and drowsiness, care should be taken in using alcoholic beverages along with carbamazepine.

## INTERACTIONS WITH OTHER DRUGS

See Individual Drug Listings.

## HOW MUCH WILL IT COST?

The brand name form costs approximately thirty cents per 200 mg pill. The generic form is about half that price.

## HOW TO AVOID ADDICTION

There is no evidence of abuse associated with carbamazepine, nor is there evidence of psychological or physical dependence.

## EFFECTS OF OVERDOSE

See Individual Drug Listings.

## LABORATORY EXAMINATIONS REQUIRED WHILE TAKING THIS DRUG

- liver function tests
- white blood cell count
- complete blood counts
- platelet counts

# Chapter 7

# Antipsychotic Drugs

THE word *psychotic* is popularly used as a synonym for *crazy, insane,* or *bizarre*. Mental health professionals use this term in a more technical sense—to indicate that a given individual has difficulty telling the difference between the unreal and the real. Psychiatrists call the process of distinguishing the real from the unreal *reality testing*. A person whose reality testing is impaired is said to be in a *psychotic state*. Although a psychotic state, or psychosis, designates a mental illness, it does not in any way specify the underlying cause or illness. Psychosis is frequently seen in people with a schizophrenia, but a psychotic state can also be a part of many other mental and physical illnesses, e.g., major depression, manic depression, infections, drug side effects, reactions to toxic effects of substances, brain tumors, and many more.

A person's ability to perform adequate reality testing can be impaired by hallucinations, delusions, or thought disorders. These states are important indications of impaired reality testing, and therefore suggest a psychosis that may require psychiatric evaluation and care.

# Hallucinations

Hallucinations are sensations that a person experiences as real, even though they are not perceived by others and cannot be confirmed by any objective standard. Hallucinations can involve any of the five senses: seeing (visual hallucinations), hearing (auditory hallucinations), tasting (gustatory hallucinations), smelling (olfactory hallucinations), and feeling (tactile hallucinations).

### Mary Ann Crowder: Auditory Hallucinations

Mary Ann, a depressed young woman, came into the emergency room with a long cut on her left arm. The emergency room doctor asked what had happened.

"I've been hearing these voices for several days," she explained. "They told me that I was evil. I was no good. This morning, when I was washing the dishes after breakfast, they told me to stab myself. So I did."

No other family members had heard the voices, even though two of them had been standing next to Mary Ann when she heard them. Her psychiatrist concluded that Mary Ann had been experiencing auditory hallucinations.

### Florence Brown: Visual and Tactile Hallucinations

Florence Brown, a frail woman of eighty-three, was admitted to the hospital with pneumonia and back pain. While in the hospital, she received large doses of meperidine, a powerful pain medication. After taking this drug for several days, Florence became extremely confused. She neither recognized her nurses nor knew where she was. She also became agitated. Florence's doctor asked a psychiatrist to evaluate her.

When the psychiatrist came to see her, Florence took his hand and began talking in a rapid, agitated voice: "Oh, Doctor, can't you please do something about these terrible people?" When asked to explain, she continued, "Every night I see men out of the corner of my eye. They come out of the wall into my room. They float down from the ceiling and come up through the floor. They hit my feet with sticks. I can feel the electricity going up my legs."

No one had been seen entering her room. No one had been hitting her. Florence was experiencing both visual hallucinations (seeing the men) and tactile hallucinations (feeling electricity). Her hallucinations turned out to be side effects of her pain medication.

### Juan Ramirez: Gustatory and Olfactory Hallucinations

A twenty-six-year-old construction worker was brought to the hospital emergency room by his concerned family after he had experienced what they described as an epileptic fit. Juan had had severe headaches for the previous ten days. During this time, he told his family that he smelled burning rubber and tasted raw fish. These hallucinations turned out to be the result of a benign brain tumor, which caused a type of seizure called temporal lobe epilepsy or partial complex seizures. The smell of burning rubber was an olfactory hallucination and the taste of raw fish was a gustatory hallucination.

## Delusions

A delusion is a fixed idea that a person continues to believe in spite of all proof that the idea is false. Delusions are much more common than hallucinations. Indeed, a number of things that might fit this definition—like the belief in a lucky charm, a lucky number, a good luck necktie—are quite common indeed but are not considered delusions. An unverified belief is considered a delusion only if the belief in question is not shared by members of the individual's culture. For instance, many people believe that cold air causes disease; many people in Caribbean countries believe in zombies; and the adherents of virtually every religion believe in certain truths that cannot be verified by objective testing. Because such ideas are widely shared in the person's culture, they are not considered delusions.

A belief is considered a delusion only if it is objectively untrue, is not widely accepted by a person's culture, and if a person continues to hold it in spite of all evidence to the contrary.

Other beliefs can suggest the presence of a mental disorder. Most psychiatrists would probably conclude that a woman who believes that flying saucers are sending her special messages, a depressed woman who believes that maggots are eating her intestines, or an older woman who is convinced that her nurses can read her thoughts are all suffering from mental disorders. Occasionally, however, it is quite difficult for the psychiatrist to ascertain whether or not a belief is delusional. For example, if an office worker believes that a co-worker dislikes her and is out to sabotage her job, there is a possibility that this perception may be fully or partially true. The psychiatrist will evaluate the *effect* of the belief on the individual's thinking and activities to gauge whether or not this belief is, in fact, a delusion—a symptom of a mental disorder. If, for example, the office worker is preoccupied with her co-worker to the extent that she thinks of nothing else, if she sleeps only two hours per night because of thoughts about how to protect herself, and if she buys a gun for "retaliation," there is a strong likelihood that the belief is delusional. The reaction to the belief is clearly excessive and all-consuming—two hallmarks of responses to delusional thoughts.

Psychiatrists often call upon close family members to help determine whether or not an unusual belief is a delusion. For example, if deeply religious family members are greatly concerned about their sister's belief that Jesus wants her to leave her husband and small children to work for the poor in India, it is likely that this belief is more than a religious and altruistic conviction.

## Paranoid Delusions

Individuals with paranoid delusions believe that other people (or in some cases other beings or things) are out to harm them. A person with delusions may feel as if he or she is being followed, is being watched, or is being defamed by vicious rumors. Paranoid delusions are the most common delusions of all.

Paranoid delusions are common in people suffering from one of the schizophrenias and may include:

• *Thought broadcasting*. The person is convinced that his or her thoughts are somehow transmitted into the external world so that other people can read his or her mind.

• *Thought insertion*. The person believes that thoughts—not his or her own—are being placed into their brains by some external force.

• *Thought withdrawal*. The person feels that his or her thoughts are being removed by some outside force.

• *Delusions of control*. The person believes that impulses, thoughts, or actions are not his or her own, but are imposed by some external agent or force.

## Miriam Goldenberg: Paranoid Delusion

Miriam, a seventeen-year-old high school student, suddenly began to lock her bedroom door at night. When her parents questioned her about this new behavior, she told them that Ralph, her eighteen-year-old brother, had been sneaking into her room at night to give her cocaine while she slept. When asked if she had actually seen her brother in her room at night, Miriam replied, "No, I just know he's doing it."

Ralph vigorously denied that he had ever entered Miriam's room at night or given her drugs. When Miriam's parents expressed doubts that it would be possible for Ralph to make her inhale drugs while she was asleep, Miriam became agitated and angry. "I don't *have* to see him," she insisted. "I just know that he is doing it to me!" Miriam was experiencing a paranoid delusion, a false belief that someone was harming or persecuting her.

# Thought Disorders

The term *thought disorder* is used to describe a situation in which an individual's thought processes are chaotic and illogical. This disorder involves the form and structure of thinking. It may at first seem that the person is talking normally, but upon listening more closely, it becomes apparent that the person's comments make little or no sense. Often the thoughts do not hang together logically, or they ramble on without making any clear point. This disordered thinking may also be reflected in the person's behavior.

### FREDERICK BARKER: THOUGHT DISORDER

Frederick, a thirty-year-old unemployed house painter, came into the emergency room to have some stitches removed. While removing the stitches, the emergency room physician noted that Frederick's speech was bizarre and incoherent, so he requested a psychiatric consultation.

When the staff psychiatrist asked Frederick why he had come to the emergency room, Frederick replied, "Well, well, I live in Hyde Park. Um, um, do you read the Koran? Don't you think India is a wonderful country?"

He went on like this for several minutes, veering from one disjointed thought to another without ever responding to the psychiatrist's original question.

The psychiatrist called Frederick's parents and learned that Frederick had been diagnosed as having schizophrenia nine years earlier. He had been taking fluphenazine (Prolixin), an antipsychotic drug, but had recently stopped taking his medication. His father told the psychiatrist that whenever Frederick had stopped taking his medication in the past, his behavior had become erratic and his verbal communication had become difficult or impossible to understand.

### FRIENDS AND FAMILY

The delusions, hallucinations, and thought disorders that accompany a psychotic episode are usually extremely baffling and alarming to friends and family members. When the affected person is a young adult who is in the process of separating from his or her parents, it can be especially difficult for the parents and other family members to sort out whether the patient's unaccustomed speech and action represent a healthy reaction to normal adjustment problems, a normal expression of individuality, the use of drugs, or a serious mental health problem (e.g., schizophrenia) that may require hospitalization and treatment. People with delusions and hallucinations hold strongly to their faulty beliefs and misperceptions, and they often become hurt or angry if a family member or friend attempts to refute them. The loved ones often feel caught in a bind—on one hand, they wish to support and comfort (through encouragement and agreement) a person they recognize as ill; but, on the other hand, they do not wish to confuse reality testing even further by lending support to psychotic ideas and perceptions. A common example is the patient with schizophrenia who entreats his parents, "You must help protect me from the Andromeda strain. They are trying to poison me with it. You believe me, don't you? You don't think I'm crazy like the doctors at the hospital do?" One helpful suggestion is to offer support, love, and protection without responding directly to the content of the delusion or hallucination: "You know that your father and I love you deeply. We will do everything possible to keep you safe, healthy, and protected."

## WHAT CAUSES PSYCHOSIS?

A seemingly bewildering variety of factors can produce psychosis: mental illnesses like schizophrenia, mania, or depression; a stroke; a tumor; a head injury; seizures; fever; infections; alcohol; medications (see Sidebar 1); legal or illegal drugs (see Sidebar 2); and a wide variety of toxic substances. In some cases, the signs of psychosis can help in diagnosing a life-threatening medical condition. Psychosis is a symptom—not a disease. Thus physicians approach psychosis as they would any other sign or symptom, by carefully evaluating the individual to determine the underlying cause.

## PSYCHIATRIC ILLNESSES THAT CAN CAUSE PSYCHOSIS

Psychosis is a component of many psychiatric illnesses. Delusions and hallucinations may accompany either mania or severe depressions. When a patient suffers from both depression and psychosis, the risk of suicide is very high indeed. If this combination of symptoms does not respond to treatment by antidepressants alone, it usually may be brought under control

## Sidebar 1: Medications That Can Cause Psychosis

| Generic Name | Reaction |
|---|---|
| albuterol (Proventil; Ventolin) | hallucinations, paranoia |
| amantadine (Symmetrel) | visual hallucinations |
| amphetamines | hallucinations, paranoia |
| dextroamphetamine, methamphetamine | |
| anticonvulsants | tactile, visual, auditory |
| phenytoin (Dilantin), primidone (Mysoline) | (ethosuximide) hallucinations; delirium; confusion |
| antihistamines | hallucinations, delirium |
| bromodiphenhydramine HCL, brompheniramine maleate, chlorpheniramine maleate, diphenhydramine maleate, hydroxyzine HCL, phenyltolaxamine citrate, pyrilamine maleate, triprolidine HCL, diphenyl pyraline HCL, azatadine HCL, tripelennamine HCL, tripelennamine citrate, cyproheptidine HCL, terfenadine promethazine HCL, dexchlorpheniramine maleate, carbinoxamine maleate, methdilazine, pyrilamine tannate, trimeprazine tartrate, clemastine fumarate, hydroxyzine pamoate, chlorpheniramine polistirex | |
| antihypertensives | delirium; visual and auditory hallucinations |
| propranolol, timolol maleate, clonidine hydrochloride, methyl dopa | |
| antidepressants | delirium |
| MAO inhibitors: isocarboxazid, pargyline, phenelzine, tranylcypromine | |
| atropine | delirium; paranoia; auditory and visual hallucinations |

## Sidebar 1: Medications That Can Cause Psychosis (*continued*)

| GENERIC NAME | REACTION |
|---|---|
| baclofen | hallucinations, paranoia |
| barbiturates | visual hallucinations |
| aprobarbital, butalbital, butabarbital sodium, mephobarbital, pentobarbital sodium, thiopental sodium, phenobarbital sodium, secobarbital sodium | |
| benzodiazepines | delirium, confusion, hallucinations |
| flurazepam HCL, lorazepam, chlordiazepoxide HCL, diazepam, alprazolam, triazolam | |
| benztropine mesylate | confusion, visual hallucinations |
| bromocriptine | delusions, visual hallucinations, paranoia |
| cimetidine | hallucinations, paranoia, delirium |
| clonazepam | hallucinations, paranoia |
| clonidine | delirium, hallucinations |
| cocaine | psychosis, paranoia |
| corticosteroids | paranoia, hallucinations |
| prednisone, cortisone | |
| diazepam | hallucinations |
| digitalis | delusions, paranoia, visual hallucinations |
| disulfiram | delirium, paranoia, auditory hallucinations |
| ephedrine | hallucinations, paranoia |
| heterocyclics (tricyclics) | hallucinations, disorientation, delusions, agitation |
| amitriptyline HCL, desipramine HCL, imipramine HCL, maprotiline, nortriptyline HCL, protriptyline HCL, trimipramine | |

## Sidebar 1: Medications That Can Cause Psychosis (*continued*)

| GENERIC NAME | REACTION |
|---|---|
| indomethacin | hallucinations, paranoia |
| levodopa | delirium; paranoia; visual and auditory hallucinations |
| methylphenidate | hallucinations, paranoia |
| procaine penicillin | hallucinations |
| propranolol | hallucinations, paranoia |
| pseudoephedrine | hallucinations, paranoia |

---

**Sidebar 2: Recreational Drugs That Can Cause Psychosis**

1. phencyclidine (PCP, angel dust, mint leaf, sherm)
2. amphetamines (speed)
3. marijuana (pot, reefer, THC)
4. cocaine (coke, blow, crack, snow)
5. hallucinogens such as LSD (acid), mescaline, and psilocybin (mushrooms)
6. alcohol and alcohol withdrawal
7. over-the-counter drugs (sedatives, antihistamines)

---

by combining an antidepressant with an antipsychotic. In some such cases, electroconvulsive therapy may prove even more effective. Psychosis is a fundamental condition of the mental illnesses called the schizophrenias.

## About the Schizophrenias

Schizophrenia is not one single disorder but a whole category of conditions that have some features in common. It is thus more accurate to speak of *the schizophrenias.*

The schizophrenias can affect virtually every aspect of psychological functioning: content and form of thought, perceptions, feelings, willpower, sense of self, interpersonal relationships, and bodily coordination. A patient with a schizophrenia will usually pass back and forth between two stages: an *active phase* during which the person experiences active delusions, hallucinations, loosening of associations, incoherence, and catatonic behavior; and a *residual or treatment phase* in which a patient's delusions or hallucinations recede, moods become more stable, and feelings become less intense.

### DISORDERED AFFECT

In addition to hallucinations, delusions, and thought disorder, a person with a schizophrenia often exhibits inappropriate emotions. This means their emotions are not consistent with what is currently happening, what they are talking about, and what seems to be on their minds. For example, a person may laugh hysterically while describing an event that would be considered by most to be quite disturbing or sad. Patients with a schizophrenia will often seem remote or detached, because they show little evidence of emotion.

## DISORDERS OF EGO BOUNDARY

People with schizophrenia often have great difficulty with their identity or sense of self. They sometimes complain that they do not feel real or do not feel like themselves. They may experience great difficulty in understanding the meaning or purpose of their existence. In extreme cases, a person may have difficulty distinguishing himself or herself from other individuals or even inanimate objects. One aspect of this symptom may be the overidentification with another individual or a cause. People with these disorders are often exploited by charismatic individuals who supply a modicum of identity in return for blind obedience and material resources.

## DISORDERS OF RELATIONSHIPS

Impaired *interpersonal relationships* are the rule rather than the exception among individuals with a schizophrenia. They may become so intensely preoccupied with objects, ideas, even parts of their bodies that they may totally avoid involvement with other people. The end result is often social isolation, withdrawal, and detachment. This is often the most difficult aspect of the disease for family members to cope with.

The relations a person with a schizophrenia has with his or her family members are usually intense and chaotic. Overdependencies, violent interchanges, dramatic shifts from intimacy and trust to distress and distrust are common. The family is thus a victim of the illness just as much as is the individual with a schizophrenia. It is therefore very important that the family be closely involved with the process of assessment and treatment.

## DISTURBED BEHAVIOR

In the active phases of the disease, a person with a schizophrenia may become extremely active and agitated. At other times, he or she will move slowly, if at all. At such times, a person with a schizophrenia may be unaware of or uninvolved in his or her own social environment and may assume odd postures or mannerisms.

Individuals with a schizophrenia may have great difficulty in initiating purposeful or goal-directed activity. They may thus appear extremely unmotivated, and are often accused of being "lazy" or "stupid." This callous attitude makes their symptoms worse and ignores the realities of an illness that affects the brain and its many functions.

## How and When Does Schizophrenia Begin?

The schizophrenias usually appear for the first time during adolescence or early adulthood. This illness only very rarely appears in childhood. Certain types of schizophrenia may also occur, for the first time, during middle age or, under very rare circumstances, after the age of fifty.

## How Common Is Schizophrenia?

About 1 percent of the American population suffers from schizophrenia; it thus comprises one of the most common chronically disabling medical illnesses.

## Is Schizophrenia Hereditary?

The child of a person with a schizophrenia has a 5 to 6 percent risk of developing the disorder. The brother or sister of a schizophrenic person has a 10 percent risk of developing schizophrenia. (A person whose parents and siblings do not have schizophrenia has only a 1 percent chance of having the disorder.) The relatives of people with a schizophrenia should consider seeking advice from a genetic counselor if they plan to have children.

## Do People with a Schizophrenia Have a Chemical Imbalance in the Brain?

Most experts now believe that schizophrenia is biologically based, and therefore involves problems with brain cells and brain chemistry. Recent research suggests that people with schizophrenia may be deficient in an enzyme that breaks down dopamine in the brain. Dopamine is a chemical messenger (or neurotransmitter) that brain cells use to communicate with one another.

There is a good deal of experimental evidence to support this so-called dopamine model of schizophrenia, and most of the drugs that have been found to help control schizophrenia (e.g., the phenothiazines, the butyrophenones, and most other medications described below) work by blocking certain dopamine receptors in the brain.

At present, however, this is still a theory, not a fully accepted explanation. There are still many, many missing pieces to the puzzle of schizophrenia. However, most researchers now believe that as our tools improve and as we gain in experience, we will ultimately identify more precisely what causes schizophrenia, and where in the brain the lesions that result in the symptoms of schizophrenia are located.

## ROBERT CARSON: SUCCESSFUL DRUG TREATMENT FOR SCHIZOPHRENIA

As a child, Robert Carson was talented and active. He showed no evidence of emotional illness until the age of seventeen. He was popular with the other children and was an excellent student from kindergarten through junior high school. His teachers described him as inquisitive, affectionate, and sensitive to the feelings and needs of others.

After entering high school, Robert continued his social and academic success. He won many awards in math and science and was a member of several scholastic honor societies. Although he showed little interest in team sports, he was a passionate and excellent tennis player. He had two close male friends. He dated occasionally but had no regular girlfriend.

Robert graduated at the top of his high school class, did very well on his college entrance exams, and was offered a full scholarship to the University of Wisconsin. During his first semester as a college freshman, he did well, although he did not get along well with Dan, his dormitory roommate.

During the second semester of his freshman year, Robert's thinking and behavior began to change. Although he had signed up to play on the college tennis team, he stopped attending practice after several sessions. He gradually withdrew from all the friendships he had made. He made a point of avoiding all women—students and teachers alike.

For the first time in his life, Robert lost interest in school. He began to skip classes. He became more and more isolated, and spent most of his time in his room. He ignored Dan completely. He also stopped cleaning his room, changing his clothes, bathing, and even stopped washing his hands. He would stay up most of the night, talking and laughing quietly to himself and listening to the same music tape over and over.

One day at 4:00 A.M., Robert shook Dan awake.

"I've put the whole scheme together," he said. "I finally know how they are doing it."

"Doing what?" asked Dan, who was surprised that Robert was speaking to him after six weeks of complete silence.

"They're using microwave technology to monitor our thoughts," Robert insisted. "They're controlling our thoughts, too. They're trying to get us to do the violations."

"Violations? What kind of violations are you talking about?" asked the bewildered Dan.

"Why violations of women, of course," Robert replied. "And you'd better be careful, unless you do to Betty what happened in Bridgeview."

"Robert, calm down. You're not making any sense. I'm not following you."

"Oh, yes, you are," Robert insisted. "You know *exactly* what I'm talking about. I know for a fact that the Ruler has been keeping you up to date on the changes as well."

Dan talked with Robert for several hours without gaining any additional clarity on what Robert was trying to tell him. As the morning light appeared outside their dorm window, Robert stood up, giving his roommate a pitying look. "I'm sorry, Dan. The Ruler has told me to stop talking to you. You've become one of the aliens."

He went back to his side of the room and put on his favorite tape. And although they shared the dorm room for the rest of the spring semester, Robert never spoke another word to Dan.

When Robert came home for his spring vacation, his parents were alarmed by his disheveled appearance and incoherent speech. Over Robert's vehement objections, the family took him to see Dr. Carol Kent, a psychiatrist their family doctor had recommended. Dr. Kent spent an hour and a half alone with Robert. After that session, she told Robert's parents that she was worried about Robert's psychological health.

"Robert has been hearing voices for the past seven months," she explained. "The voices keep up a running commentary on his behavior. The voices are now beginning to take control of his thoughts and activities.

"Although Robert has never met the people who are 'speaking' to him, he feels that they have some special knowledge about him. And they seem to have a great deal of power over him. They have been critical of his sexual thoughts and urges. They have been threatening extraordinary physical punishment, if he should fail to follow their demands.

"The voices have been telling Robert not to go to class and not to trust any of his friends or family members. Within the last four weeks, the voices have begun to order Robert to perform a number of harmful, self-destructive acts. When I was performing the physical examination, I noticed two dozen parallel scars on Robert's upper arm. When I asked Robert about the scars, he had told me that 'the Ruler' had instructed him to cut himself there each time he had a disgusting thought.

"The Ruler recently told Robert that he does not deserve to go on living. I asked Robert what he would do if the Ruler told him to take his own life.

Robert said that he would probably obey any order the Ruler gave him."

Dr. Kent went on to say that she felt that there was a grave risk that Robert might try to kill himself. She felt that he should be admitted to a local psychiatric hospital—for his protection and to give her an opportunity to provide a full assessment of Robert's illness and to propose a course of treatment. Robert entered the hospital the next day. He received a complete physical and neurological examination and a battery of laboratory tests. There was no evidence of any physical illness, drug use, or toxic reaction. Dr. Kent concluded that Robert was suffering from a schizophrenic disorder. Although Robert did report some depressed feelings, he did not meet the criteria for a depressive disorder (see Chapter 3).

Robert was placed on the antipsychotic agent chlorpromazine (Thorazine)—25 mg three times a day plus 50 mg at bedtime. His dose was gradually increased to 100 mg four times a day and 200 mg at bedtime.

Robert participated in multiple daily therapeutic activities and group activities designed to encourage socialization and enhance his ability to interpret reality. Robert also met with Dr. Kent three times a week. During these sessions, they discussed Robert's day-to-day problems in adjusting to his medications. They also talked about Robert's interactions with the other patients and with hospital staff members. Dr. Kent did not delve into Robert's childhood or probe any other sensitive issues in his past. She openly discussed Robert's delusions with him and tried to reassure him as he learned to adopt a more realistic point of view. This type of support and encouragement is called *supportive* therapy, as opposed to the analytical, uncovering, or probing type of psychotherapy that might be used for patients with other disorders.

After three weeks in the hospital, Robert had stopped hearing voices. While he said he still believed that it was possible for the Ruler to control his mind and actions, he was not so preoccupied with the Ruler as he had been before.

Dr. Kent also met regularly with the whole family: Robert, his brothers and sisters, and their parents. She explained to the family that Robert was suffering from an illness called schizophrenia. She explained that this was a physical disease that affected brain function, but that it could also be triggered by psychological conflicts and other stresses. She told the family that they should not feel responsible for having caused Robert's illness, and strongly recommended that all family members join one of several local support groups for family members of people with a schizophrenia. The family joined a local chapter of the National Alliance for the Mentally Ill (NAMI).

She also referred the family to the National Alliance for Research on

Schizophrenia and Depression (NARSAD). Through their interactions with Dr. Kent, the staff of the inpatient unit, and the patient advocacy groups, Robert's family was able to learn a great deal about schizophrenia.

During his fourth week in the hospital, Robert's medications were gradually reduced to a 25 mg dose of chlorpromazine three times a day plus 75 mg in the evening. Dr. Kent found that this was the lowest dose sufficient to control his hallucinations and delusions.

After five weeks in the hospital, Robert was discharged. He enrolled in a junior college near his home and saw Dr. Kent once a week. She checked up on his response to the medication, and they discussed his current problems—at home and school. Although he still showed little interest in dating, Robert was able to make friends with several young men and women he had met during his group therapy. Two main focuses of group therapy were (1) the awareness of the effects of Robert's behavior on other people in the group, and (2) the interpretation of the action, words, and motivations of others in the group. Robert successfully completed college and found a job as a computer programmer.

Several months later, after Robert's father suffered a heart attack, Robert stopped taking his medications and refused to see Dr. Kent or go to his other outpatient treatment programs. Within three weeks, his hallucinations and delusions had returned, and he had to return to the hospital. Within one week after being placed back on his medications and with intensive supportive care, his symptoms were markedly reduced and Robert was discharged from the hospital.

## RICHARD SMITH: PSYCHOSIS RESULTING FROM AMPHETAMINE ABUSE

Richard Smith, a twenty-two-year-old dishwasher, was a heavy user of amphetamines. On one occasion, he injected amphetamines intravenously several times daily for three days in a row. After these binges, he would become extremely restless and agitated and go without sleep for more than forty-eight hours.

Following one of these episodes, Richard developed the delusion that the police wanted to kill him because he had assassinated President Kennedy. He became preoccupied with thoughts of the police and spent most of his time trying to devise ways to hide from them. At a shopping mall, Richard believed one of the security guards had recognized him. He hid in a bathroom stall and stayed there until after closing time. When he was finally discovered by a security guard, he tried to escape; he had to be forcibly subdued. Richard was experiencing paranoid delusions from large doses of amphetamines.

## ELLA MAE SMITH: DELIRIUM RESULTING FROM A DRUG SIDE EFFECT

Ella Mae, a sixty-nine-year-old woman who developed severe chest pain, was admitted to the hospital with a possible heart attack. Her physician prescribed diphenhydramine to help her sleep and prochlorperazine to treat her nausea.

Two days later, Mrs. Smith became confused and agitated. She thought she was at the police station and demanded to be released. She pulled out her intravenous lines and tried to hit the nurses who came to assist her. She began screaming and talking to people no one else could see. The hospital psychiatrist determined that the delirium was a side effect of the drugs she was taking. When the drugs were stopped, and with brief low-dose treatment with haloperidol, her hallucinations and delusions disappeared in three days.

## ARNOLD BECKER: MANIC PSYCHOSIS

Arnold was a twenty-one-year-old college student who belonged to the ROTC. While he was living at home the summer after his junior year, Arnold's family began to notice changes in his behavior. He became excessively active, stayed up all night without feeling tired, and began to speak rapidly and with great emotion. He often expressed the opinion that America's national security was under attack and that he needed to take things in his own hands. He wore his army fatigues on a regular basis and began to purchase medals and to refer to himself as "the Commander in Chief." He spent all of his savings on uniforms, medals, and weaponry.

He also began to hear voices from "The President," who was instructing him to develop a "master plan" for the nation's defense. Arnold worked continuously on his master plan and filled hundreds of pages with handwritten strategies. Against Arnold's protestations, the family finally brought him to the hospital, where he was admitted. A thorough evaluation turned up no evidence of a physical problem or drug use. Arnold's psychiatrist concluded that his changes in behavior and thought were the result of manic-depressive illness. (For more on manic-depresssive illness, see Chapters 3 and 6.)

## BEATRICE BLANCHARD: PSYCHOTIC DEPRESSION

Beatrice Blanchard was a fifty-one-year-old woman who had been hospitalized several times over the past twenty years for depression. On a recent visit, she told her family physician that life didn't seem worth living anymore. She had been feeling sad and hopeless for about a month. She had difficulty falling asleep and would often wake up at 3:00 or 4:00 A.M., unable to fall back asleep. Mrs. Blanchard had no interest in eating and had lost ten pounds over the last month. She found that she no longer enjoyed her weekly bridge game, which had formerly been the highlight of her week. She felt hopeless; she had considered ending her life with an overdose of sleeping pills. Her family physician referred her to a psychiatrist, who advised immediate hospitalization.

Once in the hospital, Mrs. Blanchard became highly suspicious. She began to "hear" people screaming for help on other floors of the hospital. Neither her roommates nor staff members heard the screams. She was certain these people were being held hostage by the hospital staff and she was convinced that she would be next. Mrs. Blanchard called her family and begged them not to visit. "Please don't come," she told them. "The nurses are planning to kill you, too." Mrs. Blanchard's psychiatrist determined that she was having a depression with psychotic features. Because prior treatment with antidepressants combined with antipsychotic agents had not helped when she had experienced similar symptoms ten years before, and because she had had an excellent response previously to electroconvulsive therapy, her family persuaded both the psychiatrist and Mrs. Blanchard to agree to repeat that treatment. After three electroconvulsive treatments, Mrs. Blanchard was no longer experiencing psychotic symptoms and her mood was dramatically improved. (For more on electroconvulsive [shock] therapy, see Chapter 13.)

## Nondrug Treatments for Psychosis

For all patients with a schizophrenia, nondrug interventions are an essential part of treatment. Such nonmedication interventions include individual psychotherapy, family therapy, group therapy, recreational therapy, occupational therapy, and vocational therapy. A central component of most non-medicinal treatments of schizophrenia involves reducing social or environmental stresses and assisting the patient in interpreting reality. A vital component of nondrug treatment of schizophrenia is to encourage the patients to refrain from taking substances of abuse and other types of psychoactive substances, which usually makes their illnesses much worse. Assisting patients in decisions requiring judgment is also an important intervention. An example: counseling a patient with a schizophrenic illness not to travel to New Orleans for Mardi Gras. Increased visual and auditory stimulation as well as confusing social interchanges are often stressful to individuals with a schizophrenia.

Special living arrangements such as those provided in halfway houses are also important nondrug treatments of people with a schizophrenia. In such arrangements, counseling and group support are important features. All the aforementioned treatments also work well with and are vital to successful treatment of the psychosis with medications. For example, group support in halfway houses often encourages those individuals who require continuous treatment with antipsychotic agents to take their medications as prescribed. Finally, support groups and advocacy groups provide support, information, and help to all people with severe mental illness and their families.

When a psychotic episode is caused by a legal or an illegal drug, providing a quiet, supportive environment can often be sufficient treatment to see the patient safely through the psychotic episode. In some rare cases, especially with a phencyclidine-induced psychosis, treatment with low doses of antipsychotic medication may be necessary. The affected individual should be maintained in a safe environment. This often means around-the-clock observation from hospital staff; a delirious individual may harm himself or herself—either deliberately or accidentally. Other methods of treatment include reassuring the individual, who is likely to be frightened and anxious as a result of distorted perceptions or beliefs. Frequent explanations to the individual about where he or she is, what the date is, what time it is, and why he or she is in the hospital are helpful. The presence of a family member or friend in the patient's room is often reassuring. Psychotherapy alone is usually not effective in treating acute psychotic symptoms or preventing relapses in most patients.

## Drugs Used to Treat Psychosis

Drugs used to treat psychosis are called antipsychotic drugs. The antipsychotic drugs can help organize chaotic, disorganized, psychotic thinking, and reduce or remove delusions and hallucinations. These drugs are sometimes called *major tranquilizers,* but this is a misnomer; the tranquilization or sedation produced by some of the antipsychotics is a side effect, not their primary action. These drugs may also be referred to as *neuroleptics;* their side effects can sometimes imitate a neurological illness such as Parkinson's disease.

These drugs are usually classified into three groups:

- the low-potency antipsychotics
- the high-potency antipsychotics
- the intermediate-potency antipsychotics

All three groups are equally effective in treating psychotic symptoms. The term *potency* refers not to therapeutic effectiveness but to the dose of the drug received to produce a therapeutic effect. They also tend to differ in the side effects that they produce. Clozapine is a special, new class of antipsychotic agent that doesn't cause involuntary movement; thus it is not considered a neuroleptic.

## How Do Antipsychotics Work?

Although we are not completely sure just how antipsychotic drugs work, many researchers now believe that psychotic symptoms, in part, result from an excess of the brain's chemical messenger dopamine or an increased sensitivity of the dopamine receptors. This theory is supported by the fact that increasing brain dopamine (by giving L-dopa) almost always makes psychotic symptoms much worse. Antipsychotic drugs apparently prevent molecules of dopamine from binding to the dopamine receptor sites.

## Who Should Take Antipsychotic Drugs?

*People Who Experience Sudden, Short-Lived Psychotic Episodes*

In many cases of psychosis, small doses of antipsychotics can be very helpful in reversing an episode. They are usually necessary only for a short period. An example would be the use of 1 mg of haloperidol three times a day for three days to treat the psychosis of Ella Mae Smith that was a medication side effect.

*Psychosis Resulting from a Medical Illness*

When the psychosis is a part of an underlying medical illness, an antipsychotic can often be helpful in controlling the psychotic features (see Sidebar 3). Low doses of high-potency antipsychotic drugs usually produce the best results.

*Psychotic Depression*

For depressed patients with delusions, treating with an antidepressant alone may be insufficient. Antidepressants usually take several weeks to work, and these drugs may not affect the psychotic features of disorder. Only 40 percent of patients with psychotic depression respond to antidepressants

## Sidebar 3: Medical Illnesses That Can Cause Psychosis

Neurological causes
  seizures*
  strokes*
  brain hemorrhages
  tumors
  hydrocephalus
  head trauma*
  infections of the brain
    (especially with AIDS)*
  Alzheimer's disease*
  Pick's disease
  Huntington's disease*
  Parkinson's disease*
Endocrine disorders
  adrenal disorders
  diabetes mellitus
  parathyroid disorders
  pituitary disorders
  thyroid disorders
Metabolic abnormalities
  cardiac failure
  hypoglycemia, hyper-
    glycemia
  hepatic failure
  porphyria
  renal failure
  Wilson's disease
  fluid and electrolyte
    imbalances (such as
    hyponatremia and
    hypernatremia)
Nutritional deficiency diseases
  beriberi
  pellagra

  pernicious anemia
  Wernicke-Korsakoff
    syndrome
Systemic illness
  carcinomatosis
  collagen and autoimmune
    diseases (such as
    systemic lupus
    erythematosus)
  heatstroke
  infections (bacterial,
    fungal, parasitic)
  starvation
Withdrawal states
  alcohol withdrawal
  barbiturate withdrawal
  narcotic withdrawal
Intoxications
  alcohol
  barbiturates
  hallucinogens (ampheta-
    mines, LSD, mescaline,
    THC, phencyclidine
Environmental and industrial
  intoxications
  bromide
  carbon disulfide
  carbon monoxide
  heavy metals (such as lead)
  organic phosphates
    (insecticides)

* Indicates the most common causes.

alone, but over 80 percent respond when antidepressants and antipsychotics are combined. Once the patient's symptoms are gone, the antipsychotic medication may gradually be withdrawn over several weeks. The antidepressant medication should be maintained for a period of six months or longer.

### Manic Psychosis

People who have a manic-depressive illness and are experiencing acute mania with psychotic features may benefit from a brief period of treatment with an antipsychotic drug. The antipsychotic drug can calm the patient (via its sedative side effects) beginning on the first day of treatment, while lithium may require several weeks to be effective. The antimanic and antipsychotic actions of the drug may also take effect before the lithium is fully effective in treating the manic.

### Schizophrenia

The antipsychotic drugs are most frequently used to treat people with schizophrenia. Antipsychotics do not "cure" schizophrenia, but can help to control such symptoms as hallucinations, delusions, and thought disorders.

Once a treatment has reduced or eliminated psychotic symptoms, continued use of the antipsychotic medication may help prevent a return of schizophrenic symptoms.

### Other Uses of Antipsychotic Medication

Antipsychotics are sometimes used to treat a neurological disorder called Gilles de la Tourette's syndrome. This disease is characterized by vocal outbursts, often consisting of profanity, and physical tics or jerky movements of the body over which the patient has little control. Other disorders, from intractable hiccups to severe nausea, are sometimes treated by antipsychotics.

### TESTS REQUIRED PRIOR TO TAKING ANTIPSYCHOTIC MEDICATIONS

Before starting any antipsychotic medication, you will need to undergo a thorough history and a complete physical exam. These are to ensure that no treatable cause of the psychosis is overlooked. It also allows the physician to evaluate your ability to tolerate the drug and to establish a baseline of body functions against which physical changes due to treatment can be compared.

The following parts of the medical history and exam are especially important:

• *Blood pressure and pulse.* Both can be affected by antipsychotic medications. It is important to evaluate these functions before starting the medication. If your blood pressure is either too high or too low, particular antipsychotic agents may be selected so as not to aggravate these conditions. For example: The drug Thorazine (chlorpromazine) lowers blood pressure substantially, while haloperidol has less of an effect on blood pressure and the cardiovascular system.

• *Eye exam.* Antipsychotic medications (particularly thioridazine) have been associated with deposits of pigment in a part of the retina. This side effect, called *retinitis pigmentosa,* can in some cases lead to blindness. It is important to examine the eye, particularly the retina, for any pigmenting changes present prior to starting the medication. In addition, because certain properties of all antipsychotics can cause a worsening of glaucoma, it is important to test your eyes for glaucoma. Any patient with glaucoma should be treated appropriately by an ophthalmologist prior to starting an antipsychotic medication. The ophthalmologist and the psychiatrist prescribing the antipsychotic drug must communicate regularly with each other before and during treatment to be sure the patient's glaucoma is being monitored and treated.

• *A neurological exam.* Neurological side effects of antipsychotics are quite common. It is important to establish a baseline of sensorimotor function prior to starting medication so that an existing neurologic condition, such as mild Parkinson's disease, is not overlooked and made worse by the medication.

• *Prostate exam in men over forty.* A side effect of most antipsychotics is difficulty urinating. This is more likely to cause problems in someone with an enlarged prostate gland, to the point that he may become unable to urinate and may need a catheter inserted to relieve bladder pressure.

• *A complete blood count.* Some antipsychotics can lower the count of white blood cells (the infection-fighting cells). It is thus necessary to check the cell count first to make sure it is within the normal range. The special laboratory monitoring of patients taking clozapine (Clozaril) will be addressed separately.

• *Kidney and liver tests.* Antipsychotic drugs are broken down and removed from the body by the liver and kidney. If these organs are not functioning properly, removal of the antipsychotics from the body may be impaired, and the drug levels may rise to dangerously high levels.

• *Electrocardiogram*. This test provides information about electrical functions of the heart. It can also show evidence of preexisting heart damage. Since some antipsychotics affect the heart's performance, it is important for the physician to know what, if any, preexisting heart condition is present prior to starting an antipsychotic.

## How Can These Drugs Be Misused?

### Misused for Agitation and Violent Behavior

Antipsychotics are sometimes used to treat people with agitation and violent behavior. If the violent behavior results from psychotic ideas or perceptions, this may be necessary and effective. But in many cases violence and agitation have sources other than psychosis, e.g., traumatic head injury resulting in neurologically induced violence. Although the sedating side effects of the antipsychotics may at first decrease agitation or violent behavior in such patients, other medications available can be used to treat these patients without oversedation and without the risk of developing the side effects associated with the antipsychotics—especially the potentially irreversible movement disorder, tardive dyskinesia (see p. 186).

### Misused for Insomnia and Anxiety

The sedating side effects of the antipsychotics also lead them to be misused as antianxiety drugs or as sleeping aids. Once again, there are other, much safer, medications available for these conditions. In those cases in which violence, agitation, anxiety, or sleeplessness results from a psychotic state, antipsychotics are appropriate treatment.

We believe that the combination drugs—i.e., those in which an antipsychotic is combined with other drugs in a single tablet or capsule to treat a wide variety of disorders—should not be used. Use of such combinations is imprecise and unnecessary.

## Precautions to Observe While Taking Antipsychotic Medications

The most disabling and difficult to treat side effect of antipsychotics is tardive dyskinesia. Read the tardive dyskinesia section thoroughly (see p. 186). A common side effect of most antipsychotics is sedation. Therefore, it is very important to use particular care and caution when driving while taking antipsychotics. It may be necessary for some individuals to avoid driving altogether. An individual taking antipsychotic medications must also employ extreme caution while using any machinery or equipment. Similarly, because of the blood pressure–lowering properties of most antipsychotics, caution should be taken when driving, operating heavy machinery or equipment, or when engaging in sports that are potentially dangerous, such as football, mountain climbing, or diving.

Antipsychotics (and all other medications) must be used with extreme caution in patients who have medical illnesses or who are taking medications for conditions other than psychosis. Sidebar 4 lists drugs that interact dangerously with antipsychotic agents.

Caution should be used, as well, with smoking. After taking a dose of a very sedating antipsychotic such as Thorazine, it is possible to become very drowsy and to fall asleep while a cigarette is burning. The consequences could be fatal for the patient and others.

Individuals on antipsychotic medications must also be careful about using other medications or substances, such as alcohol, that are also sedating, as the sedative side effects of an antipsychotic may be compounded. In general, alcohol makes psychotic symptoms worse, so we recommend that you refrain from drinking alcohol if you have a history of psychosis.

## Side Effects

A person experiencing a psychotic state usually begins taking one of these drugs under emergency conditions. At the beginning of treatment, a person is often too agitated or upset to concentrate on the risks, benefits, and dosing requirements, so the psychiatrist must communicate this information to family members. Once the patient is more calm and lucid, he or she is in a much better condition to acquire a knowledge base about medications and other treatment approaches.

### DROWSINESS

Some antipsychotics are more sedating than others. The low-potency antipsychotics such as chlorpromazine (Thorazine) are especially sedating. Individuals usually become adjusted to this side effect over a period of

## Sidebar 4:  Drugs That Interact with Antipsychotics

| DRUGS INTERACTING WITH ANTIPSYCHOTICS | EFFECT |
| --- | --- |
| anticholinergics<br>  benztropine<br>  biperiden<br>  diphenhydramine<br>  ethopropazide<br>  orphenadrine<br>  procyclidine<br>  trihexyphenidyl | increased anticholinergic effects |
| antacids | oral absorption delayed |
| lithium | may increase central nervous system toxicity |
| narcotics<br>  codeine<br>  meperidine | increased sedation, hypotension,<br>    anticholinergic effects |
| antidepressants | cardiac effects and respiratory depression,<br>    especially with heterocyclic antidepressants |
| MAO inhibitors | hypotension |
| beta blockers | increased blood levels of antipsychotics |
| barbiturates | increased sedation |
| levodopa | may decrease effectiveness of antipsychotics |
| benzodiazepines | increased sedation (especially with<br>    phenothiazines) |
| guanethidine | chlorpromazine decreases antihypertensive<br>    effect |
| clonidine | chlorpromazine decreases antihypertensive<br>    effect |
| antihypertensives | hypotension (especially with phenothiazines) |
| vasodilator drugs<br>  epinephrine | hypotension (especially with phenothiazines) |
| antihistamines | increased sedation (especially with<br>    phenothiazines) |
| quinidine | thioridazine causes cardiac arrythmias and<br>    cardiac muscle depression |

weeks. Taking the medication around bedtime or using an antipsychotic with less sedating effects can help control this problem.

### DRY MOUTH, BLURRED VISION, CONSTIPATION, DIFFICULTY URINATING

Certain side effects of the antipsychotics are due to their blocking of another chemical messenger, acetylcholine. These so-called anticholinergic side effects include dry mouth, constipation, difficulty in urination, and blurred vision. The anticholinergic side effects usually appear early in treatment (the first several days) and are more common with the high-potency antipsychotics such as trifluoperazine and haloperidol. The body often adapts to these side effects over a period of weeks. Self-help measures that can be taken to lessen these effects: If your mouth is dry, sip water or suck on sugar-free candies. (But be aware that the candy ingredient sorbitol can cause gas, abdominal bloating, cramping, and diarrhea in some people.)

If constipation is a problem, be sure to drink at least eight glasses of water a day and eat lots of fresh fruit, vegetables, and whole grain products. Eating a bowl of high-fiber cereal in the morning can be especially helpful. If constipation persists, products such as Metamucil (which add fiber bulk to the diet) may be useful. Stool softener products such as Colace (docusate sodium) may also be used. Laxatives that work by stimulating the bowel are not recommended.

Difficulty in urination can range from problems initiating urination to complete inability to urinate. The latter condition necessitates prompt medical care.

Blurred vision may occur during the first few weeks, but it will usually disappear as you become accustomed to the drug. In rare circumstances, eye drops or corrective glasses may be required.

### CARDIOVASCULAR REACTIONS

Antipsychotic medication may cause an increase in your heart rate or pulse. This must be monitored carefully by your doctor, as this increased work load for the heart may lead to chest pain and possibly even myocardial infarction (heart attack) in susceptible individuals. Patients with preexisting cardiovascular abnormalities (either high or low blood pressure) should be careful not to stand up suddenly. Doing so can produce fainting or, in rare cases, a stroke.

## ACUTE DYSTONIC REACTIONS

An acute dystonic reaction is a sudden occurrence of a twisting and stiffening of a group of muscles. It often involves the neck and jaw or may involve muscles running up both sides of the spinal cord or vertebrae (backbones). The affected individual's neck and jaw may be twisted to one side, and any motion of the head becomes very difficult. Acute dystonic reactions may also, for example, involve other muscle groups—such as the eye muscles. This highly disturbing side effect may require emergency treatment. It can be relieved almost immediately by an injection of an anticholinergic medication such as benztropine mesylate.

An acute dystonic reaction usually occurs within the first hours or days of treatment with an antipsychotic, but it can occur at any time. Acute dystonic reactions occur most commonly in young men. However, dystonic reactions are sufficiently frequent in all patients to cause some psychiatrists to recommend that all patients started on antipsychotic medication be simultaneously started on anticholinergic medication to prevent this frightening side effect.

## PSEUDOPARKINSONISM

The parkinsonianlike side effects of antipsychotic drugs include a loss of facial expression (the individual's face will appear unmoving, like a mask), rigidity of the joints, slow body movements, drooling, small handwriting, and a tremor or shaking of the hands. These side effects usually begin days to weeks after the antipsychotic medication has been started, and respond to anticholinergic medications (and the drug amantadine).

## AGITATED RESTLESSNESS

Agitated restlessness (akathisia) is a physical reaction to antipsychotic medications in which the individual constantly feels like moving. An affected individual might pace up and down to relieve the sensation that has been described by some as "Needing to jump out of my skin." If required to sit, the individual will feel very uncomfortable and may move his or her legs up and down rapidly in an attempt to gain relief. This is a common side effect. One study showed that 40 percent of individuals experienced akathisia after one dose of haloperidol. The percentage increased to 75 percent if the haloperidol were continued for one week. If this side effect becomes too bothersome, it may be necessary to discontinue that medication. Switching to another type of antipsychotic may provide relief. The medication propranolol has been shown to be effective in the treatment of akathisia for some individuals.

## TARDIVE DYSKINESIA

Tardive dyskinesia, a neurological syndrome caused by most antipsychotic drugs, with the sole exception of clozapine (Clozaril), is one of the most serious side effects of any psychiatric medication. It is alarmingly common—20 to 25 percent of chronically hospitalized psychiatric patients show signs of tardive dyskinesia. In some cases, it is irreversible.

Tardive dyskinesia refers to a group of involuntary movements that can affect any muscle group of the body, but it is more common in certain muscle groups, especially the facial muscles (see Sidebar 5). These abnormal movements usually disappear while the person is sleeping. In the early stages of tardive dyskinesia, the affected individual may not even be aware of the abnormal movements. A family member or a mental health professional is often the first to notice. There is no known cure for tardive dyskinesia, and it may be permanent. Occasionally, this disorder becomes so severe that it makes walking, eating, and even breathing difficult; its disfiguring qualities are most embarrassing to the patient. It is important to be aware of the onset of these movements and report them to the physician prescribing the antipsychotic. Frequent (every six months) examinations should be conducted to check for early signs of tardive dyskinesia. The earliest signs of tardive dyskinesia often involve small wormlike movements under the surface of the tongue.

Since there is no cure for tardive dyskinesia, prevention must be the goal. It is recommended that people be maintained on the lowest possible dose of antipsychotic medication and that periodic attempts be made to lower the dosage. Attempts should also be made to discontinue antipsychotic medications whenever possible, especially in individuals with manic-depressive illness or those being treated for psychotic depression. People with manic-depressive illness may, in fact, have a higher risk of developing tardive dyskinesia, making it especially important for them to stop antipsychotic medications as early as possible.

Increasing age as well as prior brain damage are also associated with an increase in the incidence of tardive dyskinesia. Increased length of time on an antipsychotic as well as an increased dose of an antipsychotic may also increase the risk of developing tardive dyskinesia.

Once tardive dyskinesia has developed, the only consistently successful treatment is discontinuation of the antipsychotic medication. In one study, there was a 50 percent reduction in the abnormal movements in most patients within eighteen months of discontinuing the antipsychotic drug. The development and treatment of tardive dyskinesia is an area of much investigation. Although many drugs have been used to treat tardive dyskinesia, none has proved consistently effective.

Some antipsychotics such as pimozide are less likely to cause tardive dyskinesia; but since all antipsychotics, except clozapine, can cause tardive dyskinesia, therapeutic benefits of the antipsychotic medication must always be weighed against the possibility of developing tardive dyskinesia.

---

**Sidebar 5: Characteristic Features of Tardive Dyskinesia**

I. Movements of the face and mouth
   a. involuntary movement of the forehead, eyebrows, and cheeks; frowning, blinking, grimacing
   b. involuntary smiling, pouting, puckering, smacking of lips
   c. biting, clenching, chewing, mouth opening; may interfere with eating
   d. tongue movements, tremor, protrusion, and small wormlike movement within mouth
II. Movements of arms and legs
   a. involuntary movements of the arms, hands, and fingers; can be rapid, irregular, or slow and snakelike; tremor
   b. involuntary movements of legs, knees, toes, such as tapping, squirming
   c. trunk movements involving the neck, shoulders, hips; rocking, twisting, and squirming may at times interfere with breathing

---

## CASE STUDY: TARDIVE DYSKINESIA

Myron Washington was diagnosed as having a schizophrenia when he was seventeen years old. His symptoms included auditory hallucinations that called him disparaging names and, on occasion, directed him to harm himself. Once, when Myron stopped taking his antipsychotic drug Prolixin, a voice instructed him to stab himself in the stomach. Myron complied, and his father had to rush him to the hospital where emergency surgery and the removal of Myron's spleen were required to stop the bleeding and save his life. On every occasion that Myron stopped taking his medication, his symptoms (including agitation and violence) became so pronounced that psychiatric hospitalization was required.

When Myron was twenty-six years old, his psychiatrist, Dr. Taylor, first noted the emergence of tardive dyskinesia. Myron would occasionally purse his lips and protrude his tongue, which upon close inspection, showed fine contraction movements called fasciculations. Myron had little or no ability to control these movements. When Dr. Taylor tried to taper off Myron's Prolixin, Myron began to be plagued by auditory hallucinations and became irritable and occasionally violent. The counselor at the halfway house where Myron had lived for six years said that Myron was far too disruptive to remain when the antipsychotic was reduced. Neither treatment with propranolol nor any other medication reduced the tardive dyskinesia. Myron, Dr. Taylor, and the family were left with a difficult but clear choice—either Myron would stop taking Prolixin and have to remain indefinitely in a state hospital, or the Prolixin would be continued and Myron's tardive dyskinesia would certainly get worse. After lengthy discussions, the latter choice was agreed upon. Two years later, Dr. Taylor learned of a research project at the University of Chicago in which a new antipsychotic drug, clozapine, was being tested. The drug was reported not to carry the risk of tardive dyskinesia. Myron was enrolled in the study (after full informed consent from Myron and his family) and, to everyone's delight, not only did Myron's psychotic symptoms and behavioral problems respond better to clozapine than they had to Proxilin, not only did he become less socially withdrawn, but his symptoms of tardive dyskinesia went away completely while he was taking the clozapine. Trials of reducing the dose of clozapine were marked by the return of his psychosis and his tardive dyskinesia.

## NEUROLEPTIC MALIGNANT SYNDROME

A life-threatening side effect of antipsychotic treatment is the neuroleptic malignant syndrome. In this syndrome, the affected individual becomes rigid, develops a fever, a rapid heartbeat, abnormal blood pressure, rapid breathing, heavy sweating, and changes in mental state ranging from confusion to coma. The muscles release a chemical that can cause kidney failure. This condition is a major medical emergency and requires prompt hospitalization. The syndrome can occur with any antipsychotic medication, although it is most common with high-potency antipsychotics such as haloperidol. Neuroleptic malignant syndrome can also occur at any time during the treatment with antipsychotics.

If neuroleptic malignant syndrome is suspected, hospitalization is required. All antipsychotic medication (as well as most other medications) must be stopped immediately. Treatment options are varied, as no one treatment has been shown to be clearly superior over others. Supportive treatment is always necessary, and this includes intravenous fluids to help prevent kidney failure, and cooling blankets. Dantrolene sodium, a muscle relaxant, and bromocriptine, a dopamine agonist, have been used individually and together in the treatment of neuroleptic malignant syndrome.

## ORTHOSTATIC HYPOTENSION (LOW BLOOD PRESSURE ON STANDING OR SITTING UP)

Antipsychotics can lower your blood pressure. This can cause dizziness. Orthostatic hypotension is especially common when a person rises from a lying or sitting position. People on an antipsychotic medication should exercise care when changing positions. When getting up in the morning, instead of *jumping* out of bed, *sit* up in the bed for a few minutes, then dangle your legs over the side of the bed for a few moments. Once you get up, it is a good idea to take your bearings. Before starting to walk, make sure you are not dizzy.

## HORMONE CHANGES

Antipsychotic medications affect many hormones in the body, especially those pertaining to sexual characteristics and drives. Both men and women may develop enlargement of the breasts, and, occasionally, discharge fluid from the nipples. Breasts may become taut and tender. The medication amantadine may sometimes be effective in alleviating these side effects.

Antipsychotics may make you uninterested in sex. Some men have problems achieving or maintaining an erection. One antipsychotic, thioridazine, is associated with a condition called retrograde ejaculation. When this painful condition occurs, sperm is forced back into the man's bladder rather than out of the penis. Priapism, also very painful, is prolonged involuntary erection that can occur with the use of antipsychotic medication—especially with thioridazine and chlorpromazine. Both men and women on antipsychotic medications may have trouble achieving orgasm. Women may have menstrual period irregularities or even a cessation of their menstrual periods altogether.

It is important to discuss sexual side effects with the prescribing physician. Studies have shown that often the physician will not ask about changes in sexual functioning. Do not let your embarrassment (or even that of your physician) prevent you from receiving the proper care of sexually related side effects of any psychiatric drug. Reducing the dosage of the antipsychotic or changing the antipsychotic medication usually reverses these sexual side effects.

## DERMATOLOGICAL SIDE EFFECTS

### Sunburn

The skin of most individuals who are on antipsychotics becomes especially sensitive to the sun. A person can develop a severe sunburn after a very brief period of exposure to the sun. Any individual on antipsychotics should use a sunscreen with high ultraviolet ray–blocking properties on all exposed surfaces when out in the sun, especially during the summer. Although people with highly pigmented skin are less susceptible to this side effect, they also should take similar precautions to prevent skin irritation from the sun.

### Rash

Some individuals who are on antipsychotic medications will develop a rash. Discontinuation of the antipsychotic is the usual treatment for the problem. If the rash itches, an antihistamine such as diphenhydramine (Benadryl) may be used. If further antipsychotic medication is necessary, an antipsychotic from a different chemical family should then be used.

### Pigmentation

As mentioned previously, the antipsychotic agent thioridazine has been associated with the deposit of pigments (color molecules) in the retina of the eye. This can lead to visual impairment, and even blindness. For this reason, it is recommended that the daily dose of thioridazine not exceed 800 mg daily and that blood levels of thioridazine be drawn if it is used with other medications such as propranolol. Propranolol may cause blood levels of thioridazine to rise.

## METABOLIC SIDE EFFECTS

Antipsychotics can occasionally affect the function of the liver with a subsequent rise in certain blood-related chemicals, such as bilirubin. The patient often feels itchy or detects a yellow cast to the skin or whites of the eye. This abnormality can be detected through lab tests, and when it occurs the antipsychotic should be discontinued. Thereafter, if necessary, an antipsychotic from another chemical family must be substituted.

## Heat-Regulating Disturbances

Individuals on antipsychotics may become especially sensitive to heat. The individual's temperature regulation may not cool the body as it usually would, and his or her temperature can rise to a dangerously high point. This fever may be accompanied by destruction of muscle tissue, and even by kidney failure. Individuals on antipsychotics must take care to protect themselves from prolonged exposure to hot, humid weather. People taking an antipsychotic should also drink ample quantities of fluids, such as cold water, when exposed to warm weather.

## Blood Count Changes

Antipsychotics can have an effect on the body's white blood cell count (the infection-fighting cells of the body). This effect is usually a transient decrease in the number of white blood cells and is rarely associated with any ill effects. However, if the white blood cell count becomes very low, the body may even stop producing the white blood cells altogether. If this occurs, it constitutes a medical emergency and may even be fatal. The highest risk of discontinuation of the production of white blood cells is among middle-aged white women. This condition, called *agranulocytosis*, is also more closely associated with low-potency antipsychotics such as chlorpromazine. It is also highly associated with the drug clozapine (Clozaril).

Studies have been unable to predict which individuals will develop agranulocytosis. Periodic blood counts have *not* usually been helpful in predicting its onset, except in the case of clozapine.

Agranulocytosis usually occurs in the first three or four weeks of treatment; however, it can occur up to three months after treatment has started. Early symptoms are a high fever with listlessness or tiredness, a painfully inflamed mouth, a sore throat, and swollen lymph nodes. Immediate consultation with a physician is essential if these symptoms arise.

The antipsychotic clozapine has a 1 to 2 percent risk of agranulocytosis, the cessation of the production of white blood cells. This condition usually will resolve when the medication is stopped; however if it is not detected in time, the patient may die. More information on this side effect of clozapine appears later in this chapter.

## Weight Gain

Antipsychotics can lead to weight gain in many individuals. The explanation of this side effect is that antipsychotics both increase the appetite and reduce the metabolism, or the rate at which a person burns calories. Molindone is the antipsychotic least likely to cause weight gain.

## Seizures

Antipsychotic medication can make seizure-prone individuals more likely to have seizures. Two antipsychotics, molindone and fluphenazine, are the least likely to cause seizures in a seizure-prone individual. In rare cases, people with no previous history of seizures may have a seizure while on an antipsychotic. The two antipsychotics most likely to initiate seizures are bupropion (Wellbutrin) and clozapine (Clozaril).

## Conclusion

The many serious side effects associated with antipsychotic use should not make us forget the many benefits these drugs may offer. Without medications, hospitalizations may be prolonged. Untreated individuals can have a much poorer quality of life with disturbing, frightening, disruptive hallucinations and delusions. If our reality testing is sufficiently impaired, we might come to harm by acting on the hallucinations or delusions; for example, by jumping out of a window when auditory hallucinations command us to do so. We advise using antipsychotic agents when psychosis is present—especially during active or acute periods of a schizophrenic illness—and attempting to taper or discontinue the drugs during calmer phases.

# Drug Interactions

1. Antacids may inhibit the absorption of antipsychotics taken by mouth. Antacids should not be taken for two hours before or after taking an antipsychotic medication.

2. Heterocyclic antidepressants can increase the plasma levels of antipsychotics. This is especially important when adverse effects are associated with a higher blood level of antipsychotic (e.g., sedation). Antipsychotics can also increase the blood level of antidepressants. Heterocyclic and related antidepressants have anticholinergic properties similar to anti-

psychotics. This can cause a more severe degree of anticholinergic side effects. Their use together must be carefully monitored—especially in the elderly among whom the side effects of oversedation, confusion, and low blood pressure are common and dangerous.

3. MAOI antidepressants can cause lowering of blood pressure. Care should be used and careful monitoring should be instituted when adding an antipsychotic to an MAOI. An antipsychotic with a lower degree of hypo-teantipsychotic to an MAOI. An antipsychotic with a lower degree of hypotensive effect should be chosen (for example, haloperidol) when combining with an MAOI.

4. Antihypertensive drugs. Antipsychotics such as chlorpromazine, mesoridazine, and thioridazine have potent blood pressure–lowering properties. They should be used carefully with individuals receiving antihypertensive (high blood pressure) medications. A dangerous lowering of blood pressure can also occur when combining antipsychotics with vasodilators (medications that dilate blood vessels). There should be careful monitoring when these medications are used together.

Chlorpromazine taken concurrently with the antihypertensives clonidine or guanethidine can cause the blood pressure–lowering effect of clonidine or guanethidine to be decreased.

5. Over-the-counter drugs. Some over-the-counter cold remedies, tranquilizers, and sleeping aids have potent anticholinergic properties. These can be addictive with anticholinergic side effects of the antipsychotics. It is important to let your physician know about any over-the-counter medications you take.

6. Other types of drugs. Thioridazine used with the heart medication quinidine can cause irregular heart rhythms.

Individuals with Parkinson's disease who take L-dopa with an antipsychotic will find that the L-dopa has a decreased effect on their illness. (L-dopa can also make the psychosis much worse.)

Epinephrine is a medication often used in emergency rooms for the treatment of asthma attacks. When epinephrine is injected into an individual taking phenothiazine antipsychotics, blood pressure may drop severely. Any individual with asthma should inform the treating physician if he or she is on a phenothiazine antipsychotic.

## How These Drugs Make You Feel

Antipsychotic medication makes most psychotic individuals feel more comfortable and in control of themselves. Psychotic symptoms such as hallucinations and delusions are often frightening and intrusive, and interfere with most life activities. People often say that they feel more relaxed on antipsychotics. Antipsychotic medication usually causes a lessening of the symptoms—which then allows the individual to participate in life more fully. Often, a symptom such as a delusion can be eliminated completely with antipsychotic medications. For others, the treatment allows the symptoms to have less disruptive effects in their lives. For example, when Robert Carson was started on the antipsychotic chlorpromazine, he became less preoccupied with the "commands" of "the Ruler." He began to talk with other patients and with his family when they visited. Over a period of several weeks, he talked less about being controlled by others. Robert began to enjoy being with other patients in the hospital and with his family and was able to return home and participate in his family life. On the other hand, some individuals despise the feelings they experience while on antipsychotics. They state that they feel overcontrolled, foggy, or "doped-up." Patients whose manic symptoms are treated by antipsychotics may miss the euphoria or energized sensations associated with this condition. Understandably, parkinsonian side effects result in many patients disliking antipsychotic drugs.

## Differences Among Antipsychotic Drugs

All antipsychotic medications have been found to be helpful in reducing or eliminating psychotic forms of thinking. As a whole, no one antipsychotic has been shown to be better than another in its antipsychotic properties. However, certain individuals may respond better to one antipsychotic than to another; but there is no sure way of predicting which antipsychotic will be helpful for an individual without trying it.

Antipsychotics are divided into chemical families that derive from the molecular building blocks that compose the medication (see Table 1). The similarities within a chemical family may be useful for predicting treatment responses. For example, if an individual has a poor response to an antipsychotic in one family, it is likely that the individual will also have a poor response to another member of that particular family.

Another way of categorizing the antipsychotic medications is by *potency*: how much of a drug is necessary to achieve a desired effect. Chlorpromazine is called a low-potency antipsychotic, because more milligrams are required to achieve a similar therapeutic response when compared to other antipsychotics (see Sidebar 6). Haloperidol is called a high-potency antipsychotic, because less haloperidol is required to achieve reduction of antipsychotic symptoms (see Sidebar 7). Chlorpromazine, thioridazine,

TABLE I

**Differences Among Antipsychotic Drugs**

| CLASS | TRADE NAME | POTENCY | SIDE EFFECT PROFILE (*most prominent effects and special features*) |
|---|---|---|---|
| *Generic name* | | | |
| *Thioxanthenes* | | | |
| chlorprothixene | Taractan | low | |
| thiothixene | Navane | high | |
| *Butyrophenones* | | | |
| haloperidol | Haldol | high | high extrapyramidal symptoms |
| *Indole Derivatives* | | | |
| molindone HCl | Moban | intermediate | low incidence of weight gain: caution in seizure-prone individuals |
| *Dibenzoxapines* | | | |
| loxapine | Loxitane | intermediate | |
| clozapine | Clozaril | intermediate | seizures; agranulocytosis |
| *Diphenylbutyl* | | | |
| pimozide | Orap | high | lower association with tardive dyskinesia |
| *Phenothiazines* | | | |
| chlorpromazine | Thorazine | low | high sedation; hypotension; photosensitivity |
| thioridazine HCl | Mellaril | low | high sedation; hypotension; retrograde ejaculation; sexual dysfunction; dosage not recommended to exceed 800 mg a day because of risk of pigmental retinopathy |

TABLE I (*continued*)

**Differences Among Antipsychotic Drugs**

| CLASS | TRADE NAME | POTENCY | SIDE EFFECT PROFILE (*most prominent effects and special features*) |
|---|---|---|---|
| *Phenothiazines* | | | |
| mesoridazine besylate | Serentil | low | high sedation; hypotension |
| trifluoperazine | Stelazine | high | extrapyramidal symptoms |
| fluphenazine HCl | Prolixin Permitil | high | high extrapyramidal symptoms; less likely to induce seizures in seizure-prone individuals |
| perphenazine | Trilafon | intermediate | (as above) |
| acetophenazine maleate | Tindal | intermediate | (as above) |

mesoridazine, and chlorprothixene are considered low-potency antipsychotics. Haloperidol, trifluoperazine, fluphenazine, and thiothixene—among others—are considered high-potency antipsychotics. Trifluopromazine, perphenazine, and loxapine are considered intermediate-potency antipsychotics.

While all the antipsychotics have been shown to be equally effective against psychotic symptoms, their side effects vary. High-potency antipsychotics have an increased degree of *extrapyramidal* side effects such as dystonic reactions, parkinsonian features, and akathisia; but the high-potency antipsychotics are less sedating and cause fewer problems with low blood pressure. The low-potency antipsychotics tend to be quite sedating and often cause lowered blood pressure; but they have a low incidence of extrapyramidal side effects. The intermediate-potency antipsychotics, in general, have side effects between those of high- and low-potency antipsychotics.

For an otherwise healthy young person who has become psychotic and agitated and who is difficult to control physically, a sedating antipsychotic such as chlorpromazine may be helpful in the early part of treatment. The sedating effects are helpful in controlling the physical agitation that could lead to harm to the individual or to those treating him or her. However, as discussed earlier in this chapter, antipsychotic agents should not be used to sedate the chronically violent individual for a long period of time.

---

### Sidebar 6: Chlorpromazine (Thorazine), a Typical Low-Potency Antipsychotic

**Brand name:** Thorazine.

**Common street name:** none.

**Drug family:** phenothiazine.

**Availability:** By prescription only.

**Tablets:** 10 mg, 25 mg, 50 mg, 100 mg, 200 mg.

**Spansules** (sustained-release capsules): 30 mg, 75 mg, 150 mg, 200 mg, 300 mg.

**Syrup:** Available in this form in 4 fl oz bottles (10 mg/5 ml)

**Suppositories:** Available in this form in boxes of 12 (25 mg or 100 mg doses)

**Other routes of administration:** This drug may also be given by either intravenous (IV) or intramuscular (IM) injection.

**Generic name:** chlorpromazine. Two drug companies manufacture generic tablet and liquid forms of this medication. Two other drug companies manufacture generic injectable forms of the medication. Thorazine is the trade name for the chlorpromazine manufactured by the Smith, Kline & French pharmaceutical company.

**Type of antipsychotic:** Chlorpromazine (Thorazine) is a low-potency antipsychotic. It was the first antipsychotic used widely in this country. It is a sedating antipsychotic and is often used for this side effect as well as its antipsychotic actions. As a low-potency antipsychotic, it has fewer movement-involved side effects such as acute dystonic reactions. It can also have a significant effect on an individual's blood pressure. It can cause blood pressure to be lowered to a point that an individual may become light-headed or faint if he or she stands or sits up. Care must be taken, especially when this medication is first used, to avoid falling.

---

# Clozapine

## SPECIAL BENEFITS OF CLOZAPINE (CLOZARIL)

Clozapine (Clozaril) is an antipsychotic newly available in the United States. It is unique in both its biochemical structure as well as its side effect profile. Although it was first found to be an effective antipsychotic drug

## Sidebar 7: Haloperidol (Haldol), a Typical High-Potency Antipsychotic

**Brand name:** Haldol.

**Common street name:** none.

**Drug family:** Butyrophenone.

**Availability:** By prescription only.

**Tablets:** ½ mg, 1 mg, 2 mg, 5 mg, 10 mg, 20 mg.

**Concentrate:** Available in this form.

**Other routes of administration:** This drug can be administered intramuscularly (IM). This drug is also available in a long-acting injectable form, Haldol decanoate.

**Generic name:** haloperidol.

Haldol is a trade name for haloperidol products manufactured by McNeil Pharmaceutical, a drug manufacturer. Haloperidol comes in tablet, liquid, and injectable forms. Haloperidol is available from six other pharmaceutical companies in its generic form.

**Type of antipsychotic:** Haloperidol is a high-potency antipsychotic. This means that 1 to 2 mg haloperidol has the same antipsychotic effect as about 100 mg chlorpromazine (Thorazine). High-potency antipsychotics such as haloperidol have a relatively high risk of causing extrapyramidal side effects such as acute dystonic reactions. Many psychiatrists recommend that an anticholinergic medication such as benztropine mesylate (Cogentin) be given with haloperidol to reduce these extrapyramidal side effects. Haloperidol can cause sedation, but less so than most low-potency antipsychotics. It also has less of an effect on blood pressure. Haloperidol is available in several different forms— tablets, liquid, and injection—which makes it useful in different settings.

One relatively unusual feature of haloperidol is that it is available in a long-acting injectable form called a *depot* injection, that is, in a heavy oil that is injected into a muscle. The drug is slowly released into the body over a period of weeks. This method of giving an individual antipsychotic medication is especially useful when an individual has difficulty in taking medication daily or has a history of noncompliance with his or her physician's treatment plan.

twenty-five years ago, it was not made generally available until 1990. Potentially fatal blood-related side effects have necessitated prolonged investigation of this medication as well as the development of an extensive monitoring system to reduce dangers of these side effects.

Repeated successful studies have shown clozapine to be effective in the treatment of individuals with so-called "treatment resistant" schizo-phrenia. This group of patients suffers from a form or degree of schizo-phrenia that is relatively unresponsive to all other types of antipsychotics. They have often been treated with one type or brand of antipsychotic after another with very little effect. They are often hospitalized for extensive periods of time with florid hallucinations, delusions, and other psychotic symptoms that make it impossible for them to function in society indepen-dently. Clozapine has been shown to be useful in the treatment of people with this category of schizophrenia, with approximately 30 percent show-ing significant improvement.

Clozapine has other therapeutic features that make its use attractive. It is rarely associated with the movement disorders common with other types of antipsychotics. These include akathisia (restlessness), rigidity, and dys-tonia (sudden muscle contractions). In clinical studies thus far, no new cases of tardive dyskinesia have been reported (see p. 188). Individuals with tardive dyskinesia prior to treatment with clozapine have tended to show improvement of their tardive dyskinesia with clozapine treatment.

## SPECIAL RISKS OF CLOZAPINE

### Agranulocytosis

Clozapine's use has been limited by the relatively high risk (1 to 2 percent) of the development of agranulocytosis, a potentially fatal blood-related condition. Agranulocytosis is a failure of the body to produce certain white blood cells (granulocytes), which fight infection.

The agranulocytosis can occur at any time during the treatment, making monitoring the white blood count necessary throughout the treatment. In general with this condition, there is a gradual decrease in the white blood count over a course of several weeks. If the medication is stopped promptly once the white blood count begins to decline, the white blood count returns to normal. For this reason, weekly monitoring of the white blood count is mandatory.

Individuals on clozapine should be aware of signs of infection such as fever, malaise, or flulike symptoms, which may reflect a low white blood count. However, the white blood count can also be dangerously low with no physical symptoms.

While any individual on clozapine may develop agranulocytosis at any time, middle-aged individuals as well as those people in the first six months of treatment appear to be at higher risk for this side effect.

*Other Side Effects of Clozapine*

Other troublesome side effects that occur in a significant percentage of individuals taking clozapine include increased rate of seizures, increased heart rate, low blood pressure, sedation, and heavy salivation.

## WHO MAY BENEFIT FROM CLOZAPINE

The risk of agranulocytosis as well as the extensive blood monitoring required limit the patient population for whom clozapine treatment is currently warranted. Nevertheless, we believe this to be an important new drug in our regimen to treat psychosis. Currently, a trial of clozapine is indicated for individuals who have failed to respond to adequate courses of more typical antipsychotic medication, or who cannot tolerate other antipsychotic drugs because of side effects such as tardive dyskinesia.

## THE SIDE EFFECTS MONITORING SYSTEM

Sandoz, the drug manufacturer that currently distributes clozapine (under the brand name Clozaril), has set up an elaborate system that is the only route through which patients can receive clozapine in the United States. This system includes laboratory, pharmacy, and administrative services. Patients must have a white blood count taken weekly through a specified service established through Sandoz. If the white blood count is in a safe range, a week's worth of medication is given. If the test shows problems with the white blood count, the psychiatrist is notified and decisions are made about whether the clozapine can safely be prescribed in the future. One major drawback is that it currently costs approximately $9,000 per year for the drug and the blood monitoring system. Other systems for monitoring the side effects of clozopine are being established and approved, and the price for medication has been reduced somewhat, but treatment is still expensive.

The use of clozapine requires considerable effort and cooperation on the parts of the patient, family, physician, and mental health system. The potential benefits for people with chronic psychotic disorders are so large that the effort is worthwhile.

# Antipsychotic Drugs: User Guidelines

## HOW ANTIPSYCHOTIC DRUGS ARE TAKEN

Antipsychotic drugs are most frequently administered by mouth as tablets or capsules. Some antipsychotics are available in a liquid form. This is helpful for individuals who prefer not to take pills, who have difficulty swallowing pills, or cannot swallow. For example, a delirious individual who has had a stroke and cannot swallow may have a feeding tube. A liquid antipsychotic easily can be given through the feeding tube.

Some antipsychotics are available in an injectable form. This form is most often used in emergency situations with very psychotic individuals who need immediate treatment and who are often unwilling to take medication orally.

A second type of injectable antipsychotic drug is called a *depot* antipsychotic. After the injection, the antipsychotic is released into the body over a period of weeks. This form of administration is very helpful in the treatment of people who are unable or unwilling to take their oral medications regularly as prescribed. Depot antipsychotic drugs can reduce family stress considerably, as family members often enter into power struggles with people suffering from psychosis who are unwilling to take their medications. Fluphenazine HCl (Prolixin) and haloperidol (Haldol) are both available and have extensive use in the depot form.

## WHEN AND HOW TO TAKE THESE DRUGS

The antipsychotics are available by prescription only and should be taken according to the directions of the prescribing physician. Doses may vary. Many times it is possible to take the entire daily dose of medication at bedtime. Sometimes antipsychotics must be taken two, three, or even four times daily.

It is best to take antipsychotics on an empty stomach. These and any other medications should be taken with a full glass of water to ensure that they reach the stomach.

Antacids, such as Maalox, that contain aluminum or magnesium, should not be taken for two hours before or two hours afterward, because they may interfere with the absorption of antipsychotics into the bloodstream.

Liquid forms that can be mixed in juice are also available. The liquid forms are often more expensive than tablet forms. Injectable antipsychotics are also available if a patient is not allowed, for medical reasons, to take food or liquids orally, or if a person is too confused or agitated to accept drugs by an oral route. Both intramuscular and intravenous antipsychotic agents are available.

## HOW TO STORE THESE DRUGS

These drugs should be stored in tight, light-resistant containers. These and other drugs should be kept away from children. The liquid forms do not require refrigeration. If the liquid form is to be combined with juice or carbonated beverages, wait until the last minute to mix them and then drink the beverage immediately. If the antipsychotic is mixed into the beverage much earlier, it may become unstable and less effective.

## BEGINNING DRUG THERAPY

Individuals receiving an antipsychotic medication for the first time generally will be hospitalized for the underlying disorder. When an antipsychotic is first prescribed, a small dose is given. Physicians call this small dose a test dose. After this test dose is given, important body functions are monitored, especially blood pressure and heart rate.

The medication is then prescribed in small doses (for example, 25 mg chlorpromazine or 1 mg haloperidol) three to four times daily. Many psychiatrists recommend that individuals also be started on an anticholinergic medication at the same time to prevent or lessen the side effects involving movement. This preventive measure is especially important when high-potency antipsychotics are prescribed. Anticholinergic medications are also considered when an individual under forty years of age is experiencing delusions of a paranoid nature. If an individual with paranoia has a reaction such as an acute dystonic reaction to an antipsychotic, he or she may later refuse to take the medication.

People taking antipsychotics should be examined frequently by a physician and should have their blood pressures and pulse rates monitored regularly during treatment. The dose of medication can be increased by small amounts every few days until the desired effect is achieved or until a certain maximum dose is reached. The maximum dose varies with the antipsychotic prescribed and the physical condition of the person being treated.

## HOW TO TELL IF THE ANTIPSYCHOTIC IS WORKING

When an antipsychotic medication is effective, it will reduce the psychotic symptoms. If a psychotic individual is suffering from hallucinations, the hallucinations begin to recede and may eventually disappear. If an individual's language is incoherent because of psychotic thinking, once the antipsychotic begins to work, his or her communications will become more organized and focused. If the person is preoccupied with delusions, the person will be far less distracted by these false beliefs—even if they do not go away completely.

Family and friends will notice changes in the medicated individual as the antipsychotic agent begins to work. A psychotic individual who used to sit alone for hours talking and laughing quietly to himself might talk more with others. Occasionally, the beneficial effects of an antipsychotic agent are more apparent to others than they are to the affected person. Encouragement from others to continue with a sound treatment plan is often required for a person with psychosis to keep taking his or her drug. Usually, the patient experiences less irritability and agitation after the antipsychotic is initiated.

## LONG-TERM USE

*Antipsychotic medications, like any medication, should only be used when necessary and for as brief a period of time as possible.* In some cases, the need for an antipsychotic medication is limited. For example, if an individual requires an antipsychotic during a period of delirium related to uremia (kidney failure), once the uremia has resolved, the antipsychotic is usually tapered off or discontinued.

In other disorders, such as depression with psychotic features, mania, and schizophrenia, longer use of antipsychotics may be necessary. Schizophrenia is a chronic illness for which there is currently no cure. Risks and benefits of treating the symptoms of schizophrenia must be thoroughly evaluated and periodically reviewed by the individual, his or her family, and his or her physician.

## RECOMMENDED PERIODIC EXAMINATIONS WHILE TAKING ANTIPSYCHOTICS

Regular physical examinations, with the physician paying particular attention to check for the development of extrapyramidal side effects and tardive dyskinesia, are recommended. These should be conducted at least every six months, but more frequent exams are desirable.

Periodic eye examinations are also recommended to detect early, irreversible changes in the retina. While these early changes are most specifically associated with thioridazine, periodic eye exams are recommended for all individuals on antipsychotics. In general, no routine blood tests are recommended, except for patients receiving clozapine, for whom weekly blood tests are required.

## TREATMENT OF EXTRAPYRAMIDAL SIDE EFFECTS

The use of antipsychotic medications often leads to the development of a group of symptoms known collectively as *extrapyramidal symptoms*. These include acute dystonic reactions and pseudoparkinsonian reactions.

These symptoms can be very uncomfortable and disturbing for the affected individual as well as to those around him or her.

These side effects can be treated either by discontinuing the antipsychotic agent or changing to a drug with different side effects. In clinical practice, the side effects often are treated once the side effects occur. However, many psychiatrists believe that since these side effects are so common, they should be treated prophylactically; that is, an anticholinergic medication should be given simultaneously with the initiation of an antipsychotic treatment to prevent the emergence of extrapyramidal side effects. See Sidebar 8 for a list of the anticholinergic medications used most frequently for this purpose.

While anticholinergic medications can relieve extrapyramidal symptoms, they also have their own set of side effects, including dry mouth, blurred vision, constipation, difficulties with urination, worsening of glaucoma, and the central anticholinergic syndrome (described on p. 184).

As antipsychotic medications also have a tendency to produce anticholinergic side effects, the addition of another drug with anticholinergic properties can cause a worsening of these side effects.

Many over-the-counter preparations have anticholinergic properties that may also be additive to the side effects of anticholingeric medications (see Sidebar 8).

---

### Sidebar 8: Commonly Prescribed Anticholinergic Medications Used to Treat Parkinsonian Side Effects of Antipsychotics

| GENERIC NAME | TRADE NAME |
| --- | --- |
| benztropine mesylate | Cogentin |
| biperiden | Akineton |
| diphenhydramine HCl | Allerdryl, Benadryl |
| orphenadrine citrate | Myotrol, Norflex |
| procyclidine HCl | Kemadrin |
| trihexyphenidyl HCl | Artane |

---

#### How to Avoid Overdose

Taking antipsychotic medications exactly as prescribed by a psychiatrist or other physician is the best way to avoid overdosage. Checking the dosage dispensed by a pharmacy against the physician's prescription can also help avoid the rare accidental overdosage. Clear communication between physician and patient about how to take antipsychotic medication and what drugs cannot be combined with the antipsychotic will also help to avoid an overdose. If you don't know how much or how often to take a medication, contact the prescribing physician.

If concentration, memory problems, or confusion makes taking the medication exactly as prescribed difficult, charts documenting dates, doses, and drugs can be helpful. Family members can help make sure a patient receives the proper amount of medication at the proper time intervals. Drug stores often carry *reminder boxes* with compartments for daily medications.

## How to Avoid Addiction

Antipsychotic medications are *not* addicting. Stopping an antipsychotic medication does not usually lead to the development of physical symptoms of withdrawal nor does stopping an antipsychotic medication lead to a craving for the antipsychotic.

Occasionally, discontinuing an antipsychotic medication abruptly can lead to a flare-up of psychotic symptoms such as hallucinations or delusions. This increase or reemergence of symptoms is short-lived and will resolve spontaneously in a few days. For this reason, it is recommended that antipsychotic medication be tapered slowly.

## Use of Antipsychotics During Pregnancy and Breast-Feeding

There is an increased risk of birth defects in infants born to women taking antipsychotics. However, there is also an increased death rate in fetuses of psychotic mothers. It is generally believed that psychotic pregnant women should be treated with antipsychotics only if their symptoms make it absolutely necessary (for example, to ensure the safety of the fetus and the mother).

Jill Price, six months pregnant, with a history of schizophrenia, came to the emergency room and insisted that her baby be "cut out." Jill said that she could feel the baby eating its way through her belly and that the baby would soon reach her heart. She was certain that the baby would then eat a hole in her heart, and this would kill her. When the doctor in the emergency room would not agree to such an operation, Jill beat her fists against her pregnant belly and screamed. In this case, in order to allow Jill to continue her pregnancy safely, she was admitted to the hospital and a small dose of Haldol was prescribed, which successfully treated her delusion.

When antipsychotic medication must be taken by a pregnant woman, it is recommended that she be on the lowest dose possible for the briefest possible time.

Antipsychotic medication is found in the breast milk of women taking such drugs. Because the effects on the baby are unknown, women on antipsychotics are advised not to breast-feed their babies.

## PRECAUTIONS FOR THOSE OVER SIXTY

Individuals over the age of sixty are more likely than younger people to have preexisting medical problems such as glaucoma that can be aggravated by antipsychotic medication. Older individuals are also more likely to have heart conditions, which can be worsened by antipsychotics.

Older men often have enlarged prostate glands and this can result in their being unable to empty their bladders when taking antipsychotic drugs. This is a particular danger in the very old in nursing homes who have difficulty in communicating about their symptoms and discomfort. An examination to determine if the prostate gland is enlarged is important, as is frequent monitoring of urination ability for elderly males taking antipsychotics.

In general, individuals over the age of sixty should be started on a very low dose of antipsychotics; this dose should be increased slowly, with careful monitoring for the development of side effects.

## THE ECONOMICS OF ANTIPSYCHOTIC DRUGS

It is estimated that the *cost* of schizophrenia in the United States is about $11 billion to $20 billion a year. Part of this amount is for the *direct* cost of schizophrenia. This includes the cost of medication, hospitalization, as well as physician and mental health care workers' fees. *Indirect* costs are also part of the cost of schizophrenia. Loss of income of the affected individual, lost work time and decreased productivity of the individual's family, personal and property damage caused by the affected individual, all contribute to this indirect cost of schizophrenia. The treatment of those suffering from schizophrenia with antipsychotic medication has been shown to be massively effective and *cost effective*. In other words, both the reduction of human suffering and a decrease in the costs associated with untreated schizophrenia are remarkable. Studies show that schizophrenia can be treated at much lower cost with antipsychotic medication than with psychotherapy without medication. However, we believe in combining many modes of treatment with our drug therapy, particularly family, group, vocational, and individual supportive care. People with a schizophrenia have a lower chance of being rehospitalized and their hospitalizations tend to be briefer when they are treated with antipsychotic medication. Antipsychotic medication thus has a beneficial effect on the economic costs of schizophrenia as well as the emotional toll that the illness takes on the affected persons, their families, and society.

## Recommended Reading on Psychosis

Torrey, E. Fuller. *Surviving Schizophrenia: A Family Manual*. New York: Harper and Row, 1988.

Walsh, Maryellen. *Schizophrenia: Straight Talk for Families and Friends*. New York: William Morrow and Company, Inc., 1985.

Wender, Paul H. and Donald F. Klein. *Mind, Mood, & Medicine: A Guide to the New Biopsychiatry*. New York: Meridian Books, 1981.

# Chapter 8

# Sedatives and Sleeping Pills

W E spend roughly a third of our lives asleep. By age seventy, most of us will have devoted nearly a quarter of a million hours to sleep. Yet more than one hundred million people in the United States alone have trouble falling asleep. For some, this is only an occasional problem; others experience it virtually every night.

Sleep is a more active state than one might think. When we are asleep, our muscles tense and relax. Our pulse, temperature, and blood pressure rise and fall. The hormones that control our growth and development are secreted into our bloodstreams.

Researchers divide sleep into distinct stages:

• Wakefulness is stage zero.
• Stage one is the twilight zone between sleeping and waking, a stage you might experience if you fell asleep at a lecture, while watching TV, or while performing some repetitive task. During stage one sleep, your muscle tension decreases and your breathing becomes deep and regular. A variety of half-processed thoughts may flow through your mind.

• In stage two, you are definitely asleep. If someone spoke to you or touched you softly, you would probably not wake up. An EEG (electroencephalogram) would reveal occasional bursts of electrical activity in your brain.

• In stage three, your body functions slow down even more. You are sound asleep. An EEG would show large and slow brain waves.

• Stage four is your deepest sleep, the most profound level of unconsciousness. The journey down into stage four sleep usually takes about an hour. Your brain waves are large and slow, similar to stage three. These brain waves are called *sleep spindles*. It is during this stage that you receive your greatest rest.

After you reach stage four, you will begin to drift back upward to the lighter stages (stages one and two), not all the way to full wakefulness but into a more active state called REM sleep. During this state, the pupils move back and forth, producing the so-called *rapid eye movement* that gives this stage its name. In summary, there are five stages of sleep: stages one and two (the lightest stages of quiet sleep), stages three and four (the deepest stages of quiet sleep), and REM, the active, dreaming stage of sleep.

The four stages of quiet sleep described previously are referred to collectively as *non-REM sleep*. During REM sleep, the brain waves resemble those of someone awake. Your large muscles are inactive but your fingers and toes may twitch. Your breathing becomes quick and shallow. During REM sleep, you may have vivid dreams. After spending about ten minutes in REM sleep, you will descend again into the quiet stages of sleep (stages three and four). The entire cycle of REM and non-REM stages takes about ninety minutes. We spend most of the first half of the night in non-REM stages three and four—the deepest stages of quiet sleep. We spend more of the second half in REM sleep. We may go through four or five such REM/non-REM cycles during a normal sleep period.

As we grow older, most of us will need less and less sleep (see Table 1). A newborn may spend as many as eighteen hours per day sleeping, while a child of three or four may spend only nine to ten hours asleep. For an adult, seven or eight hours are usually sufficient. After age sixty-five, six hours a night is usually adequate.

Older people spend less time in REM sleep. By age sixty-five, the lighter sleep stages (stages one and two) increase and your proportion of REM sleep (in contrast to what it was in your teens or twenties) decreases to about a fifth of your total sleep time. Also, as they grow older, most people experience more frequent nighttime awakenings.

TABLE 1

**Patterns of Sleep**

**A Model Night's Sleep in Children, Young Adults, and the Elderly**

CHILDREN

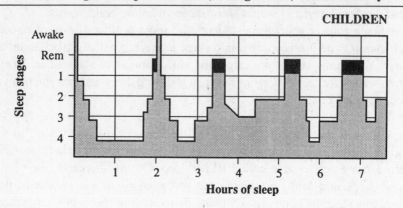

YOUNG ADULTS

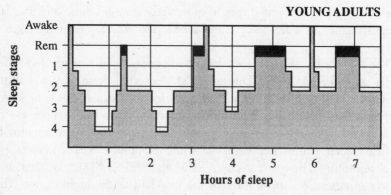

ELDERLY

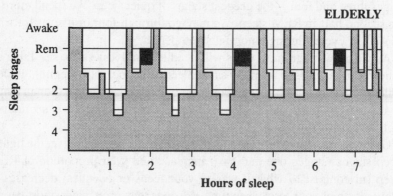

**Source:** Adapted from Kales, A. "Sleep and Dreams: Recent Research on Clinical Aspects." *Annals of Internal Medicine* 68 (May 1968): 1081.

# Sleep Disorders

Sleep disorders fall into four categories:

• Ordinary insomnia: difficulty in falling asleep and staying asleep. Insomnia is one of the disorders of initiating and maintaining sleep (DIMS).
• Disorders of excessive sleepiness (DOES): sleepiness during the day.
• Disorders of sleep/wake schedule (DOSWS). This is common for people who travel across time zones (jet lag) or shift workers. They have problems going to bed or waking up at the desired time.
• Parasomnias are disorders of sleep that occur either during sleep or at the threshold between sleep and wakefulness. Complaints are usually about the anxiety associated with dreams. Nightmares are the most common type of parasomnia. Because medications are not usually prescribed for the other sleep disorders, only insomnia will be discussed in this chapter.

# Insomnia

Most people with sleep problems experience insomnia. Sleep experts have defined three types of insomnia:

• Transient insomnia—affects nearly everyone at least occasionally, e.g., before a trip, an exam, or some other special event. It typically lasts for only one night or, at most, up to three or four nights.
• Short-term insomnia—may last from three or four days to a few weeks. It may occur during particularly stressful times: during moves, after the death of a loved one, following a divorce, loss of a job, while working hard at a new job, or during some other particularly stressful period.
• Chronic or long-term insomnia—may last for months or even years. It can begin at an early age and may last throughout one's life.

Approximately 70 percent of all the insomnias are either transient or short-term. For the 30 percent of insomnia sufferers who experience chronic insomnia, two-thirds can benefit from treatment.

## PSYCHIATRIC DISORDERS ASSOCIATED WITH INSOMNIA

Insomnia is sometimes a symptom of a more extensive medical or psychiatric disorder:

• People who are depressed often experience severe insomnia.

• Those with chronic anxiety, panic attacks, or obsessive-compulsive disorder may find themselves plagued with persistent ideas, thoughts, or impulses that interfere with their ability to fall asleep.

• Other disorders often associated with insomnia include the following:

adjustment disorder with depressed mood
amphetamine withdrawal
cocaine addiction or withdrawal
generalized anxiety disorder
heavy caffeine intake
loss of a loved one (uncomplicated bereavement)
manic-depressive disorder (or bipolar disorder)
mild, chronic mood swings (cyclothymia)
phencyclidine (PCP)-induced mood disorder
posttraumatic stress disorder
premenstrual syndrome (PMS)
schizoaffective disorder
schizophrenic disorder
withdrawal from pain medications
withdrawal from sleeping pills

## MEDICAL DISORDERS ASSOCIATED WITH INSOMNIA

In addition, many medical disorders may cause sleep disturbances. Among the most common problems are:

Alzheimer's syndrome or other primary degenerative dementia
anemia
cancer (many different types)
congestive heart failure
diabetes mellitus
emphysema (chronic obstructive pulmonary disease)
epilepsy and other seizure disorders
heart attack (myocardial infarction)
hepatitis
hyperfunction or hypofunction of the thyroid, parathyroid, pituitary, or
    adrenal gland
irregularity of the heartbeat (cardiac arrhythmias)
kidney disease
malaria

migraine headaches
multiple sclerosis
Parkinson's disease
pheochromocytoma
pneumonia
postoperative states
stroke
systemic lupus erythematosus
tuberculosis

## TREATMENT

If you or a family member or someone you know is having problems sleeping, and it is interfering with either your work or relationships, talk to your physician. He or she will conduct a careful physical exam and rule out medical problems or medications that may be producing the insomnia. Your physician can then refer you to either a sleep specialist or a psychiatrist for further evaluation and treatment.

# Sleeping Pills

Insomnia is not a disease, and sleeping pills are not a cure, as they do not produce normal sleep. Sleeping pills do work, at least in the short term, but those who use them inappropriately may pay a considerable price. Most experts agree that sleeping pills are one of the most overused types of psychiatric drugs.

Chances are that you have taken a sleeping pill at least once in your life. Residents of the United States take enough sleeping pills annually to put every American man, woman, and child to sleep for 200 hours. Nearly thirty million doses of sleep-producing medication, both prescription and over-the-counter, are taken each night.

About eight million people in the United States use prescription sleeping pills. Even greater numbers (twenty to twenty-two million people) use nonprescription sleep medications.

A typical sleeping medication will speed the onset of sleep in people with insomnia by five to twenty minutes, decrease the number of nighttime awakenings, and extend total sleep time. But in the long run, people who take sleeping pills for more than a few days usually end up sleeping less and complaining more about their sleep problems.

Sleeping pills are often mistakenly prescribed. Physicians give about 30 percent of prescriptions for sleeping pills to people whose primary problem is psychiatric, about 25 percent to patients with physical medical problems, and 18 percent to people with ill-defined, vague symptoms. Only about 15 percent of prescriptions for sleeping medications are given to people with primary sleep disorders.

If you are hospitalized, you may be given a sleeping pill whether you want it or not. Roughly 50 percent of hospital patients are routinely given sleeping medications. An estimated 20 percent of those given a sleeping pill while in the hospital will later become dependent on that medication.

Most sleeping pills suppress the deepest, most restful stages of non-REM sleep (stages three and four), as well as REM sleep, even when taken as directed. When these drugs are misused, they can completely destroy normal sleep patterns.

Sleep researchers believe that 50 percent of the patients who take sleeping pills for their insomnia become *worse* as a result. Unfortunately, the negative effects may not stop immediately when you stop taking the pills. Even after withdrawal, your healthy sleep patterns can be disrupted for several weeks. An estimated 20 percent of all cases of insomnia are caused by withdrawal from sleeping medications.

Sleeping pills should not be considered a long-term solution for insomnia. They are effective only when used for a few nights at a time. After three to seven nights, most sleeping pills lose their punch. People who take sleeping pills for more than a week take just as long to fall asleep, wake up just as often, and sleep no longer than someone with the same problem who has *not* taken any medication. A major study of health habits demonstrated that people who use sleeping pills regularly face a 50 percent higher risk of accidental death. Taking sleeping medication is the third most common means of suicide. And sleeping pills are implicated in a third of all drug-related suicide attempts or deaths.

## WHO SHOULD USE SLEEPING PILLS?

These medications should be used only for a specific reason, such as episodic emotional turmoil associated with a traumatic life event—the death of a loved one, a major move, a new job, etc. They should be taken for no more than one to seven days.

## YOU SHOULD NOT USE SLEEPING PILLS IF:

• You have a chronic breathing problem. Sleeping medication can decrease your brain's ability to regulate your breathing.

• You have kidney or liver disease. In most cases, sleeping pills are metabolized by your liver and excreted by your kidneys. Problems with either of these organs mean that drugs will stay in your body longer. This may cause serious difficulties.

• You are pregnant. Some sleeping medications have been associated with birth defects.

• You are over sixty-five. The older you are, the more time it takes to metabolize and excrete medications. Some longer-acting sleeping medications remain in your body for even longer periods of time, causing confusion and daytime drowsiness. Use of sleeping medications in the elderly is a frequent cause of falls and broken bones.

• You have been drinking alcohol. The effects of sleeping pills and alcohol are increased when combined. This dangerous combination can result in overdose, medical complications, and even death.

## WHAT ARE THE DANGERS OF SLEEPING MEDICATIONS?

There are some very real dangers of relying on either prescription or nonprescription sleep medications. These include:

• Fatal overdoses, especially when combined with alcohol or other drugs that act on the central nervous system.

• Harmful interactions with other prescription medications.

• Interference with breathing, especially in people with chronic respiratory problems.

• Impairment of daytime coordination, memory, driving skills, and thinking.

• Development of physical or psychological dependence.

• Development of tolerance: you need to take larger and larger doses of the drug to achieve the same effect.

• Disruption of normal sleep stages.

• Worsening of your initial sleep problem.

• Potentially harmful effects on your kidneys, liver, and lungs.

• Confusion, hallucinations, and other psychiatric disturbances, especially if you are elderly.

• Possible birth defects.

• Difficulty in awakening to a fire alarm, a crying child, or any other nighttime crisis.

## EVALUATING SLEEPING MEDICATIONS

To evaluate the potential benefits and drawbacks of a sleeping medication, you should ask your doctor several key questions:

• *How long will this drug remain in my body?* The term *half-life* refers to the amount of time it takes for half of the drug that you have taken to leave your body. If the drug has a half-life of six hours, as does triazolam (Halcion), for example, half of the drug will still be in your body six hours later. Some sleeping pills, e.g., flurazepam (Dalmane), can have half-lives of up to seventy-two hours. These drugs are especially likely to produce lingering aftereffects, since half or more of the medication will remain in your body for several days. Some of the barbiturates and the long-acting benzodiazepines have half-lives of up to four days. These drugs can impair your daytime functioning, making you drowsy and unable to concentrate. This is a special problem in the elderly, whose livers and kidneys don't function as effectively as in younger people.

• *What kinds of drug interactions should I be concerned about?* Two or more different medications can combine within your body to enhance, slow, or oppose one another. For instance, alcohol and sleeping pills, taken together, can depress your ability to breathe. Sleeping pills may also interact with medications taken for medical problems. Barbiturates stimulate liver enzymes that metabolize other drugs. If you are taking propranolol (Inderal), a drug used to treat high blood pressure, taking a barbiturate may decrease the amount of Inderal in your blood, causing your blood pressure to rise to dangerously high levels.

• *How will this drug be eliminated from my body?* If you know how a medication is eliminated from your body and how much of it leaves unchanged, you can identify the organs involved in metabolizing the substance. The liver and kidneys play vital roles in eliminating sleeping pills from the body. Most of the sleeping medications are metabolized in the liver and excreted by the kidneys in the urine. Any problem with either of these organs may slow the rate of elimination, resulting in higher blood levels. The sedative effects of these drugs will thus be prolonged.

# Benzodiazepines

The benzodiazepine antianxiety drugs are used to treat generalized anxiety disorders, panic disorder, and insomnia. (The benzodiazepine drug family is discussed in detail in Chapter 4.) The first of the benzodiazepines approved for use as a sleeping pill was flurazepam (Dalmane). Two recently developed benzodiapines are also used principally as sleeping pills: temazepam (Restoril) and triazolam (Halcion). Many other benzodiazepines have sleep-producing properties, even though they are usually prescribed to treat anixety. Benzodiazepines are metabolized by the liver and excreted by the kidneys.

## FLURAZEPAM (DALMANE)

Flurazepam has a half-life of between two and four days, but it tends to build up in the body with successive daily use. Some patients report that flurazepam works better on the second or third night than on the first night. Flurazepam may also continue to have sleep-producing effects for a night or two after you stop taking it. If you take flurazepam consecutively for seven to ten nights, the cumulative blood levels of flurazepam on the seventh or tenth mornings will be four to six times higher than on the first morning. With continued use, people taking flurazepam will have as much of the drug in their systems during the day as they have at night.

## TEMAZEPAM (RESTORIL)

The principal advantage of temazepam is its shorter half-life, approximately twelve hours. But since temazepam is absorbed very slowly, people taking this drug may not fall asleep rapidly afterward. Temazepam is excreted from the body very quickly, with less effect on the user the following day.

## TRIAZOLAM (HALCION)

This drug is rapidly absorbed, producing the quick onset of sleep. Like temazepam, triazolam (with a half-life of between three and six hours) is cleared quickly from the body. Some clinicians recommend triazolam to prevent transatlantic or transpacific jet lag. A major problem with triazolam is that patients may experience memory problems the morning following a dose. For instance, one executive who took triazolam on a plane to Europe didn't remember renting a car or checking into his hotel the next day. For information on the controversy about Halcion, see pages 570–71.

## COMPARISONS AMONG THESE THREE DRUGS

Both flurazepam and triazolam can speed the onset of sleep in people with insomnia. All three of these drugs (1) reduce body movements and total awakenings at night, and (2) lower the number of shifts in sleep stages. However, all three suppress dreaming (REM stage) and produce a lighter than natural sleep (decrease stage three and four sleep). Triazolam and temazepam impair daytime function less severely than flurazepam. Since daytime drowsiness is often particularly severe in older people, flurazepam should not be taken by those over sixty-five.

## Who Should *Not* Take These Drugs?

• Do not take benzodiazepines if you are pregnant. These drugs produce an increased risk of birth defects, especially if taken during the first three months of pregnancy.

• These drugs should not be used by children. There have been no studies of the effects of these drugs on children.

## Use with Alcohol

None of the members of the benzodiazepine family—this includes flurazepam, triazolam, and temazepam—should be used with alcohol. This combination has a profoundly negative effect on both behavior and thinking—and especially on driving.

## Can These Drugs Be Misused?

Suicide by overdose of flurazepam, triazolam, or temazepam is relatively rare. A few reported deaths have been attributed to extremely high doses. However, these drugs can kill you if they are combined with alcohol.

As with all the benzodiazepines, the long-term use of triazolam, temazepam, and flurazepam can lead to psychological dependence and physical addiction. Stopping these medications after several weeks may produce severe withdrawal symptoms, e.g., nervous agitation and severe anxiety. Those who have been taking high doses of these medications for a long period of time will need to taper off these drugs gradually. This should be done under a physician's care. If you have been taking high doses for some time, do not simply discontinue these drugs on your own. Stopping these medications abruptly can produce seizures and delirium.

If you use these drugs for a week or more, you may find that when you stop the drug, your sleep is even more gravely disturbed than it was before you first took the drug. This is called *rebound insomnia*. If rebound insomnia occurs, taking benzodiazepines again will not solve the problem. Nondrug treatments or a gradual tapering of the benzodiazepine will be required.

## BENEFITS

Benzodiazepines do not depress breathing, blood pressure, and other vital functions as much as the barbiturates do. They are much less likely to cause damage or death in the case of overdose.

# Barbiturates

Barbiturates are classified by their duration of action in the body. The short-acting barbiturates, such as methohexital (Brevital), have half-lives of three to eight hours and are used primarily as anesthetic agents. Butabarbital (Butisol) and phenobarbital are used mainly as anticonvulsants and, to a much lesser extent, antianxiety agents. The intermediate duration barbiturates amobarital (Amytal), pentobarbital (Nembutal), and secobarbital (Seconal) have tradionally been used as sleeping pills. However, their use has greatly diminished with the development of benzodiazepines. These three drugs have half-lives of approximately one to two days.

## DRUG INTERACTIONS

The barbiturates can diminish the effectiveness of normal doses of many medications that are metabolized by the kidneys. This includes many blood-thinning drugs (anticoagulants), antidepressants, antiseizure medications, and many others. If you are taking a barbiturate, be sure it does not interact with any other drug.

## RISKS

There are a great many risks involved in taking barbiturates. Most experts currently believe that these risks are so great that barbiturates should not be used as sleeping pills. Although they usually produce less of a drug hangover than the longer-acting benzodiazepines, they have great addiction potential. In large doses, they can cause respiratory depression, kidney failure, circulatory collapse, and coma. This combination can be deadly. If barbiturates are taken with alcohol, their toxic effects on the body are greatly enhanced.

## WHAT TO DO IF YOU ARE ADDICTED TO BARBITURATES

If you are addicted to barbiturates, you will need a doctor's help. Since there is some risk of delirium, or even death, withdrawing from these drugs is often best accomplished in the hospital.

## BENEFITS

The only currently recommended use of barbiturates instead of benzodiazepines as a sleeping pill is in elderly people who require sleep medication for a brief period of time (less than a week) and in those elderly patients who were successfully treated with barbiturates in the past.

# Nonbarbiturate Hypnotics

Some of the nonbarbiturate hypnotics—methaqualone (Quaalude), ethchlorvynol (Placidyl), glutethimide (Doriden)—were developed principally in the hopes of avoiding some of the adverse effects of the barbiturates, particularly the high capacity for addiction. Unfortunately, except for chloral hydrate, nonbarbiturate hypnotics turned out to be just as addictive as the barbiturates.

## METHAQUALONE (QUAALUDE)

Methaqualone will usually produce sleep within thirty minutes. It provides sleep that lasts for five to eight hours with little drug hangover the next day. It is not effective for more than two weeks. Drug dependence develops quickly, and this substance is frequently abused. The pills are sold on the street as *ludes*, or *quads*.

Methaqualone is believed to cause birth defects if taken by pregnant women. It is not recommended for use by children. Even a short period of use (one month) can produce serious dependence. Taken with alcohol, methaqualone can seriously impair vital functions and may depress a person's ability to breathe. Methaqualone should not be used as a sleep medication because of its high addiction and abuse potential and because of the severe and often deadly complications associated with alcohol and overdose. Fortunately, methaqualone is no longer commercially available in the United States.

## GLUTETHIMIDE (DORIDEN)

Glutethimide was introduced in the mid-1950s as a potential replacement for the barbiturates. It has proved to be just as toxic and addictive. Glutethimide is absorbed poorly and somewhat erratically from the intestinal tract. Although it may be used to treat insomnia for three to seven days, it causes daytime sleepiness and may severely impair next-day ability to drive or to engage in other activities requiring mental alertness or physical coordination. The usual adult dose is 250 to 500 mg. Doses of 5 g may produce severe intoxication, and doses from 10 to 20 g can be deadly.

Like the barbiturates, glutethimide can impair a person's ability to breathe. It also has severe effects on the heart. Glutethimide can cause muscle spasm and convulsions. A person who has taken an overdose and who has apparently recovered from a coma may suddenly lapse into unconsciousness again. Of those who take a deliberate overdose and reach the emergency room alive, the mortality rate is thirteen times higher than for barbiturates. In one series of over two hundred nonnarcotic drug overdoses, glutethimide was the number-one cause of death. Because of the serious dangers of addiction and overdose, glutethimide should not be routinely used as a sleeping medication. Because of its high addiction potential and its potentially deadly side effects, many physicians believe that glutethimide should not be used under any circumstances.

## ETHCHLORVYNOL (PLACIDYL)

This widely used prescription medication may improve sleep onset, but the sleep-inducing effects last for only five hours. People taking ethchlorvynol frequently experience confusion and severe emotional distress the next morning.

Ethchlorvynol is highly addictive and can be toxic in doses only slightly above a therapeutic dose. Toxic symptoms include coordination problems, tremor, confusion, slurred speech, and muscle weakness. Withdrawal from the medication may produce delirium, seizures, memory disturbance, tremor, nausea, and vomiting.

Because of its relatively limited and short-lived benefits and its high potential for addiction and toxic effects, ethchlorvynol is not recommended for routine use. It is specifically contraindicated in pregnant women, children, people taking anticoagulant drugs, people with impaired kidneys or a damaged liver, and in the elderly and the debilitated.

### CHLORAL HYDRATE

Chloral hydrate is the oldest sleeping medication currently in use. It is one of the ingredients in a Mickey Finn, the supposed knock-out drink surreptitiously slipped to a whole generation of detective heroes in movies made in the 1930s and 1940s. Chloral hydrate does in fact produce sleep, although not as quickly as Hollywood writers would have us believe. And Humphrey Bogart notwithstanding, it rarely produces a drug hangover the next day.

The usual therapeutic dose of 500 mg to 1 g produces few side effects and rarely if ever produces daytime drowsiness. Chloral hydrate can be mildly habit-forming if taken on a regular basis, but dependence is much less of a problem today than it was in the 1800s, when chloral hydrate abuse ran to epidemic proportions. Because chloral hydrate may increase the action of certain anticoagulant medications, it must be prescribed with great caution to patients taking these drugs. It should not be used by those with impaired kidney or liver function.

#### WHO SHOULD TAKE THIS DRUG

Chloral hydrate can be a useful drug of second choice for patients who need a sleeping pill but cannot take benzodiazepines. This includes the young, the elderly, or those whose physical conditions preclude the use of other drugs. Some physicians prefer chloral hydrate over the benzodiazepines; it is less addictive, and less likely to produce daytime drowsiness.

#### RISKS

Doses of chloral hydrate as low as ten times the therapeutic dosage may result in severe or lethal complications. Alcohol drastically increases the danger associated with this medication.

## Antihistamines

Antihistamines were originally used to treat allergies, motion sickness, Parkinson's disease, and the side effects of antipsychotic medication. Many antihistamines produce drowsiness; this makes them ideally suited for use as sleeping pills.

Two antihistamines frequently used as sleeping pills are hydroxyzine (Atarax, Vistaril) and diphenhydramine (Benadryl). Some clinicians feel that these medications are safer or milder than other sleeping pills, such as the benzodiazepines or barbiturates. Others disagree, insisting that the safety of antihistamines used as sleeping pills has not been adequately studied.

## RISKS

Antihistamines can produce nausea, vomiting, headaches, dizziness, coordination problems, blurred vision, tightness of the chest, wheezing, and occasional disturbances of the heartbeat (arrhythmias).

## BENEFITS

As sleeping pills, antihistamines do offer certain advantages: Unlike most other sleeping medications, they pose no risk of addiction. They are rapidly absorbed and metabolized, typically inducing sleep soon after they are taken. Because they are cleared from the body quickly, there is little daytime drowsiness.

Many physicians use antihistamines as the short-term sleeping pill of first choice for patients with minor sleep difficulties and for those who have trouble falling asleep while in the hospital. However, some psychiatrists feel that they are not as effective as benzodiazepines in inducing sleep.

# Nonprescription Sleep Aids

## L-TRYPTOPHAN

L-tryptophan is not a drug in the ordinary sense. It is an amino acid found naturally within the body. High concentrations of tryptophan are found in milk and other common food products.

A recent review of its effectiveness as a sleeping pill found that L-tryptophan may induce sleep if taken in doses ranging from 1 to 15 g shortly before bedtime. For patients with chronic insomnia and for those who require long-term treatment, doses of approximately 2 g should be taken. At this dose, L-tryptophan has relatively few adverse side effects and is usually well tolerated. However, at higher doses, above 5 g, some people may experience nausea and vomiting. Some patients with chronic insomnia find that they can fall asleep easily if they switch back and forth between a 2 g dose of L-tryptophan and a hypnotic medication (such as Halcion) on alternate nights.

L-tryptophan takes a bit longer to induce sleep than other sleep medications. You should take it about forty-five minutes before you want to fall asleep. L-tryptophan is eliminated from the body quite rapidly, has little effect on sleep stages, and does not produce daytime drowsiness. It is not addictive. Like other sleep medications, L-tryptophan is not recommended for regular use. It should only be used for a short period of time until more permanent solutions are found.

Some people suggest that drinking a warm glass of milk or eating foods rich in L-tryptophan before bedtime is equally effective. However, you would have to drink more than six glasses of milk to achieve a dose of 1 g of L-tryptophan, the amount formerly recommended in dietary supplement form to induce sleep. Nonetheless, many people find that much smaller amounts in natural forms are just as effective in inducing sleep.

*Note of caution:* For many years, L-tryptophan was manufactured and sold as a dietary supplement in pharmacies and health food stores around the country. Tens of thousands of Americans took L-tryptophan in the dietary supplement form for a variety of purposes including its effects as an antidepressant and sleeping aid. Recently, however, L-tryptophan was directly linked to a nationwide outbreak of a relatively rare blood disorder called eosinophilia-myalgia syndrome (EMS). At the time of the writing of this book, the Food and Drug Administration has removed L-tryptophan completely from the American market—the direct result of over fourteen hundred cases of L-tryptophan–related EMS that have resulted in approximately twenty deaths. At the present time, we do not know the exact cause of this outbreak; some have suggested that the problem could derive from impurities in the chemicals that go into the manufacture of L-tryptophan. If the outbreak of EMS turns out to be the result of a contaminant or a manufacturing impurity, it is likely that once the problem is eradicated, L-tryptophan will be returned to the market. At the present time and until such time as the exact cause of this L-tryptophan–related side effect is understood and corrected, our readers are advised not to take L-tryptophan in the dietary supplement form.

## NONPRESCRIPTION ANTIHISTAMINES

Like Benadryl and Atarax, the nonprescription antihistamines may help induce sleep by producing drowsiness. Although originally developed to relieve hay fever and allergic reactions, they may have some limited benefit as a sleep aid. The most common antihistamine used in over-the-counter (OTC) sleep aids is pyrilamine maleate. Most OTC sleep aids contain a very low level—25 mg—of this substance. Another OTC product contains doxylamine succinate, an antihistamine also associated with the production of drowsiness.

The adverse side effects of the OTC sleep medications and some OTC antihistamine sleep aids are similar to those of Benadryl and Atarax. They may produce nausea, vomiting, hallucinations, delirium, and convulsions if taken in very high doses. See Table 2 for a list of the most commonly prescribed OTC sleep medications.

TABLE 2

**Over-the-Counter Nonprescription Sleep Aids**

| BRAND NAME (MANUFACTURER) | ACTIVE INGREDIENTS PER TABLET |
|---|---|
| Compōz (Jeffery Martin) | pyrilamine maleate (antihistamine) 25 mg |
| Nervine (Miles) | diphenhydramine hydrochloride 25 mg |
| Nytol (Block) | diphenhydramine hydrochloride 25 mg |
| Quiet Tabs (Commerce) | pyrilamine maleate 23 mg |
| Quiet World (Whitehall) | acetaminophen 162.5 mg |
| | aspirin 227.5 mg |
| | pyrilamine maleate 25 mg |
| Relax-U-Caps (Columbia Medical) | pyrilamine maleate 25 mg |
| Sedacaps (Vitarine) | pyrilamine maleate 25 mg |
| Sleep-Eze (Whitehall) | diphenhydramine hydrochloride 25 mg |
| Sominex 2 (Beecham Products) | diphenhydramine hydrochloride 25 mg |
| Somicaps (Beecham Products) | pyrilamine maleate 25 mg |
| Unisom (Leeming) | doxylamine succinate, 25 mg |

*Note:* None of these medications is indicated for prolonged use, or for use in children under twelve, in women who are pregnant or nursing, in men with an enlarged prostate gland, and in people with asthma or glaucoma. Avoid drinking alcohol. If taking a prescription medication, consult your physician before using.

## OTHER NONPRESCRIPTION SLEEP AIDS

If you watch television late at night, you have probably seen those commercials in which an actor takes a brand name nonprescription sleeping pill, yawns once or twice, shuts off the light, and immediately falls asleep. Such commercials notwithstanding, a recent FDA review concluded that except for nonprescription antihistamines, described above, there were no safe and effective OTC sleeping pills. The FDA concluded that certain ingredients in the OTC preparations have *not* been generally recognized as safe and effective. These ingredients are:

• Bromides. These drugs displace the normal chloride ion in the body with a bromide, which may produce depression of the central nervous system. They tend to accumulate in the body when used regularly and pose a serious hazard to health.

• Methapyrilene. This has been identified as a factor in the development of cancer in laboratory rats. The data are inconclusive but frightening. Methapyrilene may be effective in inducing sleep, but may also interfere with brain impulses that regulate basic bodily functions.

• Scopolamine. This occurs naturally as a derivative of belladonna and is frequently abused by people who are addicted to illicit drugs. Even in small doses, scopolamine can cause delusions and delirium. Other side effects include dryness of the mouth, blurred vision, sensitivity to light, cardiac arrhythmias, worsening of acute glaucoma, constipation, urinary retention, walking problems, and difficulty in regulating body temperature.

• Miscellaneous compounds. Other OTC sleep medications contain acetaminophen, aspirin, passion flower extract, vitamin $B_I$ (thiamine), and other medications. There are no data to support the efficacy of these agents in enhancing sleep.

As a result of these findings, the FDA ordered changes in the advertising for OTC sleeping pills containing these ingredients. No longer can a package insert state that the drugs help you relax so you can fall asleep, are nonhabit-forming, or are guaranteed to act fast. They also cannot state that they produce sleep that is natural, normal, or sound.

# Prescription Medications Not to Be Used as Sleeping Pills

### ANTIPSYCHOTICS

Occasionally, antipsychotic medications may be prescribed as sleeping pills. Among those producing the greatest degree of sedation are mesoridazine (Serentil) or chloropromazine (Thorazine). These and other antipsychotic medications should not be used as sleeping pills.

These medications can produce severe side effects, such as tardive dyskinesia (see Chapter 7), hypotension (a rapid drop in blood pressure when attempting to stand up), inability to pass urine, dry mouth, blurred vision, and confusion. Yet antipsychotic medications are frequently prescribed to elderly patients because of their sleep-producing properties. They are also sometimes used to treat mental confusion in elderly people with mild dementia. Antipsychotic medication should not be used in such situations.

Elderly people are frequently brought to the emergency room because of confusion, delirium, and other problems that turn out to be the adverse side effects of antipsychotic drugs they were given as sleeping pills. These drugs may also produce low blood pressure; this can, in turn, cause dangerous falls, especially during the night.

### ANTIDEPRESSANTS

People with severe depression frequently have trouble sleeping through the night. They may also experience early morning awakening and, to a lesser extent, problems falling asleep (especially those with anxiety symptoms). While some antidepressants—e.g., amitriptyline (Elavil), doxepin (Sinequan), and trazodone (Desyrel)—can have profoundly sedating effects, these drugs should not be used as sleeping pills. Low doses are ineffective and high doses pose a substantial risk of side effects (e.g., dry mouth, blurred vision, urinary retention, confusion, and delirium). There is also a considerable risk of overdose with these drugs.

## Sedatives and Sleeping Pills

### WHEN AND HOW TO TAKE THESE DRUGS

Table 3 lists the most commonly used sedatives and sleeping pills. The dosages shown are those for a healthy middle-aged adult of normal size. If you are over sixty-five, you may need a smaller dose. Only the antihistamine sleeping pills—Atarax, Vistaril, and Benadryl—should be given to children. When using these medications with children between the ages of six and twelve, a pediatrician should be consulted. Sleeping pills should not be given to children less than six years of age.

Most sleeping pills should be taken thirty minutes before bedtime. Exception: Restoril is absorbed slowly and should be taken approximately one hour before retiring.

### HOW TO STORE THESE DRUGS

All these medications should be kept away from children. They should be kept in a sealed container.

### OVERDOSE

When taken in overdose, the benzodiazepines have not usually been associated with death or serious side effects. The barbiturates are lethal, as are the

## TABLE 3
### Sedatives and Sleeping Pills

| Brand Name | Generic Name | Dosage Form | Usual Daily Dosage | Approximate Half-Life |
|---|---|---|---|---|
| *Benzodiazepine Hypnotics* | | | | |
| Dalmane | flurazepam | capsules 15, 30 mg | 15–30 mg | 3–4 days |
| Restoril | temazepam | capsules 15, 30 mg | 15–30 mg | 9–12 hours |
| Halcion | triazolam | tablets 0.125, 0.25 mg | 0.125–0.25 mg | 3–6 hours |
| *Barbiturates* | | | | |
| Amytal | amobarbital | tablets 15, 30, 50, 100 MG<br>capsules 65, 200 mg<br>concentrate 44 mg/5 cc | 50–200 mg | 1–2 days |
| Nembutal | phenobarbital | capsules 30, 50, 100 mg<br>concentrate 20 mg/5 cc<br>suppositories 30, 60, 120, 200 mg | | |
| Seconal | secobarbital | capsules 50, 100 mg<br>suppositories 30, 60, 120, 200 mg | 100–200 mg | 1–2 days |

| | | | | |
|---|---|---|---|---|
| *Nonbarbiturate Hypnotics* | | | | |
| Quaalude | methaqualone | no longer available | | |
| none | chloral hydrate | capsules 250, 500 mg<br>concentrate 500 mg/cc | 500–1,000 mg | 8–12 hours |
| Placidyl | ethchlorvynol | capsules 100, 200, 500, 750 mg | 500–750 mg | 10–20 hours |
| Doriden | glutethimide | tablets 250, 500 mg | 250–500 mg | 10–20 hours |
| *Antihistamines* | | | | |
| Atarax | hydroxyzine hydrochloride | tablets 10, 25, 50, 100 mg<br>concentrate 10 mg/5 cc | 75–400 mg | 4–6 hours |
| Vistaril | hydroxyzine pamoate | tablets 25, 50, 100 mg<br>concentrate 25 mg/5 cc | 200–400 mg | 4–6 hours |
| Benadryl | diphenhydramine | capsules 25, 50 mg | 50–100 mg | 4–6 hours |

nonbarbiturate hypnotics. The antihistamines, if taken in high doses, can cause confusion, delirium, and agitation.

## BEGINNING DRUG THERAPY

Your sleep environment should be conducive to sleep. Loud noises, light, and other distractions may still make it difficult to fall asleep.

Do not expect the medication to put you to sleep if taken during the day. If taken at a time other than your normal sleep time, it will merely make you drowsy. These drugs work most effectively when taken shortly before your normal sleep time.

## LONG-TERM USE

Withdrawal from the benzodiazepine, barbiturate, and nonbarbiturate hypnotic sleeping pills listed in Table 3 can be as difficult as withdrawal from narcotics. If you have taken one or more of these pills for a long period of time (or even for as little as several weeks), you may well be physiologically and psychologically addicted. Sudden withdrawal is dangerous. It may not be wise to stop the drug abruptly. Withdrawal guidelines for the various categories of drugs are given below, but these are only guidelines. If you are taking an addictive sleeping pill, we strongly advise you to seek professional advice on the proper means of withdrawing from the drug.

If you have been taking one of the barbiturates for a long period of time, this medication needs to be withdrawn quite slowly to prevent seizures or delirium. In some cases, if you have been taking a barbiturate for a long period at a high dose, your physician may hospitalize you. The shorter-acting benzodiazepines—especially triazolam (Halcion), and the antianxiety benzodiazepine Xanax (alprazolam; see Chapter 4)—have been associated with seizures if withdrawn too quickly. Sudden withdrawal after prolonged use of a barbiturate or benzodiazepine can also produce other symptoms: insomnia, anxiety, stomach cramps, nausea, vomiting, weakness, hallucinations, hypertension, and nightmares. You should never stop sleeping medications on your own. Consult your physician, who will stabilize your dosage at a consistent nightly dose and who will withdraw you from it very gradually. For instance, for the faster-acting benzodiazepine agents (Halcion or Xanax), a recommended decrease in dosage is 10 percent per week. A more rapid withdrawal rate may be achieved with other medications, usually a decrease of one therapeutic dose per week. For instance, if you were taking 60 mg of flurazepam (Dalmane) or 60 mg of Nembutal a night, a reduction of 15 mg per week may be used.

Even if you have been taking a benzodiazepine or barbiturate for a short period of time, you will experience some worsening of sleep disturbance within the first two or three nights after stopping it. For the longer-acting benzodiazepines, such as flurazepam (Dalmane) or barbiturates (Seconal), the sleep problems may last for as long as a week. Instead of restarting the benzodiazepine, try an antihistamine such as Vistaril or Benadryl for a few days. If this is not successful, then the benzodiazepine or barbiturate may have to be restarted and slowly tapered.

## SYMPTOMS OF WITHDRAWAL FROM SLEEPING PILLS

During each stage of the withdrawal process, you should anticipate sleep problems. Since benzodiazepines and barbiturates would have been suppressing REM sleep, you may experience vivid and bizarre nightmares. They will not be permanent. They are just temporary signs that you are weaning yourself from the medication. This process may take four to six weeks, depending upon the dosage and type of medication. Although this may be a long process, approximately 20 percent of cases of insomnia may be cured by simple withdrawal from medication.

## RECOMMENDED EXAMINATIONS PRIOR TO TAKING SEDATIVES AND SLEEPING PILLS

If you have a medical record, your physician should obtain it and read it thoroughly.

*History and Physical*
- complete medical history
- complete physical examination
- mental status examination
- neurologic assessment

*Urine Tests*
- urinalysis
- urine drug screen
- twenty-four-hour urine catecholamines

*Blood Tests*
- complete blood count
- serum electrolytes
- blood urea nitrogen

- calcium
- uric acid
- alkaline phosphatase
- total bilirubin
- SGOT
- SGPT
- T3
- T4
- TSH (if warranted by positive findings)
- serum catecholamines

*Other Tests*
- sleep-lab referral
- chest X ray
- EKG
- thyroid scan

## RECOMMENDED PERIODIC EXAMINATIONS WHILE TAKING THESE DRUGS

As emphasized previously, long-term use of these drugs is not recommended; therefore, periodic examinations should not be needed.

## USE OF SLEEP MEDICATIONS IN THE ELDERLY

As we grow older, we spend less time sleeping. When we do sleep, we sleep less soundly—and dream less.

Sleep problems are most common in older people. An estimated 20 to 45 percent of all sleeping pills are prescribed for people over sixty. Because of the physical changes involved in aging, sleeping pills have a much stronger and more prolonged effect on older people. Older people are often given sleeping pills they do not need. This is indeed unfortunate, for when sleeping pills are routinely and uncritically prescribed for older people—as they are in many nursing homes—underlying and often treatable physical and psychiatric illnesses are frequently ignored.

## SLEEP MEDICATION AND SLEEP APNEA

An estimated 5 to 10 percent of all cases of insomnia are caused by a breathing problem called sleep apnea. In this condition, the brain fails to send impulses through the nervous system to the diaphragm to maintain breathing. People who have sleep apnea may complain of lighter, fragmented sleep during the night. Since the control centers in the brain are not functioning properly to begin with, the use of sleep medication may further suppress the body's ability to breathe. This can be fatal.

Sleep apnea is most common in the elderly. Some experts believe that the recent increase in deaths of the elderly is a result of prescribing sleeping pills for people with sleep apnea.

People who have respiratory problems due to lung disease, such as emphysema or other chronic obstructive pulmonary disease, should not be prescribed sleep medication. Studies have shown that the respiratory drive in these patients is significantly reduced if sleep medications are used.

## Who Should Receive a Sleep Laboratory Evaluation

There are now modern, up-to-date sleep laboratories in most major cities. The Association of Sleep Disorders Centers, in Rochester, Minn., was organized in 1976 to establish standards and to act as a certifying body for these facilities and their staff. Sleep centers have the sophisticated equipment needed to perform night-long recordings of various physiological functions (polysomnograms). Physicians are usually on call during these tests.

Your physician may refer you to a sleep center if you have a sleep problem that cannot be attributed to either physical or psychiatric problems and if your problem has not been relieved by drug treatment or non-drug treatment. See Sidebar 1 for information on what to expect at a sleep center.

## How to Avoid Overdose and Addiction

The best way to avoid overdose is to take any sleep medication in the doses prescribed and for only one to seven days. The longer you use the medication, the higher the dose you will need to achieve the desired effect. *You should never drink alcohol with a benzodiazepine, barbiturate, nonbarbiturate hypnotic, or antihistamine sleeping pill.*

These same procedures will help you avoid addiction.

## Use During Pregnancy and Breast-Feeding

Benzodiazepine, barbiturate, nonbarbiturate hypnotic, and antihistamine sleeping pills should not be used during pregnancy, especially during the first trimester. Several of these medications are associated with birth defects. Even though some of these agents are *not* associated with birth

## Sidebar 1: What to Expect at a Sleep Center

Sleep medicine is one of the newest medical specialties. Two decades ago, there were only a few special facilities for people with sleep problems. Now there are more than one hundred clinical sleep disorders centers in the United States where experts in a variety of fields—psychiatry, neurology, respiratory medicine, urology, and ear, nose, and throat surgery—work together to solve sleep problems.

Sometimes your sleep history alone—for example, years of waking up screaming in the night—will pinpoint exactly what the problem is. If your primary complaint is excessive daytime sleepiness, you might undergo a daytime procedure called a *Multiple Sleep Latency Test*. At two-hour intervals throughout the day, you will be hooked up to a polysomnograph—a machine that monitors brain waves, heart rhythm, respiration, and other bodily functions—and allowed to nap.

For other sleep complaints, you may have to undergo an all-night sleep evaluation. This test involves no injections, no anesthetics, no incisions, no X rays, and no discomfort other than the slight initial irritation of the electrodes attached to your face and scalp. All you have to do is sleep. If you're afraid that you won't be able to sleep in an unfamiliar setting, be assured that many others have felt the same way. Sleep specialists can recognize and discount most "first-nighter" effects.

You will come to the sleep center in the late evening, several hours before your usual bedtime. Your bedroom will be comfortable and quiet, with an intercom so that you can speak to a technician at any time in the night. You can bring your own pajamas, pillow, and nighttime reading material.

Once you're ready for bed, technicians will attach several electrodes to your face and body. These are placed on the skin, usually over an ointment dabbed on the skin to form a better seal. All are arranged in pairs, so that if one falls off during the night, the other will serve as a backup. While they don't hurt, the electrodes may feel irritating at first, like insects that have landed on your face.

Two electrodes are placed on the chin to record muscle tension; two at the corner of the eyes to measure eye movements; two on the scalp to detect brain waves. Other electrodes on the upper right and lower left chest measure heartbeats. One on each leg records movements. A temperature-sensitive device may be taped under your nostrils and at your mouth to record your breathing rate and the volume of inhaled air. A beltlike gadget around the lower chest monitors the movements of your diaphragm.

The electrodes will be hooked up to the central line of the polysomnograph equipment. Although the wires are firmly secured, they are not confining. You will be able to sit up, turn to either side, and, usually with the technician's help in "unplugging" yourself, get up and go to the bathroom.

The technician will make note of when you turn out the light and, by watching the brain waves recorded on the polysomnogram, when you fall asleep. All night long, the electrodes will send signals to the polysomnograph; these are converted into electrical impulses that appear as wavy lines on continuous sheets of paper. In the course of a single night, squiggles and waves will cover half a mile of paper.

In the morning, you will be asked questions about how you slept, including estimates of how long it took for you to fall asleep, how often you awakened, and how this night compared with a normal night's sleep. With the aid of a computer, a trained polysomnographer will assess the data recorded from your sleeping body and brain. Some centers may ask you to spend an additional night in order to supply further information.

The costs of an all-night sleep evaluation vary, but two nights of polysomnography and a complete analysis of your sleep patterns can run as much as $1,000. Medicare, Medicaid, and many insurance companies cover such fees, but you should always check your policy before undertaking the tests.

### FINDING A SLEEP CENTER

Most major medical centers, particularly those affiliated with medical schools, have some physicians with expertise in sleep medicine on their staff. You can check with the departments of psychiatry and neurology.

defects, it is prudent to avoid using them. Any medication that the mother takes will cross the placenta and affect the fetus. Even if they are minimal, as with the benzodiazepines, the respiratory depressant effects of sleep medication will affect the fetus. Additionally, the medication and most of its metabolic products will be found in various concentrations in the mother's milk; consequently, breast-feeding mothers should refrain from using hypnotic medication.

## RHONDA RUSSELL: UNSUCCESSFUL USE OF SEDATIVES AND SLEEPING PILLS

Rhonda Russell, a thirty-nine-year-old divorced woman, is the treasurer of a small manufacturing company. She received her B.A. and M.B.A. from Harvard. She describes herself as a hardworking go-getter. It has always been her ambition to become the president of a large company.

Rhonda joined her current firm soon after she graduated from her M.B.A. program. She was immediately placed on the fast track and was relocated to a different city every three years. She was the first woman in her firm to become a senior executive.

Rhonda met her exhusband when she was thirty-two. He too was a fast-rising star at the same company. Their courtship lasted less than a month. Following the wedding, they immediately began to have problems. He was frequently gone for several weeks at a time on business trips. She frequently worked from five in the morning until eight or nine o'clock at night, eating breakfast, lunch, and dinner at her desk.

Their marital problems grew worse when she was promoted ahead of him, and he was offered a job in another city. Rhonda's sleep problems became worse as their marital difficulties intensified. She started getting up in the middle of the night, unable to fall asleep. The company physician prescribed 30 mg of flurazepam (Dalmane), to be taken thirty minutes before bedtime. The drug helped her sleep through the night. She did not seek further help for her marital problems. She and her husband were divorced six months later.

After taking flurazepam (Dalmane) for two years, she consulted a psychiatrist because she noticed that she was having problems concentrating during the day. Over the preceding two years, she had gradually increased her dose from 60 to 90 mg per day. She stated that she felt drowsy all the time. This difficulty grew worse when she drank alcoholic beverages. And despite the pills she was taking, she had begun waking up at night again. Sometimes she used alcohol to help her get to sleep.

Rhonda was being considered for the position of vice president of finance in the company; she had decided to consult the psychiatrist only because of her concern about her job performance. She drank coffee throughout the day and had begun smoking at least a pack of cigarettes per day. She explained that the combination of coffee and cigarettes helped her stay alert. Rhonda had no real friends outside of work. She spent all her time either working or on job-related social activities.

Rhonda's problem with long-term flurazepam use is very common. Her situation exemplifies some of the frequent difficulties in using sleep medications:

• *Chronic use of sleep medication.* Rhonda took the medicine not for several days or a week to treat a specific sleep disturbance, but for a long period of time—two years. Her company physician should have given her only enough medication for one week and should have seen her in follow-up. If her sleep problems had persisted, he should have talked to her about her current life situation. If the physician had thought that he could not assist her (in recognizing her overly intense involvement in her work, marital problems, or later self-medication with caffeine and nicotine), he should have referred her to a psychiatrist.

• *Increasing the dose of the medication.* Rhonda had doubled and sometimes tripled the dose of her sleep medication in the hopes that this would improve her sleep. This only increased the amount of daytime drowsiness and impaired her ability to concentrate further.

• *Use of stimulants to counteract the effects of the sleep medication.* When increasing the dose of the sleep medication did not work, Rhonda began to use stimulants during the day to counteract her feelings of drowsiness. Taking caffeine and nicotine can help you stay awake; unfortunately, they can also interfere with your ability to fall asleep.

• *Use of alcohol to assist with sleep.* Rhonda further compounded her problem by using alcohol to help her fall asleep. Although alcohol may make you feel sleepy, it decreases your total sleep time by disrupting your normal sleep pattern and making you wake up early.

• *Failure to see more global problems.* Neither Rhonda nor her physician realized that her sleep disturbance was only a symptom of long-standing difficulties: being a workaholic, not developing any significant personal relationships, and being goal-driven to the exclusion of everything else. Since she was a high-ranking person in the company, the company physician may have understandably been hesitant to offer unsolicited advice or suggest a referral to a psychiatrist.

*Epilogue*

Rhonda eventually consulted a psychiatrist who recommended a number of changes. She slowly decreased her caffeine intake and stopped smoking. She took 15 mg less flurazepam each week.

After four weeks, she stopped taking flurazepam altogether. She did experience a worsening of her sleep problems during this period; however, by using Benadryl (100 mg the first week and 50 mg the second week), she was able to get enough sleep so that she felt reasonably effective during the day.

Rhonda saw the psychiatrist once a week for approximately one year. The focus of the therapy was on her driven behavior and her inability to relax. She learned to use the stimulus-control methods and relaxation training to assist with her sleep. She was also given various cognitive-focusing techniques.

Rhonda continued to work hard, but she began to spend less time working and more time on other activities, jogging, dating, and regular vacations. Her sleep problems did not return. She eventually met and married another male executive at her company and has received several additional promotions.

In her final session with her psychiatrist, Rhonda remarked that it seemed ironic that as she learned to relax and develop a life of her own, people actually seemed to like her more, she began to do better work, and she enjoyed work and leisure time more than she ever had before.

### JIM O'BRIEN: SUCCESSFUL USE OF SEDATIVES

Jim, a sixty-six-year-old retired electrician, came to his family physician's office complaining of insomnia that had been getting worse for the past six months.

His sleep problems had begun after his wife had died suddenly of a heart attack. Shortly before her death, they had both retired and moved to Florida. They had been married for forty-one years; and Jim still felt distraught. He had been "wandering around in a daze" since his wife's death.

During this time, Jim had lost thirty pounds. He felt that he was no longer capable of experiencing pleasure. He could not enjoy his friends, he had no interest in attending social gatherings, and he could no longer enjoy his former passion—fishing. Instead, he stayed home alone—thinking of death and considering suicide.

Jim's doctor suggested that he try taking a sleeping pill for a few nights. As Jim seemed severely depressed, his doctor recommended taking an antidepressant also. Jim agreed to give these two drugs a try. His doctor gave Jim a prescription for triazolam (Halcion). He also gave Jim a second prescription for an antidepressant. Jim took triazolam (0.125 mg per night at bedtime for six nights) and began taking the antidepressant trazodone (Desyrel). For the first few days, he took 150 mg of this antidepressant at bedtime. Later, his physician gradually increased the dose until he was taking 400 mg a night.

One week after trazodone was started, Jim's sleep patterns had returned to normal. He experienced some sedation from the trazodone, but felt slightly less depressed. At the end of one month, he had returned to his normal mood and once again had a healthy, enthusiastic outlook on life. He began socializing more frequently and visiting his children and grand-children regularly. Jim continued taking 400 mg trazodone per day for approximately six months. This drug was tapered to a lower dose (200 mg) for another six months, then stopped by his physician after one year.

Jim's case illustrates the appropriate use of sleeping pills. As in Jim's case, sleep problems are often a symptom of some other disturbance. Had his physician not asked what was going on in Jim's personal life, he might not have learned that Jim's sleep problem was the result of a major depression, not just a transient sleep disturbance.

Like Jim's doctor, physicians will frequently advise the short-term use of a sleeping pill when beginning antidepressant therapy. As in Jim's case, the sleeping pill frequently helps the person reestablish his or her normal sleep patterns. And as sleep patterns return to normal, the person's mood will usually improve. The sleeping pill also helps the person sleep through the initial period of antidepressant treatment, when side effects from the medication are most pronounced.

Jim's physician prescribed triazolam, a relatively short-acting benzodiazepine. This was a good choice for Jim. When older people are given a longer-acting benzodiazepine, they frequently experience residual daytime drowsiness.

Prior to beginning medication, Jim's doctor conducted a complete physical examination and ordered a number of laboratory tests to make sure that Jim's depression did not have a physical cause—such as a malignant tumor or an adverse side effect from a drug. He also obtained a good medical history to make sure Jim was not drinking heavily and was not taking benzodiazepines or other medications that could interfere with sleep. And in addition to prescribing medication, Jim's doctor spent several hours speaking with Jim about his feelings for his wife and his plans for the future. Although these discussions were sometimes painful, they enabled Jim to begin to work through some of his grief.

Jim is currently alive and well, and he is looking forward to celebrating his seventieth birthday with his children and grandchildren.

## Nondrug Alternatives for Insomnia

Prescription sleeping pills, if they are used at all, should be used for only a few days at a time. Long-term use of sleeping pills—either prescription or OTC—frequently produces physical and/or psychological problems. If you have a sleep problem, you should consider one or more of the following nondrug alternatives as a long-term solution:

• *Progressive muscular relaxation.* You systematically tense, then relax, each of the major muscle groups in your body. Begin by tightening all the muscles in your hands and arms for ten seconds. Then allow these muscles to become completely relaxed. Continue the same process for all the other

## Sidebar 2: Progressive Relaxation

1. Make sure you're comfortable.
2. When tensing your muscles, do so vigorously—but not so vigorously that you develop a cramp. Hold the muscle in its tensed position for five to seven seconds, counting "one thousand one, one thousand two," and so on. Then relax for fifteen to twenty seconds.
3. Concentrate on what is happening. Feel the buildup of tension; notice the tightening of the muscles; feel the strain and then the release; relax and enjoy the sudden feeling of limpness.
4. You will be tensing and relaxing each muscle group twice. If any part of your body still feels tense after completing the exercises, go back and tense and relax those muscles again.
5. Try to keep all the other muscles relaxed as you work on a specific group.
6. To begin, take three deep breaths, holding each one for five seconds.
7. Clench your right fist if you're right-handed, your left fist if you're left-handed. Hold, and count for five to seven seconds. Relax, and repeat.
8. Flex the bicep of your right arm if you're right-handed, your left if you're left-handed. Tense. Relax. Tense. Relax.
9. Clench your other fist. Relax. Repeat. Tense your other bicep. Relax. Repeat. Take a couple of deep breaths and notice how relaxed and warm your arms feel. Enjoy the sensation.
10. Tense up the muscles of your forehead by raising your eyebrows as high as you can. Hold for five seconds. Relax. Repeat. Let a wave of relaxation wash over your face.
11. Close your eyes tightly. Release and notice the relaxation. Repeat.
12. Clench your jaw very tightly and make an exaggerated smile. Release. Repeat.
13. Take a couple of deep breaths and notice how relaxed the muscles of your arms and head feel.

muscle groups in your body. Sidebar 2 provides guidelines for using the progressive relaxation method. (Don't worry if you fall asleep before finishing the process: Sleep is the goal of the exercise.)

• *Autogenic training*. Begin by telling yourself, "My hands are growing heavier and heavier," then imagine that your hands are indeed becoming so heavy that you can no longer hold them up. Repeat for your arms, legs, feet, head, chest, abdomen, pelvic area, and all the other parts of your body.

14. Take a deep breath and hold it for a few seconds. Release slowly. Repeat.
15. Try to touch your chin to your chest but use counterpressure to keep it from touching. Release. Repeat.
16. Try to touch your back with your head, but at the same time push the opposite way with the opposing muscles. Notice the tension building up. Release quickly. Repeat. Let your neck muscles become completely relaxed.
17. Push your shoulder blades back and try to make them touch. Notice the tension across your shoulders and chest. Relax. Repeat.
18. Try to touch your shoulders by pushing forward as far as you can. Hold. Repeat.
19. Shrug your shoulders, as if trying to touch them to your ears. Hold. Release. Repeat.
20. Take a very deep breath. Hold for several seconds and release slowly. Do this again, noticing a wave of relaxation overtaking your body.
21. Tighten your stomach muscles and hold for several seconds. Relax. Repeat, noticing the relaxed feeling in your abdomen.
22. Tighten your buttocks. Hold. Release. Repeat.
23. Tense your thighs. Release quickly. Repeat.
24. Extend your feet so your toes point away from your body. Notice the tension. Return to normal position. Repeat.
25. Point your toes toward your head. Notice the tension. Return to normal position. Repeat.
26. Point your feet outward left and right. Release quickly. Repeat.
27. Just let your body relax for a few minutes. Notice and enjoy the good feeling.

Practice this routine twice a day. When you become proficient, schedule a practice session for bedtime. Don't worry if you fall asleep before finishing. That's the whole point.

**Source:** Hales, D.R. *How to Sleep Like a Baby, Wake Up Refreshed, and Get More Out of Life.* New York: Ballantine Books, 1987, pp. 78–79. Used with permission.

*Systematic desensitization.* Imagine a series of very pleasurable, relaxing scenes immediately before you go to bed. The goal is to associate bedtime with sensory relaxation and to overcome anxiety that can interfere with sleep.

• *Transcendental Meditation.* This technique uses the repetition of a word or other sound, called a mantra (e.g., the word *relax, one,* or *om,* or any other word or phrase that may appeal to you). You sit upright with your eyes closed, repeating your chosen mantra again and again, either aloud or silently to yourself. If other thoughts come into your mind, let them go; return your attention to your mantra. When a mantra is repeated in this way for five to ten minutes (or more), it will gradually bring about a state of alert, relaxed restfulness.

During this relaxed state, oxygen consumption drops dramatically, the heartbeat slows, and respirations are reduced. This technique works best when it is performed for twenty-minute periods in the morning and afternoon, and in the evening as a prelude to sleep. Its ability to assist with sleep and treat insomnia appears to be related to its ability to relieve daytime stress that may interfere with sleep.

• *Yoga*. Yoga is a system of mental and physical exercises based on various bodily postures. When done in the prescribed manner, these exercises can promote both physical fitness and mental well-being. Three yoga exercises that may be particularly useful in relaxing at bedtime—the tension reliever, the sponge, and deep breathing—are described in Sidebar 3.

• *Cognitive refocusing*. Many people have trouble falling asleep because they find themselves obsessed with a succession of ideas, fears, plans, or regrets about events that occurred during the day. Cognitive refocusing can be used to refocus your mind, using imagery to help you relax. Counting sheep is one such visualization exercise. Studying the surroundings in your bedroom is another. You might try counting the ceiling tiles, the floor boards, or the number of threads in your blanket. You might count backward from one hundred to zero. If you get all the way to zero and are still awake, begin again, counting backward by twos, then by threes, etc. You might try to name all fifty states, the seven dwarfs, or to remember all the houses you have ever lived in. You can pretend you are Noah preparing for the boarding of the Ark; think about all the types of animals you are bringing aboard. There are many mind games you can play to refocus your thoughts from your daytime worries to simple repetitive tasks that may help you sleep.

• *Stimulus control*. Developed by Richard Bootzin, Ph.D., of Northwestern University, this is a classic behavioral approach to sleep. The goal of this method is to condition yourself to associate your bed with rest. Some fundamental guidelines are:

1. Go to bed only when you are sleepy.
2. Do not read, eat, watch television, knit, or chat with your bed partner in bed.
3. If you do not fall asleep within ten minutes, get up and leave the bedroom.
4. Stay in another room until you feel sleepy, then go back to bed.

## Sidebar 3: Yoga Exercises

### TENSION RELIEVER

1. Lie flat on your back. Inhale to a count of five. Raise your arms over your head until your hands touch the bed. Make two fists.
2. Raise your buttocks. Tense and stretch every muscle in your body, including those of your face.
3. Hold for a count of five.
4. Release your breath and relax your body, keeping your arms over your head. Relax your fingers. With eyes closed, let the tension drain out of your body.
5. Each time you do this exercise, slowly increase the amount of time you hold this position.

### SPONGE

1. Lie on your back, feet slightly apart, hands at your sides, palms upward. Close your eyes. Breathe normally.
2. Check your body for hidden tension in your legs, hands, face, shoulders.
3. Concentrate on removing all negative feelings, such as tiredness, restlessness, or tension. Mentally replace these feelings with feelings of lightness and serenity.
4. Relax each part of the body, starting at your toes and working up to your forehead. Do not rush.

### DEEP BREATHING

1. Exhale, breathing through your nose with your mouth closed.
2. Inhale. Expand your abdomen, middle rib cage, and then the upper lungs. Hold. (Relax your face.)
3. Exhale. Release air slowly. Exhale air from the upper lungs, then from the middle rib cage. Contract your abdominal muscles slightly. Squeeze all the air out of your body.
4. Repeat six times.

**Source:** Hales, D.R. *The Complete Book of Sleep*. Reading, Massachusetts: Addison-Wesley, 1981, pp. 117–118. Used with permission.

5. If you do not fall asleep within ten minutes, get up again and repeat the process.
6. Do this as often as necessary until you fall asleep within ten minutes of returning to bed.
7. Regardless of how many times you commute to and from your bedroom and how little you sleep, get up in the morning at a fixed time.
8. Do not nap during the day.
9. Keep a sleep log for each night. Include the total number of times you went to bed and got out of bed and the total time you spent out of bed.

You may find yourself getting out of bed five or even ten times the first night. This may continue for several nights. You may be tempted to give up. Don't. Within two to three weeks you should find yourself falling asleep more and more easily, and within one to two months, you should be able to sleep through the night without getting up at all. Many people who have suffered from chronic sleep problems have benefited from this approach. The key ingredient is to comply with the sleep-in-bed-or-get-up rule.

• *Biofeedback*. This technique can help you relax by providing detailed feedback on certain measures of relaxation (e.g., hand temperature, sweating, brain waves, or muscle tension). Once you have this feedback, you can easily learn, by trial and error, how to bring about the physiologic changes desired. If you are interested in trying biofeedback, ask your physician to refer you to a local expert trained in this technique.

• *Hypnosis*. The use of hypnotic suggestions to relax can be very effective in individuals who choose to use this technique, but you must have faith in the hypnotist and must be willing to heed his or her commands. Studies show that hypnosis can help a person fall asleep more quickly and can even prevent sleepwalking. Some hypnotists use direct suggestion to help people overcome a fear of insomnia and to give the person a feeling of confidence and mastery in sleeping. The key to hypnosis is to think positively about yourself.

Many people use self-hypnosis without realizing it, by telling themselves: "I am falling asleep, I am falling asleep." People with insomnia may play a tape recording giving hypnotic commands at bedtime. Self-hypnotic suggestions can easily be combined with other relaxation techniques.

• *Paradoxical intention*. Concentrate on staying awake instead of trying to fall asleep. This may sound like a contradictory approach, but it can be dramatically effective. In one study, people with insomnia who had unsuccessfully used relaxation therapy to help them fall asleep were told by researchers that they needed more information about their before-sleep thoughts. These patients were instructed to remain awake as long as possible in order to describe these thoughts more accurately. After receiving these instructions, the subjects fell asleep twice as quickly as they had when they were trying to fall asleep. One woman, who had taken seventy minutes to fall asleep after using relaxation techniques, dozed off in less than six minutes after she was directed to stay awake.

• *Sleep restriction*. Some people with insomnia may spend eight or nine hours in bed even though they are only able to sleep for five or six hours. Research suggests that they would probably fall asleep more quickly if they spent less time in bed. If you go to bed at 10:00 P.M., get up at 6:30 A.M., but do not fall asleep until 11:00 or 11:30 P.M., try getting into bed thirty minutes later each night—but getting up at the same time as usual—until you find that you are spending most of your time in bed asleep.

• *Exercise*. People who exercise regularly are less depressed, sleep better, and have fewer medical and physical ailments. Brisk walking, swimming, jogging, bicycling and many other exercise routines have all proved effective. You should begin exercising at a very modest level; increase the time and intensity of your exercise very gradually. You might, for instance, begin with a ten-minute walk every afternoon, increasing your walking time by one minute per day until you have worked your way up to a forty-five-minute daily walk. For the first two to three months of a new exercise program, regularity is much more important than intensity. If you are over forty years of age or have a history of heart problems, you should consult your physician before beginning an exercise program.

• *Restrict daytime napping*. Taking a nap during the day, or after work, can interfere with your ability to fall asleep at night. If you find yourself falling asleep watching T.V. after dinner, then tossing and turning when you finally do get into bed, you may need to give up your nap and save your sleeping for bedtime.

# Chapter 9

# Antiaddiction Drugs

DRUG addiction and drug use—including nicotine and alcohol use—are extremely widespread. Twenty-nine percent of American adults are addicted to nicotine. Fourteen percent are addicted to, or abuse, alcohol. A rapidly growing portion use such illicit drugs as cocaine, crack, heroin, marijuana, and PCP—and millions of Americans are currently addicted to drugs that are legally available by prescription.

## Why Do People Take Drugs?

A full discussion of this question is beyond the scope of this book. People abuse alcohol and smoke, snort, or inject illegal substances for many reasons. Some take drugs such as alcohol to forget their problems or to help themselves deal with anxiety. Some researchers believe that human beings have an innate need to get high. For adolescents, peer pressure often contributes to drug use. This youthful experimentation sometimes leads to dependence, especially when the drugs are potent and addicting, such as cocaine.

Others (of any age) may take cocaine or other stimulants to make themselves feel better when they are depressed or sad. Some individuals become addicted to the drugs prescribed by their physicians.

Joan, a forty-year-old housewife, received a prescription for alprazolam (Xanax), an antianxiety drug, as part of her treatment for panic disorder. She subsequently became addicted to this medication, required higher and higher doses, and eventually had to be hospitalized to withdraw from the drug.

Herb, a fifty-five-year-old construction worker, sustained a back injury at work. While hospitalized, he became dependent on meperidine (Demerol), a drug for intense pain. To reduce the unintentional misuse of prescription drugs, you should ask yourself the questions shown in Sidebar 1 before leaving your physician's office.

---

### Sidebar 1: Avoid Prescription Drug Misuse

Be sure you know the answers to the following questions before leaving your physician's office:
• What is the name of the drug, and what is it supposed to do?
• When should it be taken, and for how long?
• What foods, drinks, other medicines, or activities should I avoid while taking this drug?
• Are there any possible side effects?
• Is there any written information on the drug?
• Is there any alternative or any other treatment that might be equally effective?
• Can I become dependent on or addicted to this drug?

**Source:** Hales, D.R. *An Invitation to Health*, 4th ed. Redwood City, California: Benjamin/Cummings, 1989, p. 325. Used with permission.

---

## How Do You Know If You Are Addicted to a Drug?

Psychiatrists' official term for drug dependence is *psychoactive substance dependence*. To receive this diagnosis, a person must meet three of the following nine criteria:

• *The person has been taking larger and larger amounts of the drug over a longer period of time than originally intended.* For instance, Barbara, a thirty-one-year-old physician, originally began taking dextroamphetamine (Dexedrine) to stay alert while studying for her medical examinations. She subsequently required higher and higher doses, and later found that she just could not stop taking the drug.

• *The person has tried without success to reduce drug use.* Peter, a forty-seven-year-old lawyer, tried unsuccessfully five times over the last year to stop drinking. He concluded he could not accomplish his goal on his own. He was finally able to stop drinking, but only after entering an alcohol treatment unit.

• *The person spends a lot of time obtaining the substance, taking the substance, and recovering from the effects of the substance.* For example, Chris, a thirty-five-year-old stockbroker, lost his position with a prestigious brokerage firm because he was spending most of his day at a local crack house getting high on cocaine.

• *The person frequently becomes intoxicated or experiences withdrawal symptoms when expected to be at work or school, or expected to fulfill responsibilities at home.* He or she may use the drug even when it is hazardous to health. Joe, a twenty-one-year-old construction worker, was involved in two serious automobile accidents after drinking excessively and smoking marijuana. He subsequently died of injuries sustained in the second accident. Melinda, a sixty-two-year-old retired schoolteacher, continued to smoke two packs of cigarettes a day even after she had two heart attacks, a stroke, lung cancer, and emphysema.

• *The person will tend to withdraw from normal social, job-related, or recreational activities because of his or her preoccupation with the abused drug.* Bill, a forty-one-year-old salesman, turned down a job promotion with a substantial pay increase because it would mean he would have to move to a new city—away from his current supplier of cocaine.

• *The person may continue to use the abused substance in spite of social, psychological, or physical difficulties that the drug causes them or their families.* Marjorie, a twenty-nine-year-old divorced real estate agent with a two-year-old daughter, continued to spend large amounts of money on cocaine in spite of her limited income, large mortgage, and substantial child-care expenses.

• *The person requires larger and larger doses of the drug in order to become intoxicated or to experience a high.* Bob, a forty-nine-year-old naval officer, found that he had to drink half a quart of scotch or three six-packs of beer a day to become intoxicated. Users of cocaine, barbiturates, and opiates may end up using amounts that produce adverse effects powerful enough to kill them.

• *The person develops withdrawal symptoms when the medication is discontinued.* Joan, the housewife mentioned above, suddenly stopped taking her daily 6 mg dose of alprazolam. Within twenty-four hours, she experienced two severe seizures. When Bob, the alcoholic naval officer, failed to drink his accustomed half a quart of scotch per day, he would experience a wide range of withdrawal symptoms: tremors, restlessness, agitation, irritability, increased heart rate, and rapid breathing. Fortunately, he sought medical attention and was eventually able to stop drinking.

• *The person takes his or her drug of choice to help relieve withdrawal symptoms.* Before he quit drinking altogether, Bob would have a couple of drinks in the morning to relieve his alcoholic withdrawal symptoms.

The term *substance abuse* is used to refer to those individuals who continue to use the substance despite clear evidence that it is causing severe problems for themselves and others. James continued to smoke in spite of having emphysema, a disease that made it difficult for him to breathe. Cheryl, a fifty-two-year-old high school teacher, continued to drink heavily even after her physician told her that she had severe liver disease. The term *abuse* is usually used to refer to people who have a severe problem but do not meet the criteria for psychoactive substance dependency (see Sidebar 2).

---

### Sidebar 2: How Can You Tell If Someone Is Abusing Drugs?

The National Institute on Drug Abuse lists the following behaviors as indications of a drug problem:
• An abrupt change in attitude, including a noticeable lack of interest in activities once enjoyed
• Frequent vague, withdrawn moods
• A sudden decline in work or school performance, or the regular skipping of classes
• Sudden resistance to discipline or criticism
• Secret telephone calls and meetings, and a demand for greater privacy of personal possessions
• Increased frustration levels
• Changes in sleeping and eating habits
• Sudden weight loss
• Evidence of drug use (smell of marijuana, drug paraphernalia)
• The frequent borrowing of money
• Stealing
• A disregard for personal appearance
• Impaired relationships with family and friends
• The ignoring of deadlines, curfews, or other regulations
• Unusual flare-ups of temper
• Associating with new friends, especially known drug users, and strong allegiance to these friends

**Source:** Hales, D.R. *An Invitation to Health*, 4th ed. Redwood City, California: Benjamin/ Cummings, 1989, p. 328. Used with permission.

## Friends and Family

The most important thing that family and friends can do is to get their loved one into treatment. People addicted to drugs will vehemently deny that they have a problem. Friends or family must confront the person and insist that he or she see a physician. Once an appointment is made, it is important for a family member to accompany the patient to document the severity of the addiction and to provide missing information, especially about times when the person may have been intoxicated or experiencing withdrawal symptoms.

## Denial

A key characteristic of most substance abusers is denial. People who use drugs often believe that they can *handle* the drug; they may express little concern about developing dependency.

• John, a successful business executive, began having more and more martinis at lunch, in the evening, and eventually even at breakfast. Even though his boss referred him to an inpatient alcohol detoxification program, John still denied that he had a problem.
• Joe, a high school student, began smoking marijuana in the parking lot after school, and then progressed to smoking it throughout the day. Next, he started taking PCP in the evening. He also began experimenting with LSD over the weekend. Prior to his hospitalization, he too felt that he was completely in control.
• Stephanie, a college student, lost her job and was finally kicked out of school because of her alcohol and drug abuse problems. Even so, she insisted on blaming others for her difficulties rather than admitting her drug dependency.

The best way to avoid being addicted to drugs is not to use them in the first place. Sidebar 3 gives you some tips to follow if you are offered a drug.

## Drug Treatment of Drug Dependence

Within the last few years, clinicians have found several medications that help people stop taking a drug to which they are addicted. These medica-

---

### Sidebar 3: Suggestions for Saying *No* to Drugs.

If people offer you a drug, here are some ways to say no:
- Let them know you are not interested.
- Tell them that you have something else to do: "No, I'm going for a walk now."
- Be prepared for different types of pressure. If your friends tease you, tease back. If the pressure seems threatening, simply walk away.
- Keep it simple: "No, thanks," "No," or "No way" gets the point across.
- Give them the cold shoulder; ignore them.
- Change the subject.
- Hang out with people who don't use drugs. They won't ask you questions you have to say no to.

**Source:** Hales, D.R. *An Invitation to Health*, 4th ed. Redwood City, California: Benjamin/Cummings, 1989, p. 327. Used with permission.

---

tions reduce the severity of withdrawal symptoms from alcohol and from heroin and other opiates. Others can help treat the feelings of depression people often experience when they withdraw from a drug. There is even an effective drug to help people who wish to quit smoking. Such treatments can make the process of stopping a drug much less unpleasant.

## Overcoming Alcohol Addiction

### EARLY SIGNS

The early signs of alcohol dependence may be quite subtle. Sometimes, the spouse of an alcoholic person will contact a physician or psychiatrist to complain about problems in the marriage—for example, frequent arguments with the partner. A wife may complain of her husband's lack of interest in sex or his frequent absence from the home at night when he goes to bars or clubs. A boss may complain that an employee fails to show up at work, especially on Mondays. Frequent absences from the job may be noted. (For other early warning signs of alcoholism, and what to do if someone close to you drinks too much, see Sidebars 4 and 5.)

Alcohol abusers may have a history of automobile accidents or an arrest record for driving while intoxicated. During a routine physical examination, the physician may note an enlarged liver, or the person may complain of stomach pains. Sometimes these individuals will admit to having blackouts (periods when they do not remember what occurred).

## Sidebar 4: Early Warning Signs of Alcoholism

Because no one is immune to alcoholism, everyone should recognize its early characteristics:
- Experiencing the following symptoms after drinking: frequent headaches, nausea, stomach pain, heartburn, gas, fatigue, weakness, muscle cramps, or irregular or rapid heartbeats
- Needing a drink in the morning to start the day
- Denying any problem with alcohol
- Doing things while drinking that are regretted afterward
- Dramatic mood swings, from anger to laughter to anxiety
- Sleep problems
- Depression and paranoia
- Forgetting what happened during a drinking episode
- Changing brands or going on the wagon to control drinking
- Having five or more drinks a day

**Source:** Hales, D.R. *An Invitation to Health*, 4th ed. Redwood City, California: Benjamin/ Cummings, 1989, p. 361. Used with permission.

## Sidebar 5: What to Do If Someone Close to You Drinks Too Much

- Try to remain calm, unemotional, and factually honest in speaking about the drinker's behavior and its day-to-day consequences.
- Discuss the situation with someone you trust: a clergyman, a social worker, friends, or an individual who has experienced alcoholism directly.
- Try to include the drinker in family life. Encourage new interests and participate in leisure-time activities that the drinker enjoys.
- Be patient, and live one day at a time. Try to accept setbacks and relapses calmly.
- Refuse to ride with the drinker when he or she is intoxicated.
- Never cover up or make excuses for the drinker, or shield him or her from the consequences of drinking.
- Don't assume the drinker's responsibilities; that takes away dignity and a sense of importance.

**Source:** Hales, D.R. *An Invitation to Health*, 4th ed. Redwood City, California: Benjamin/ Cummings, 1989, p. 365. Used with permission.

## Medical Risks of Alcohol Abuse

Heavy drinking can produce many harmful physical effects. Alcohol can irritate the stomach lining, leading to occasional bleeding, ulcers, or severe stomach pain. People who are dependent on alcohol frequently have liver problems, generally cirrhosis or alcoholic hepatitis, and may also experience chronic inflammation of the pancreas. Alcohol may damage the heart muscles, leading to a condition known as cardiomyopathy, in which the heart's ability to pump blood is markedly reduced. Alcohol may decrease the body's ability to fight disease, leading to episodes of pneumonia, tuberculosis, or other infections. Men may complain that they are unable to have an erection. Alcohol may lower testosterone levels and cause atrophy of the testicles. In women, it may decrease the ability to produce normal quantities of female hormones, leading to reduced menstruation and infertility.

If women abuse alcohol while pregnant, their fetuses may develop fetal alcohol syndrome. In this syndrome, the baby may have abnormal facial features and a small head circumference. The baby may also have a decreased IQ, be mentally retarded, or later develop behavioral problems. Woman who drink while pregnant have a higher rate of spontaneous abortion.

## Alcohol Withdrawal Symptoms

People addicted to alcohol who suddenly stop drinking may exhibit a wide range of withdrawal symptoms.

### Alcohol Withdrawal

Several hours following cessation of drinking, people addicted to alcohol will experience a tremor that is made worse when they attempt to move their hands or perform a precise task. They may also exhibit increased blood pressure, rapid heart rate, profuse sweating, nausea, vomiting, and a general feeling of malaise. These symptoms usually begin within several hours after a person has stopped drinking and become worse over the next one to two days. During this time, the person may complain of nightmares, sleep problems, and auditory or visual hallucinations. Other common withdrawal symptoms include anxiety, depressed mood, and irritability.

### Alcohol Withdrawal Seizures

An alcoholic who stops drinking may begin to experience seizures within twelve to forty-eight hours after the last drink. Seizures may be caused by the direct or by the secondary effects of alcohol, e.g., low serum magnesium levels, low blood sugar, or serum electrolyte abnormalities.

### Alcohol Hallucinations

Heavy drinkers who stop drinking suddenly may experience auditory or visual hallucinations. The auditory hallucinations are usually unpleasant and disturbing voices. Hallucinations usually begin within two days after the person has stopped or reduced his or her drinking and may last a few weeks or months. The condition usually occurs after ten years of heavy drinking in people forty years or older.

### Delirium Tremens (Alcohol Withdrawal Delirium)

Patients who develop this condition may experience confusion, disorientation, visual or auditory hallucinations, illusions, a disturbance in their level of consciousness, and disorganized thinking. They may become either very agitated or very withdrawn. Patients who exhibit delirium tremens may report that real objects appear smaller or larger than they really are. They may report seeing small animals or other objects in their room. They may also complain of a sensation of bugs crawling under their skin.

Delirium tremens is a disorder that can cause death due to medical complications. People with preexisting physical illnesses are at highest risk. Symptoms of delirium tremens usually begin two to three days after the cessation of alcohol and become most intense after four to five days. These patients also may experience irregularities of the heartbeat, pneumonia, or bleeding in the brain as the result of a fall or from liver failure.

### Wernicke-Korsakoff Syndrome

This syndrome is caused by thiamine deficiency, usually due to the failure of the patient with alcoholism to maintain an adequate diet. It is frequently seen in chronic alcoholics who are unemployed and live on the streets. This disorder may include long- and short-term memory disturbances. These people may not remember the names of their doctors, what they had for breakfast, the name of their hospital, and other events requiring adequate short-term memory. Other symptoms include ophthalmopelgia (eye movement abnormalities), confusion, ataxia (difficulty walking), and peripheral neuropathy (decreased sensation to touch in the extremities).

### ALCOHOL DETOXIFICATION

Patients may be withdrawn from alcohol or detoxified either as outpatients or inpatients. Most alcoholic patients, usually 75 percent to 95 percent, can be treated as outpatients. Patients with serious medical problems—such as dementia, a history of trauma, neurologic disturbances, severe liver disease, a history of alcohol withdrawal seizures, alcohol hallucinosis, delirium tremens, or other complications—should be treated in an inpatient setting. People abusing alcohol and other substances (such as alcohol and barbiturates) simultaneously should also be treated in an inpatient setting.

The overall goal of detoxification is to prevent the occurrence of serious complications: alcohol-withdrawal seizures, delirium tremens, alcohol hallucinosis, and Wernicke-Korsakoff syndrome.

## Use of Benzodiazepines in Alcohol Detoxification

The drugs most frequently used to treat alcohol dependence are the benzodiazepines. (These drugs are discussed at length in Chapter 4.) These drugs produce less respiratory depression and are rarely associated with serious complications because of overdose. In treating the alcohol abuser with these drugs, the physician substitutes the benzodiazepine for alcohol, gets the person intoxicated on the benzodiazepine, then withdraws the benzodiazepine from the patient.

The benzodiazepines used most frequently for alcohol detoxification are chlordiazepoxide (Librium) and diazepam (Valium). As discussed in Chapter 4, these relatively long-acting benzodiazepines are metabolized by the liver and excreted by the kidneys. For patients with liver damage, shorter-acting agents such as lorazepam (Ativan) or oxazepam (Serax) may be used. Ativan can be given by injection.

Different physicians may employ different treatment approaches. Hospitalized patients may initially receive 25 to 100 mg of chlordiazepoxide orally, every six hours, on the first day. Additional doses of between 25 and 100 mg may be given if the patient develops agitation, tremors, or an increase in heart rate, respirations, or temperature. Chlordiazepoxide is then gradually tapered over the first week, with a reduction in daily doses not to exceed 20 to 25 percent of the initial (first day) dose. Most physicians will write orders for extra doses of the drug as needed if withdrawal symptoms reoccur.

For people who are not hospitalized, a lower dose of chlordiazepoxide is used, usually from 25 to 50 mg four times a day on the first day, with a gradual decrease in dose over a week. This should prevent the most severe withdrawal symptoms: seizures and delirium tremens.

To prevent the occurrence of Wernicke-Korsakoff syndrome, thiamine (vitamin $B_1$) is also given, in a dose of 50 to 100 mg four times a day. Hospitalized patients may also receive multivitamins and folic acid. Individuals who have not been eating well-balanced meals may require vitamin supplementation, especially thiamine, for a week or more.

Benzodiazepines are usually quite useful in helping people withdraw from alcohol. They help prevent nausea, vomiting, and hyperactivity, and reduce the risk of serious complications such as convulsions or delirium tremens.

## OTHER DRUGS USED IN ALCOHOL DETOXIFICATION

Some clinicians will use either the alpha-adrenergic blocker clonidine (Catapres) or one of the beta-adrenergic blockers, propranolol (Inderal) or atenolol (Tenormin), sometimes in combination with a benzodiazepine, to treat alcohol withdrawal. These uses are still experimental, but results to date are encouraging.

Other medications—e.g., barbiturates, paraldehyde, and chloral hydrate—are occasionally used in special situations.

## REHABILITATION

Once a patient has successfully withdrawn from alcohol, the rehabilitation process begins. For those who go through this process in a hospital or treatment center, these programs provide a high degree of structure and support. Emphasis is placed on self-help. Patients learn a great deal about alcoholism and its treatment. They also have an opportunity to participate in discussion groups and therapy sessions.

These programs insist on complete abstinence from alcohol. They provide a warm, supportive environment and emphasize the use of a medical model that does not attempt to blame the patient for his or her problem.

Since many alcoholic patients have become socially isolated because of their heavy alcohol use, they often lack the social skills necessary to help them reestablish their connections with friends and co-workers. Most treatment programs emphasize group interaction to help patients develop these skills.

Similar programs are available to those who are not hospitalized. These programs may last anywhere from several hours a day for a week to daylong-plus-evening sessions for a month. Family members are usually asked to participate. Outpatient treatment may be directed either by individual physicians or by specialized addiction treatment facilities.

## USE OF AVERSIVE DRUGS IN ALCOHOL DETOXIFICATION

An aversive drug combines with alcohol to make the user sick. Aversive drugs block the liver's ability to metabolize acetaldehyde, a major metabolic product of ethyl alcohol. This leads to a significant increase in blood acetaldehyde—which in turn produces the unpleasant effects of the alcohol-drug reaction. These symptoms include facial flushing, headache, nausea, vomiting, sweating, thirst, palpitations, increased pulse rate, weakness, dizziness, and sometimes confusion. These symptoms can occur even with small amounts of alcohol, e.g., from cough syrup or absorbing alcohol in shaving lotion through the skin. If the person consumes a large amount of alcohol, extremely severe reactions may occur: cardiac arrhythmias, myocardial infarction (heart attack), seizures, and even death. Reactions generally last from around thirty minutes to several hours.

The most frequently used aversive medication is disulfiram (Antabuse). This is given in a single daily dose of 125 to 500 mg. Within twelve hours after the administration, disulfiram will inactivate the key enzyme described above. This enzyme inactivation lasts for up to two weeks. If the patient consumes *any* alcoholic beverage during this period, he or she will become violently ill.

Because of their potential for very serious consequences, aversive treatments are usually reserved for those patients in whom all other treatment approaches have failed. These techniques should be used only under the close supervision of qualified professionals—and only if provided as a part of a well-organized and comprehensive alcohol treatment program.

## TESTS REQUIRED PRIOR TO TAKING DISULFIRAM

*Medical History*
- Recent ingestion of alcohol (to include cough syrups, tonics, etc.) within twelve hours?
- Liver disease?
- Currently taking phenytoin (Dilantin)?

*Physical Exam*
- Emphasis upon liver exam

*Blood Tests*
- Blood alcohol level
- Liver function tests
- If taking Dilantin, serum dilantin level

*Other*

- EKG (if a history of cardiac disease or if the person is over forty years of age)

## How Can This Drug Be Misused?

Antabuse is not associated with abuse or dependence. In the past, soon after taking Antabuse, patients received at least one supervised alcohol-drug reaction to emphasize the adverse consequences of alcohol ingestion. Because these reactions were sometimes quite violent—even life-threatening—such practices have been abandoned and should not be tried.

## Precautions to Observe While Taking This Drug

Patients taking Antabuse need to be fully aware of the Antabuse-alcohol reaction: flushing, headache, nausea, vomiting, sweating, thirst, chest pain, palpitations, breathing problems, racing heart, dizziness, weakness, and blurred vision. The intensity of the reaction varies with individuals. Patients taking this drug should be warned to avoid contact with alcohol in every form: sauces, cough medication, after-shave lotions, perfume, tonics, etc.

## Possible Drug Interactions

Because Antabuse decreases the rate of metabolism of certain drugs, it should be used with caution with other medications. Especially at risk are people taking phenytoin (Dilantin) for a seizure disorder, since the metabolism of Dilantin by the liver may be decreased considerably—leading to increased (and possibly toxic) Dilantin blood levels.

# Overcoming Addiction to Sedatives and Antianxiety Drugs

As indicated in Chapter 4, benzodiazepines, barbiturates, and non-benzodiazepine antianxiety agents are frequently prescribed to treat anxiety disorders and sleep disturbances. Benzodiazepine abuse is especially widespread (see Sidebar 6). An estimated 15 percent of adults in the United States have used a benzodiazepine within the past year. There are two common patterns of abuse:

• A physician prescribes a benzodiazepine, barbiturate, or similar medication to treat anxiety or insomnia. The person taking the drug gradually
increases the dose to the point of using the drug not just to treat the
symptoms but to continue functioning normally. The person may then go to
several different physicians in various specialties seeking additional supplies of the medication. As time goes by, higher and higher doses are
required.

• Teenagers or young adults obtain benzodiazepines or barbiturates
illegally. They use these drugs to get high. They may combine them with
other illegal drugs, such as cocaine, to counteract some of cocaine's stimulant properties. After a few episodes of brief use, they become addicted.

## SYMPTOMS OF SEDATIVE OR ANTIANXIETY DRUG ABUSE
## OR DEPENDENCE

Many aspects of benzodiazepine abuse are quite similar to those of alcoholism. The user may become intoxicated, experience withdrawal, and even
exhibit delirium and amnesia. With high doses, seizures may occur. Since
the effects of the benzodiazepines last much longer than those of alcohol,
withdrawal symptoms may not occur until a week to ten days after the
person stops taking the drug. The newer, shorter-acting agents such as
alprazolam (Xanax), if stopped, can produce marked withdrawal symptoms within twelve to twenty-four hours. When benzodiazepines are taken
with alcohol, the blood level of the benzodiazepines is usually increased
considerably. On a long-term basis, memory, learning, and coordination
may be impaired.

The barbiturates amobarbital (Amytal), pentobarbital (Nembutal), phenobarbital, and secobarbital (Seconal) can interact with alcohol to produce
an increase in adverse effects: impaired coordination, respiratory depression, and memory impairment. People addicted to barbiturates and other
sedatives may be at greater risk of becoming depressed and extremely
anxious when they withdraw from these drugs.

## DETOXIFICATION FROM SEDATIVES OR ANTIANXIETY DRUGS

Addicted patients are withdrawn from these drugs in much the same way
that patients are withdrawn from alcohol. Most patients can be safely
withdrawn from these drugs without being hospitalized. For those who are
addicted to very large doses of medication or have other medical complications, hospitalization may be necessary and these drugs must be discontinued gradually. Abrupt withdrawal may lead to seizures or even death. In

## Sidebar 6: Frequently Abused Drugs

| Class | Trade Name | Street Name |
|---|---|---|
| *Benzodiazepines* | | |
| diazepam | Valium | barbs, candy, dolls, goofers, peanuts, sleeping pills |
| chlordiazepoxide | Librium | |
| alprazolam | Xanax | |
| oxazepam | Serax | |
| lorazepam | Ativan | |
| *Barbiturates* | | |
| secobarbital | Seconal | pink lady, red devils, red, seccy, pinks |
| amobarbital | Amytal | blue angels, bluebirds, blue devils, blues, lilly |
| pentobarbital | Nembutal | nebbies, yellow bullets, yellow dolls |
| phenobarbital | Luminal | phennies, purple hearts |
| amobarbital/secobarbital | Tuinal | Christmas trees, double-trouble, rainbows, tooie |
| *Other sedative-hypnotics* | | |
| methaqualone | Quaalude | sopors, ludes |
| glutethimide | Doriden | CIBAs, packs (with codeine) |
| methyprylon | Noludar | |
| ethchlorvynol | Placidyl | |
| chloral hydrate | Noctec | |
| paraldehyde | Paral | |
| meprobamate | Miltown | |
| scopolamine | Sominex | truth serum |

## Sidebar 6: Frequently Abused Drugs (*continued*)

| CLASS | TRADE NAME | STREET NAME |
|---|---|---|
| *Opioids* | | |
| morphine | morphine sulfate | dope, M, Miss Emma, Morpho, white stuff |
| heroin | none | H, junk, skag, smack, boy, hard stuff, horse |
| hydromorphone | Dilaudid | DLs |
| oxymorphone | Numorphan | blues |
| oxycodone | Percodan, Percocet | Percs |
| meperidine | Demerol | |
| methadone hydrochloride | Dolophine | dollys, done |
| pentazocine | Talwin | |
| tincture of opium | paregoric | PG, licorice |
| cough preparations with codeine | Elixir terpin hydrate, Robitussin A-C | schoolboy, blue velvet, Robby |
| hydrocodone | Hycodan | |
| *Nonnarcotic analgesic* | | |
| propoxyphene | Darvon | |
| *Central nervous system stimulants* | | |
| cocaine hydrochloride | cocaine | coke, blow, toot, girl |
| cocaine freebase | | crack, rock, base |
| dextroamphetamine | Biphetamine | black beauties |

## Sidebar 6: Frequently Abused Drugs (*continued*)

| CLASS | TRADE NAME | STREET NAME |
|---|---|---|
| *Central nervous system stimulants* (continued) | | |
| amphetamine sulfate | Benzedrine | A's, beans, bennies, cartwheels, crossroads, jelly beans, hearts, peaches, whites |
| amphetamine sulfate/amobarbital | Dexamyl | greenies |
| dextroamphetamine sulfate | Dexedrine | brownies, Christmas trees, dexies, hearts, wakeups |
| methamphetamine hydrochloride | Methedrine | bombit, crank, crystal, meth, speed |
| *Hallucinogenic drugs* | | |
| lysergic acid diethylamide (LSD) | synthetic derivative (ergot fungus) | acid, pink wedges, sandos, sugar cubes |
| psilocin/psilocybin | mushroom (*Psilocybe mexicana*) | businessman's acid, magic mushroom |
| dimethyltryptamine | synthetic | DMT, DET, DPT |
| morning glory seeds | bindweed (*Rivea corymbosa*) | flower power, heavenly blue, pearly gates |
| mescaline | peyote cactus | barf tea, big chief, buttons, cactus, mesc |
| methyldimethoxy-amphetamine (DOM) | synthetic (derivative) | STP |
| myristicin | nutmeg | MMDA |
| muscarine | mushroom (*Amanita muscaria*) | fly |
| phencyclidine | | angel dust, dust, PCP |

## Sidebar 6: Frequently Abused Drugs (*continued*)

| CLASS | TRADE NAME | STREET NAME |
|---|---|---|
| *Cannabis* | | |
| marijuana | *Cannabis sativa* (leaves, flowers) | grass, hay, joints, Mary Jane, pot, reefer, rope, smoke, weed |
| hashish | *Cannabis sativa*, resin | hash |

Source: Stone, E. M., ed. *American Psychiatric Glossary* Washington, D.C.: American Psychiatric Press, 1989, pp. 122–124. Used with permission.

263

some cases, the patient's physician may provide another, less addictive sedative medication. Once a patient is stabilized on a substituted medication, the substituted medication is gradually decreased by approximately 10 percent per *day*. The only exception to this rule is Xanax (alprazolam), for which an even more gradual reduction is necessary, approximately a 10 percent reduction in dose per *week*.

### JANE ALBERT: SUCCESSFUL WITHDRAWAL FROM DIAZEPAM (VALIUM)

Jane, a thirty-two-year old housewife, became dependent upon diazepam after receiving a prescription from her gynecologist. Because she also had some medical problems, she chose to withdraw from the drug in a hospital setting. After a thorough medical evaluation, she was given 50 mg chlordiazepoxide (Librium) every two hours until she became sedated. Subsequently, she required a dose of 200 mg Librium the first day. This was then gradually reduced to 10 percent a day. After ten days, she was successfully withdrawn from diazepam without serious complications or acute withdrawal symptoms. While being withdrawn from the benzodiazepine, her vital signs were carefully monitored for withdrawal symptoms (increases in her pulse rate, blood pressure, and temperature—profuse sweating). Because chlordiazepoxide was withdrawn gradually, there were no significant withdrawl symptoms.

### REHABILITATION

Older patients are often referred to rehabilitation programs similar to those used for alcoholics since the characteristics of those dependent on benzodiazepines are quite similar. For people with psychiatric disorders, individual psychotherapy, family therapy, or group therapy may also be useful. Young people who have abused benzodiazepines or barbiturates may respond best to residential treatment programs that use intensive group therapy. For both older and younger abusers, participation in drug counseling and self-help programs similar to Alcoholics Anonymous is usually extremely helpful. For those patients who develop depressive symptoms following withdrawal of medication, antidepressants are frequently prescribed. Doses used are similar to those used in the treatment of major depression.

# Overcoming Addictions to Heroin and Other Opiates

Opiates include naturally occurring compounds, such as heroin and morphine, and synthetic agents frequently prescribed in the hospital, such as codeine, meperidine (Demerol), methadone, oxycodone (Percocet), and others. Synthetic opiates, usually taken as pills, are sometimes administered intravenously. Heroin is almost always used intravenously, but may also be smoked or inhaled. High levels of tolerance may develop after chronic use.

As with the benzodiazepines, two patterns of use characterize opiate dependence and abuse:

• The use of opiates often begins when someone is hospitalized for a surgical procedure or medical problem and a physician prescribes analgesic pain medication, frequently an opiate. People may become dependent upon the opiate medication while in the hospital and then require increasing doses once they are discharged.

• Teenagers or young adults may purchase opiates illegally in order to get high. Young people frequently use opiates in combination with other illegal substances: amphetamines, marijuana, or sedatives. These drugs are used to counteract or enhance the effects of the opiates. For such uses, opiates are frequently just one of several classes of abused substances.

Heroin or morphine, when injected, will produce euphoria within two to five minutes. The period of euphoria may last up to thirty minutes. This is followed by a two- to six-hour period of lethargy, sleepiness, and impaired functioning. While in an intoxicated state, a person's pupils become constricted. Speech may be slurred. Memory may be impaired. If taken in an overdose, opiates may cause severe respiratory depression, coma, and death.

## OPIATE WITHDRAWAL

Withdrawing from the opiate drugs produces flulike symptoms: sweating, diarrhea, fever, sleep disturbance, increased heart rate, and a mild elevation in blood pressure. In addition, the person may become intensely restless, irritable, and depressed. Withdrawal symptoms begin from six to twelve hours after the last dose and typically become most severe in two to three days. In contrast to alcohol or barbiturate withdrawal, opiate withdrawal is usually not life threatening.

## OPIATE DETOXIFICATION

Methadone is frequently used to detoxify patients who are dependent on more addictive opiates. Methadone is a long-acting opiate that can be administered once a day without causing severe withdrawal symptoms. It is especially useful in patients who have been using intravenous heroin. Methadone treatment allows the patient to take his or her medication in pill form once a day. The patient does not have extreme changes in opiate blood levels and does not experience the euphoria associated with heroin use.

The patient usually begins with an initial dose of 10 to 20 mg of methadone. Some heavily addicted patients may require doses of up to 60 mg per day. Once an adequate dose is reached, the hospitalized patient begins withdrawing from methadone at a rate of 1 mg per day. This normally takes twenty days. For patients who are not in the hospital, methadone is optimally reduced 10 percent per week until a daily dose of 10 to 20 mg of methadone is achieved. The remaining dose is then decreased by approximately 3 percent per week. This slow detoxification program reduces the likelihood of relapse.

For patients addicted to codeine or oxycodone (Percocet), detoxification may begin at a methadone dose of approximately 20 mg, with a reduction of 1 mg per day over a two- to three-week period.

Those addicted to both heroin and alcohol are usually first withdrawn from heroin with methadone. They are then withdrawn from alcohol using a benzodiazepine. Their methadone dose is then gradually reduced.

A newer antiopiate drug, L-alpha acetylmethadol (L-AAM), is longer-acting than methadone. This drug can be taken three times per week. The patient does not need Saturday and Sunday doses. The Friday dose will last for the whole weekend. Thus L-AAM reduces the risk of the patient's selling the medication on the street and ending up using an addictive street drug.

## OTHER PHARMACOLOGICAL TREATMENTS FOR OPIATE DETOXIFICATION

Clonidine (Catapres), an alpha-adrenergic blocker, is sometimes used to aid opiate withdrawal. While this drug can reduce some withdrawal symptoms, especially hyperactivity, it is less effective in reducing subjective discomfort. Once the methadone dose is stabilized at 20 mg or less, methadone is stopped abruptly and clonidine is substituted. Usually, clonidine is begun three times daily in a dose starting at 0.1 to 0.3 mg. It is then gradually increased 0.2 to 0.7 mg three times a day over an eight- to fourteen-day period. Although clonidine is not currently FDA-approved for opiate detoxification, it is used by both outpatient and inpatient treatment centers. Clonidine may produce dry mouth, drowsiness, fatigue, headache, dizziness, and sedation.

Another drug used by some special programs in treating opiate withdrawal is naltrexone (Trexan). This opiate antagonist blocks opiate receptors in the central nervous system, preventing euphoria if opiates are taken. If used on a long-term basis, naltrexone may gradually extinguish drug-seeking behavior. Naltrexone does not produce dependence, has few side effects, and reduces the likelihood of overdose if opiates are used. Success rates in using naltrexone have been quite variable, with high refusal and dropout rates in some outpatient clinic populations, in particular those treating hard-core addicts. However, in highly motivated patients who have reasons to continue treatment, naltrexone has proved extremely helpful.

# Overcoming Addiction to Cocaine

Cocaine is derived from the coca plant *Erythroxylon coca*, which is cultivated in several Central and South American countries. Various coca preparations may be used to achieve euphoria: The coca leaves may be chewed, or a coca paste may be smoked in a pipe. Both these forms of use are usually restricted to the Central and South American countries where the plant is grown.

In the United States, the usual form of use is cocaine hydrochloride powder, which is either inhaled via the nose or injected intravenously. When mixed with heroin, the combination is called a speedball. More recently, cocaine has been distributed in its alkaloid form, called crack, or freebase cocaine. This form may be purchased and smoked in crack houses and is associated with intense addiction.

### SYMPTOMS OF INTOXICATION

Symptoms of cocaine intoxication include euphoria, sexual arousal, disinhibition, and elation. The intensity of the *rush* is much greater if cocaine is used intravenously in crack or freebase form. In higher doses, people may exhibit agitation, grandiosity, paranoid thinking, and impaired judgment. Increased heart rates, pupillary dilation, elevated blood pressure, and even hallucinations may occur. Cocaine is usually abused in a binge fashion, with a typical binge lasting from a few hours to several days.

Cocaine's half-life, if snorted intranasally, is approximately ninety minutes. The euphoric effects last from fifteen to thirty minutes. When stopped abruptly, cocaine may produce depression, characterized as the *crash*.

## MEDICAL COMPLICATIONS

Intravenous injection of cocaine with dirty or contaminated needles may produce damage to the heart valves (endocarditis), inflammation and damage to the liver, hepatitis, AIDS and HIV infection, and damage to the lungs (emphysema and pulmonary infections). Because the drug can produce abnormal heartbeats that impair the heart's ability to pump blood to the brain, death can occur, especially when the freebase form is smoked. Heart attacks, seizures, and respiratory arrest can also occur.

## COCAINE WITHDRAWAL

Cocaine withdrawal consists of three phases:

1. The *crash* consists of depression, insomnia, anxiety, irritability, and an intense craving for more cocaine. Pronounced depression or suicidal thoughts may occur during this period. This phase may last for up to three days.
2. Lasting from three to ten days, the second phase is characterized by low-level cocaine craving, with irritability, anxiety, and lack of pleasure in the person's usual activities. During this period, memories of the crash decline, and desire for more cocaine is increased.
3. For several weeks, a milder craving for cocaine may develop.

## DRUGS USED TO TREAT COCAINE WITHDRAWAL

Heterocyclic antidepressants have been successfully used to treat the depression associated with withdrawal from cocaine. The mechanism of action of the antidepressants is not known, but may be related to the heterocyclics' ability to turn off norepinephrine receptor sites, making them less sensitive to, and thus less in need of, cocaine and its euphoric properties. The dosages are similar to those used to treat major depression. The antidepressants found most promising to reduce craving are desipramine and imipramine. For more on these drugs, see Chapter 3.

Researchers have also used other medications to reduce cocaine craving. Bromocriptine (Parlodel), a drug used to treat Parkinson's disease, mimics the action of dopamine by stimulating dopamine receptors and, hence, down-regulating the receptors. This may lead to reduced craving for cocaine. L-tryptophan (before it was taken off the market—see Chapter 8) and L-tyrosine have also been used with some success. These naturally occurring amino acids can apparently help replenish the patient's depleted dopamine neurotransmitter storage sites caused by repeated cocaine use.

# Overcoming Addiction to Amphetamines and Stimulants

Amphetamines such as dextroamphetamine (Dexedrine) and methylphenidate (Ritalin) are medications used to treat narcolepsy and attention-deficit disorders in children. In rare cases, these drugs are used to treat depression in the medically ill. Other forms of these drugs can be found in appetite suppressants—the so-called *diet pills*. When abused, these substances can be inhaled, injected intravenously, or taken orally.

Symptoms of amphetamine abuse include an increase in heart rate, elevated blood pressure, pupillary dilation, and agitation. With increasing dosages, more severe side effects such as irritability, confusion, hostility, and sleep disturbances may occur. With even higher doses, patients may exhibit bizarre thoughts, delusions, agitation, and extreme suspiciousness—symptoms indistinguishable from schizophrenia. People intoxicated with amphetamines may be indistinguishable from those with an acute manic episode or delirium. Some people become addicted to amphetamines as a result of trying to lose weight quickly or to remain alert while studying for exams.

### TREATMENT OF AMPHETAMINE WITHDRAWAL

The principal symptoms of amphetamine or methylphenidate (Ritalin) withdrawal are fatigue, insomnia or hypersomnia, and agitation. Withdrawal can usually be accomplished on an outpatient basis. Inpatient hospitalization is required only for those patients who (1) abuse the medication intravenously, (2) who have been severely depressed and had suicidal thoughts, or (3) who have completely lost touch with reality. Haloperidol (Haldol) or other antipsychotic medications may help treat psychotic symptoms (delusions, hallucinations, agitation, and confusion) associated with amphetamine intoxication. For patients who experience severe depression following withdrawal, heterocyclic antidepressants may be helpful. Patients may be quickly withdrawn from stimulants without any serious adverse medical complications.

## Overcoming Marijuana Abuse

Marijuana is a mixture of leaves, stems, seeds, and flowering tops of the plant *Cannabis sativa*. Marijuana has been used frequently as a recreational drug. The active component of marijuana is delta-9-tetrahydrocannabinol (THC). Marijuana use peaked in the late 1970s, with regular marijuana use dropping to 42 percent of Americans in 1983 and daily use to 5 percent. Unfortunately, the increasing disapproval of marijuana use has been supplemented with an increase in the popularity of cocaine, especially in young people of high school and college age.

When smoking marijuana, intoxication levels occur within ten to thirty minutes and last approximately two to four hours. When ingested, marijuana produces a slower onset of intoxication, from forty-five to sixty minutes. The marijuana high is characterized by a slowed sense of time; increased appetite; a keener sense of color, sound, and other sensory stimuli; euphoria, a relaxed feeling, and an increase in confidence.

### ADVERSE EFFECTS

The most common adverse effects reported by marijuana users are anxiety, depression, and paranoid thinking. Long-term use may produce passivity and lack of motivation. Even after the acute effects of marijuana subside, the drug itself remains in the fat cells fifty hours or more. Some people may have problems concentrating, remembering things, and even speaking coherently over the next two to three days. Marijuana may impair motor coordination, a particularly serious problem if one is driving an automobile while intoxicated on marijuana or immediately after marijuana use.

There is no convincing evidence that marijuana produces permanent central nervous system or behavioral changes. However, there is some evidence that heavy, chronic marijuana use may predispose individuals to chronic obstructive lung disease or lung cancer—roughly on the order of the risk of tobacco smoking. Although many investigators believe that an *amotivational syndrome* may develop in chronic marijuana users, the studies done to date have not established the existence of this syndrome.

### POSITIVE BENEFITS

Cannabis extract has been used in medical settings to treat nausea and vomiting in cancer patients who were unresponsive to traditional treatments, such as droperidol (Inapsine). In patients with glaucoma, cannabis may help decrease intraocular pressure. However, in both circumstances, long-term use of cannabis does not appear justified because of the other potential adverse medical consequences.

### TREATMENT OF MARIJUANA ABUSE AND DEPENDENCE

Drugs are not used to withdraw people from marijuana. Inpatient treatment is rarely necessary. Outpatient treatment programs usually resemble the alcohol rehabilitation programs discussed above: self-help groups, group therapy, individual therapy, family therapy, and education programs.

Most treatment programs include urine drug testing. Cannabis may be detected in the urine up to twenty-one days after cessation of use. Urinalysis detection is an inexpensive and quick way to monitor marijuana use.

The most effective interventions focus on prevention and cessation of later drug use. It is important to encourage adolescents to avoid people or places where marijuana or other drugs are being abused. Active parental involvement is very important in preventing further abuse.

## Overcoming Nicotine Addiction

Tobacco addiction is a very serious medical problem. Smoking causes heart disease, lung cancer, and a variety of severe medical problems (see Sidebar 7).

The principal active ingredient in tobacco is nicotine, which produces euphoric effects similar to those produced by cocaine and the amphetamines. Cessation of prolonged cigarette smoking will lead to withdrawal symptoms: craving, irritability, anxiety, concentration problems, and restlessness. Tobacco has been shown to increase the liver's metabolism of various medications, thereby causing lower levels of not only heterocyclic antidepressant medications but others that are metabolized by the liver. Women who smoke while pregnant have been shown to have low–birthweight children.

### TREATMENT

Most people who stop smoking are able to do so using self-help measures without the aid of any drug. Certain smokers seem to have a harder time quitting—especially those under great stress, those with poor social supports, those with a family member who smokes, those who lack educational information, women with low self-confidence, and those with poor motivation.

## Sidebar 7: Selected Statistics About Deaths from Smoking (1984)

| | MEN | | WOMEN | |
| DISEASES | TOTAL DEATHS | PERCENTAGE ATTRIBUTABLE TO SMOKING | TOTAL DEATHS | PERCENTAGE ATTRIBUTABLE TO SMOKING |
| --- | --- | --- | --- | --- |
| Cancer of lung, trachea, and bronchus | 82,459 | 80 | 36,227 | 75 |
| Cancer of larynx | 2,959 | 80 | 664 | 41 |
| Heart disease, under age 65 | 78,340 | 29 | 27,000 | 18 |
| Heart disease, over age 65 | 211,003 | 16 | 224,756 | 8 |
| Disorders of brain circulation | 59,185 | 10 | 88,285 | 14 |
| Pneumonia and influenza | 28,774 | 21 | 28,935 | 9 |
| Chronic bronchitis and emphysema | 10,708 | 85 | 5,517 | 70 |
| Chronic airway obstruction | 31,240 | 85 | 16,625 | 69 |

Adapted from Hales, D. R., *An Invitation to Health*, 4th ed. Redwood City, California: Benjamin/Cummings, 1989, p. 378. Used with permission.

A new pharmacological treatment using nicotine gum (Nicorette) has been found to increase significantly a smoker's chances of long-term quitting. It should be emphasized that nicotine gum should not be taken unless the person also employs a variety of other stop-smoking techniques, e.g., an exercise program, a weight control strategy, educational seminars, behavioral modification, self-help books.

## NICOTINE GUM

Although nicotine is the pharmacologically active substance in tobacco smoke, nicotine itself, in the doses taken by smokers, is relatively harmless. It is the *tar, carbon monoxide, and other toxic gases* that produce virtually all tobacco-related disease.

Nicotine gum provides smokers a way of breaking the quitting process down into two manageable stages: In stage one, you will smoke your last cigarette and will begin getting your nicotine from Nicorette. In stage two, you will gradually taper down and discontinue the Nicorette. Guidelines for the effective use of Nicorette include the following:

• You cannot chew Nicorette like regular chewing gum. Chewing Nicorette like regular gum makes it much less effective and greatly increases the risk of side effects—such as heartburn, nausea, or hiccups.

• Nicotine is released from the Nicorette when a freshly exposed surface comes in contact with saliva. You will only need to chew a new piece of Nicorette for a few seconds (approximately ten to twelve chews) after you begin using a new piece. This is enough to moisten and soften the resin and to initiate release of the nicotine. As soon as you begin to feel a spicy taste or tingling, stop chewing. Park the Nicorette in your cheek.

• The nicotine is absorbed through the membrane on the inside of the cheek. Nicotine that is swallowed is broken down in the stomach and may cause side effects.

• Keep the Nicorette in your cheek until the spicy taste disappears. Bite the Nicorette gently once or twice to restart the release of nicotine. *Vigorous chewing is not necessary*. Stop chewing when you feel the tingle. Again, you should park the Nicorette in your cheek.

• Repeat this process until you no longer feel the tingle when you bite or chew the Nicorette. Each piece lasts for approximately 25 to 30 minutes, although this varies from person to person.

• Do not drink acidic beverages (e.g., sodas, coffee, orange juice) while you have Nicorette in your mouth.

Using Nicorette appears roughly to double a smoker's chances of successful long-term quitting. In addition, the gum significantly decreases the severity of such withdrawal symptoms as irritability, anger, frustration, restlessness, impatience, sleepiness, and food cravings. The gum can also significantly reduce, though it does not completely eliminate, the craving for cigarettes.

Nicorette appears to be particularly effective in decreasing withdrawal symptoms during the afternoon and evening hours. This makes the gum especially useful, since withdrawal symptoms characteristically become more intense during the later part of the day.

What Nicorette does *not* eliminate is the need for alternative healthful activities, new thinking patterns, and intense social and psychological support for the six to twelve months after quitting. Here are some of the kinds of support that seem to be most important:

- Reviewing and recording the pattern of Nicorette use.
- Learning and using new stress management skills.
- Getting together with a key support person to discuss potential problems and brainstorm possible solutions.
- Avoiding high-risk relapse situations.
- Reinforcing the commitment to continue Nicorette use. (Smokers who use Nicorette for less than four months are more likely to relapse.)
- Beginning again immediately if slips do occur.

### NICOTINE DEPENDENCE QUIZ

The Swedish smoking researcher Karl-Olov Fagerstrom has developed a self-scoring quiz (see Sidebar 8) to help you determine how addicted you are to nicotine. Most researchers would agree that the more addicted a smoker is, the more the nicotine gum will help.

### HOW TO GET A PRESCRIPTION FOR NICOTINE GUM

Any licensed physician or dentist can write a prescription for Nicorette. Ask your doctor or dentist for a prescription, or ask your local pharmacist to recommend a doctor or dentist who is knowledgeable in using this medication.

We suggest that you ask your physician or dentist to write a prescription that you can refill as needed over the next twelve months.

# Sidebar 8: Nicotine Addiction Questionnaire

| QUESTIONS | ANSWERS | POINTS | SCORE |
|---|---|---|---|
| 1. How soon after you wake do you smoke your first cigarette? | Within 30 minutes | 1 | — |
| | After 30 minutes | 0 | — |
| 2. Do you find it difficult to refrain from smoking in places where it is forbidden? | Yes | 1 | — |
| | No | 0 | — |
| 3. Which cigarette would you hate to give up most? | The first one in the morning | 1 | — |
| | Any other | 0 | — |
| 4. How many cigarettes a day do you smoke? | 15 or fewer | 0 | — |
| | 16–25 | 1 | — |
| | 26 or more | 2 | — |
| 5. Do you smoke more frequently during the early morning than during the rest of the day? | Yes | 1 | — |
| | No | 0 | — |
| 6. Do you smoke if you are so ill that you are in bed most of the day? | Yes | 1 | — |
| | No | 0 | — |
| 7. What is the nicotine level of your usual brand of cigarettes? | 0.9 mg or less (low) | 0 | — |
| | 1.0–1.2 mg (medium) | 1 | — |
| | 1.3 mg or more (high) | 2 | — |
| 8. Do you inhale? | Never | 0 | — |
| | Sometimes | 1 | — |
| | Always | 2 | — |

Total ___

Scoring:
0–5  Low dependence level
6–7  Medium dependence level
8–11  High dependence level

## How to Use Nicorette

Zero to four months: Chew Nicorette whenever desired, but do not exceed thirty pieces per day. (Moderate smokers usually experience best results if they chew eight to twenty pieces per day. Heavy smokers may find they need to chew twenty to thirty pieces per day.)

Four to six months: Gradually begin to taper down on the gum. To maximize chances of success, continue using Nicorette at a maintenance level for at least four months.

Six to twelve months: Taper down to one to four pieces of gum per day. You should feel free to discontinue the gum after six months of use—if you feel ready to do so. You may wish to carry a few pieces with you at all times as a security blanket—and to use it if you feel an overpowering urge to smoke.

One year and beyond: Discontinue Nicorette except for emergencies. Keep a few pieces in a convenient place—for intense cravings.

Keep Nicorette away from children. If a child accidentally chews or swallows a piece of Nicorette, contact a physician or the local poison control center immediately.

## Nicotine Gum: What Does It Cost?

If you fill your prescription at a discount pharmacy, Nicorette will probably cost just a bit more than you're now spending for cigarettes. As we go to press, prices for a ninety-six-piece box of Nicorette range from a high of $32.30 at our neighborhood pharmacy to a low of $18.45 at our local Wal-Mart. That works out to between 19 and 34 cents per piece. Thus, the pack-a-day smoker who quit and began chewing twelve pieces of gum a day would switch from a daily cigarette bill of $1.50 to a daily Nicorette bill of $2.25.

One of us (Ferguson) has written a book for smokers who wish to quit on their own. This paperback may have the longest title of any book in recent memory: *The No-Nag, No-Guilt, Do-It-Your-Own-Way Guide to Quitting Smoking* helps smokers design their own stop-smoking method, choosing from the tools and strategies that have been found most effective.

# Choosing the Right Treatment

In deciding on the proper treatment for a person with a substance abuse or dependence problem, physicians usually consider several important factors: severity of any coexisting medical or psychiatric illnesses, a patient's personal characteristics, cultural factors, finances, and availability of treatment programs.

Inpatient treatment is indicated if a person has major medical or psychiatric problems; a history of serious withdrawal symptoms, such as delirium, withdrawal seizures, or other medical complications; failure of successful outpatient treatment; lack of a supportive family, friends, or a social network to encourage continued abstinence; a previous history of addiction to multiple substances; or a previous history of inpatient detoxification or rehabilitation treatment.

Sometimes people may be detoxified on an inpatient basis, then undergo rehabilitation in an outpatient setting. More rarely, they may initially be detoxified on an outpatient basis followed by later inpatient rehabilitation. The most successful treatment programs on an outpatient basis are those that offer comprehensive services including individual psychotherapy, psychoeducational programs, group psychotherapy, family therapy, recreational programs, occupational therapy, and other support services.

## INDIVIDUAL PSYCHOTHERAPY

People with substance dependence frequently respond well to individual psychotherapy. Those who are psychologically minded, have a history of being able to establish an intimate relationship (i.e., are married or have a significant other), are of average or above average intelligence, and are highly motivated are the best candidates for psychotherapy. Psychotherapy may deal with both individual and interpersonal issues that may contribute to their addiction. Psychotherapy may also help the addicted person learn to recognize anxiety and depressive symptoms.

## GROUP PSYCHOTHERAPY

Groups are frequently used in both inpatient and outpatient settings to treat people with addiction problems. Groups enable individuals to enter into normal social settings from which they may have become isolated. Group settings also may foster development of improved impulse control and may enhance a person's sense of self-esteem. Groups of patients with substance abuse disorders are very effective in that individual group members will cut through attempts at hiding distasteful situations or emotionally charged material. These groups also help people realize that others have similar problems. Drug abusers are generally much more willing to listen to others who have experienced similar addiction problems than to nonaddicted individuals.

## FAMILY THERAPY

Many patients who have substance abuse problems may benefit from family therapy. Children of alcoholics may especially benefit from such approaches. Confrontation by other family members frequently will force patients into continuing treatment and remaining abstinent. Family treatments focus on the resolution of problems within the family, especially problems relating to other family members. These treatments are advised for patients who have been frequently intoxicated or isolated from other family members.

## SELF-HELP APPROACHES

The most well-known and successful self-help programs are Alcoholics Anonymous, Al-Anon, and many other related groups—such as Substance Anonymous, Narcotics Anonymous, Cocaine Anonymous, etc. Alcoholics Anonymous was established in the 1930s and currently includes over two million members. Its message is that people with an addiction to alcohol can, through recognition that alcoholism is an illness, achieve sobriety. The twelve-step program addresses spiritual issues, including the alcoholic's acceptance that he or she lacks power in overcoming alcohol dependency without help from others. Most members attend four to five meetings each week, although during the early stages, they may attend nightly. The meetings vary greatly in style; however, a sense of acceptance and understanding usually pervades most groups.

The meetings emphasize self-help through helping others with a similar problem. Important aspects of membership include the generosity, time, and energy of its members. Experienced Alcoholics Anonymous attendees sponsor new members and help them overcome initial reluctance to share their plight with the group. Alcoholics Anonymous provides an opportunity for people to practice relating to others, to be honest, to test judgments, to find acceptance, and to regain hope.

# Addicted Patients Who Are Also Mentally Ill

Anywhere from one-fourth to one-half of all patients who seek psychiatric treatment also have a substance abuse disorder. Since the treatment approaches for their two problems are often vastly different, such a situation presents special problems for both the patients and the clinicians. Special Alcoholics Anonymous groups have been established for such dual-diagnosis patients. It has been reported that patients who abuse substances and who also have psychiatric disorders may benefit from the addition of individual psychotherapy. Those with severe psychiatric disorders may require hospitalization. In most cases, they should be treated by a substance abuse specialist.

## WHO RESPONDS BEST TO TREATMENT?

Generally speaking, those people who respond best to treatment for a substance use disorder are those with a good employment history, high socioeconomic status, a low rate of antisocial personality difficulties, no psychiatric or medical problems, and no family history of alcoholism. Other factors that may contribute to a positive outcome are a productive work history; attendance at Alcoholics Anonymous meetings; a relatively stable marriage; and few if any arrests.

## PREVENTING RELAPSE

Addictions are similar to other diseases in that people may have episodic relapses. It has been estimated that 90 percent of patients in any twelve-month period following abstinence will again abuse psychoactive substances. Nearly half will reexperience the same problems that led them to treatment in the first place.

Recovering substance abusers should avoid high-risk situations that may contribute to repeated episodes of abuse: unpleasant emotions, emotionally charged situations, physical discomfort, testing one's ability to control oneself, urges and temptation, conflict with others, and social pressure to drink or abuse drugs. The importance of each of these factors may vary according to the individual and type of substance being abused. During such difficult times—for instance, when in conflict with a fellow worker—assistance from a psychotherapist or family member can be helpful.

The recovering addict must learn to recognize the thoughts and feelings that may occur during these high-risk situations, and, finally, the recovering addict must develop behavioral, cognitive, and emotional techniques to deal effectively with the thoughts and feelings that may occur during these high-risk situations.

John, forty-seven years old, was a recovering alcoholic. He was also the director of development at a charitable organization, and frequently had to attend evening fund-raising receptions where alcohol was served. When he felt the urge to have a drink, he wouldn't. Instead, he would make an effort to meet someone new or would go out of his way to greet or socialize with prospective contributors. Not only did he remain abstinent, but his fund-raising efforts improved dramatically.

### JAMES CASSADY: UNSUCCESSFUL TREATMENT OF DRUG ADDICTION

James was a forty-two-year-old married man, a successful stockbroker who worked for a large Wall Street brokerage firm. In his late thirties, he became very successful and earned a great deal of money. He found himself going to various parties after work with clients and other business associates. A good friend advised him to try cocaine. James experienced a brief period of euphoria "not like anything I have ever previously felt." He began to experiment more and more frequently with cocaine at parties. He would use cocaine either given to him by or purchased from colleagues. Unfortunately, such episodic use did not satisfy James. He developed an intense craving for more cocaine. He began purchasing larger and larger quantities over the next year until he was spending $200 per day on the drug. He needed to take cocaine the first thing in the morning and even during his lunch hour to prevent himself from experiencing the crash associated with cocaine withdrawal.

James found himself spending less and less time at home with his wife and children, and more and more time engaged in efforts to obtain new sources of the drug. He also began to visit crack houses and to spend more and more money on his drug habit. He obtained a second mortgage on his house and spent nearly all the money in his savings account on cocaine. After approximately eighteen months, he began experimenting with intravenous injections of cocaine. Sometimes he combined cocaine with heroin.

It was about this time that his productivity at the office dramatically plummeted. James would frequently miss scheduled appointments and fail to return phone calls from clients. His immediate supervisor received many complaints about his absences and nonavailability. James became suspicious of his co-workers and blamed them for taking away his clients. His wife unsuccessfully tried to get him into treatment. When she brought him to a psychiatrist, he refused treatment, denying that he even had a problem. Marital therapy was unsuccessful and his wife left him. His employer eventually fired him because of many mistakes and lapses on the job.

Now unemployed, James spent almost all his time on the street, either in crack houses or obtaining supplies of cocaine or heroin for intravenous use. He also began spending more time with prostitutes and drug abusers. His house was foreclosed and nearly all his money was gone. He became increasingly despondent and isolated from his usual friends. He moved into a cheap boardinghouse where he ate little and spent most of his time looking for cheaper sources of cocaine. He was found dead one morning by the landlord, the result of an apparent heart attack from a massive injection of cocaine.

James's story, although dramatic and tragic, is unfortunately common. The user's intense craving for cocaine should not be underestimated. James's preoccupation with cocaine and his isolation from his loved ones and co-workers represent a natural progression of the disease. A dramatic and untimely death is also all too common.

What makes the treatment of such people so difficult is the intense denial they exhibit concerning their dependency. Repeated confrontations by his wife, physician, and colleagues were completely unsuccessful. After prolonged cocaine use, paranoid symptoms frequently develop. James, for instance, came to believe that others were trying to ruin his career. A combination of denial and paranoid behavior makes it very difficult to successfully engage such people in treatment.

## Brenda Hanson: Successful Treatment of Drug Addiction

Brenda was a forty-two-year-old married housewife with two grown children. While working around the house one day, she sustained a back injury that required her to be hospitalized. She subsequently underwent repair of a ruptured lumbar disk. She was prescribed meperidine (Demerol) at a dose of 75 mg four times a day. While in the hospital, she found that it was very difficult for her to stop the medicine. When the physician tried to taper her off the meperidine, she complained that she needed more medication. The surgeon was busy and did not feel this was a serious problem. Consequently, he continued to allow her to receive meperidine, now at a dose of 100 mg five times a day, while in the hospital. He indicated that he would try to get her off the meperidine after discharge and during her follow-up visits. He gave her a limited prescription: enough for approximately one week. The next time she went to his office, he indicated that he planned to stop the medicine that day. Brenda became very upset with him. To stave off what he feared would be a nasty incident from occurring in his office, he gave her another prescription for one week and told her that she should stop the medicine as soon as possible. He did not arrange any follow-up for her.

She continued to take the meperidine every four hours. Her daily dose gradually increased to 800 mg. Brenda then told her internist (who had originally referred her to the orthopedic surgeon) that she was still having back pains and wanted a second opinion. He gave her a prescription for meperidine and referred her to another orthopedic surgeon. This orthopedic surgeon, in turn, gave her a new supply of meperidine—which she hoarded with her other pills.

Her husband noticed that she was becoming increasingly lethargic. She wasn't interested in her usual activities—gardening, tennis, volunteer work. She was sleeping a great deal, and when she drank alcohol in the evening she would slur her sentences and fall asleep early. Her husband thought that some of these symptoms might be related to her recent surgery and continued pain. Brenda began to shop around to other physicians to obtain more doses of meperidine. She also made periodic visits to an emergency room at a nearby hospital and to acute care clinics located in the city. She then became increasingly isolated from her husband and friends.

One day, her husband discovered several hundred meperidine tablets in various containers with labels of eight different physicians. He confronted her with this evidence and demanded that she see her physician. She admitted taking 200 to 300 mg of meperidine six to seven times a day. Because of the high dose to which she was addicted, her internist referred her to a psychiatrist who in turn admitted her to an inpatient detoxification program. After a thorough physical and laboratory evaluation to rule out any serious medical problems, she was begun on methadone, which was gradually reduced by 1 mg a day over a ten-day period. Included in this detoxification program were therapy sessions with her psychiatrist.

She participated in group psychotherapy as an inpatient. She also began attending Narcotics Anonymous meetings that were held each evening. She and her husband began a marital therapy program in conjunction with her detoxification.

Upon discharge, following her two-week hospital stay, she was referred to an outpatient substance abuse rehabilitation program. It focused on educational programs, a continuation of marital therapy sessions, and weekly individual psychotherapy sessions with her psychiatrist. She also attended Narcotics Anonymous meetings approximately five times a week.

Two months after she was first admitted, Brenda was able to begin returning to a normal routine. She continued her individual psychotherapy sessions and attended Narcotics Anonymous approximately once a week. She also began to contribute time to the outpatient treatment program—to help other people who had developed addiction problems.

Brenda met many of the criteria generally associated with successful outcome: no previous psychiatric or medical problems, no family history of substance abuse, relatively high socioeconomic status, and a stable family and personal environment. She also attended Narcotics Anonymous meetings regularly and was actively involved in the program. She had a supportive husband who took the initiative to direct her to seek treatment. She was then referred to an effective inpatient detoxification program that combined many treatment modalities. It is important to note that she then began treatment in a rehabilitation program to continue the gains that she had achieved during her inpatient experience. Inpatient detoxification seeks principally to get the person off the drug and begin individual and group psychotherapy. Abstinence will not endure if participation in a comprehensive rehabilitation program is not begun.

Brenda, and many others like her, have successfully overcome drug dependency. Substance dependency often begins when a person is hospitalized, and his or her physician prescribes either sedative medications or opiates. Patients should be very cautious about the dosages and amounts of medications prescribed by their physicians. If they notice that they are requiring higher or more frequent doses, they should let their physicians know. Family members should also be kept informed of pharmacologic treatment recommendations so they may provide assistance if a drug-abuse or drug-dependency problem develops.

# Recommended Reading on Addiction

Frances, Richard J., and John E. Franklin, Jr. "Alcohol and Other Psychoactive Substance Use Disorders," *The American Psychiatric Press Textbook of Psychiatry*. Edited by John A. Talbott, Robert E. Hales, and Stuart Yudofsky. Washington, D.C.: American Psychiatric Press, 1988, pp. 313–355.

Frances, Richard J., and John E. Franklin, Jr. *Concise Guide to Treatment of Alcoholism and Addictions*. Washington, D.C.: American Psychiatric Press, 1989.

# Chapter 10

# Drugs for Attention-Deficit Hyperactivity Disorder

MANY children are too active for their parents' comfort—so active that it is difficult for any parent or teacher to deal with them. Researchers and clinicians use the term *hyperactive* to describe these children.

Hyperactive children are almost constantly on the move, far more than usual for their age. They run and move almost continuously. They have great difficulty keeping still or even remaining in their seats for more than a few minutes. Hyperactive children are also impulsive in their actions: They act without thinking, talk out of turn, and cannot wait in line. They need more supervision from adults to keep them from disrupting playmates and classmates.

Children with attention-deficit disorder may have great difficulty completing activities. They are unusually distractible and may find it difficult or impossible to concentrate on school tasks, on games—even on their own self-initiated activities. They appear not to hear—or want to hear—teachers, parents, or other adults. This problem is frequently so severe that parents, teachers, and health professionals all agree that the child has a psychiatric disorder. If parents believe that inattentiveness, impulsivity, and hyperactivity are at the heart of their child's problems, they should discuss this possibility with the child's teachers, the school principal, or with experts in this disorder.

# Attention-Deficit Hyperactivity Disorder

## THE CONTROVERSY OVER ATTENTION-DEFICIT HYPERACTIVITY DISORDER

Attention-deficit hyperactivity disorder is a relatively new diagnosis. The diagnostic concept has been a godsend for many children—for it implies that the reason they have had trouble in school is not that they are "bad," lazy, or stupid but that they have a medical problem that makes it extremely difficult for them to learn material that is presented in the traditional lecture-and-textbook format. This syndrome has forced educators to rethink some of their basic assumptions about education.

Attention-deficit disorder is still considered a controversial diagnosis in some schools. Some educators contend that there is no such thing as attention-deficit hyperactivity disorder or any other such psychiatric disorder of children. They believe it to be merely an invention of the psychiatric profession, and are concerned that physicians might damage a child by applying such a diagnostic label. Others fear that children might be harmed by the drugs used to treat these disorders. We suggest that parents make the effort to hear all sides of this controversy before making decisions that might affect their child's well-being.

## HOW COMMON IS ATTENTION-DEFICIT HYPERACTIVITY DISORDER? WHEN, IN WHOM, AND WHY DOES IT OCCUR?

Attention-deficit hyperactivity disorder and conduct disorders are the two most common groups of childhood psychiatric disorders. An estimated 7 percent of American children meet the criteria for these diagnoses (see Sidebar 1).

Attention-deficit hyperactivity disorder is five times more common in boys than girls. The first signs of this condition frequently appear before the age of four. This condition does seem to run in families. Many researchers believe that it may be associated with a type of minimal brain dysfunction, but this has not been conclusively proved.

### Sidebar 1:  DSM-III-R Diagnostic Criteria for Attention-Deficit Hyperactivity Disorder

A. A disturbance of at least six months during which at least eight of the following are present (listed in order of diagnostic specificity) in the child, who:

1. often fidgets with hands or feet or squirms in seat (in adolescents, may be limited to subjective feelings of restlessness)
2. has difficulty remaining seated when required to do so
3. is easily distracted by extraneous stimuli
4. has difficulty awaiting turn in games or group situations
5. often blurts out answers to questions before they are completed
6. has difficulty following through on instructions from others (not due to oppositional behavior or failure of comprehension), e.g., fails to finish chores
7. has difficulty sustaining attention in tasks or play activities
8. often shifts from one uncompleted activity to another
9. has difficulty playing quietly
10. often talks excessively
11. often interrupts or intrudes on others, e.g., butts into other children's games
12. often does not seem to listen to what is being said to him or her
13. often loses things necessary for tasks or activities at school or at home (e.g., toys, pencils, books, assignments)
14. often engages in physically dangerous activities without considering possible consequences (not for the purpose of thrill-seeking), e.g., runs into the street without looking

B. Onset before the age of seven.

C. Does not meet the criteria for a Pervasive Developmental Disorder.

## TREATMENT OF ATTENTION-DEFICIT HYPERACTIVITY DISORDER

### Evaluation

Any child suspected of having this disorder should have a thorough medical and psychiatric evaluation. This evaluation should include an assessment of the child's psychosocial functioning in a variety of different settings—at home, at school, in social settings with other children and adults, and with the extended family (see Sidebar 2). In many cases, a child will behave differently in each setting. These differences may have important implications for the treatment plan.

Thus, assessment should include:

• A thorough evaluation by a pediatrician. This should include a physical examination and a medical history.

• A psychiatric evaluation by a child psychiatrist. This should include screening for problems related to vision, speech, hearing; evaluation of intellectual capacity; and other standard measures of achievement.

• Other laboratory testing and educational testing may be indicated.

• An assessment of the child's living situation. This may include one or more visits to the home to observe family patterns.

---

### Sidebar 2:  Criteria for Severity of Attention-Deficit Hyperactivity Disorder

• *Mild:* Few if any symptoms in excess of those required to make the diagnosis *and* only minimal or no impairment in school and social functioning

• *Moderate:* Symptoms or functional impairment intermediate between "mild" and "severe"

• *Severe:* Many symptoms in excess of those required to make the diagnosis *and* significant pervasive impairment in functioning at home and in school and with peers

---

*Establish a Treatment Plan*

Attention-deficit hyperactivity disorder typically requires several years of treatment. Many different people must be included in the process of developing the plan. These should include:

• parents
• the child
• the pediatrician
• the child's psychiatrist
• the child's present and future teachers
• the child's school principal
• a family therapist

Open communication among all involved parties is essential. We recommend formulating a symptom list and a problem list. The goal of the treatment plan should be to choose specific interventions for each problem. For example, if distractibility in the home setting is a major problem for a child, establishing a quiet work setting may be an important part of the treatment.

The plan should include several levels:

• Special classroom arrangements may need to be made. Sometimes a change of school or of class size can have dramatic effects on the child's adjustment, as can special educational interventions like tutoring or intensive remedial programs.

• Family psychotherapy may be required even for well-functioning families. Attention-deficit hyperactivity disorder can cause marital discord even in the most solid relationships.

• Individual psychotherapy to help restore the child's self-esteem is frequently useful. Failure at school, at home, and in activities with friends can do extraordinary damage to a child's sense of self-worth, particularly in a success-oriented, status-conscious culture (like ours!).

• Group and/or recreational activity therapy to promote the development of social skills (such as the ability to understand the feelings of others). For example, participating on a soccer team or a baseball team will help the child understand that rules and appreciation of the rights of others are as important as individual skills and talents.

• The parents should receive "postgraduate" training in parenting skills and techniques. This may include reading printed material, working with a family therapist, or participating in a support group of parents with other hyperactive children. We are often told that it is hard enough to parent children without psychiatric disorders; a child with any illness—particularly psychiatric—requires special skills, patience, knowledge, and communication.

• Parental education about attention-deficit hyperactivity disorder symptoms, the clinical course, and the prognosis for children with the disorder.

• Information for the child about attention-deficit hyperactivity disorder and about its treatment in a form that he or she can understand. This should help identify for the child those problems that are a result of the illness.

• Collaboration among teachers, principals, school counselors, and others (with parental consent) in all aspects of the child's assessment and treatment.

• Counseling with parents and with school personnel about an educational plan that takes attention-deficit hyperactivity disorder into account (e.g., appropriate school and class placement, classroom size, seating arrangements).

• A clear recommendation about medication with sufficient information about benefits and side effects, so that parents can make an informed decision about their child.

• An ongoing "master plan" that includes precise documentation of symptoms, guidelines for medication, periodic pediatric evaluations, and regular meetings (every three months) to measure progress, monitor side effects, and reassess the treatment plan.

## NONDRUG APPROACHES TO ATTENTION-DEFICIT HYPERACTIVITY DISORDER

While drugs are often extremely helpful in the treatment of attention-deficit hyperactivity disorder, no drug will solve the problem by itself. Children with this condition frequently exhibit other psychological problems, especially low self-esteem. Problems in the family, failure at school, and inability to maintain friendships are common.

In some cases, a child can benefit immensely from psychotherapy. Other problem patterns (e.g., alcoholism) in the family must be identified and discussed; they can make it more difficult for the family to deal with a hyperactive learning-disabled child.

The nondrug alternatives to the treatment of attention-deficit hyperactivity disorder are well summarized in the American Psychiatric Association's manual *Treatments of Psychiatric Disorders* (pp. 377–381). The reader is also referred to this excellent chapter for bibliographies and references on each alternative type of treatment—behavioral treatment, cognitive therapy, social skills training, psychotherapy, special education, and others.

## HYPERACTIVITY MAY BE CAUSED BY SCHIZOPHRENIA OR DEPRESSION

Not all hyperactivity is caused by or related to attention-deficit hyperactivity disorder. When hyperactivity is part of another psychiatric illness, such as one of the schizophrenias, it is the underlying illness that must be treated. Children who suffer from schizophrenia or other psychotic disorders should not be given stimulants. These drugs may make their symptoms worse. When hyperactivity and attention-deficiency are associated with symptoms of depression, antidepressant medication may be useful. Antidepressant medications have also been used with positive results in special cases where there was no depressive illness. However, most practitioners will use antidepressant medication to treat attention-deficit hyperactivity disorder only when depression is present, or as a second choice when the stimulant medications have not proved useful.

## THE USE OF STIMULANT DRUGS TO TREAT ATTENTION-DEFICIT HYPERACTIVITY DISORDER

The drugs most often used to treat attention-deficit hyperactivity disorder are the stimulants dextroamphetamine (Dexedrine) and methylphenidate (Ritalin) (see Sidebar 3). For those children who have problems with attention and concentration, but show few signs of hyperactivity, methylphenidate is usually the drug of first choice. If hyperactivity is present, dextroamphetamine is usually the drug of first choice. However, since dextroamphetamine may cause bothersome side effects, methylphenidate is often an equally acceptable alternative. Magnesium pemoline (Cylert) is used as a medication of first choice for attention-deficit hyperactivity disorder by some child psychiatrists even though clinical improvement may not be noticeable for as long as three or four weeks. Magnesium pemoline may be given in once-per-day doses, and its great advantage is that it usually produces the fewest side effects—even fewer than methylphenidate.

---

### Sidebar 3: Psychostimulants

*Brand names*
    Dexedrine, Benzedrine, Ritalin, Cylert
*Generic names*
    amphetamine, methylphenidate, magnesium pemoline
*Street names*
    pep pills, diet pills, speed, bennys, crystal, uppers

**Source:** Reproduced with permission of the American Psychiatric Association.

---

## HOW DO THESE DRUGS WORK?

More is understood about *where* stimulants work to treat attention-deficit hyperactivity disorder than about *how* they work. Dextroamphetamine, methylphenidate, and magnesium pemoline (Dexedrine, Ritalin, and Cylert) all act on a part of the brain called the *brain stem* to improve attention, concentration, and task performance. This makes it easier for children with attention-deficit hyperactivity disorder to focus on the task at hand and to organize their activities. Exactly how they work is the subject of much research and considerable controversy. As is true for most drugs that treat dysfunctions of the brain, we do not understand the mechanism of actions.

These drugs also stimulate other parts of the brain, which may lead to these effects and some of the side effects described below.

## WHO SHOULD TAKE THESE DRUGS?

There are an estimated five million children with attention-deficit hyperactivity disorder in the United States. Since this condition is frequently accompanied by some degree of learning disability, this constitutes a major problem for our school systems. Thus, it is not surprising that pressures mount "to do something quick" to correct the problems.

However, no child should be rushed into taking any medication. The decision to employ medication must be made in a deliberate manner and only after a full medical and psychological evaluation. Parents must consider the severity of their child's symptoms, their own feelings, their preference about using or not using medication, the ability of the child to understand the problems and cooperate with the treatment, the flexibility and awareness of teachers and other school figures, and the failure or success of previous efforts.

Regrettably, despite years of study and research, it is still not possible to predict with any degree of certainty which children with attention-deficit hyperactivity disorder will respond to medication and which will not. Children who have tics should be given stimulants only if the potential benefits outweigh the risks of the drug: stimulants may bring out Gilles de la Tourette's syndrome. For more on the side effects of stimulants, see p. 293.

## HOW CAN STIMULANT DRUGS BE MISUSED IN THE TREATMENT OF ATTENTION-DEFICIT HYPERACTIVITY DISORDER?

### Failure to Establish a Cohesive Treatment Plan

No medication is completely harmless. The stimulants used to treat attention-deficit hyperactivity disorder can be dangerous to one's physical health (if taken in large amounts) because of their effects on the nervous system, blood pressure, and heart rate. Still, it is very rare for a person to suffer serious physical harm as the result of taking an overdose of these medications. The most common medically related misuse of the stimulants is to use them for the treatment of hyperactivity or attention-deficit disorder without employing other therapeutic and educational strategies at the same time.

## CAN THESE DRUGS BE ABUSED?

Because psychostimulants rarely cause euphoria in children with attention-deficit hyperactivity disorder, they are rarely abused by these children. However, these drugs do have powerful euphoric effects in older adolescents and adults; there is thus substantial potential for abuse by persons other than the designated patient. In fact, the addictive potential of these drugs is so high that the use of amphetamines and other stimulants has become highly regulated and restricted by the Food and Drug Administration. When these drugs are illegally used by adults for their euphoric effects or to maintain alertness or to stay awake, there is often a tendency to use increasing amounts to achieve the initial alerting or euphoric effects. If high doses are taken for a prolonged period of time, the adult user may experience many side effects, including severely pronounced paranoia and other psychoses. Therefore, caution must be taken to protect the supply of drugs prescribed for your child from anyone who might abuse the drug.

## PRECAUTIONS TO TAKE WHILE USING THESE DRUGS

All children require an extraordinary amount of attention and care. The child with a diagnosed illness who is undergoing further assessment or treatment will require even more intense attention. The psychiatrist, teacher, and other professionals should be keeping records of their observations and impressions as the treatment progresses. We recommend that parents also keep a journal or diary of their child's major events and experiences each day. This can include a symptom checklist, school reports, and the effects, both positive and negative, of medication and treatment. Keeping such a record will also help you educate your child about his or her responsibility for the outcome of treatment—e.g., "Your drug diary says that you have one more pill to take today." You should keep careful records about the numbers and doses of medications prescribed and compare these with the amount that has been taken by your child. In this fashion, you will be able to detect whether your child fails to take his or her medication as prescribed, and will know if any drugs are missing. To keep these drugs from being stolen, you should keep them in a locked drawer, safe, or cabinet. You should know, and record, the number of pills in your home at all times.

You should also record regular measurements of your child's height and weight, changes in appetite or food preference, and changes in sleeping patterns while taking these drugs. In addition, you should record any unusual illness, aches, pains, or other physical complaints your child may experience while taking these drugs.

## POSSIBLE SIDE EFFECTS OF STIMULANTS

There is very little risk involved in taking the three main stimulant drugs so long as they are taken exactly as directed. None of the side effects of the stimulants is life-threatening. Initially, the most common side effects are loss of appetite and difficulty falling asleep at night.

Weight loss, abdominal pain, and/or headaches are less common side effects of these drugs, and usually become less troublesome within a few weeks as the side effects wear off. They are rarely severe enough to require stopping the medication. Some infrequently observed side effects are drowsiness, dizziness, mood changes (typically weepiness), disturbances of coordination, and a state of extreme emotional and behavioral agitation (psychosis). These drugs suppress the production of growth hormones. This can result in a suppression of weight and height gain in growing children. This lag in growth is temporary, except in those children who take large dosages of stimulants for long periods of time. This suppression of growth may be of special significance for those children who are unusually short to begin with, and must be taken in consideration when weighing the risks and benefits of this therapeutic approach.

The long-term effects of stimulants on a child's growth and physical and mental states are extremely controversial. On one extreme are those who believe that no drug of any type should ever be utilized to treat behavioral disorders of children and that it is unwise or even unethical to prescribe a drug for which all the short- and long-term effects are not known. We strongly advise you to raise these issues related to the use of drugs in children with your pediatrician, child psychiatrist, and other trusted professionals.

## POSSIBLE ADVERSE REACTIONS

In rare cases, these drugs may suppress a child's ability to produce blood cells, and this condition is reversed by discontinuation of the drug.

A small (less than 2 percent) but significant number of children develop tics in response to stimulant medication. When this happens, the medication is usually discontinued, and an assessment is made of the risk of developing Tourette's syndrome before reinstituting the drug.

## POSSIBLE DRUG INTERACTIONS

Children with seizure disorders who are taking antiseizure medication should not be given any other medication without consultation with their pediatrician and neurologist. This is particularly true for stimulants, which are thought to increase vulnerability to seizure disorders.

## HOW THESE STIMULANTS MAKE YOU FEEL

If you are an adolescent or adult without any history of attention-deficit hyperactivity disorder, if you take a stimulant drug you will feel increased energy, increased interest level, excitement, euphoria, and perhaps some slight impairment of judgment. Children with attention-deficit hyperactivity disorder who take these medications do not report any such feelings. In fact, they will typically deny that they feel anything at all from taking the medication. If they notice anything, it is that they are calmer and better able to pay attention. When the faster-acting medications are effective, adults observing the child will usually report some degree of improvement almost from the moment the medication is first taken. Even when adults notice dramatic improvement, the child will typically not be impressed with the medication's impact.

## COMMONLY USED DRUGS FOR ATTENTION-DEFICIT HYPERACTIVITY DISORDER

Methylphenidate (Ritalin) is by far the most commonly prescribed medication for attention-deficit hyperactivity disorder. Dextroamphetamine (Dexedrine) is sometimes used when methylphenidate has not produced an adequate effect. Magnesium pemoline (Cylert) is used most commonly in milder cases of attention-deficit hyperactivity disorder when an immediate response is not required and when a once-a-day dose is particularly desirable. A sustained-release form of methylphenidate is now available so that this drug can now be taken once a day as well. Antidepressants are sometimes used if the stimulants are not effective or are contraindicated. Antipsychotic drugs are used only rarely—in special circumstances.

## HOW TO STORE THESE DRUGS

The principal concern in storing these drugs is to protect them from accidental or intentional abuse. Since many children will take these drugs for at least a year, prescriptions are usually written for a month at a time. We advise parents to store these drugs in a small lockable cash box or safe with a strong lock that can be hidden out of reach and knowledge of children and others.

## DOSES, FORMS, AND STRENGTHS

Medications are usually measured in milligrams (thousandths of a gram). Methylphenidate doses for a child with attention-deficit hyperactivity disorder may range from 5 to 60 mg per day. Doses of magnesium pemoline range from 18.75 to 112.5 mg per day. A few children may require lower doses.

The effects of methylphenidate last, perhaps, three to four hours. It must thus be given two or three times each day (at home in the morning, at school before lunch, and, if necessary, at home in the early afternoon). A recently introduced sustained-release form of methylphenidate comes as a 20 mg capsule. This long-lasting form can be given only once a day. Unfortunately, it seems to work as designed for some children but not for others.

Dextroamphetamine is available in short-acting tablets (three to six hours) and in long-acting capsules (eight to sixteen hours). For some children, the release of medication may be uneven—too much initially, followed by too little later on. The medication needs to be taken several times a day to maintain ideal blood levels.

The duration of action of magnesium pemoline can also be variable; it must be given twice a day to some children, even though it appears to last twelve to eighteen hours in others, and may even carry over to the next day or longer for some children.

## BEGINNING DRUG THERAPY

### Assessment

The assessment of school-aged children (ages six to twelve years) for the treatment of attention-deficit hyperactivity disorder will almost always begin with an interview of the parents. This interview will emphasize the child's developmental history, a family history (including any other developmental, learning, or psychiatric disorders), the family's general style of coping with the world, and its personal and economic resources.

Both parents and psychiatric consultants will need to work with appropriate school staff such as the principal and administrative assistants, teachers, and the school nurse. Good communication among all parties involved is essential; and the parties must help the child to understand what the assessment and treatment are all about.

The child's active involvement in the process is also required for success. A clinical interview of the child by an experienced clinician is a part of the initial assessment. It can sometimes be useful to make use of standardized rating scales of symptoms and problems, which are completed by both parents and teachers, to ensure that a valid diagnosis is made. Referral for intelligence testing, psychological assessment, speech and language evaluation, and testing for learning disability may also be included. The medical evaluation of the child must include a recent, complete physical exam, vision and hearing check, and appropriate evaluation of other medical and neurological conditions. If there is a history of tics, a neurological exam should be included.

If an antidepressant is used, baseline studies of the heart and blood pressure should be done before the medication is started; they should be repeated at regular intervals (e.g., every six months) if the drug is continued for a prolonged period. This is done because, at high dosages in children, antidepressants used for treating attention-deficit hyperactivity disorder can interfere with the regularity of the heartbeat. Antidepressants are rarely used if there is any preexisting problem with the child's heart. If taken in an overdose, antidepressants can be fatal and, like all medications, should be kept under lock and key, accessible only to responsible adults.

## Treatment

When parents, consultants, and school staff all agree that the symptoms of attention-deficit hyperactivity disorder are interfering with the child's functioning and that the risks of medication are justified, a trial of a low dosage of the chosen medication can be started. Although the child's understanding of the disorder and of the treatment's risks and benefits may be limited, every effort should be made to make the child an active participant in both the assessment process and the treatment planning.

In rare cases, a child may be so out of control that both parents and consultants agree to begin the medication before the assessment has been completed. However, the physical examination and laboratory testing should always precede drug treatment.

## HOW TO TELL IF THE DRUG IS WORKING

There should be an improvement in the target symptoms of hyperactivity, impulsivity, and inattention within a few days or a few weeks of beginning medication. If there is no response within eight weeks, the treatment must be considered ineffective. In milder cases, it may be necessary to do regular standardized ratings of behavior at home and in school in order to determine if the medication is effective. A diary (kept by parents) focusing on academic performance, school behavior, emotional growth, relationships with friends, leisure-time activities, and the quality of family interactions will usually show significant improvement shortly after beginning medication. If it does not, parents and professionals must ask themselves whether other factors may be present, e.g., low intelligence, mental retardation, or another learning disability. Parents, school staff, and psychiatric consultants should review the child's progress after one month and reassess the treatment plan.

## LONG-TERM USE

Most child psychiatrists believe that the risks incurred by long-term use of stimulant medication are very low. Before the recent governmental restrictions on the use of stimulants, millions of adults took these drugs regularly without any evidence of irreversible physical effects. Allergic reactions are so rare that blood testing to detect them is unnecessary. Dextroamphetamines and methylphenidate appear to be as safe as, or safer than, aspirin or penicillin with regard to allergic and other unusual physical reactions.

The risk of development of Tourette's syndrome is probably even less than that of an allergic reaction. The slowing of the growth rate appears to be the most important common side effect. This is of most concern to parents of children who are already shorter than normal.

## PERIODIC EXAMINATIONS NECESSARY WHILE TAKING THESE DRUGS

The child should be examined every four to six months while taking these drugs. The pediatrician should monitor height and weight, look for the presence of tics, measure blood pressure and pulse, and ask about the child's appetite, mood, and any side effects—such as dizziness or abdominal cramps. Blood studies should be done at the time of the periodic physical examination, but are not required more frequently. The level of care is only slightly more intense than that which the average child should be receiving under ordinary circumstances.

## HOW TO AVOID OVERDOSE

These drugs are typically taken for long periods. For convenience and economy, parents may wish to keep substantial amounts of the medication on hand. While not so dangerous as many other medications if taken in overdose, the stimulants can cause illness and could be life-threatening to people with heart disease or high blood pressure. When heterocyclic antidepressants are used, there is substantial risk of a lethal overdose (see Chapter 3). These medications should therefore be kept in a locked medicine cabinet, box, or safe.

## ABOUT ADDICTION TO STIMULANTS

Amphetamines produce profound feelings of euphoria and excitation when taken in large doses by adults—especially if injected directly into the blood. The federal government places amphetamines and methylphenidate in the same category as morphine, which means that they cannot be prescribed in amounts in excess of that required for treatment for more than a month at a time. Although they are not so likely to be abused as the opiates (morphine, heroin, etc.), dextroamphetamines, and to a lesser extent methylphenidate, have been widely abused. Having heard about this abuse potential, some parents object to the stimulant medications for fear that their child will become dependent upon them. The fact is that although children may be happy about the improvement in their lives subsequent to taking these medications, they do not get high from them, nor do they especially enjoy taking them. Thus, dependency or addiction among children with attention-deficit hyperactivity disorder who receive stimulants is extremely rare. As with all psychiatric drugs, we suggest tapering the dose when it is time to discontinue use. Withdrawal effects rarely occur if the dose is tapered off over several weeks.

## USE DURING PREGNANCY AND BREAST-FEEDING

In the event that an adolescent girl or young woman taking either a stimulant or a heterocyclic antidepressant becomes pregnant, the medication should be stopped for the duration of the pregnancy and for as long as she is breast-feeding.

## USE OF THESE DRUGS IN ADULTS

Little is known about the number of people who might need to continue taking a medicine for attention-deficit hyperactivity disorder in later life, although it stands to reason that a number of such persons must exist. Interestingly, magnesium pemoline was originally used in an attempt to improve the cognitive functioning of older persons, and methylphenidate has been used for transient and mild depression in the elderly. It may be that future research will find an increased place for these medications in the elderly, as has been the case in their use in young adulthood and middle age.

## How Much Do These Drugs Cost?

The stimulants are not particularly expensive compared with some other medications or treatments. The usual dosage of methylphenidate can be expected to cost between $30 and $40 per month. Sustained-release stimulants (longer-acting forms) are twice as costly or more. When compared with the other costs of such special education and psychological treatment for children, and when compared with the costs of long-term psychological dysfunctions that can stem from unresolved attention-deficit hyperactivity disorder, the cost of an effective medication regimen is modest.

## Recommended Reading on Attention-Deficit Hyperactivity Disorder

Wender, Paul H. *The Hyperactive Child, Adolescent, and Adult.* New York: Oxford University Press, 1987.

# Chapter 11

# Drugs for Alzheimer's Disease and Other Dementias

DEMENTIA, the loss of previous mental capabilities, can be the result of either a reversible physical problem in the brain or a permanent loss of brain function. The former is potentially curable, the latter is not.

About 15 percent of older Americans develop dementia. Sixty percent of these men and women suffer from Alzheimer's disease, a progressive deterioration of brain cells and mental capacity. About 20 percent have *multi-infarct dementia*, in which the brain suffers a series of small strokes that leads to loss of blood flow in the affected regions. Other dementias are diseases of the brain cells themselves, such as Korsakoff's psychosis (a consequence of lifelong alcoholism) and Huntington's disease (a genetic disorder). Dementia pugilistica—the "punch-drunk" syndrome—develops after the repeated head traumas inflicted in a boxing career. Slow-acting viruses may be responsible for the dementias linked with Creutzfeld-Jakob disease and Kuru. In Parkinson's disease, a deficiency of the neurotransmitter dopamine appears to be the culprit. Pernicious anemia, a blood disorder caused by inability to use B vitamins, can also sometimes cause dementia.

Victims of dementia suffer decreased intellectual ability, memory loss, disorientation, and impaired judgment. In the early stages, they may repeat what they've just said, get lost in unfamiliar locations, and find it impossible to keep track of appointments. On a vacation trip, Brian, a sixty-seven-year-old retired teacher, wandered away from his tour group in a national park and became lost. A search party of park rangers found him several hours later. Two years later, he was diagnosed as suffering from Alzheimer's disease.

As dementia advances, patients may not recognize family members. They may become disoriented in their own homes or be unable to think in coherent fashion. They may withdraw from loved ones, losing interest in everyone and everything and becoming increasingly self-centered and dependent on others.

## Alzheimer's Disease

The most common form of dementia, first described by the German psychiatrist Alois Alzheimer in 1907, is the fourth leading cause of death in America. One million people over sixty-five have severe Alzheimer's. Another two million are moderately affected. The chance of developing this illness is roughly one in a hundred, but the risk is four times as great if a family member has the disease. The longer we live, the greater our likelihood of developing Alzheimer's. Over 40 percent of those who live past eighty-five show brain and behavior changes that can be traced to the disease!

Alzheimer's disease produces an abnormal number of changes inside and outside the brain's nerve cells. Normal fibers within brain cells become tangled around each other. Bits of nerve cells and protein, called neuritic plaques, form outside brain cells. The plaques and tangles are the key to the mental changes of Alzheimer's disease.

The signs of Alzheimer's usually appear quite slowly. The first symptom is frequently the loss of short-term memory, such as forgetting recent events. The first problem that Peter, a seventy-seven-year-old retired engineer, noticed was that he would get in the car to run an errand and not be able to remember what he was about to do or where he was going to go. Mild personality changes, such as apathy or withdrawal, also may occur. Peter, for instance, began staying home more. Because he found it hard to keep track of conversation, he said little and walked away when family members tried to engage him in a conversation. As Alzheimer's progresses, the person may have difficulty thinking abstractly, working with numbers, understanding what he or she is reading, or in organizing the day. The person may also become agitated, quarrelsome, irritable, or slovenly in appearance, or may say or do inappropriate things. Peter was referred to a psychiatrist after he was found naked in a neighbor's yard.

In advanced Alzheimer's, patients become confused or disoriented about time and year and may not remember where they live. Ultimately, they may stop talking, or stop caring for themselves and may become uncooperative. In some cases, people with Alzheimer's may lose control of bladder and bowel functions. About a third of those with Alzheimer's have other medical or psychiatric problems. Alzheimer's can reduce life expectancy by one-half; 95 percent of victims over age seventy die within eight years of diagnosis.

In the early stages, Alzheimer's patients still have moments of clarity—which can be profoundly depressing for them and for their families. Eventually, these episodes become less and less frequent. While no treatment can restore the personality and mental powers Alzheimer's patients once had, they can be made comfortable and, in many cases, content.

### DRUG THERAPY

When impaired blood flow is the cause of mild dementia, vasodilators—drugs that widen blood vessels—can have some limited effectiveness. But there is no evidence that these drugs can reverse the damage of Alzheimer's disease.

Ergoloid mesylates (Hydergine) may be somewhat more effective than other vasodilators. In a study of treatment with doses of up to 7.5 mg a day for twelve weeks, patients receiving ergoloid mesylates showed less confusion, memory impairment, depression, and mood swings than other Alzheimer's patients who received a placebo. Improvements continued for six months, and none of the patients deteriorated (as many of those on the placebo did). Side effects include sublingual irritation (if tablets placed under the tongue are used), nausea, and digestive disturbances.

Antipsychotic drugs in low doses can reduce such symptoms as paranoia, hallucinations, hostility, or agitation if they should occur. These symptoms—sometimes called *sundowning*—typically occur at night. Benzodiazepines can have the paradoxical effect of increasing agitation. Thus, they should not be used in patients with Alzheimer's disease.

Antidepressant drugs can improve appetite, sleep patterns, energy, and interest. They help the family as well as the patient by enabling them to get their loved one up and around again.

Various experimental treatments—all still unproven—have been used for dementia. Because Alzheimer's patients have lower levels of choline, a substance necessary for synthesizing the neurotransmitter acetylcholine, researchers have given choline (found naturally in eggs, organ meats, or fish) and drugs that boost acetylcholine to older patients with mild to moderate impairment. Others have tried lecithin, another precursor of acetylcholine. The results have been disappointing so far. Physostigmine, an anticholinesterase drug, seemed to produce some brief improvement in cognition in some patients, but causes troubling side effects.

## NONDRUG ALTERNATIVES

Poor nutrition can contribute to mental confusion. Some studies have found that hospitalized elderly patients have diets low in folate and vitamin $B_{12}$; daily vitamin supplements can help. Regular exercise, good blood pressure control, and quitting smoking also can help by enhancing blood flow to the brain. The interaction of drugs or the use of alcohol while on drugs can lead to confusion, mood changes, and other symptoms of dementia. Curtailing alcohol and careful supervision of drugs may also help.

Environmental factors also can be beneficial. "Reality orientation," a technique developed by James Folsom of the Veterans Administration Hospital in Tuscaloosa, Alabama, formalizes an approach that family members have long used intuitively. The disoriented elderly are given numerous visual and verbal clues as to time and place: calendars, clocks, and bulletin boards. Each day follows a set routine, with consistent times for getting up, eating meals, and going to bed. If a person makes an observation that is not true—such as mistaking a visitor for a long-dead relative—a staff member points out the features of the visitor's face and helps the patient realize that this is a different person. Kindness and respect are essential components of environmental therapies and may provide greater benefits than do the structure or specifics of a program.

## Chapter 12

# Psychiatric Drugs and Older People

AMERICA is turning gray. Thirty million women and men are over age sixty-five, and the number is growing daily. By the year 2000, 13 percent of our population will be over sixty-five.

Today's sixty-five-year-olds are much healthier than their parents and grandparents who survived to that age. In fact, they can expect to live nearly twenty years longer. The fastest growing segment of society today is made up of the so-called *old-old*: those over seventy-five.

For some of these men and women, life's final decades are indeed golden. But sometimes the golden years are less relaxing and more tedious than one had hoped. Long life can bring many losses: physical vitality, productive work, cherished friends, social networks, intimacy, and emotional support. Many elders are troubled by illness, poverty, or loneliness. The loss of a spouse can take an enormous toll at any age: Grieving spouses are hospitalized much more often and use more alcohol and more antianxiety drugs. Isolation from others and a narrowing sense of the borders of one's life can provide a breeding ground for emotional distress. An estimated 15 to 25 percent of the elderly have significant symptoms of mental illness.

Elderly individuals are two-and-a-half times more likely to suffer from a mental illness than younger people. Older men are most likely to suffer severe cognitive impairment, phobias, alcohol abuse, and chronic mild depression. Older women are especially prone to phobias, severe cognitive impairment, chronic mild depression, and major depression. Among older people hospitalized for medical or surgical reasons, as many as half may also have psychiatric difficulties.

Severe organic mental disorders afflict one million older people. Another two million suffer mild to moderate organic mental disorders. About 10 percent of hospitalized patients over sixty-five show signs of dementia. Another 30 to 50 percent develop delirium while hospitalized. Thirty percent of all hospitalized older people are depressed, usually as a result of their physical problems. Older Americans have the highest suicide rates in our society; each year some 8,500 elderly persons kill themselves, and the number is increasing.

Unfortunately, older people usually suffer these problems alone. Seniors are among the least likely to get the help they need. Only 4 percent of patients seen at community mental health centers and 2 percent of patients seen by private practitioners are over sixty-five. Many older men and women simply don't understand mental illness or don't believe they can get better. They—and their family members—all too frequently fail to recognize the symptoms of mental illness and mistakenly think of distressing behavior or personality changes as an inevitable consequence of old age.

## Drug Use Among the Elderly

Older Americans are the most highly medicated individuals in the world. Elderly Americans, who currently make up 10 to 12 percent of the population, consume 25 percent of all drugs prescribed in the United States. Elders are particularly likely to take several medicines at the same time. Some use ten or more different medications per day. These drugs frequently interact, producing a baffling array of symptoms and reactions.

One in every seven elderly men and women uses tranquilizers. Half are psychologically dependent on these drugs and feel they could not get along without them. Others take sleeping medications every night.

Older people may have special problems in monitoring their drug use: Those with poor vision have problems reading labels and may mistake one pill for another. Those with arthritis may have difficulty opening a child-proof cap, cutting a pill in half, or measuring out a liquid preparation. (It should be noted that you can request regular, nonchild proof medication containers.) And the more medications a person takes, the greater the chance of error.

Joe Webber, a seventy-six-year-old retired truck driver, was taking thirteen different drugs for his various ailments. Unfortunately, he confused some of the drugs, taking too much of one and not enough of another, and became delirious. Only after he was admitted to the hospital for tests did he and his doctor realize that he had inadvertently overdosed on his digoxin.

Because of internal physical changes, the elderly may react differently to drugs than they did when they were younger. A drug that is completely cleared from the body of a thirty-year-old within twenty-four hours may remain in the bloodstream of a seventy-year-old several days after it was taken. Older people frequently have fewer intestinal cells to absorb drugs, and decreased blood flow through the intestines, liver, and kidneys. All these factors interfere with the body's ability to break down and excrete drug molecules.

The basic principle of psychiatric drug therapy for the elderly is to start with a low dose and increase it slowly, with careful monitoring for symptoms and side effects. With close supervision, many older patients can take full therapeutic doses. Others, especially those over age seventy, may require smaller doses. And older people should take a drug only for the shortest possible time.

The abuse of illegal drugs is extremely rare among older Americans; but the misuse and abuse of prescription and over-the-counter medications (including psychoactive drugs) are quite common. The most commonly misused are sleeping pills, tranquilizers, and pain medications.

Matilda, a seventy-three-year-old widow, experienced severe withdrawal symptoms, including delusions and visual hallucinations, when she was admitted to the hospital's orthopedic surgery service for the replacement of her right hip joint. The psychiatrist who was called in on her case discovered that she had been taking 60 mg flurazepam at bedtime for ten years to help her sleep. This drug should be used for no more than one week at a time. If you have been taking an addictive drug for a long period of time, you will need a physician's help to withdraw from it.

## FRIENDS AND FAMILY

It is very important for family members to know what medications their elderly parents or grandparents are taking. Frequently, older people are placed on multiple medications by different medical specialists. Unless you check on them by asking them to show you all the medications they are taking, you won't know. Also, older people frequently neglect their health by not getting physical exams or checkups. You may help them by ensuring that they get regular checkups and see their primary care physician on a regular basis.

# Depression

While the majority of elderly individuals do *not* become depressed, a significant proportion—as high as 27 percent in some studies—develop mild or severe depressive symptoms. Depression late in life is sometimes hard to recognize because older patients may not display the typical symptoms, and the symptoms of depression are frequently mistaken for normal signs of aging. In one recent study of 150 older patients admitted to a hospital for medical reasons, the examining physicians did not detect a single case of depression. But when a psychiatrist interviewed the same patients, he found that 15 percent were severely depressed.

Depression is extremely common among older people with one or more physical problems. Some signs of depression—particularly appetite changes or a gain or loss of 5 percent of body weight in a month, insomnia, or excessive sleep, fidgeting or extremely slow movements or speech, and fatigue or loss of energy—often are attributed to medical problems or medications. Sometimes depression is a reaction to illness, but if undetected and untreated, it can hinder the person's speedy recovery from a physical problem.

The greatest risk of failing to treat depression is suicide. The suicide rate at age sixty-five is five times higher than the rate for younger individuals. Depressed older men and women also are more likely to die of other causes. With treatment, more than 70 percent of the depressed elderly improve.

## DRUG TREATMENT FOR DEPRESSION

In selecting an antidepressant for an older person, the psychiatrist will want to know about any previous bouts with depression, which medications were used, whether they led to serious side effects, and how effective they were. The psychiatrist will ask similar questions about any family members who have been treated for depression.

The psychiatrist also needs to know which other drugs a patient may be taking. In cases of multiple prescriptions, it is usually a good idea for the patient or a family member to bring all current medicines to the doctor's office. The physician will also need to know about nonprescription drugs and alcohol use.

Since elderly patients sometimes show a partial response to a single medication, your physician may suggest a combination of antidepressive drugs.

### Heterocyclic Antidepressants

These drugs, the mainstay of antidepressive treatment in younger patients, require special attention in the elderly. Amitriptyline (Elavil), doxepin (Sinequan), and imipramine (Tofranil) can produce serious problems in older patients: confusion, delirium, urinary retention, impotence, constipation, an abnormally rapid heart rate, and intestinal problems that can lead to bowel obstruction. Amitriptyline (Elavil), doxepin (Sinequan), trazodone (Desyrel), trimipramine (Surmontil), and maprotiline (Ludiomil) tend to have sedating effects. Individuals with heart failure or electrical problems of the heart (arrhythmias) are particularly vulnerable. Nortriptyline (Aventyl) is least likely to alter the heart's conduction patterns.

Some antidepressants lower blood pressure, particularly when a person gets up from a reclining position. This is called *orthostatic hypotension.* Low blood pressure can be dangerous in older patients because they could fall and suffer fractures or other injuries. The danger may be greatest when the patients have low blood pressure prior to treatment, take other medications that affect blood pressure, or are given a large dose.

Older patients should avoid taking the entire dose of their medication at bedtime since they could waken at night and fall getting out of bed. For instance, many psychiatrists recommend taking antidepressants three or four times a day to avoid a large nighttime dose. Patients who are taking antidepressants can help prevent side effects by drinking adequate amounts of fluid—e.g., six to eight glasses of water a day—changing position slowly, ingesting caffeine, and using ephedrine (Sudafed, an over-the-counter decongestant). Ephedrine and caffeine stimulate the nervous system and increase blood pressure, reducing the risk of potentially dangerous reductions.

Antidepressant heterocyclics always carry a small risk of seizures: about 1 in 1,000 if the person has no other risk factors. The risk is somewhat higher with maprotiline and clomipramine. Overdoses of amoxapine, maprotiline, and desipramine can increase the likelihood of seizures.

Other possible side effects of the antidepressants include skin rash (especially with maprotiline), liver damage, ringing in the ears, and involuntary muscle spasms (which can be treated with quinine, a reduced dose of the drug, or switching to another medication). Since heterocyclics alter the normal electric activity of the heart, many physicians suggest an ECG before any elderly patient starts on an antidepressant.

Elderly patients taking imipramine or nortriptyline should be tested regularly to be sure they are receiving adequate blood levels of these drugs. This test enables physicians to make sure that the dose is neither too high nor too low. Doctors are most likely to test blood plasma levels if patients are not responding to typical doses, if the patient does not seem to be complying or has suffered an overdose, if side effects have developed, if the doctor is considering a higher dose or an additional drug that could affect plasma levels or metabolism of the antidepressant, or if the patient's condition changed after switching to a generic brand of the same medication.

Starting doses for patients over sixty-five should be low. For those over seventy-five, in poor health, or known to be sensitive to drug side effects, the initial dose may be as low as 10 mg for a heterocyclic. Your doctor should check your pulse and blood pressure (while you stand and while you lie down), test for signs of confusion, and make sure your urinary and bowel functions are normal. Typically, the dose is increased gradually every two to three days until improvement begins or side effects develop.

In some cases, it may be several weeks before you notice a dramatic change. Side effects may develop before any beneficial signs appear. But in depressed individuals of all ages, various symptoms (including depressed mood, anxiety, hostility, and depressed appearance) usually show improvement within a week. Often family members notice these changes before the patient does. If you show no improvement at all within three weeks, your physician should switch you to another drug.

There is no evidence that any one heterocyclic works faster than the others. Some indication of response within two weeks is a good predictor of eventual improvement. If patients show no improvement at all within three weeks, the medication usually is not working, and the physician will switch to another drug.

Sometimes another drug has to be added to a heterocyclic to make it more effective. Full doses of lithium, an antimania agent that is relatively safe for the elderly, can enhance response, particularly for older patients. Lithium is usually continued for three or four weeks, or until improvement is obvious. Some physicians add triiodothyronine (a thyroid medication) or L-tryptophan (an amino acid most often used as a sleep aid, when it was available). Methylphenidate (a stimulant) increases the blood levels of heterocyclics but can cause insomnia and agitation.

Depression tends to linger late in life. After age fifty, untreated depression can persist for three to five years, compared with nine to eighteen months in younger adults. Older patients must continue antidepressant treatment longer than younger individuals. Reducing doses or stopping medication can lead to a relapse.

### Monoamine Oxidase Inhibitors (MAOIs)

These drugs, which block or inhibit monoamine oxidase, an enzyme that regulates various biologic activities, are usually not the first choice for elderly patients because they are potentially more dangerous than heterocyclics. However, they can be beneficial in patients who fail to respond to heterocyclic antidepressants. They also may help when elderly patients develop phobic anxiety, agitation, somatic anxiety, a profound lack of energy, depression triggered by the antihypertensive medication reserpine, or have a history of panic attacks or chronic anxiety. Phenelzine (Nardil) has clearly been shown to be effective in older depressed patients. Some psychiatrists feel that tranylcypromine (Parnate) is the most effective MAOI in the elderly.

The risk of liver damage with phenelzine and the related drug isocarboxazid (Marplan) is very low. Both medications seem equally effective, but some individuals respond better to one or the other. They do not have the same side effects as heterocyclics, which is why they are sometimes used when patients on heterocyclics develop problems such as urinary retention, constipation, blurred vision, abnormal heartbeats, or impaired sexual arousal. High doses of MAOIs can produce these effects, as can combinations of MAOIs with heterocyclics, antihistamines, or antiparkinsonian drugs.

MAOIs can cause orthostatic hypotension, creating dizziness, weakness, or an inability to stand up. This may not occur immediately, but symptoms may develop after three weeks of treatment. With isocarboxazid, the problem is usually related to dose. Sometimes sodium chloride helps—but is not an option for patients who must restrict salt or who have heart or kidney disease. Drinking fluids and taking extra care when sitting or standing can prevent harm.

Patients who are taking MAOIs and drugs that increase blood pressure (such as tyramine, phylephrine, phenylpropanolamine, pseudoephedrine, and amphetamine) run the risk of a hypertensive crisis, in which their blood pressure can surge dramatically. For 1 in 100,000 patients, this reaction is fatal. Prompt treatment with intravenous medications to lower pressure is critical.

Other side effects of MAOIs are sleep problems, weight gain, involuntary muscle spasms, impaired memory, headache, restlessness, and loss of appetite. Patients may have to restrict their diets and drug intake.

## Other Antidepressant Medications

Sometimes physicians select other drugs to treat depression in the elderly because of individual needs or risks. Among these agents:

• *Trazodone (Desyrel)*. This drug does not produce the troubling side effects of heterocyclic antidepressants; however, it can cause sleepiness, low blood pressure, dizziness, and, rarely, a persistent erection in males (priapism). Generally, the initial dose is low and is increased gradually. Often, patients begin to sleep better before reaching the dosage level needed for improvement of depression, and they may be tempted not to continue increasing the dose to the optimal therapeutic level.

• *Carbamazepine (Tegretol)*. This drug, used primarily to treat seizures, is being tried for patients who do not respond to other treatments. However, before taking carbamazepine, all patients should undergo a complete blood count, tests of liver function, an ECG, and measurement of serum electrolyte levels. In rare cases, carbamazepine has been associated with aplastic anemia and liver damage. Frequent monitoring of blood levels is critical. The medication should be stopped if patients develop mouth ulcers, fever, bleeding, sore throat, or any infection.

• *Stimulants (Ritalin, Dexedrine)*. Rarely used in younger patients, stimulants such as dextroamphetamine (Dexedrine) or methylphenidate (Ritalin) can help elderly patients who suffer strokes, undergo surgery, or develop chronic medical illnesses, and who become apathetic, listless, and dependent. Stimulants also can help when heterocyclics or other drugs produce dangerous side effects.

Often within forty-eight to seventy-two hours, stimulants improve motivation, mood, sleep, appetite, and performance. Amphetamines cannot be used in patients with cardiovascular disease, high blood pressure, or kidney disorders. Insomnia can be a side effect, particularly if the last dose is taken late in the day. However, stimulants generally do not produce harmful side effects in the elderly and can be discontinued shortly after the patient shows sustained improvement. Stimulants also can be effective in combination with a heterocyclic or to counteract the blood pressure–lowering effects of antidepressants.

## Lithium

Mania is rare in the elderly, but lithium, generally used to treat manic states, also can regulate and prevent depression. Lithium's effects last longer in the elderly because elderly people's kidneys take longer to clear it from the body.

Most physicians perform several tests before initiating lithium therapy, including a complete blood count, urinalysis, tests of thyroid function, electrolytes, creatinine, and ECG. In patients with possibly impaired kidney function, a twenty-four-hour creatinine clearance test may be performed (see Chapter 6).

Initial lithium doses are low and slowly increased. Desired blood levels are higher for patients suffering from mania than those who are receiving lithium as a preventive treatment. Many physicians check lithium levels monthly or bimonthly in older patients.

Soon after starting lithium therapy, patients may develop relatively harmless side effects, such as fine tremor, nausea, headache, fatigue, and frequent urination. More serious complications are impaired memory, weight gain, enlarged thyroid, decreased thyroid hormone production, diabetes insipidus, psoriasis, skin infection, and heart arrhythmia. At high blood levels, lithium can cause pronounced tremor, slurred speech, double vision, peculiar eye movements, hyperreflexia, weakness, drowsiness, muscle twitches, and vomiting. If unchecked, they can progress to impaired consciousness, seizures, coma, and eventual death. Prompt recognition and treatment (including stopping lithium) can prevent such dire complications.

Lithium interacts with various drugs, including nonsteroidal anti-inflammatory agents (except aspirin), thiazide diuretics, spironolactone, triamterene, and possibly tetracycline. Any of these agents can increase lithium to toxic levels. Other drugs, such as theophylline, may lower lithium levels. Various combinations also can cause toxic effects, including lithium and neuroleptic drugs, lithium and phenytoin, lithium and carbamazepine, and high doses of MAOIs and lithium.

Sometimes elderly patients require a combination of lithium and a diuretic. If so, physicians will check blood levels, lower the lithium dose, monitor lithium levels and electrolytes at least twice a week initially, and adjust the dose to minimize complications.

Because of the complexity and potential seriousness of lithium's effects, patients and their families should learn as much as possible about this drug to obtain optimal benefits. Good dietary habits, monitoring of other medications, and appropriate care of any medical problems are important. Notify your physician of any digestive upsets and changes in salt intake or diet.

## Anxiety in the Elderly

Anxiety (the most widespread psychological problem in our society) can affect individuals of all ages. However, the rate of anxiety generally decreases with age. The older the individuals in the NIMH Epidemiologic Catchment Area program, the less likely they were to report ever suffering a serious anxiety disorder. In a six-month period, prevalence rates for anxiety were lower in those over age sixty-five than in younger age groups. However, anxiety can and does occur in the elderly, causing the same distress that it does in younger men and women.

Hazel, a retired librarian who lived alone in an apartment in a big city, first found herself becoming anxious whenever she walked to the bank to deposit her Social Security check. Several elderly women in her neighborhood had been mugged by gangs of young boys who grabbed their purses, pushed them to the sidewalk, and ran. Even when she wasn't carrying a check or a large amount of cash, Hazel began feeling anxious when walking in certain areas. Her anxiety steadily grew, making it harder for her to leave her apartment. Her daughter urged her to move into her large suburban home. Hazel hated the prospect of giving up her independence but realized that she had become a prisoner in the city.

Hazel's primary physician referred her to a psychiatrist. Through a combination of benzodiazepines and behavior modification therapy for approximately three months, Hazel gradually overcame her phobic anxiety. (See Chapter 5 for detailed information on the treatment of phobias.) Some practical strategies, such as having checks mailed directly to the bank and never carrying more than ten dollars in her purse, helped alleviate her justifiable fears of being robbed.

## DRUG THERAPY FOR ANXIETY

Some older patients who have been taking barbiturates for decades with great success can continue to do so; however, the benzodiazepines have largely replaced barbiturates in treating anxiety disorders. Other options include antidepressants, antihistamines, neuroleptics, beta blockers, and buspirone.

### Benzodiazepines

These medications are the first choices for anxiety. All are equally effective, but there are differences in metabolism and side effects. Triazolam (Halcion) is a short-acting drug with a half-life of two to four hours. Alprazolam (Xanax), lorazepam (Ativan), oxazepam (Serax), and temazepam (Restoril) are intermediate-acting. Flurazepam, diazepam (Valium), chlordiazepoxide (Librium), clorazepate (Tranxene), and prazepam (Centrax) are long-acting medications. Short-acting benzodiazepines are less likely to produce cumulative side effects, but have the disadvantage of withdrawal effects, rebound insomnia, and the need for divided doses.

All of the benzodiazepines can produce side effects, including: sleepiness, lethargy, impaired memory and thinking, ataxia, hostility, increased breathing difficulty during sleep, nightmares, hallucinations, slurred speech, double vision, peculiar eye movements, weakness, and depression. If the drugs interfere with breathing, patients may feel more anxious rather than less. Alcohol, sedatives, anticonvulsants, antihypertensives, sedating heterocyclics or neuroleptics, and MAOIs can enhance or magnify the effects of the benzodiazepines.

Usually the benzodiazepines are prescribed for generalized anxiety, posttraumatic stress disorder, panic disorder, acute anxiety or agitation, and alcohol withdrawal. They can help in treating depressed patients suffering from anxiety or impaired sleep and can relieve insomnia triggered by MAOIs. Alprazolam and clonazepam have been especially helpful in controlling panic attacks.

Starting doses are low for elderly patients and are raised every few days until improvement or side effects occur. Generally, benzodiazepines are a short-term treatment and are discontinued or reduced after a few weeks. In patients with chronic anxiety, they may be used intermittently, along with other approaches. Daily, long-term therapy in the elderly could produce cumulative harmful effects, including withdrawal symptoms and psychosis. Usually, the dose is tapered at the rate of 10 percent per day.

Elderly people with brain disorders such as Alzheimer's disease may be especially sensitive to the effects of benzodiazepines. If these drugs are used, the dose should be as low as possible, and the patients should be monitored closely.

### Other Drugs

Buspirone is a nonsedating antianxiety agent that does not interact with alcohol, has no potential for abuse, and does not cause sedation. Consequently, it may be especially effective in elderly patients. Most important, it does not interfere with a person's ability to perform complex motor tasks such as driving a car. However, patients may feel that improvements take somewhat longer than with other drugs. Starting doses are low and gradually increased.

Low doses of heterocyclic antidepressants often can relieve anxiety. Beta-adrenergic blockers (drugs that inhibit the receptors in the brain and nervous system that modify our reactions to stress) have been used to relieve the physical symptoms of anxiety, such as a racing heartbeat, sweating, or nervous stomach, but their side effects (dizziness, low blood pressure, depression, respiratory distress, diabetes, slowed heart rate, and heart failure) can be serious in the elderly. These agents also may not be as effective in relieving anxiety in older patients as they are with younger adults.

Antihistamines, which have mild effects on anxiety, may work best in patients with chronic obstructive pulmonary disease. The two most often used are hydroxyzine or diphenhydramine.

# Sleep Disorders in the Elderly

At sixty, men and women don't look or feel twenty—nor do they sleep the same. A typical twenty-year-old falls asleep in eight minutes, spends 95 percent of the night asleep, sinks into deep non-REM sleep for half an hour or more, and dreams for almost two hours of the night. Total sleep time comes to 7.5 to 8 hours. A typical eighty-year-old takes eighteen minutes to fall asleep, spends 80 percent of the night asleep, and dreams for a little more than an hour. Total sleep time is about six hours, with only a few minutes—if any—in the deepest sleep stage. These changes are normal consequences of aging. However, some elderly individuals develop true sleep disorders that may require treatment.

### Drug Therapy

No sleeping pill provides a long-term solution to the problem of sleeplessness at any age. Many sedating medications lead to physical and psychological dependence and create lingering side effects. Some could be fatal. Sleeping pills interfere with the brain's signals to the body to resume breathing—an impairment that occurs with sleep apnea, which is more common in the elderly. Older people who take sleeping pills may wake up confused in the middle of the night, fall, and hurt themselves. The ingredients in various pills may cause complications in people with high blood pressure, heart disease, and other chronic medical conditions.

In older patients with chronic insomnia, a low-dose heterocyclic antidepressant may be a better choice than a benzodiazepine. Often these patients also suffer from a mood disorder or sleep apnea, in which breathing stops for brief periods during the night, which could worsen with benzodiazepines. Antidepressants also carry less risk of tolerance, daytime impairment, or withdrawal problems. In older patients with diagnosed depression as well as sleep problems, the heterocyclic antidepressants nortriptyline, trimipramine, or trazodone have been shown to improve the quality of sleep.

As a short-term solution, low doses of intermediate-acting benzodiazepines, particularly oxazepam, taken thirty to sixty minutes before bedtime can help some older persons with troubled sleep. The key in selecting a benzodiazepine is how long it stays in the body. Flurazepam, which has an extremely long half-life in the elderly, can lead to intoxication, dramatic drops in blood pressure, restlessness, and aggression. Psychiatrists recommend a dose no higher than one-third to one-half the usual amount.

Patients taking benzodiazepines for sleep should skip medication at least one or two nights a week (aiming for fewer than twenty doses in a month) and should monitor themselves for daytime effects, including "fogginess," forgetfulness, and hangover. Ideally, they should discontinue treatment within three months and rely on nondrug alternatives for better sleep.

Benzodiazepines should not be used in older patients who have dementia or a history of substance abuse; snore heavily; have impaired kidney, liver, or lung function; are ingesting other drugs or alcohol; work in jobs requiring alertness; or may be suicidal.

## NONDRUG ALTERNATIVES

The nondrug alternatives described in Chapter 8 are the best long-term solutions for poor sleep at any age. Among the basic guidelines that are especially helpful for older individuals are:

• Follow a daily routine, with regular hours for waking, mealtimes, and bedtime.
• While most people feel an increasing need to nap as they grow older, spending too much time in bed during the day may make it harder to consolidate sleep into a long period at night.
• Develop a long, soothing bedtime ritual, such as soaking in a warm tub, back massage, or listening to soft music.
• Try not to go to bed too early. If you set a consistent wake-up time and let your body determine when it's ready for sleep at night, you'll probably wake up less during the night.
• Restrict total sleep time to six and a half or seven hours. Cutting down on the quantity of time in bed often can improve the quality of sleep.
• Take care of your health: Eat light, nutritious meals. Try to get some

daily exercise. Reduce use of stimulants, such as caffeine and nicotine.

• Fill your days with activities that please and interest you, and your nights may also become more satisfying.


# Psychosis in the Elderly

Schizophrenia is rare in the elderly. However, older individuals can develop severe psychiatric impairment, including delusions and paranoia. Psychiatrists use the term *paraphrenia* to refer to paranoia and schizophreniclike symptoms that develop late in life and that are not related to depression or an organic mental disorder. Paraphrenia generally does not lead to the devastating deterioration that can occur with Alzheimer's disease.

Symptoms of paranoia are common in elderly women living alone, particularly if they have impaired vision and hearing. Because they cannot interpret or comprehend what they see and hear, they may assume that innocent stimuli represent a threat to them. Mild symptoms do not require medication. Often reassurance, correcting vision or hearing problems, treating underlying illnesses, and pointing out the consequences of voicing delusions (such as angering the neighbors by repeated accusations that they are spying) help.


### DRUG THERAPY

The primary treatment for schizophreniclike symptoms in the elderly is the dopamine-receptor-blocking neuroleptics:

• Phenothiazines (aliphatic, piperidine, and piperazine). While these medications can produce more side effects than other neuroleptics, the aliphatic and piperidine phenothiazines, such as chlorpromazine (Thorazine) and thioridazine (Mellaril), are often the most effective drugs for elderly patients. The starting dose, almost always lower than in younger adults, depends on severity of symptoms, other medications, heart status, and other factors.
• Butyrophenones (haloperidol, Haldol).
• Thioxanthenes (thiothixene, Navane, chlorprothixene).
• Dibenzoxazepines (loxapine, Loxitane).
• Dihydroindolones (molindone, Moban).

The nonphenothiazine neuroleptics are more powerful and less sedating, but they are more likely to induce movement disorders, such as tremors or spasms. All neuroleptics are equally likely to produce tardive dyskinesia, the involuntary twitching of facial muscles that is a more common complication in older people.

### Side Effects

The aliphatic and piperidine phenothiazines can produce dry mouth, constipation, impotence, urinary retention, tachycardia, impaired breathing, aggravation of narrow-angle glaucoma, impaired memory, and delirium. These can be relieved by lowering the dose, switching medicine, or adding urecholine, a noncentrally acting cholinergic compound.

Other potential problems are low blood pressure, which can be relieved by lowering the dose or switching to a more potent drug, and impaired ejaculation. In addition, neuroleptics can cause dystonia, parkinsonian symptoms (such as tremor and rigidity), drowsiness, lethargy, fatigue, muscle cramps, jitteriness, restlessness, increased risk of seizures, agranulocytosis, cholestatic jaundice, photosensitivity, damage to the eye, temperature disturbance, alterations of cardiac conduction, and neuroleptic malignant syndrome, a potentially fatal complication that consists of elevated body temperature, high blood pressure, sweating, muscular rigidity, and altered awareness.

The prognosis for patients who receive adequate treatment and maintenance is good. Follow-up studies have shown that the majority of patients remain symptom-free up to three years after initial diagnosis and therapy.

In addition to medication, patients need to develop relationships within their own environments. Family members, neighbors, police officers, and others in the community also can provide a supportive network for older men and women. Often paranoia eases as physical health improves, hearing and vision problems are corrected, and patients break out of their self-imposed isolation. Frequent social contacts, even brief interactions with relative strangers, can be extremely beneficial.

## About Delirium

Delirium is a disorder of attention that impairs ability to sustain attention, think coherently, carry on a conversation, or perform a simple task. Unable to register and retain new information, delirious individuals lose their train of thought, switch from subject to subject, or cannot recall recent events. They may be agitated or drowsy, unable to sleep, and troubled by visual and auditory hallucinations. Awareness may fluctuate, and lucid periods can occur. Usually delirium develops rapidly and does not last long (usually hours or days). Delirium can occur in someone with dementia, making it harder to diagnose.

Delirium has numerous causes, including:

• Medical illnesses, such as infection, congestive heart failure, burns, systemic lupus erythematosus, and liver, kidney, or lung problems.
• Metabolic disorders, such as hypothyroidism or hypoglycemia.
• Neurologic disorders, such as head trauma, stroke, or meningitis.
• Drug reactions to medications such as L-dopa, digitalis, sedatives, hypnotics, heterocyclic antidepressants, antipsychotic drugs, and corticosteroids.

Delirium can occur after surgery (particularly heart operations), while in an intensive care unit, or during withdrawal from addicting substances such as alcohol or sedatives. An estimated 30 to 50 percent of elderly patients develop delirium during their hospital stay.

The goal of treatment is to identify and correct the cause of the delirium. Reassurance and a structured environment can relieve mild anxiety in delirious patients. Ideally, physicians try to avoid adding more medications to a delirious patient's regimen. However, drug treatment may be necessary to protect the patient's safety and assure adequate care for underlying problems.

## DRUG THERAPY

For delirium triggered by withdrawal from alcohol, barbiturates, or benzodiazepines, treatment with a cross-tolerant drug of medium duration (a half-life of twelve to twenty-four hours) can help. In other cases, low doses of neuroleptic drugs may help. These medications carry a risk of orthostatic hypotension, withdrawal, seizures, and osteoporosis. In some studies, elderly patients have experienced on average 14 percent bone loss while on the drugs. Haloperidol (Haldol), a high-potency neuroleptic with few side effects, is the most useful agent in treating older patients with delirium. The starting dose should be low (0.5 mg to 1 mg every hour) until agitation or confusion subsides. Once stabilized, patients can be put on lower maintenance doses.

## CARL JACKSON: IMPROPER USE OF PSYCHIATRIC DRUGS IN THE ELDERLY

At eighty, Carl Jackson was still a charmer. He always had a twinkle in his eye, a quip on his lips, and a compliment for the ladies. "I'm a boy in an old man's body," he would say with a sly wink.

Carl's health had always been fairly good. He'd suffered a mild heart attack in his sixties and had undergone bypass surgery. He'd worn a hearing aid for twenty years. His other complaints were minor: His legs ached after a walk; his stomach "acted up" now and then. But Carl, who lived with his wife, Gloria, in a residential community for retired people, kept up a full schedule of activities.

After Carl began having problems breathing, ·particularly at night, he went to his doctor. When he learned that he had a tumor in his lungs, Carl absorbed the bad news quietly and listened to his options. "I'm not going out without a fight," he told his physician, who scheduled surgery for the following day.

Carl sailed through the operation without any problems. The following day, he appeared to be recovering well. Suddenly he began thrashing about, tore out his intravenous tubes, and shouted incoherently. The intensive care physicians immediately administered a huge intravenous dose of the benzodiazepine diazepam (Valium) to calm Carl down. It had no noticeable effect. They then repeated the dose, which so depressed Carl's respiratory system that he was in danger of respiratory arrest (cessation of breathing). As a result, they had to put Carl on a respirator.

A psychiatrist was called in to recommend further medication. She prescribed intravenous haloperidol (Haldol), gave Carl his watch, hearing aid, and glasses, and provided behavioral cues to orient him.

Hours after Carl's initial outburst, a staff member reported that the level of oxygen in his blood when he'd been on room air after surgery was insufficient—the probable reason for his bizarre behavior. After Carl was taken off the respirator, he received oxygen through a nasal tube for several days. He was placed in a room with a window so he could tell night from day. His wife and staff members helped orient and assist him.

Unfortunately, the physicians treating Carl after his operation made a common and sadly mistaken assumption: that all old people who become disoriented or incoherent must be demented. With adequate oxygen and help with orientation, he recovered quickly and returned home, where he lived for another five years.

### SADIE JIMINSKI: SUCCESSFUL USE OF PSYCHIATRIC DRUGS IN THE ELDERLY

After her husband, Neil, died of a heart attack, Sadie Jiminski, then sixty-seven, took solace in her faith and her memories of their many happy years together. She attended daily Mass, remained active in her church groups, and devoted much of her time to her two young grandchildren. Arthritis and hypertension troubled her, but medication kept both under control. "God has been good to me," she would often say.

Three years later, her older sister, Marya, learned that she had ovarian cancer, which had spread throughout her body. Realizing that there was little hope for a cure, Marya wanted only to die at home. Sadie moved into her house to care for her. Her sister's final months were long and arduous. Often Sadie was up most of the night with Marya. She dozed in a chair by her bed during the day and lived on hurried snacks. Sometimes she didn't leave the house for days at a time. After Marya's death, Sadie returned home a different woman.

"Mom's gotten so old," her daughters said as they noticed Sadie's forgetfulness, poor appetite, fatigue, and lack of interest in her garden, friends, or grandchildren. "Maybe she still hasn't gotten over Aunt Marya's death," they thought.

Months after her sister's funeral, Sadie was more withdrawn than ever. She complained that she couldn't sleep and her arthritis bothered her more than before. Her memory was unreliable. Some days she fidgeted restlessly, while on others she seemed to be moving in slow motion. An air of profound sadness and emptiness clung to her. She stopped going to church and rarely saw her grandchildren. When her son visited from the West Coast, he was shocked at Sadie's appearance. "She's demented," he said. "Her mind wanders. She doesn't bother combing her hair. The house is a mess. We have to put her in a home."

That suggestion infuriated Sadie, and she raged at her children, telling them to go away and leave her alone. A few weeks later, Sadie slipped and broke her hip. While she was in the hospital, a consulting psychiatrist diagnosed the true cause of her distress: depression.

Sadie's daughters noticed some small improvements in her behavior and mood within two weeks of starting antidepressant drug therapy. By the time she recovered from her fracture, Sadie found herself feeling more energetic. Once again, she started going to daily Mass and planning outings with her grandchildren. Within a few months, she was once more the cheerful, loving mother her children remembered.

Sadie's situation is hardly unusual. Often depression in the elderly is misdiagnosed as dementia, and psychiatrists use the term *pseudodementia* to describe dementialike symptoms in depressed, elderly patients like her. Fortunately, Sadie was properly diagnosed and treated and recovered fully from her depression.

# Chapter 13

# Drugs for Anger and Aggression

## About Rage and Violence

Although aggressive and violent behaviors are highly prevalent both in our society in general and among patients who suffer from psychiatric disorders, it must be emphasized that the vast majority of patients with psychiatric disorders are nonviolent. In fact, it has been shown that patients with severe psychiatric disorders such as schizophrenia are more likely to be victims of violence than they are to be perpetrators of such.

Nonetheless, agitation, irritability, anger, rageful affects, aggressive behavior, and violence can be significant problems for patients with psychiatric and/or neurological conditions, and these conditions are highly disruptive to families. For example, approximately 50 percent of patients with Alzheimer's disease give evidence of agitation and periodic violent behavior, and 75 percent of their families who were surveyed rated this aggressive behavior as the most serious problem due to the illness that they must confront. Often, it is agitation and aggressive behavior, not memory deficits, that result in the need to place our elderly with Alzheimer's disease in a nursing home. An example from our clinical experience is a seventy-seven-year-old wife of an eighty-two-year-old man with Alzheimer's disease. The wife said to us, "It's not my husband's bad memory that troubles me most. Rather, it's when I try to restrain him when he awakes at 3:00 A.M. to go to work. (He has been retired for eight years.) He begins to hit me and yell so loudly that he awakens all the neighbors."

## CAUSES

Invariably, the underlying causes of rageful affects and aggressive behaviors are complex. Not infrequently, these causes are a multidetermined blend of temperament, past personal experience, present areas of stress, and current neurological and medical conditions. For example, we are aware that most people who, as children, were physically and psychologically abused will have angry feelings and tendencies to react violently as adolescents and adults. Certainly, not every person who has experienced such childhood abuse will grow up to be a violent adult; but, on the other hand, a large proportion of people who are violent as adults were treated violently and psychologically abused as children. In addition, as reviewed in the next section of this chapter, certain illnesses that affect specific areas of the brain may also give rise to violent behavior. Alcohol and substances of abuse are often directly associated with violent outbursts in adolescents and adults. There are, for example, large numbers of individuals whose periodic violent behavior occurs only when they are under the influence of alcohol. Other people may be unusually sensitive to environmental stimuli and stresses and become violent only when a certain type and level of external stimulation are encountered. As a rule, multiple variables combine to lead an individual to react violently; therefore, the assessment and treatment of individuals suffering from excesses of anger and from aggressive behaviors must be comprehensive.

## ASSOCIATED MEDICAL CONDITIONS

Aggressive behavior is often associated with neurologic disorders, as well as other medical illnesses that affect the brain. Our research group has called the condition in which patients become aggressive in response to brain illness or in response to medications or drugs *organic aggressive syndrome*. Table 1 summarizes the diagnostic criteria for organic aggressive syndrome and Table 2 summarizes the characteristic features of organic aggressive syndrome. In addition, our research team has developed a scale that rates aggressive behavior, the Overt Aggression Scale (see Table

3). We often ask family members to utilize this scale to document whether or not interventions with medications and other forms of treatment are reducing the aggression in our patients. Table 4 summarizes the most commonly occurring medical and neurological causes of violence, and Table 5 includes prescribed medications, over-the-counter drugs, alcohol, and other substances of abuse that also are associated with violent behaviors.

TABLE I

## Diagnostic Criteria for Organic Aggressive Syndrome

1. Persistent or recurrent aggressive outbursts, either of a verbal or physical nature.
2. The outbursts are out of proportion to the precipitating stress or provocation.
3. Evidence from history, physical examination, or laboratory tests of a specific organic factor that is judged to be etiologically related to the disturbance.
4. The outbursts are not primarily related to personality features or disorders such as narcissistic personality disorder, borderline disorder, conduct disorder, or antisocial personality disorder.
5. Not due to schizophrenia or manic-depressive disorder.

TABLE 2

## Characteristic Features of Organic Aggressive Syndrome

| | |
|---|---|
| *Reactive* | Triggered by modest trivial stimuli. |
| *Nonreflective* | Usually does not involve premeditation or planning. |
| *Nonpurposeful* | Aggression serves no obvious long-term aims or goals. |
| *Explosive* | Buildup is *not* gradual. |
| *Periodic* | Brief outbursts of rage and aggression, punctuated by long periods of relative calm. |
| *Not justified* | After outbursts, patients are upset, concerned, embarrassed; as opposed to blaming others or justifying behavior. |

TABLE 3

## Overt Aggression Scale (OAS)

Stuart Yudofsky, M.D., Jonathan Silver, M.D., Wynn Jackson, M.D., and Jean Endicott, Ph.D.

### IDENTIFYING DATA

| Name of Patient | Name of Rater |
|---|---|

Sex of Patient:   1 Male   2 Female

Date   /  /   (mo/day/yr)

Shift: 1 Night   2 Day   3 Evening

☐ No aggressive incident(s) (verbal or physical) against self, others, or objects during the shift. (Check here)

### AGGRESSIVE BEHAVIOR (check all that apply)

*Verbal Aggression*

☐ Makes loud noises, shouts angrily.

☐ Yells mild personal insults, e.g., "You're stupid!"

☐ Curses viciously, uses foul language in anger, makes moderate threats to others or self.

☐ Makes clear threats of violence toward others or self ("I'm going to kill you") or requests help to control self.

*Physical Aggression Against Objects*

☐ Slams door, scatters clothing, makes a mess.

☐ Throws objects down, kicks furniture without breaking it, marks the wall.

☐ Breaks objects, smashes windows.

☐ Sets fires, throws objects dangerously.

Time incident began: __ __ : __ __ AM/PM

*Physical Aggression Against Self*

☐ Picks or scratches skin, hits self, pulls hair (with no or minor injury only)

☐ Bangs head, hits fist into objects, throws self onto floor or into objects (hurts self without serious injury).

☐ Small cuts or bruises, minor burns.

☐ Mutilates self, makes deep cuts, bites that bleed, internal injury, fracture, loss of consciousness, loss of teeth.

*Physical Aggression Against Other People*

☐ Makes threatening gestures, swings at people, grabs at clothes

☐ Strikes, kicks, pushes, pulls hair (without injury to them).

☐ Attacks others, causing mild-moderate physical injury (bruises, sprain, welts).

☐ Attacks others, causing severe physical injury (broken bones, deep lacerations, internal injury).

Duration of incident: __ __ : __ __
(hours/minutes)

### INTERVENTION (check all that apply)

☐ None.

☐ Talking to patient.

☐ Closer observation.

☐ Holding patient.

☐ Immediate medication given by mouth.

☐ Immediate medication given by injection.

☐ Isolation without seclusion.

☐ Seclusion.

☐ Use of restraints.

☐ Injury requires immediate medical treatment for patient.

☐ Injury requires immediate treatment for other person.

TABLE 4

## Common Neurological and Medical Causes of Aggression

1. Alzheimer's disease.
2. Stroke and other cerebrovascular disease.
3. Medications, alcohol and other abused substances, over-the-counter drugs.
4. Delirium (low blood oxygen, electrolyte imbalance, anesthesia and surgery).
5. Traumatic brain injury.
6. Chronic neurologic disorders: Parkinson's disease, Huntington's disease, Wilson's disease, multiple sclerosis, systemic lupus erythematosus.
7. Brain tumors.
8. Infectious diseases.
9. Epilepsy.
10. Metabolic disorders: hyperthyroidism or hypothyrodism, low blood sugar, vitamin deficiencies.

TABLE 5

## Medications and Drugs Associated with Aggression

1. Alcohol—intoxications and withdrawal states.
2. Hypnotic and antianxiety agents (barbiturates, benzodiazepines); intoxication and withdrawal states.
3. Analgesics—opiates and other narcotics—intoxication and withdrawal states.
4. Steroids—manic side effects in initial stages of treatment.
5. Antidepressants—especially heterocyclics and MAO inhibitors in initial phases of treatment.
6. Amphetamines and cocaine—aggression associated with manic excitement in early stages of abuse and secondary to paranoid ideation in later stages of use.
7. Anticholinergic drugs (including over-the-counter sedatives) associated with delirium and central anticholinergic syndrome.

## THE NEED FOR COLLABORATION

Often, the full picture related to the degree and implications of the person's anger and aggressive outbursts is not clear to the physician and mental health professionals without the benefit of input from family members, friends, co-workers, employers, and so forth. This is an area in which both the person who is subject to angry and violent outbursts as well as those affected by such are essential to the professional before an accurate assessment can be made or an effective treatment plan implemented. Because of the social sensitivity and embarrassment associated with excess anger and aggression, patients and their family members may not seek help for this type of problem; and many physicians are reluctant to inquire directly about these symptoms because of their concerns about alienating or irritating their patients. Nonetheless, we can think of no other clinical area in which it is more important for patients, families, physicians, and other mental health professionals to work together closely and openly. When such collaboration does occur, far-reaching benefits in understanding and caring for people with disabling aggressive behavior are achieved.

## Drug Treatment of Aggression

At the present time, there is no medication for the treatment of aggression that is approved by the Food and Drug Administration. In general, the sedative side effects of antipsychotics and benzodiazepines are used—or, in most cases, misused—for the management of aggression and agitation. Investigators have found that approximately 50 percent of the total prescriptions used by the elderly in nursing homes and Veterans Administration settings are antipsychotic agents—and these are largely used to "calm" agitated behaviors through sedation. As indicated in Chapter 7, the use of antipsychotic drugs for purposes other than treatment of psychosis is discouraged because of the severely disabling side effects of this category of medication. Table 6 summarizes the side effects of commonly used and misused drugs in the management of aggression.

Our research group has questioned the use of the sedative side effect of benzodiazepines and antipsychotic agents to "mask" aggressive symptomatologies that are secondary to a wide range of causes. We believe that this widespread practice often results in the generation of side effects that are even more dangerous and disabling than the aggressive behavior for which the medications are prescribed originally. Our practice is to treat, directly where possible, the underlying diagnoses that lead to the aggressive event. If, for example, an individual is aggressive in response to a paranoid delusion that his or her life is being threatened, we advocate using antipsychotic agents to treat the underlying psychosis. Similarly, if aggression is related to the manic excitement of bipolar disorder, we treat the underlying condition with lithium and/or carbamazepine (Chapter 6). For aggression associated with severe depression and/or anxiety disorders, we

TABLE 6

**Side Effects of Drugs Used in the Management of Aggression**

*Antipsychotic*

Oversedation
Hypotension (falls)
Confusion
Neuroleptic malignant syndrome
Parkinsonian side effects
Akathisia
Dystonia
Tardive dyskinesia

*Benzodiazepines*

Oversedation
Motor disturbances (poor coordination)
Mood disturbances
Memory impairment, confusion
Dependency, overdoses, withdrawal syndromes
Paradoxical violence

commonly use psychiatric drugs with prominent serotonin activity such as buspirone (BuSpar), fluoxetine (Prozac), and trazodone (Desyrel). Propranolol is our choice in treating chronic aggression associated with brain damage, and our protocol for the utilization of propranolol in this fashion is summarized in Table 7. Our overview for the management of aggression is summarized in Table 8. When using propranolol, it is important to note that antiaggressive effects do not appear until six to eight weeks after a patient is on a high dose of the medication (400 mg to 600 mg). In addition, as with our practice in using other psychiatric drugs, drug treatment for aggression is always used in combination with psychotherapy, behavioral treatments, family treatments, exercise, environmental restructuring, and other non-drug treatments aimed at reducing stresses that may precipitate rageful or violent responses.

TABLE 7

**Use of Propranolol for Treatment of Aggression**

1. Conduct a thorough medical evaluation, including electrocardiogram.
2. Exclude patients with the following disorders: bronchial asthma, chronic obstructive pulmonary disease, insulin-dependent diabetes, diabetes mellitus, congestive heart failure, persistent angina, significant peripheral vascular disease, hyperthyroidism.
3. In patients for whom there are clinical concerns about hypotension or bradycardia, begin with a single test dose of 20 mg per day. Increase the dose of propranolol by 20 mg per day every three days.
4. For patients without cardiovascular or cardiopulmonary disorder, initiate propranolol on a 20 mg, three-times-a-day schedule.
5. Increase the dose of propranolol by 60 mg per day, every three days.
6. Increase propranolol unless the pulse rate is reduced below 50 beats per minute, or systolic blood pressure is less than 90 mm of mercury.
7. Hold medication doses if severe dizziness, ataxia, or wheezing occurs. Reduce or discontinue propranolol if such symptoms persist.
8. Increase dose to 12 mg per kilogram of body weight, or until aggressive behavior is under control. Doses of greater than 800 mg are not usually required to control aggressive behavior.
9. Maintain the patient on the highest doses of propranolol for at least eight weeks prior to determining that the patient is not responding to the medication. Some patients, however, may respond rapidly to propranolol.
10. Utilize concurrent medications with caution. Monitor plasma blood levels of all antipsychotic and anticonvulsant medications. Propranolol has been shown to increase plasma levels of chlorpromazine and thioridazine.
11. Avoid sudden discontinuation of propranolol, particularly in patients with hypertension.
12. Taper a patient's dose of propranolol by 60 mg per day until the patient is on a total daily dose of 60 mg per day. At that point, taper the medication at a rate of 20 mg every other day (or more gradually in patients with hypertension) to avoid rebound hypertension.

TABLE 8

## Overview of the Drug Management of Aggression

| Agent | Indications | Approximate Dose | Special Clinical Considerations |
|---|---|---|---|
| Antipsychotics | Aggression directly related to psychotic ideation. Acute management of violence or aggression utilizing sedative side effects | Standard doses used in treating psychosis. | Oversedation and multiple side effects including significant risk of tardive dyskinesia when used to treat chronic aggression. |
| Carbamazepine | Aggression related to complex partial seizure disorder. | 600 mg to 1,200 mg per day in divided doses (to maintain serum levels at 4 to 12 micrograms per milliliter. | Monitor closely for evidence of bone marrow suppression or hematologic abnormalities. |
| Lithium | Aggression and irritability related to manic excitement or cyclic mood disorders. | 300 mg three times a day (to maintain serum levels at 0.6 to 1.2 millequivalents per liter). | Has been reported to be effective for aggression in prison populations, mental retardation. |
| Buspirone | Aggression associated with severe anxiety | 10 mg to 20 mg orally three times a day. | Latency period of onset of action may be four to six weeks. |
| Propranolol | Chronic or recurrent aggression in patients with organic brain diseases or injuries. | 200 mg to 800 mg per day in divided doses. | Latency period of onset of action may be four to six weeks. |

## Chapter 14

# Electroconvulsive Therapy

THE mere mention of the term *shock therapy* or *electroshock therapy* evokes for most people thoughts of archaic medical practices, loss of control, and even torture. In the novel *One Flew Over the Cuckoo's Nest*, and the movie of the same name, electroconvulsive therapy (ECT) was used to punish an individual whose only obvious "problems" were enthusiasm, rebelliousness, and having a mind of his own.

Let us assure you that this fiction does not reflect reality. The reality is that electroconvulsive therapy, when utilized for its several well-defined indications, is among the safest and most effective forms of treatment. Largely as a result of the inaccurate ways this procedure has been portrayed in movies and on television, and perhaps because of certain understandable fears that we all may share about electricity, many patients who could receive substantial benefit are fearful of even considering this form of treatment.

Much of the information in this chapter comes from the lectures on the history of ECT given at Columbia University by ECT pioneer Dr. Lothar Kalinowsky, as well as from Dr. Richard Abrams's outstanding text *Electroconvulsive Therapy*. New York: Oxford University Press, 1988.

## Professional Opinion and ECT

Surveys by the American Psychiatric Association have shown that although only 3 to 5 percent of hospitalized psychiatric patients receive electroconvulsive therapy, over 70 percent of psychiatrists believe that there are *many* patients for whom electroconvulsive therapy is the safest, least expensive, and most effective form of treatment. In the same survey, 83 percent of those who responded agreed with this statement: "Any psychiatric institute claiming to offer comprehensive care should be equipped to provide ECT." Another survey of over one thousand mental health professionals and of patients who had received ECT found that ECT was an appropriate and effective treatment. An important result of this survey was that groups of patients and professionals "agree to a striking extent on the appropriateness of using ECT for specific psychiatric conditions and on the clinical improvement associated with its use." Research scientist Dr. Max Fink has reviewed the impact of the treatment and concluded that after a half century of experience with tens of thousands of patients receiving ECT each year in the United States, experts agree that ECT is a safe, reliable, efficient, and effective treatment for people with affective disorders and certain other mental illnesses.

## The Discovery and History of Electroconvulsive Therapy

As early as the sixteenth century, the Swiss physician Paracelsus was said to have given patients with "lunacy" the chemical camphor to produce convulsions, or epileptic seizures. He believed that these seizures helped to cure their mental symptoms. Over the next three hundred years, camphor-induced seizures were episodically used to treat symptoms of mania, schizophrenia, and depression. In the mid-1930s, a group of Italian scientists introduced a technique in which grand mal seizures were initiated by passing electrical current through the brain between two electrodes placed at each temple, and the new treatment quickly became widely used. Many psychiatrists became enthusiastic about this new therapy. Until the revolution in the use of psychiatric drugs to treat mental illness in the mid- to late 1950s, electroconvulsive therapy was, without rival, the most effective biological treatment for severe depression, symptoms of schizophrenia, and mania.

In some cases, however, ECT was used excessively—both for conditions for which it was indicated and those for which it was not indicated. A few patients were injured as the result of the treatments. As a result, popular opinion turned against ECT. Today, electroconvulsive therapy is underutilized—particularly by those who are socioeconomically disadvantaged.

Since it was first developed in 1934, the techniques of administering ECT have been constantly improved. Experts in ECT can now use barbiturate anesthesia, oxygenation, muscle relaxant drugs, and brief pulse stimulation. All of these modern techniques significantly reduce the amount of energy necessary to initiate a seizure. This increases the benefit to the patient while substantially reducing the risk of side effects.

## Mechanisms of Action of ECT

No one understands exactly how ECT works, but it appears likely that electroconvulsive therapy helps to correct the impaired neuroendocrine and neurotransmitter systems that give rise to psychiatric illnesses. Electroconvulsive therapy has been shown to have important positive effects on such brain transmitters as norepinephrine, epinephrine, dopamine, serotonin, acetylcholine, and gamma-amino butyric acid (GABA), as well as on the naturally occurring opiates, the endorphins and the enkephalins.

## Indications for Electroconvulsive Therapy

### DEPRESSION

Electroconvulsive therapy is most commonly used in the treatment of severe depression—particularly for depression in which the symptoms are intense, prolonged, and accompanied by profound psychological changes that may affect the patient's sleep, appetite, sexual energy, general activity level, and perceptions. As with drug treatment, patients treated with electroconvulsive therapy have significantly lower mortality rates (not just from suicide, but also from natural causes) than those people with depression who are not treated by ECT or drugs.

Most psychiatrists use antidepressant drugs as a treatment of first choice for depression. It is only when drug treatment fails that electroconvulsive therapy is attempted. Even so, studies comparing electroconvulsive therapy to antidepressant treatment conclude that electroconvulsive therapy is just as safe as, and in some ways therapeutically superior to, antidepressant drugs. Marked improvement is generally found in 80 to 90 percent of depressed patients who receive electroconvulsive therapy. Our own practice is also to use medications first for most patients with severe depression who require a biologic intervention. We recommend ECT in the following situations:

• For patients whose severe depressions have *not* responded to adequate (appropriate dose and duration of treatment) trials with antidepressant drugs.

• For people who have delusional depression. As noted in Chapter 3, only 40 to 50 percent of patients with psychotic or delusional depression respond to heterocyclic antidepressants alone. Approximately 70 to 80 percent respond to the combination of antipsychotic agents and heterocyclic antidepressants. More than 80 percent show a positive response when treated with ECT.

• For patients, particularly elderly patients, who cannot tolerate the cardiovascular, renal, central nervous system, and other side effects of antidepressant or antipsychotic agents. ECT is occasionally indicated for pregnant women whose pregnancy may be endangered by psychiatric drugs. The safety and efficacy of ECT for the pregnant woman and the fetus are well established for these purposes.

• For a person whose acute depressive symptoms are so severe (such as people who are actively suicidal or have severe medical problems such as dehydration and starvation secondary to their depressions) that a rapid and dramatic response is required. Often, electroconvulsive therapy relieves symptoms in such individuals in briefer time periods (one to two weeks) than required for antidepressants (three to five weeks).

• For a person with a history of prior depressive episodes that did not respond to antidepressant drugs.

• For a person who has successfully responded to previous electroconvulsive therapy treatment.

## ECT FOR MANIC SYMPTOMS

Although major depression is the principal indication for the use of electroconvulsive therapy, other psychiatric illnesses and symptoms may also respond to this treatment. Acute manic symptoms (including euphoria, agitation, and irritability) are highly responsive to treatment with ECT. Although mania is usually reversed by antipsychotic agents or by lithium treatment (about 20 percent of hospitalized manics fail to remit fully), occasionally a patient's inability to tolerate the side effects of such drugs or the untoward danger of the symptoms may require the use of electroconvulsive therapy. ECT can usually be counted on to work quickly and effectively (one to three treatments) in the treatment of mania.

## ECT for Symptoms Associated with Acute Schizophrenia

ECT has powerful antipsychotic effects, and many symptoms associated with schizophrenia respond well to electroconvulsive therapy. It is clear that ECT does not treat the underlying illness of schizophrenia per se, but it may be useful:

- when individuals with schizophrenia become dangerously out of control,
- when catatonic symptoms are present and threaten the health of the person,
- when side effects associated with antipsychotics are problematic (e.g., tardive dyskinesia),
- when an individual is suffering greatly from symptoms related to schizophrenia but has not responded to adequate trials of drug treatment,
- when depressive or manic effects are prominent (schizoaffective disorder).

## Mental Illness for Which Electroconvulsive Therapy Is *Not* Indicated

Electroconvulsive therapy is indicated primarily for the treatment of depression, mania, and certain clinical situations associated with schizophrenia as described above. It is not indicated for other mental disorders such as conduct disorders, antisocial personality disorders, anxiety disorders, alcoholism or other substance use disorders, eating disorders, attention-deficit disorders, most organic mental disorders or dementias, sexual disorders, personality disorders, character disorders, or the so-called neuroses that are not complicated by major depression.

## Medical Evaluation Before Treatment with Electroconvulsive Therapy

### Laboratory Evaluation

Before receiving ECT, a patient should have a complete medical and neurological examination, complete blood count, blood chemistry analysis, urinalysis, and X ray of the lumbosacral region of the spine (in individuals over fifty years of age or if orthopedic problems are suggested), and a chest X ray. Also included in the pre-ECT workup are an electrocardiogram and an electroencephalogram. If there is clinical evidence or suggestion of a brain tumor or another type of brain lesion, a CAT scan or a magnetic resonance imaging (MRI) procedure may be required.

*Informed Consent*

Because of the high degree of fear, misunderstanding, and misinformation related to ECT, we devote a minimum of two hours to meeting with both the patient and his or her family in order to provide ample opportunity for the exchange of ideas, feelings, and information related to electroconvulsive treatment. During this time, we discuss the reasons for the consideration of electroconvulsive therapy, the risks and potential benefits, and the actual techniques. We provide copies of scientific papers that discuss the efficacy, safety, and value of ECT compared with other treatments. A full discussion of side effects, especially memory problems, is an important part of this process. We consider such discussion a necessary part of the treatment.

## Technique of Electroconvulsive Therapy

### INFORMATION ABOUT THE PROCEDURE

We explain to the patient and his or her family exactly what will be done to the patient, how it will be done, why it will be done, and what he or she should expect to feel before, during, and after the electroconvulsive therapy treatment. We give the individual the opportunity to speak with other people who have experienced this treatment. This experience inevitably makes the person feel much more comfortable about ECT. We offer our patients the opportunity to see videotapes of other patients undergoing electroconvulsive therapy and to make visits to the procedure room to examine the equipment. We feel that the more the individual knows about the procedure, the better will be his or her ability to make an informed decision. It also increases the chance of a good response to treatment.

### TECHNIQUE OF ADMINISTRATION

During ECT, an electric current passes through the brain, and initiates a grand mal seizure. Such seizures are associated with therapeutic benefits for certain mental disorders. Muscle relaxants such as succinylcholine are administered intravenously to paralyze the muscles for brief periods of time (two to three minutes) to prevent the muscle contractions that might lead to sprains and fractured bones if the seizure were not modified in this fashion.

In many cases, electroconvulsive therapy is done in the surgical suite of a general hospital or in a special area of the psychiatric center. The patient is anesthetized and is asleep during the procedure. The anesthesia is induced by an anesthetist or anesthesiologist by injecting a fast-acting intravenous barbiturate anesthetic, such as methohexital, through a vein in the back of the hand. In general, it takes half a minute to a minute for a patient to enter the required stage of anesthesia before the muscle relaxant succinylcholine can be injected intravenously. Once the patient is under general anesthesia and his or her muscles begin to relax, the patient is ventilated with 100 percent oxygen until there is an indication that all of his or her muscles are fully relaxed by the intravenous succinylcholine. At that point, electrodes about the size of silver dollars are applied to the temple and forehead regions, and a brief (approximately one-half to two seconds is standard) electrical stimulation is applied. The resulting seizure lasts from twenty-five to sixty seconds. Because the patient is fully relaxed with the intravenous muscle relaxant, there is usually little or no observable evidence that a seizure or electrical discharge of the brain is taking place. In fact, medical students and other professionals observing the procedure for the first time are frequently surprised by the lack of movement. However, the patient's brain waves are monitored during the procedure so that the physician can be certain that an electrical discharge of the brain of adequate duration (longer than twenty-five seconds) has taken place. We also monitor the patient's heart throughout the continuous recording of an electrocardiogram and check the patient's blood pressure throughout the treatment. The whole process, from the time of the first injection of anesthesia until the time when the patient is ready to be taken to the recovery room, rarely exceeds five to ten minutes. Patients remain in a recovery room for approximately one hour and then return to their rooms in the hospital, where they have breakfast and resume their normal daily activities.

## MORTALITY RATES AND ECT

Electroconvulsive therapy is an extraordinarily safe medical procedure. The risk of death from ECT is very low—about one death in twenty to forty thousand treatments. By comparison, the risk of death by suicide in severe untreated depression may be as high as 10 percent. This mortality rate of ECT is much lower than that for women during childbirth in the United States and is about the same as the risk of general anesthesia alone.

## ADVERSE EFFECTS OF ELECTROCONVULSIVE THERAPY

The two most frequent questions that psychiatrists are asked about electro-convulsive therapy are: (1) "What does it feel like to go through a course of electroconvulsive therapy—particularly, does it hurt?" and (2) "What are the side effects of this procedure—particularly, will it damage my brain?" In this section, we will review the most common adverse effects of electro-convulsive therapy and in a subsequent section review the experience of a course of treatment from a patient's perspective.

In general, side effects related to electroconvulsive therapy derive from three sources: (1) the drugs used to initiate anesthesia and block the neuromuscular effects of the seizures; (2) the electrical stimulation utilized to initiate the seizure; and (3) the effects of the seizure, or the electrical discharge of the brain per se. For the purposes of discussion, we will also divide the review of the side effects associated with electroconvulsive therapy into those that occur during a course of the treatments and those that persist after the course of a treatment.

## ADVERSE EFFECTS OF ECT OCCURRING DURING A COURSE OF TREATMENT

### Adverse Effects Associated with Drugs Used to Induce Anesthesia and to Modify Effects of ECT Treatment

Because the time required for the procedure of electroconvulsive therapy is so brief, the side effects from barbiturate anesthesia are mild and rare. Some patients report brief nausea and vomiting after barbiturate general anesthesia, others report brief headaches. There are occasional skin reactions such as a rash.

Certain patients with preexisting cardiac problems may, during the course of treatment, experience changes in heart rhythms. Using methohex-ital anesthesia instead of thiopental reduces irregularities of heart rhythm in patients with preexisting heart disorders. Again, we must understand these changes from the perspective of the extraordinary safety record of ECT that has been discussed earlier. A very small percentage of individuals have what is called *pseudocholinesterase deficiency*. What this means is that it takes longer for the muscle relaxants to wear off. This rare and unusual condition is highly unlikely to result in discomfort or danger to the patient, because the psychiatrist and anesthesiologist are familiar with this condi-tion and will simply maintain the patient's general anesthesia and oxygena-tion until the muscle-blocking properties wear off. There are no lasting effects. Finally, because a patient must restrict food and liquids for a period of twelve hours prior to electroconvulsive therapy treatment and because medications like atropine are used to dry secretions during the procedure, some people experience dry mouth for several hours following each procedure. This condition is only moderately uncomfortable and is quickly reversed once a person resumes his or her normal diet (usually within several hours after the procedure).

### Cardiovascular Effects

Changes in the heart rhythm and conduction commonly occur in patients—both during and immediately after the induction of the seizure. These changes include both slowing and increases in the rate of the heartbeat as well as a wide variety of changes in the pattern (rhythm) of the heartbeat. The changes are more common in people with preexisting heart disease, and with the use of thiopental general anesthesia as opposed to methohexital anesthesia. These heart changes are limited to the course of ECT as well as to the immediate posttreatment stage. Careful tests conducted several hours after ECT do not reveal any changes in heart rhythm or heart function, even in patients with preexisting heart diseases. There is no evidence of lasting heart changes or of heart damage as a result of electroconvulsive therapy.

### ADVERSE EFFECTS OF ECT OCCURRING AFTER A COURSE OF TREATMENT

### Confusion

All generalized seizures, whether they are induced electrically or not, are followed by a period of confusion (lasting less than an hour) during which time individuals may be uncertain of where they are, what has happened to them, what the date is, etc. Other aspects of thinking, feeling, and behaving may also be affected. For approximately 5 to 10 percent of patients receiving ECT, this confusional state becomes more pronounced. Some patients become restless, agitated, or somewhat dazed. This is called postictal or postseizure delirium and usually persists for ten to twenty minutes. In either case, the confusional state usually goes away on its own. It is not recalled by or upsetting to most patients over the long term. Some clinicians now use a newer, low-energy version of electroconvulsive therapy in which both electrodes are placed on the same side of the patient's head (called a *nondominant unilateral ECT*). This appears to reduce significantly the time and the severity of any confusion that may occur; however, some clinicians question whether this technique is as effective as more traditional electrode placement in ECT. Many clinicians in academic and other settings now use this innovative technique.

### Memory Impairment

Memory impairment constitutes the most significant side effect of electroconvulsive therapy. It is often difficult to tell whether this has occurred, as decreased attention, difficulty concentrating, and memory impairment are frequently prominent features of severe depression. While certain individuals may complain of memory impairment, careful testing of their memories only occasionally documents any change.

If memory loss does occur, it principally involves those memories recorded during the period of treatment. Earlier and later memories are not usually affected. Placing both electrodes on the nondominant side of the brain, using the lowest possible quantity of energy to initiate the seizure, and providing supportive care of the patient both before and after treatment will keep memory loss to a minimum.

In general, most patients suffer loss of memory for the events that occur immediately before and after the treatment process, but *very* few have lasting impairment of memory of important life events or of their ability to learn and remember new things. Thus, although patients may experience transient memory disturbances for events immediately before and after treatment, or, in the most rare and extreme cases, may even have gaps in memory that extend for over six months after treatment, they can be assured that their memory function, or their ability to learn and retain new information, will not be impaired. And other mental functions, such as cognitive function, intelligence, reasoning, judgment, comprehension, and abstract thinking are rarely affected by ECT. Because of the dysfunctions in these realms caused by depression, they are usually improved after ECT.

## Frequent Questions About ECT

**Q.** *Is there any physical pain associated with ECT?*

**A.** There is rarely any physical pain associated with electroconvulsive therapy beyond the needle stick required to put in place the intravenous line through which anesthetics and muscle relaxants are injected. Occasionally, some patients complain of headaches after treatment. These are generally responsive to aspirin and rarely last for more than several hours after each treatment.

**Q.** *Is ECT dangerous?*

**A.** As has been discussed earlier in this chapter, ECT has one of the best safety records of any treatment in all of medicine. The mortality rate from the procedure is so low that in California only two deaths were recorded over a six-year period, even though many of the 18,627 patients treated during that time had serious preexisting medical illnesses in addition to their depression.

**Q.** *Is it safe for me to have ECT even though I have a serious medical condition in addition to my depression?*

**A.** In the vast majority of cases, ECT may be used safely even though a person has a significant medical illness in addition to the psychiatric condition for which ECT is being used. For example, ECT has been used safely for people who have had depressions immediately following major heart surgery; it is used safely for patients with pacemakers; it is used safely for pregnant women, for individuals with epilepsy, for people with histories of stroke, for people with recent histories of traumatic brain injury, for people with Alzheimer's disease and other dementias, for individuals with a wide range of heart diseases, for people with Parkinson's disease (in fact, it has been reported to even benefit the movement disorder associated with Parkinson's disease), and for people with a wide variety of other medical conditions. Of course, every individual who is to receive ECT, whether or not he or she has a coexisting medical disorder, must be evaluated individually and thoroughly for the ability to benefit from the procedure and to tolerate its side effects and adverse effects. We feel that the greatest risk associated with electroconvulsive therapy is in utilizing the treatment for individuals who have had recent myocardial infarctions or for those who have brain tumors or other brain lesions that increase pressure on the brain and its fluids.

**Q.** *How many ECT treatments constitute an ideal course?*

**A.** In general, six to eight treatments are usually sufficient to treat depression. Occasionally, patients may require ten or more treatments to achieve a response. Even though patients may improve with the third or fourth treatment, we often give a full course of six to eight treatments in order to attempt to prevent relapse. We hasten to emphasize that for each individual patient, clinical judgment is required to determine the exact number of treatments that is most likely to be beneficial. This judgment is best derived from a physician who has extensive experience in using electroconvulsive therapy as well as other treatment modalities, such as psychotherapy and drugs.

**Q.** *Should my psychiatric medications be continued during my course of ECT?*

**A.** We usually recommend that antidepressants be discontinued during ECT. Careful studies by many investigators have not found that the presence of psychiatric drugs enhances the effects of ECT when given during a course of ECT. Some investigators have found, in fact, that these drugs reduce the benefit of the treatments. Lithium, especially, should be discontinued during a course of ECT, as it may cause confusion. It is known, however, that adding antidepressants or lithium *after* a successful course of ECT significantly reduces the recurrence of mood disorders (both mania and depression). We routinely readminister antidepressants and lithium (when indicated) following successful courses of ECT, and usually maintain these drugs at treatment doses for at least six months.

**Q.** *Do I have to be in the hospital to receive ECT, or may I receive ECT as an outpatient?*

**A.** In this country, a complete course of ECT is usually administered while a patient remains in the hospital. The advantages of this are the facilitation of the pre-ECT medical workup, the assessment, the treatment, and monitoring of coexisting medical illnesses, the protection of the patient from self-destructive impulses, and the overall enhanced care and comfort of a person with a severe depressive illness. However, ECT is routinely administered on an outpatient basis in the United Kingdom and often delivered in the United States in surgicenters for patients who require maintenance treatments (or occasional individual treatments to prevent relapse). We anticipate that outpatient ECT will become increasingly frequent over the years to come, primarily because of cost. In the cases where outpatient treatment is delivered, special care must be taken to monitor the patient during the posttreatment confusional stage as well as to be sure that those memory impairments or thinking impairments that do occur around the time of treatment do not place an individual at risk (e.g., while driving a car, or on the job).

**Q.** *I am eighty years old. Does this mean I am too old to have treatments?*

**A.** Because of its great safety and efficacy, ECT is often the safest treatment for mood disorders of the elderly. The authors have successfully administered ECT to individuals in their early nineties with highly beneficial results and with no significant side effects.

**Q.** *What is the difference between unilateral and bilateral ECT?*

**A.** Unilateral and bilateral ECT refer to the placement of the electrodes through which the electrical stimulation is delivered to the brain to initiate a seizure. It has been proved that unilateral administration (or administering the impulse to one half of the brain) on the nondominant side (i.e., to the right side of the brain for a right-handed individual) significantly reduces the immediate confusion and memory impairment associated with ECT. On the other hand, some investigators and clinicians think that bilateral ECT may be more potent in the treatment of those psychiatric disorders that have been proven to be responsive to ECT. In general, we tend to use unilateral nondominant ECT in most patients, except for those whose psychiatric symptomatologies are so severe that they require the most rapid of interventions.

**Q.** *Will ECT damage my brain?*

**A.** Although this is a very simple and direct question, there is no easy answer to it. As has been described throughout this book, the brain is a highly complex entity, and it is affected both beneficially and adversely by a wide variety of substances and conditions. Whether or not ECT results in lasting changes in the brain remains a controversial question. Carefully conducted scientific studies using such imaging techniques as CAT and MRI scans and other devices do not provide evidence that structural brain damage occurs. In addition, investigations of animals receiving ECT and the examination of the tissues of the brains of people who have received ECT do not substantiate lasting brain injury associated with the procedure. In addition, the use of modern techniques including general anesthesia, muscle relaxation, oxygenation, and low-dose electrical initiation of seizures reduces the possibility of brain damage. Nevertheless, it remains possible that ECT has lasting effects on the brain that we cannot currently document. The important question is, "How does this possible risk compare with the benefit of ECT?" The answer is clear: For most people who have psychiatric disorders for which ECT has been proved effective, the benefits of this treatment far outweigh any associated risks.

No single therapeutic measure (including medication) has been shown to be superior to electroconvulsive therapy (ECT) in the treatment of depression. In fact, few approaches have been shown to be safer. For persons who are severely depressed and suicidal, who cannot tolerate the side effects of the antidepressants, who have psychotic aspects to their depression, or are unresponsive to adequate trials of medication, ECT is often the treatment of choice.

## Recommended Reading on Electroconvulsive Therapy

For those wishing a more extensive presentation and critical review of the mechanisms of action of electroconvulsive therapy, please refer to the chapter by Dr. Harold A. Sacheim in Volume 7 of the *American Psychiatric Press Annual Review of Psychiatry* (1988, pp. 436–457). Also recommended is an outstanding book by Richard Abrams, M.D., *Electroconvulsive Therapy* (New York: Oxford University Press, 1988).

# Chapter 15

# Psychiatric Drugs of the Future

ALTHOUGH the last quarter of a century has seen a revolution in the extraordinary public health benefits of psychiatric drugs, we believe that future discoveries will be even more dramatic and far reaching. Research in all aspects of science and medicine is now being applied to psychiatric illness, and the results will be the development of more specific and effective biologic treatment for most mental illnesses. In this chapter, we will outline some of the present directions of research in psychopharmacology and other biologic treatments and speculate on the future implications of these efforts.

In this chapter, we will first review those developments and advancements that are certain to come about for the assessment and biologic treatment of various psychiatric disorders. Then we will also speculate about other scientific innovations that have far-reaching implications, but may or may not result in clinical treatments. This latter speculative approach is a wide departure from the conservative, data-based approach that we have taken throughout this book. However, many of our colleagues in psychiatry, as they reviewed and critiqued this book, told us that we were far too conservative, and had understated the relative advantages and potentials of psychopharmacological and other biologic interventions. Perhaps our indulgence in some speculation in this chapter will provide balance and optimism to offset our therapeutic conservatism.

We believe that the most realistic hope for those people whose mental illnesses are not currently treatable lies in biologic research. Therefore, we conclude this chapter and this book with facts about psychiatric research, and encourage our readers to support it and participate in it.

In the preceding chapters of this book, we have described the ways in which current medications are highly effective in the treatment of many psychiatric illnesses. Nevertheless, many psychiatric disorders and symptoms remain prevalent and disabling, so new psychopharmacologic treatments are necessary. For example, some patients may not have an optimal response to (or cannot tolerate the side effects of) the currently available medications—for example, a patient with schizophrenia who had developed tardive dyskinesia but still required an antipsychotic medication to treat paranoid delusions. The advent of clozapine in the United States in February 1990 provides for the first time an antipsychotic agent that is not associated with tardive dyskinesia. We expect the imminent development and testing of many newer generation derivatives of clozapine that are even more effective, without its dangerous side effects. In addition, many psychiatric disorders currently have no approved drug therapy—for example, antisocial personality disorder, in which people have patterns of behavior that are exploitive of and damaging to others, without respect for the law, the rights of others, or feelings of guilt. Some recent evidence shows hereditary and biologic features of this disorder and, therefore, gives increased hope for pharmacologic interventions.

The development of new methods of drug administration, such as small pumps that can safely inject drugs directly into the brain, the use of electrical devices to stimulate discrete regions of the brain, and even transplants into the brain of living tissue that will produce and secrete chemicals to affect mood and behavior, may open new corridors that lead to vast horizons of potential for biologic interventions of psychiatric disorders. We will summarize these advances in relation to the disorders that may potentially benefit from discoveries; we will then review technological advances and describe the process of clinical research in psychopharmacology.

# Depression

### NEW HETEROCYCLIC ANTIDEPRESSANTS

Although depression currently can be effectively treated with medications, up to 20 percent of the patients may not respond to these drugs. In addition, many people have difficulty in tolerating the side effects of the antidepressants. New antidepressant drugs being developed differ from the standard heterocyclic antidepressants (HCAs) such as imipramine and amitriptyline in their "side effect profile." All the HCAs can cause blurry vision, dry mouth, and constipation because of anticholinergic effects. New antidepressants that are specific for the serotonin neurotransmitter system effectively treat depression without causing anticholinergic side effects. Trazodone (Desyrel), fluoxetine (Prozac), and bupropion (Wellbutrin) are the first of many new drugs of this type. Drugs of this genre that are currently under investigation include fluoxamine and citalopram.

### NEW MONOAMINE OXIDASE INHIBITORS

One category of antidepressant medications, the monoamine oxidase inhibitors (MAOIs), may particularly benefit those depressed people with "atypical features" that include oversleeping, overeating, anxiety, and sensitivity to interpersonal rejection. Unfortunately, treatment with MAOIs requires that the patient strictly comply with a diet that is tyramine-free, so that sudden elevations of blood pressure can be avoided. Foods that contain tyramine include cheeses, wines, aged meats, and smoked fish. When a patient who is taking an MAOI eats one of these foods, tyramine is not metabolized by enzymes in the intestines as it usually is, but remains and causes the buildup of epinephrine, which may result in a sudden and potentially hazardous elevation in blood pressure. This is called a "hypertensive crisis," and has the potential to cause a stroke. Although most patients are able to comply with this diet, the very thought of a hypertensive crisis is often sufficiently upsetting for patients to refuse the prescription of a MAOI. However, newly developed MAOIs such as moclobemide that are currently under investigation have minimal or no risk of producing the hypertensive crisis or sudden elevation in blood pressure when a person on an MAOI eats food containing tyramine. If such drugs are shown to be effective, they will provide an important treatment option for many patients suffering from depression.

## NEW CLASSES OF ANTIDEPRESSANTS

As we discussed in Chapter 3, most antidepressants work, in part, by affecting the neurotransmitters through which one brain cell communicates with another. The currently available antidepressants, although highly effective, involve only a few transmitter systems. Recently, research has identified over one hundred chemical compounds that meet the definition of neurotransmitters, and we can be certain that new, better antidepressants will be developed that involve these distinct chemical messengers. We have also learned that messages are transmitted within each neuronal cell itself. This message transmission may involve channels within the membranes of cells and many other complex processes of the cell. As understanding of the processes at the single cell level improves, researchers will see new opportunities for intervention in depressive illness. We may anticipate, therefore, the development of new drugs that work by affecting clinical transmission in between cells (or intercellular messengers) as well as by involving intracellular message systems, that is, messenger systems that work within the cell.

## LIGHT THERAPY

For those patients who suffer episodes of depression that occur specifically during the winter months (called Seasonal Affective Disorder, SAD), treatment with special lights has been shown to be beneficial. For this treatment, the patient sits in front of a panel of high-intensity lights for up to one-half hour per day in the early morning (e.g., 6:30 to 7:00 A.M.). Elevations in the mood of depressed patients have been reported in studies of the National Institute of Mental Health, and the results have been confirmed by several other prominent research teams throughout the country. The effectiveness of this type of "natural" treatment is important because it stimulates research into alternative mechanisms of antidepressant action. For example, light therapy may alter the abnormal circadian rhythms or sleep/wake cycles in people with depression. The effect of light therapy for those patients who have depression without SAD has yet to be demonstrated but, in our opinion, is highly promising.

# Psychosis

The currently available drug treatments for patients with schizophrenia are effective for treating "positive" psychotic symptoms, such as delusions and hallucinations. "Negative" symptoms, such as apathy, withdrawal, and flatness of mood and expression are not so responsive to treatment with these drugs. It is generally accepted that antipsychotic drugs work, in part, through their ability to block dopamine receptors in the brain. Unfortunately, several side effects are produced by dopamine blockade, including parkinsonism (tremor, rigidity, and restlessness) and tardive dyskinesia. The search for new drugs that treat schizophrenia is focused on two major areas: (1) drugs that can treat negative symptoms as well as positive symptoms and (2) drugs that work specifically in those regions of the brain that involve psychosis, but do not cause side effects by acting on other brain sites. Efforts are thus currently concentrated on developing antipsychotic drugs that work only on dopamine receptors involved in psychosis, as opposed to dopamine receptors elsewhere in the brain, such as those involved with the regulation of movement.

## CLOZAPINE

Clozapine (Clozaril) is an antipsychotic drug that has just become available in the United States for the treatment of patients with schizophrenia who have not responded to other antipsychotic drugs. As has been discussed in Chapter 7, carefully performed studies demonstrate that one-third of patients with schizophrenia who have been "drug-refractory" show significant improvement after treatment with clozapine. In addition, clozapine does not appear to cause parkinsonian side effects or tardive dyskinesia. Unfortunately, a number of patients may develop difficulties with the production of white blood cells (agranulocytosis), which can predispose them to serious infections. Because of this complication, all patients treated with clozapine are required to have weekly blood counts for as long as they are on the medication. New drugs are currently being developed and tested that are similar to clozapine, but that do not have the side effect of agranulocytosis. Nonetheless, clozapine is regarded as a significant breakthrough in the treatment of people with schizophrenia who have not responded to traditional antipsychotic agents.

## PHENCYCLIDINE

Phencyclidine (PCP, or angel dust) can produce hallucinations and delusions. Researchers have found that phencyclidine has its own specific receptor in the brain, and that it also acts on a specific type of opiate receptor. This has opened research efforts into finding new drugs that act on this brain receptor in these systems (rather than the dopamine system) to block psychosis. New experimental drugs have been developed, such as BMY 14802 and remoxipride, that act on these receptors and may soon prove effective in treating schizophrenia without the production of parkinsonian side effects.

# Anxiety Disorders

## GENERALIZED ANXIETY DISORDER

The benzodiazepine family of drugs, including diazepam (Valium), lorazepam (Ativan), and alprazolam (Xanax), are highly effective in the treatment of acute and chronic anxiety. Although they are very safe drugs in that they have a low toxicity if taken in large amounts, there is realistic concern that people can become dependent on this class of agent. This concern has stimulated research to discover new, effective anxiolytics that do not cause dependency or addiction. The discovery and increased understanding of benzodiazepine receptors in the brain have enabled researchers not only to recognize how these drugs work, but also have allowed the development of newer types of drugs that may be even more effective in treating anxiety, without producing sedation or dependence. These drugs are called *partial agonist* benzodiazepines, and several new prototypes are currently under investigation. Lastly, an *antagonist* benzodiazepine drug, flumazenil, which will immediately reverse the effects of all benzodiazepines, is likely to be available to the public soon, and this drug will rapidly reverse the life-threatening effects of patients who have taken overdoses of benzodiazepines.

## PANIC DISORDER

Until the early 1980s, the prevalence of panic disorder was underrecognized and underappreciated. One of the stimuli to extensive research in this area was the study of efficacy of alprazolam in the treatment of this disorder. Since then, many other drugs have been investigated and are currently being developed. These include other anxiolytic drugs such as adnazolam, as well as antidepressants such as moclobemide, and many others. New methods of administration of drugs for the treatment of panic disorder may also be developed. For example, a patient with infrequent panic attacks may be able to dissolve a medicine under his or her tongue to abort impending panic attacks, in the same way that nitroglycerine is taken by someone with angina. This type of administration will likely have benefits in the treatment of other episodic anxiety disorders such as social phobia.

## OBSESSIVE-COMPULSIVE DISORDER

Until recently, it was believed that patients with compulsions (the urge to perform certain acts repeatedly, such as handwashing) or obsessions (the presence of recurrent unwanted thoughts, images, or impulses) would not improve with medication treatments. Psychologic therapies were thought to be the only effective treatment for people with these painful symptoms. It has now been found that drugs that act specifically on the serotonin system of the brain can be of great help for patients that suffer from these obsessive-compulsive disorders. One of these drugs, fluoxetine (Prozac), has recently been approved for the treatment of depression and has shown great promise in several studies investigating its efficacy in the treatment of obsessive-compulsive disorder. Clomipramine (Anafranil) is now available to American psychiatrists. Several scientific studies have substantiated that clomipramine is highly effective in the treatment of severe obsessive-compulsive disorder in many people who have not responded to other treatments. Side effects of clomipramine are similar to those experienced with other heterocyclic antidepressants, including constipation, dry mouth, sweating, and increased energy. There are several other drugs that are under investigation for the treatment of obsessions and compulsions at specific research centers, and these will also become available in the near future.

## PHOBIAS

Fear of situations, either social, such as public speaking, or of specific stimuli or objects, such as snakes, flying, or taking elevators, has usually been treated with behavioral therapy in which the person is progressively exposed to the feared situation or object. Recent research strongly suggests that several drugs used for other conditions may be effective for social phobia as well. For example, beta blockers such as propranolol are currently prescribed to ameliorate performance anxiety in musicians, actors, and public speakers (see Chapter 5). Antidepressant drugs such as phenelzine have also been shown to help those with social and other types of phobias. It is likely that more specific and effective drugs will be developed for this condition. Perhaps, someday, the large number of students who suffer from "exam nerves" may be able to take tests and demonstrate their knowledge without the distress and disadvantages of anxiety.

## Eating Disorders

Several investigators have found that patients with anorexia nervosa and bulimia show significant improvement in their abnormal eating behaviors when treated with antidepressant medications. These drugs include heterocyclic antidepressants such as imipramine, and MAO inhibitors such as phenelzine (Nardil). This effect is probably not due to treatment of undiagnosed depression, but is specific for the eating disorder. With further research and investigation, more specific and effective drugs will be developed to treat anorexia and bulimia. At present, several pharmaceutical companies are researching agents that may be appetite suppressants for people who are overweight. Hopefully, these agents will be safer and not addicting, as are the stimulants that have been misprescribed and misused as "diet pills."

Some investigators contend that fluoxetine (Prozac) has antiappetite effects, and the manufacturer, Eli Lilly Company, is pursuing FDA approval for this purpose. Our own experience in using fluoxetine to treat people with depression or panic does not confirm this action with regard to appetite suppression.

## Dementia, Alzheimer's Disease, Memory Impairment

Because of the increasing number of elderly in the population and the marked increase in memory disorders among this group, intensive investigation has been made of treatments of the dementias including Alzheimer's disease (also known as senile dementia of the Alzheimer type). Based on findings of abnormalities in brain structure and chemistry in these patients, drugs have been developed that are targeted for the specific neurotransmitter systems that are affected. For example, drugs that increase the amount of acetylcholine in the brain, such as bethanechol, have been administered in the hope that they will reverse the memory loss that may be caused by cholinergic deficiency. Drugs called *nootrophic agents*, which are hypothesized to improve memory and cognitive functioning (thinking), have also been investigated. At present, tests have been devised to identify those at risk of Alzheimer's disease. An abnormal protein found in the brains of patients with Alzheimer's disease has also been found in their skin; its presence may lead to the first tool to diagnose this dreaded disease in the living patient. It may also lead to an understanding of how this protein—amyloid—builds up in the brain and contributes to symptoms. Brilliant ground-breaking research on the biochemistry of memory and the learning processes is currently being conducted by Columbia University psychiatrist Eric Kandel and co-workers. In this work, scientists condition animals such as the California sea snail (*Aplysia*) to respond to certain stimuli and then measure the changes that result from what the snail has learned in protein and other biochemicals that are involved. Through these efforts we will understand more about the chemistry of learning. Someday, perhaps, we may be able to intervene biologically in those who suffer from learning disorders, such as mental retardation.

Although problems with one's memory are significant in patients with Alzheimer's disease and dementias, other symptoms of the illness are often most troublesome to the family and other caretakers. These symptoms include (1) irritability, (2) wandering, (3) aggressive outbursts, (4) paranoid delusions, and (5) hallucinations. Effective treatments under investigation for these disabilities include beta blockers for the first three, and antipsychotic medications for the latter two. Depression in such patients is effectively treated with antidepressants. As we learn more about the causes of and effective treatments for Alzheimer's disease, new classes of drugs may be developed to enhance learning and memory in general, even for those who do not suffer from the many illnesses that affect memory.

## Treatment of Addictions

### COCAINE

Research on the biological mechanisms of addiction to drugs has shown that certain medications can be beneficial during drug withdrawal and in the maintenance of abstinence. For example, when cocaine is taken frequently, the brain stores of dopamine are depleted. This leads to a chronic state of low energy and reduced ability to experience pleasure. The person addicted continues to use cocaine in greater frequency and at higher doses to achieve a short-lived high, with the long-term cost of depression. Investigators have found that bromocriptine, a drug used to treat Parkinson's disease that acts on the dopamine receptor, can also decrease the craving that addicts have for cocaine. Bromocriptine has been found to maintain abstinence in people with cocaine dependency. Antidepressants such as imipramine or desipramine have also been shown helpful during the withdrawal process (see Chapter 9).

Because of the incalculable public health problems encompassed by substance abuse, scientists are actively developing and testing new drugs that block the high of addicting chemicals and thus reduce the craving for those substances. Research is currently in progress at many centers, including the Drug Abuse Research Center at the University of Chicago. One experimental drug being studied is a dopamine antagonist that reduces addicted monkeys' preference for cocaine over nonaddicting substances. As has occurred in the past, drugs that have been developed for other purposes (e.g., for treating heart disorders, depression, and Parkinson's disease) will increasingly be applied to the treatment of addictive disorders.

## NICOTINE

With the recognition of the significant health hazards from cigarette smoking, addiction to nicotine is finally receiving the investigational attention it deserves. Several powerful drugs may help with cigarette withdrawal and abstinence, including clonidine, an antihypertensive drug that acts at the brain center that controls adrenergic function (the locus coeruleus). In addition, other medications may be beneficial, including antidepressant drugs and buspirone. Well-controlled research studies are necessary to confirm these initial reports.

## ALCOHOL

Alcohol has been the most frequently used and abused drug throughout the world and history. Research into the biologic effects of alcohol on brain receptors are certain to provide insight into future therapies of alcohol addiction and dependence. For example, one of the most recent diagnostic tests, called the Positron Emission Tomography (PET) scan, is able to measure regional metabolism in the brain. Utilizing such scans, investigators may isolate and pinpoint specific regions of the brain that are involved in alcoholism. We also know, for example, that brains of people who *are* dependent on alcohol react differently to alcohol from the brains of those who are *not*. Once the areas of the brain involved in alcohol dependence are better diagnosed and understood, computer-assisted technologies will be used to develop drugs that reach the brain sites involved in alcohol dependence. The development of new drugs in the treatment of the ancient scourge of humankind is one of the most exciting prospects in medical science.

## Treatment of Premenstrual Stress Syndrome (PMS)

Another new area of drug research involves the syndrome labeled *premenstrual stress* or *late luteal phase dysphoric disorder,* in official psychiatric terminology. In this disorder, there is a marked increase in anxiety, depression, and anger, along with decreased energy, sleep, and concentration in the last week of the menstrual cycle. Several studies have indicated that antidepressants, anxiolytic drugs, and hormones may treat the depression and anxiety that occur premenstrually. As we learn more about reproductive biology, a safe and effective treatment for this prevalent disorder will no doubt emerge.

## Treatment of Brain Injury and Related Disorders

### DRUGS

Over one million people each year suffer from brain injury caused by trauma or strokes. Many psychiatric disorders are associated with brain injury, and they involve virtually every aspect of mood regulation, intelligence, memory, thought, perception, and behavior. Although most research has been directed toward treating the long-term sequel of this brain damage, there has been exciting recent work on treating an individual immediately following injury in order to preserve brain functioning. When areas of the brain are deprived of glucose and oxygen (as happens during both stroke and traumatic head injury), specific toxins are released that increase damage to the brain cells (neurons). The action of these neurotoxins may be inhibited by specific drugs, leading to a decrease in the cell death and brain damage that are involved in psychiatric disorders. Examples of these types of drugs include MK-801 (Merck, Sharpe, & Dohme), dextrorphan (Hoffman La Roche), and lazeroids (Upjohn). It is hoped that the use of these drugs in the period immediately after a stroke or injury will inhibit further neuronal damage that may be involved in the development of posttraumatic memory problems, learning difficulties, and mood changes.

### TRANSPLANTATION

A variety of investigations is currently being conducted to find ways to assist the brain in regaining function after injury. For example, nerve growth factors have been discovered that help damaged brain cells to repair themselves. Brain surgery to implant cells from embryos into the brain may also assist the process of regeneration of damaged areas. To treat Parkinson's disease, experimental surgery has been performed wherein cells from one part of the body, the adrenal gland, are transplanted into the brain. The adrenal glands are capable of producing neurotransmitters, and it is hoped that increased availability of dopamine and other transmitters may treat the depression and dementia as well as the motor problems associated with traumatic brain injury.

As medicine becomes more adept in growing cells outside the body and as science becomes more adept in solving the immunologic rejection problems associated with most types of transplantation, we anticipate that transplantation will assume an increasingly important role in the treatment of psychiatric disorders. For example, if we learn that a particular type of psychosis is caused by the absence of a particular enzyme produced by a particular type of brain cell, cloning this cell for transplantation into the brain may provide an intervention that is highly specific, but without the side effects associated with most of the present-day industrially manufactured agents.

## Genetic Treatments

One benefit accrued from research on the genetic basis of psychiatric illness may be the development of new therapies. Huntington's disease, Alzheimer's disease, the schizophrenias, and bipolar disease have been linked (in some populations) to specific chromosomes. When the gene is located that accounts for the illness, specific therapies can be directed toward correcting the abnormality. This could be done with replacement of a deficiency of a gene product, or inhibition of a gene that is overproducing a toxic substance. We view this as one of the most promising areas in medical science, but the promise is long-range. Do not expect major breakthroughs that lead to practical applications for at least five years.

## New Methods of Administration

### PUMPS

At present, psychiatric drugs are given to patients to be taken by mouth in the form of pills, tablets, capsules, or liquid, or by injection into the muscle or into a vein. These drugs then must pass through several organs in the body (such as the stomach, intestines, and liver) before they reach the ultimate site of action, the brain. Because of this process, some drugs that may be potentially effective do not reach the brain in sufficient concentrations. One possible solution to this problem is the administration of drugs directly into the brain. A catheter can be inserted into the ventricles of the brain and attached to a pump that ensures a uniform delivery of the drug. Through this method, drugs can also be delivered directly to a specific site of action in the brain rather than to the whole brain through blood circulation. There has been research on the administration, in this fashion, of one drug for the treatment of Alzheimer's disease. Although the drug did not work, these studies did show that drugs can be safely and reliably administered via pump to the brain. Currently, one of the authors (Yudofsky), working with collaborators in Pittsburgh, is conducting animal research in which aggression is treated by using a small pump to deliver beta blockers into the brains of violent animals. We anticipate that progressive advances in technology will produce increasingly smaller and more efficient catheters and pumps that will allow drugs to be delivered directly and precisely to those sites where their actions are required. Although this may sound like futurology or science fiction, we only need to compare this projection with the early examples of pacemakers (large, imprecise, unreliable) that evolved into the safe, effective, miniaturized examples of today. We also predict that similar electrical devices that alter brain electrical activities in specific regions of the brain will be developed in the future to treat all types of symptomatologies, from pain to aggression, or even to stimulate so-called pleasure centers.

## DOSE SEQUENCING

When people are prescribed drugs for psychiatric disorders, they are usually advised to take the drug every day. In fact, daily doses of drugs are generally standard practice in most fields of medicine. Recent evidence shows that some drugs may not need to be administered daily: intermittent administration of drugs may be even more effective. There is at present insufficient research in psychiatric disorders to recommend intermittent sequencing for clinical practice; however, studies in animals have shown that intermittent dosing of antidepressants and antipsychotic drugs has profound and unique effects on the brain cell receptors and chemical messenger systems in the brain. These special dose-sequencing patterns may prove to be more effective than conventional daily regimens in the treatment of specific psychiatric disorders. But such sequencing may also reduce clinical efficacy for certain disorders and potentially could cause an increase in side effects such as tardive dyskinesia. As with any other innovation in medicine, along with the advantages will come new challenges and problems.


## Use of Vitamins and Nutrients for the Treatment of Psychiatric Disorders

For many years, a few psychiatrists, called *orthomolecular psychiatrists,* have advocated the use of vitamins, usually in high doses, to treat major psychiatric illness. In general, research studies have not confirmed that psychiatric illness is a result of vitamin deficiency, or that megadose vitamins treat psychiatric illness. However, there are indications that some vitamins and amino acids—which are essentially foods or nutrients—may have beneficial effects in the treatment of specific psychiatric conditions. We highlight the most compelling data in this realm below.

Tryptophan, an amino acid, can help induce sleep. This amino acid, as well as another amino acid, tryptamine, may also be beneficial in treating depression. Both amino acids are important in the production of serotonin, a neurotransmitter that is involved in depressive illness (see Chapter 3). However, recently L-tryptophan has been removed from the market because of a life-threatening, blood-related side effect. Vitamin E has also been reported to reduce the symptoms of tardive dyskinesia and to treat the early stages of Parkinson's disease. Vitamin E prevents the production of certain toxic chemicals, called oxidants, that are often released after stroke or brain injury and that can result in cell damage. Some research has suggested that Vitamin C, in combination with antipsychotic drugs, can enhance the benefit of antipsychotic drugs alone. However, there are many other studies that have failed to prove the suggested benefit. As we learn more about brain function, we will learn the specific role that vitamins and amino acids can play in the development and treatment of psychiatric illness. Only through carefully conducted research studies can we learn which therapies are truly beneficial. We must avoid the understandable inclination to become overly hopeful and overly enthusiastic when relatively simple solutions are proposed for complex problems for which we do not yet have answers. False hope results in disappointment, demoralization, and distrust that may discourage a person from trying another treatment that has been proven to have partial efficacy.

# Psychiatric Research

**Q.** *How are drugs discovered and developed?*

**A.** New drug entities have often been discovered by luck or chance. For example, Cade, an Australian physician, found that lithium had a tranquilizing effect on animals, which led him to test the use of the drug in the treatment of mania. The mood of depressed patients treated with the antituberculosis drug iproniazid was found to improve. Iproniazid is a monoamine oxidase inhibitor (MAOI), and therefore other MAOIs were developed, investigated, and applied for the treatment of depression. Chlorpromazine (Thorazine) was used as a drug that facilitated surgical anesthesia. Its calming effect led physicians to investigate its use in the treatment of schizophrenia, for which it was discovered not only to have a sedating effect but also to organize psychotic thinking (e.g., delusions) and to reduce hallucinations. After these initial discoveries, scientists then tried to develop drugs related to chlorpromazine—drugs that were structurally similar to the original compound—seeking greater efficacy with fewer side effects.

Many drugs that are beneficial in the treatment of psychiatric disorders were found by accident. Careful studies first document their efficacy and safety. Thereafter, similar drugs are developed and tested with the hope that these will be more effective, safer, have fewer side effects, and be more convenient to use (e.g., to be taken once per day instead of three times per day). The pharmaceutical company that develops this drug then submits the results of its investigations regarding the safety and efficacy of the new compound to the Food and Drug Administration (FDA). The FDA determines whether or not and for what indications the drug may legally be prescribed. Note that there are drugs prescribed in other countries that have not been approved for use by the FDA and therefore are not legally available in the United States.

**Q.** *May my doctor prescribe a drug for a use that has not been approved by the FDA?*

**A.** The FDA approves a drug for a specific use based on the studies conducted by a pharmaceutical company. Unless the company submits adequate and well-controlled studies for a specific indication (such as to treat depression), the FDA will not approve its use for that disorder. Drug companies usually will investigate the effectiveness of a medication for an illness that is common, even though it may be effective in the treatment of other more rarely occurring illnesses. The reason for this is largely the economics of the great expense entailed in bringing a drug to market and in securing FDA approval for a specific indication. Before pursuing a new indication for a drug, the manufacturer will consider several factors, such as whether it is the exclusive producer of the drug or whether generic brands of the drug are available. If the latter is true, the manufacturers have fewer economic incentives.

FDA approval limits the indications for which a drug company can *promote* its product—for example, to treat high blood pressure—however, FDA approval does not restrict the use for which the doctor prescribes the drug. The FDA has stated that "the labeling is not intended either to preclude the physician from using his best judgment in the interest of the patient, or to impose liability if he does not follow the package insert." Thus, psychiatrists may use a high blood pressure drug to treat social phobia, or antiseizure drugs to treat manic symptoms. However, patients should be informed of the scientific evidence supporting the use of a drug for any unapproved indications. Therefore, "approved" uses of a drug do not exhaust the possible effective uses of the drug. Some important examples are: the use of carbamazepine (Tegretol) to treat bipolar disorder, the use of imipramine (Tofranil) to treat panic disorder, and the use of beta blockers to treat aggressive disorders and social phobia.

**Q.** *Should I use the brand name drug or the generic copy?*

**A.** The answer to this question is: "It depends." The FDA has set standards for the approval of generic copies of the brand name drug. However, there is now considerable controversy as to whether these drug standards always ensure that the generic and brand name drugs will be identical. Cases have shown that identical dosages of generic and brand name drugs may produce differing plasma levels that may have an impact on therapeutic effect. Many of our patients have told us that they noticed important differences in efficacy when we changed them from brand name to generic drugs.

We believe that patients should not randomly switch among differing manufacturers of the same drug. Because federal regulation allows the availability of the drug in the body to differ between any generic and brand name drug by 15 percent, *any two generics may therefore differ by up to 30 percent!* Switching between two generics may thus result in large differences in the amount of drug in the body. In many states, the pharmacist substitutes whatever generic drug is least expensive at the moment, a practice that can lead to considerable variability in plasma levels of the drug and even, it seems, variability in quality control. While the cost differential between a generic and brand name drug may be great, the costs associated with a relapse of an emotional illness are dramatically higher.

# Participation in the Research of Psychiatric Drugs

**Q.** *Should I participate in research of a new drug?*

**A.** The authors of this book have been involved in psychopharmacologic research at universities and in the pharmaceutical industry. We firmly believe that studies of new drug entities and studies involving new uses of currently available drugs provide an essential foundation for safe and effective treatment. It is only through this research that we can confidently tell our patients which treatments may or may not work. Participation in research studies by patients with psychiatric illnesses may not only benefit the individual who enters such a study, but also may benefit thousands of patients in the future.

However, before any patient enters a study, we believe that he or she should be aware of all aspects of these studies. A person should not enter a study unless he or she is able to answer satisfactorily the following questions:

**Q.** *Am I giving informed consent?*

**A.** Before you participate in a study, the investigator is required to discuss the potential benefits and probable risks of the research. This is called *informed consent*. The Food and Drug Administration (FDA) has specific guidelines for informed consent. The basic elements listed here are abstracted from the published guidelines. You should be told:

1. That you will be in a research study, and the reasons this research is being conducted. You should be told how long the study will last, what the study entails (for example, weekly visits with a research psychiatrist, blood tests), and which aspects of the study are experimental.
2. Of the "reasonably foreseeable risks." The investigator does not have to tell you of all possible risks, if they are unlikely to occur.
3. Of benefits that you or others may accrue from this study, including direct therapeutic benefits (e.g., you will receive a drug that will treat your illness) or potential benefits to future patients (through the increase in knowledge about psychiatric illness).

4. Which alternative treatments are available. For example, for studies of new drugs for depression, you should be told that current treatments are available that have been shown effective. For other disorders, such as aggression, there is no FDA-approved treatment.
5. That the records of the study that can be used to identify you are confidential. Be aware that the FDA may inspect the research records and the actual patient files to ensure accuracy of any study done with FDA approval.
6. If you can receive compensation or medical treatment if you are injured during the course of the study. Most studies will provide medical treatment for complications arising from the investigational treatment, but no monetary compensation for any claimed damages of the new treatment.
7. Whom to contact if you have any questions during the study.
8. That your decision to enter the study is voluntary. You may refuse to participate or can decide to withdraw from the study at any time without penalty of any sort.

**Q.** *Is there anyone who makes sure that this study is safe?*

**A.** All research must be approved by an Institutional Review Board (IRB) of the hospital or medical school and/or university that is conducting the research. This group consists of researchers, clinicians, nonscientists (such as lawyers, clergy members, and ethicists), and at least one person who is not associated with the institution. The IRB reviews the research for potential risks and benefits to all participants, and ensures that the study is ethical, safe, and scientific.

**Q.** *Is this study likely to be scientifically valid?*

**A.** The most rigorous research study designs for testing whether medications are effective are *double-blind* and *placebo-controlled*. *Double-blind* means that neither the patient nor the people conducting the study knows which of several drugs the patient is receiving. This is done to minimize patient and investigator bias concerning the expected effects. Only at the end of the study (or during the study if unexpected side effects occur) is the code broken that disguises the exact drug being used. *Placebo-controlled* means that one of the drugs administered is an inactive drug that does not have any therapeutic effect. For most diseases, a number of patients may improve spontaneously. The inclusion of an inactive drug controls for this fact. For example, in a double-blind, placebo-controlled study of imipramine and placebo in the treatment of patients with depression, one group of patients will receive imipramine, and another group will receive identical-appearing placebo tablets. At the completion of the study, the investigator will compare the number of patients who improved on imipramine with the number who improved on the placebo. If these numbers, after statistical analysis, are significantly different from that expected by chance, the investigator concludes that the drug works. Most studies provide an opportunity for treatment with the active substance if the patient in the study has been receiving placebo tablets.

**Q.** *How many other people have received this drug?*

**A.** In some studies, the drugs that are investigated have been previously approved by the FDA and have been available for several years. In these cases, it is possible that millions of people have received the medication. In studies where new medications are being used, usually only hundreds to several thousand patients have taken the drug. You should ask and be told how many people have received this drug and what its side effects have been thus far.

## Recommended Reading on Psychiatric Drugs of the Future

Andreasen, Nancy. *The Broken Brain: The Biological Revolution in Psychiatry.* New York: Harper and Row, 1984.
Snyder, Solomon. *Drugs and the Brain.* New York: W. H. Freeman, 1986.

# PART III

# Individual Drug Listings

# Alphabetical Listing of Selected Psychiatric Drugs Currently in Use

acetophenazine
 Tindal
alprazolam
 Xanax
amantadine
 Symmetrel
amitriptyline
 Elavil
 Endep
amoxapine
 Asendin
benztropine
 Cogentin
bupropion
 Wellbutrin
buspirone
 BuSpar

carbamazepine
 Epitol
 Tegretol
chloral hydrate
 Noctec
chlordiazepoxide
 Libritabs
 Librium
chlorpromazine
 Thorazine
chlorprothixene
 Taractan
clomipramine
 Anafranil
clonazepam
 Klonopin
clorazepate
 Tranxene

*Note*: Brand names are indented.

367

clozapine
  Clozaril
desipramine
  Norpramine
  Pertofrane
dextroamphetamine
  Dexedrine
diazepam
  T-Quil
  Valium
  Valrelease
diphenhydramine
  Allerdryl
  Benadryl
  Dytuss
disulfiram
  Antabuse
doxepin
  Adapin
  Sinequan
fluoxetine
  Prozac
fluphenazine
  Permitil
  Prolixin
  Prolixin Decanoate
  Prolixin Enanthate
flurazepam
  Dalmane
haloperidol
  Haldol
  Haldol Decanoate
imipramine
  Janimine
  Tofranil
isocarboxazid
  Marplan
lithium
  Cibalith-S
  Eskalith
  Eskalith CR

  Lithane
  Lithobid
  Lithonate
  Lithotabs
lorazepam
  Ativan
loxapine
  Loxitane
maprotiline
  Ludiomil
meprobamate
  Equanil
  Meprospan
  Miltown
mesoridazine
  Serentil
methamphetamine
  Desoxyn
methylphenidate
  Ritalin
molindone
  Lidone
  Moban
nortriptyline
  Aventyl
  Pamelor
oxazepam
  Serax
pemoline
  Cylert
perphenazine
  Etrafon
  Trilafon
phenelzine
  Nardil
pimozide
  Orap
prazepam
  Centrax
promazine
  Sparine

propranolol
Inderal
protriptyline
Vivactil
temazepam
Restoril
thioridazine
Mellaril
thiothixene
Navane
tranylcypromine
Parnate
trazodone
Desyrel
triazolam
Halcion

trifluoperazine
Stelazine
triflupromazine
Vesprin
trihexyphenidyl
Artane
trimipramine
Surmontil
valproic acid
Depakene
verapamil
Calan
Isoptin

# Drug Name: **Acetophenazine**

**Brand Name:** Tindal
**For more information:** See Chapter 7, Antipsychotic Drugs.

---

**FAST FACTS** **Drug group:** Antipsychotics.      **Available as generic?** No.

**Prescription needed?** Yes.      **Habit-forming?** No.

 **Overdose:** Symptoms include light-headedness, sedation, confusion, agitation, restlessness, disorientation, convulsions, fever, and coma. Seek immediate emergency medical treatment.

---

## PRECAUTIONS

### Do not take this drug if:

- You have ever had an allergic reaction to this drug or any phenothiazine.

### Inform your physician if:

- You have ever had an allergic reaction to any drug.
- You have epilepsy or asthma.
- You are taking any other drug—prescription or nonprescription—or vitamins.
- You are on a low-salt, low-sugar, or any other special diet.
- You will be under anesthesia or undergoing surgery or medical testing in the next few months.

 **Pregnancy/Breast-feeding**

Except in unusual cases where the mother or the baby's life is endangered, this drug should not be taken by pregnant women. Women taking acetophenazine should not breast-feed.

 **Infants/Children**

Should not be given to children under six months of age.

 **Over Sixty**

Side effects, some serious, can be worse. Initial dose should be low, with careful monitoring for side effects. Special care should be taken when sitting up from a lying position, or standing from a sitting position, as blood pressure may be lowered and balance impaired.

 **Driving/Operating Machinery**

Extreme caution is advised. This medicine can impair mental alertness and coordination. If you do drive or operate machinery, this medicine should be taken at bedtime when its sedating effects are less likely to interfere with daytime activities.

---

## GENERAL INFORMATION

Acetophenazine is a moderate-potency antipsychotic used to treat people who are experiencing disorganized, psychotic thinking, and perceptions such as delusions and hallucinations. For an explanation of how this drug works, see Chapter 7.

---

## BENEFITS

- Effective in treating hallucinations, delusions, confused thinking, and mania. Sedating effects helpful in calming agitated persons.

## RISKS

- May dangerously lower white blood cell count.
- Can cause tardive dyskinesia.
- Can cause neuroleptic malignant syndrome.
- Can dangerously lower blood pressure.

## GUIDELINES FOR USERS

**How is the drug taken?** Tablets (20 mg); syrup.

**What is the usual dosage?** The initial dose should be 20 mg to 40 mg per day in the healthy young adult, with increases as needed to control symptoms. A maximum daily dose of up to 600 mg may be used if necessary. Maintenance doses should be as low as possible and still control the psychotic symptoms.

**What are the instructions for taking the drug?** It is best to take this drug on an empty stomach with a full glass of water.

**How quickly will I feel the effect of the drug?** It usually takes several weeks for you to experience the full benefit of this drug. However, you may feel more calm and relaxed after the first dose or two. The drug should also help you sleep better, if this is a problem.

**What if I miss a dose or several doses?** If you miss a dose and remember within an hour or so, take the missed dose. Otherwise, skip the missed dose and continue on your regular dosing schedule. Do not take double doses.

If you are missing doses on a frequent basis, notify your psychiatrist. A slow-release form of an antipsychotic drug may help with your compliance and help avoid a relapse.

**What if I stop taking the drug?** Do not stop taking this drug without consulting your physician. Abruptly stopping this medication will lead to uncomfortable but not dangerous physical symptoms. Should your physician and you agree that the drug should be discontinued, your medication should be tapered slowly to prevent physical symptoms of withdrawal and a reemergence of your psychotic symptoms.

**How should I store the drug?** Keep out of reach of children. Store in a dry, tightly closed, light-resistant container. Heat and moisture may cause this drug to break down. The liquid form does not require refrigeration.

## INTERACTIONS

**Alcohol:** Avoid alcohol. When combined with alcohol, this medicine can cause excessive sedation and dangerously lower blood pressure.

**Food/Beverages:** No restrictions.

**Smoking:** Smoking lowers the blood level of acetophenazine. If you do smoke, blood samples should be taken to test whether the drug is in the therapeutic range.

**DRUG NAME:** Acetophenazine (*continued*)

## INTERACTIONS (*continued*)

**Other drugs:** Antacids with aluminum or magnesium (Maalox, for example) should not be taken for two hours before or after taking acetophenazine because they may interfere with the absorption of this drug.

Heterocyclic antidepressants can increase the plasma level of this drug and cause a worsening of side effects. Conversely, this drug can increase the blood level of antidepressants. The concurrent use of these two types of drugs must be carefully monitored.

Blood pressure can be dangerously lowered when antipsychotics are combined with vasodilators (medications that dilate blood vessels).

Acetophenazine will increase the effect of medicines known as CNS (central nervous system) depressants. Examples include antihistamines, hay fever medicines, sedatives, narcotics, muscle relaxants, barbiturates, and anesthetics. Check with your physician before taking any of these drugs.

## HABIT-FORMING POTENTIAL

None.

## LONG-TERM USE

Prolonged use of acetophenazine is associated with increased risk of developing tardive dyskinesia, a potentially irreversible side effect involving disfiguring movements of the face, tongue, and limbs. For more information on tardive dyskinesia, please see Chapter 7.

## PLEASE NOTE

Not a sleeping pill: This drug, which has a sedating effect, is sometimes misused as a sleeping pill. There are much safer medications available as sleeping aids.

Not specifically antiaggressive: Because of the potential serious side effects of the antipsychotic drugs, especially over the long term, this medication should not be used to treat anxiety or chronic aggression and agitation.

Frequent examinations required: While taking this medication, your blood pressure and pulse rate should be monitored frequently. Regular checks should also be made for the early signs of tardive dyskinesia.

Classification: Acetophenazine is classified as a phenothiazine. Other antipsychotics in the same group include chlorpromazine, fluphenazine, mesoridazine, perphenazine, promazine, thioridazine, trifluoperazine, and triflupromazine. In general, if you have a poor response to one drug in this family, you will likely have a similar poor response to other drugs in the family.

| Acetophenazine | | | | | | | |
|---|---|---|---|---|---|---|---|
| | Frequency | | Discuss with Physician | | | | |
| Symptom/Effect | Common | Rare | Not Necessary | In All Cases | Only If Severe | Stop Taking Drug Now | Call Physician Now |
| lethargy/sleepiness | X | | | | X | | |
| low blood pressure | X | | | X | | | |
| dizziness | | X | | X | | | |
| dry mouth | X | | | | X | | |
| blurred vision | X | | | | X | | |
| constipation | X | | | | X | | |
| difficulty urinating | X | | | X | | | |
| racing heartbeat/ palpitations | | X | | X | | | |
| weakness | | X | | X | | | |
| sexual problems | | X | | X | | | |
| restlessness | | X | | X | | | |
| skin rash | | X | | X | | | |
| weight gain | X | | | | X | | |
| seizures | | X | | X | | X | X |
| low white blood cell count | | X | | X | | | X |
| tremors | | X | | X | | | |
| stiffness | X | | | X | | | |
| reduced urinary output | | X | | X | | | |

# Drug Name: Alprazolam

**Brand Name:** Xanax

**For more information:** See Chapter 4, Antianxiety Drugs; Chapter 3, Antidepressant Drugs; and Chapter 5, Antipanic and Antiphobic Drugs.

**FAST FACTS**

**Drug group:** Antianxiety agents (benzodiazepines).

**Available as generic?** No.

**Prescription needed?** Yes.

**Habit-forming?** Yes.

 **Overdose:** It is possible, though not easy, to overdose. Signs of toxicity include sedation, decreased breathing rate, confusion, and loss of coordination. If these symptoms are present, seek immediate emergency medical treatment.

## PRECAUTIONS

**Do not take this drug if:**

- You have had previously negative reactions to benzodiazepines.
- You have a history of drug dependence.
- You have Alzheimer's disease, have had a stroke, or have multiple sclerosis or other brain disorders.
- You are seriously depressed.

**Inform your physician if:**

- You are taking any other drug—prescription or nonprescription—or vitamins.
- You have ever had an allergic reaction to any drug.
- You will be under anesthesia or undergoing surgery or medical testing in the next few months.

 **Pregnancy/Breast-feeding**

Do not take this drug if you are pregnant, planning a pregnancy, or are breast-feeding.

**Infants/Children**

Safety and effectiveness have not been established for children and adolescents under eighteen.

 **Over Sixty**

Smaller doses are advised and should be monitored very closely.

 **Driving/Operating Machinery**

WARNING: Do not fly, drive, or operate heavy machinery since this drug can impair mental alertness and coordination.

## GENERAL INFORMATION

Alprazolam, which is used to treat anxiety, depression, and panic attacks, is currently the most commonly prescribed psychiatric drug. About one-third of all benzodiazepine prescriptions are for Xanax, manufactured by Upjohn. Alprazolam is somewhat less sedating than other members of its drug family. Side effects, including loss of coordination, loss of memory, and muscular weakness, may be less pronounced than with other benzodiazepines. Alprazolam is eliminated from the body quickly; thus, it is more likely than other benzodiazepines to produce withdrawal symptoms unless it is discontinued very gradually.

## BENEFITS

- More effective and fewer side effects than barbiturates.
- Less addictive and safer in overdoses than barbiturates.
- Relieves anxiety in about 65 percent to 70 percent of users.
- Less sedating than other benzo-diazepines.
- Has antidepressant and antipanic effects.

## RISKS

- Physically and psychologically addictive if misused.
- Makes some people feel lethargic, less able to concentrate, less alert.
- Can affect physical coordination.

## GUIDELINES FOR USERS

**How is the drug taken?** Tablets (0.25, 0.5, 1, 2 mg)

**What is the usual dosage?** The initial dose for the treatment of anxiety should be 0.25 mg to 1.5 mg per day, with increases as needed to control symptoms. A maximum daily dose of up to 10 mg may be used, if necessary, for up to eight months. Dosage may be higher or lower when alprazolam is used to treat panic.

**What are the instructions for taking the drug?** As with all benzodiazepines, if you are taking this drug for the first time, take your first dose at home and during a time when you are not required to work or drive. Your physician should tell you how often to take subsequent doses. Follow these instructions carefully. This drug can be taken before, during, or after meals. The tablets can be crushed and dissolved in water before taking, if you prefer.

**How quickly will I feel the effect of the drug and how long does it last?** Those who benefit from this drug will usually experience a reduction in anxiety within the first week. Many people feel the drug's effect the first day of treatment. The antianxiety effect is temporary, generally lasting for several hours. The antidepressant and antipanic effects of the drug take longer to feel, generally one week.

**What if I miss a dose or several doses?** If you miss a dose and remember within an hour or so, take the missed dose. However, if more than an hour has elapsed, skip the dose and continue on your regular schedule. Do not take double doses. It is important not to skip doses as anxiety or panic symptoms may reoccur or discontinuation symptoms may begin.

**What if I stop taking the drug?** If you take this drug regularly for three weeks or more, you should not stop abruptly. Your dosage should be gradually reduced. Abrupt cessation can cause psychological and physical withdrawal symptoms.

**How should I store the drug?** Keep out of reach of children, since all benzodiazepines can be extremely dangerous to children. Store in a dry, tightly closed, light-resistant container. Heat and moisture may cause this drug to break down.

## INTERACTIONS

**Alcohol:** Do not drink alcohol. Alprazolam is highly dangerous when combined with alcohol. It can dangerously lower blood pressure, decrease the breathing rate, and lead to loss of consciousness.

DRUG NAME:    Alprazolam (*continued*)

## INTERACTIONS (*continued*)

**Food/Beverages:** No restrictions on food. Control caffeine intake, as caffeine makes anxiety worse.

**Smoking:** Heavy smoking of tobacco may reduce the sedative effects of the drug. Marijuana smoking may increase many of the drug's side effects and significantly reduce mental alertness.

**Other drugs:** Narcotics (e.g., Demerol, Percodan, codeine, morphine, Talwin) may *increase* the sedative effects of this drug. The combination can be fatal. Do not use narcotics with this drug.

Barbiturates and other sedatives (e.g., phenobarbital, pentobarbital, Seconal, Tuinal) may *increase* sedation to dangerous levels. Do not combine sedatives with this drug.

Do not take other benzodiazepines when using this drug, since the combination is both unnecessary and unsafe.

Do not take sleeping pills while taking this drug. If you are having trouble sleeping, your doctor may prescribe larger doses of alprazolam.

The following drugs may reduce the liver's ability to remove this drug from the body, making the drug more powerful and increasing side effects:

- ulcer drugs
- birth control pills
- propranolol
- disulfiram (Antabuse)

## HABIT-FORMING POTENTIAL

High.

## LONG-TERM USE

Physical and psychological dependence are common problems. A clear treatment plan is important. It is possible to become dependent in as short a time span as two to four weeks. Some patients may require months of treatment for their panic disorders. Long-term use can also increase the risk of side effects.

## PLEASE NOTE

Nondrug alternatives: See Chapter 4 for a discussion of the value of exercise and a good diet in the treatment of anxiety. One of the best nondrug ways to reduce anxiety is to identify and reduce sources of stress in your life.

Correct diagnosis: You should always consult a physician to be sure that any medical causes of anxiety (such as hyperthyroidism) are diagnosed and treated. Anxiety may be a component of depression, in which case the symptoms of anxiety are treated by treating the underlying depression with antidepressants and/or other therapies for mood disorders.

Generic possible: Alprazolam may become available in generic form in the United States in 1993.

"Rebound anxiety": While alprazolam is an excellent antipanic medication, because it is quickly eliminated from the body ("short-acting"), its antipanic effects disappear rapidly. This may cause "rebound anxiety," which is panic and anxiety resulting from withdrawal.

| | Alprazolam | | | | | | |
|---|---|---|---|---|---|---|---|
| | Frequency | | Discuss with Physician | | | | |
| Symptom/Effect | Common | Rare | Not Necessary | In All Cases | Only If Severe | Stop Taking Drug Now | Call Physician Now |
| clumsiness, sleepiness | X | | | | X | | |
| abdominal cramps | | X | | X | | | |
| blurred vision | | X | | X | | | |
| dry mouth | | X | | X | | | |
| racing heartbeat/ palpitations | | X | | X | | | |
| shaking/slurred speech | | X | | X | | | |
| urination problems | | X | | X | | | |
| convulsions | | X | | X | | | X |
| hallucinations | | X | | X | | | X |
| memory loss | | X | | X | | | X |
| trouble breathing | | X | | X | | | X |
| staggering/trembling | | X | | X | | | X |
| headache | | X | | X | | | |
| confusion | | X | | X | | | |
| sore breasts/milk secretion | | X | | X | | | |
| irregular menstruation | | X | | X | | | |

DRUG NAME: **Amantadine**

**BRAND NAME:** Symmetrel
**For more information:** See Chapter 7, Antipsychotic Drugs.

**FAST FACTS**  **Drug group:** Antiparkinsonian medications.

**Available as generic?** Yes.

**Prescription needed?** Yes.

**Habit-forming?** No.

 **Overdose:** Symptoms include severe drowsiness, convulsions, trouble breathing, loss of coordination, hallucinations. If these symptoms are present, seek immediate emergency medical treatment.

## PRECAUTIONS

**Do not take this drug if:**

- You have ever had an allergic reaction to this drug.

**Inform your physician if:**

- You have ever had an allergic reaction to any drug or to any dopamine agonist.
- You are taking any other drug— prescription or nonprescription —or vitamins.
- You have epilepsy.
- You have a kidney disorder, as special precautions must be taken.
- You have heart or liver disease.
- You will be under anesthesia or undergoing surgery or medical testing in the next few months.

 **Pregnancy/Breast-feeding**

Except in unusual cases where the woman's life or the pregnancy is endangered, this drug should not be taken by pregnant women. Women taking amantadine should not breast-feed. Amantadine passes into the breast milk and may cause vomiting, difficult urination, and skin rashes in nursing babies.

 **Infants/Children**

May be used in children in lower doses. Child psychiatrists frequently prescribe this to children with parkinsonian side effects of other psychiatric drugs, with careful monitoring for side effects.

 **Over Sixty**

Side effects, some serious, can be worse. Initial dose should be low, with careful monitoring for side effects. Special care should be taken when sitting up from a lying position, or standing from a sitting position, as blood pressure may be lowered and balance impaired. If you experience confusion, a memory loss, urinary problems, or vision changes, check with your doctor at once.

 **Driving/Operating Machinery**

This drug may impair mental alertness and coordination. Do not drive or operate machinery until you are certain this drug will not affect your performance.

## GENERAL INFORMATION

Amantadine is in a class of drugs referred to as *antidyskinetics*. It is used to treat Parkinson's disease and to control movement side effects that occur fairly commonly with antipsychotic drugs. Amantadine improves muscle control and decreases stiffness and tremors. This drug also belongs to the antiviral family of medicines and is used to treat type-A flu infections.

## BENEFITS

- Generally effective in controlling the symptoms of Parkinson's disease and movement side effects of antipsychotic drugs.

## RISKS

- In some cases, this drug does not alleviate movement symptoms and may even aggravate them.
- May aggravate seizures in patients with a history of epilepsy.
- May result in heart failure in people with preexisting heart disease.

## GUIDELINES FOR USERS

**How is the drug taken?** Capsules (100 mg); syrup.

**What is the usual dosage?** The initial dose should be 100 mg a day in healthy young adults, with increases as needed to control symptoms. The average daily dose is 200 mg, and the usual maximum daily dose is 400 mg in divided doses.

**What are the instructions for taking the drug?** Your dose should be taken with meals to prevent stomach upset. The syrup may be mixed with water or juice to improve the taste and prevent stomach upset. If dry mouth is a problem, it is often better to take amantadine before meals.

**How quickly will I feel the effect of the drug and how long does it last?** Some people will notice a benefit from this drug within a few days. However, it can take up to two weeks before the full effect of the drug is felt.

**What if I miss a dose or several doses?** If you miss a dose and remember within an hour or so, take the missed dose. Otherwise, skip the missed dose and continue on your regular dosing schedule. Do not take double doses. It is extremely important not to miss doses because this medicine works best when there is a constant amount in the blood.

**What if I stop taking the drug?** Do not stop taking this drug without consulting your physician. Your medication should be tapered slowly to prevent a reemergence of your symptoms.

**How should I store the drug?** Keep out of reach of children. Store in a dry, tightly closed, light-resistant container. Heat and moisture may cause this drug to break down.

## INTERACTIONS

**Alcohol:** Do not drink alcohol. Alcohol increases the side effects of amantadine and can cause circulation problems, dizziness, fainting, and confusion.

**Food/Beverages:** No restrictions.

DRUG NAME:   Amantadine (*continued*)

---

## INTERACTIONS (*continued*)

**Smoking:** No restrictions.

**Other drugs:** Amantadine will *increase* the effect of other CNS (central nervous system) depressants. Examples include hay fever medicines, sedatives, narcotics, muscle relaxants, barbiturates, and anesthetics. Check with your physician before taking any of these drugs.

---

## HABIT-FORMING POTENTIAL

None.

---

## LONG-TERM USE

Poses no danger.

---

| Amantadine | | | | | | | |
|---|---|---|---|---|---|---|---|
| | **Frequency** | | **Discuss with Physician** | | | | |
| **Symptom/Effect** | **Common** | **Rare** | **Not Necessary** | **In All Cases** | **Only If Severe** | **Stop Taking Drug Now** | **Call Physician Now** |
| dizziness/ light-headedness | X | | | | X | | |
| dry mouth | X | | | | X | | |
| spots or blotches on skin | | X | | X | | | |
| confusion | | X | | X | | | |
| hallucinations | | X | | X | | X | X |
| mood changes | | X | | X | | | |
| change in appetite | | X | | X | | | |
| nausea | X | | | | X | | |
| nervousness | | X | | X | | | |
| disturbed sleep | | X | | X | | | |
| constipation | | X | | | X | | |
| blurred vision | X | | | | X | | |
| headache | | X | | X | | | |
| unusual tiredness | | X | | | X | | |
| skin rash | | X | | X | | X | |
| depression | | X | | X | | | |
| memory loss | | X | | X | | | |
| problems urinating | | X | | X | | | |

# DRUG NAME: **Amitriptyline**

**BRAND NAMES:** Elavil, Endep
**For more information:** See Chapter 3, Antidepressant Drugs.

---

**FAST FACTS** **Drug group:** Antidepressants.   **Available as generic?** Yes.

**Prescription needed?** Yes.   **Habit-forming?** No.

 **Overdose:** The danger of an overdose, which can be lethal, is extremely high. Symptoms include difficulty breathing, shock, agitation, delirium, and coma. Seek immediate emergency medical treatment.

---

## PRECAUTIONS

### Do not take this drug if:

- You have ever had an allergic or negative reaction to any drug in this group.

### Inform your physician if:

- You have ever had an allergic reaction to any drug.
- You have epilepsy.
- You are taking any other drug—prescription or nonprescription—or vitamins.
- You will be under anesthesia or undergoing surgery or medical testing in the next few months.

 **Pregnancy/Breast-feeding**

If you are pregnant or planning a pregnancy, you should, if possible, use non-drug alternatives for treating your depression. This drug has not been demonstrated to be safe during pregnancy. Nursing mothers should not take this drug since it is passed on to the baby in the mother's milk.

 **Infants/Children**

Not recommended for children under age twelve. Adolescents should be given lower doses. Its use in the treatment of depression in children and adolescents must be under the guidance of a child psychiatrist.

 **Over Sixty**

In general, lower doses are required. Side effects may be worse, and some older patients may experience confusion. Elderly people may fall after standing up because of the drug's hypotensive (blood pressure lowering) side effects.

 **Driving/Operating Machinery**

Extreme caution is advised. This medicine can impair mental alertness and coordination. If you do drive or operate machinery, this medicine should be taken at bedtime, when its sedating effects are less likely to interfere with daytime activities.

**DRUG NAME:**    Amitryptiline (*continued*)

## GENERAL INFORMATION

Amitriptyline is one of the heterocyclic drugs used to treat depression. In addition, it is sometimes prescribed for patients with chronic pain. It works by inhibiting the nerve cell's ability to reabsorb the neurotransmitters norepinephrine and serotonin (see Chapter 3). Amitriptyline is more sedating than most antidepressants. This may be helpful if insomnia is a problem, but it also may cause daytime drowsiness—especially early in the course of treatment. Brands include Elavil, manufactured by Merck, Sharpe, & Dohme; and Endep, made by Roche Products. Almost a dozen generics are available. This medicine also is available in combination with drugs that are not antidepressants. These combination products are not recommended (see Chapter 3).

## BENEFITS

- Helps 75 percent to 80 percent of people with major depression.

## RISKS

- Produces annoying side effects.
- Potential for use in suicide attempts.

## GUIDELINES FOR USERS

**How is the drug taken?** Tablets (10, 25, 50, 75, 100, 150 mg); intramuscular.

**What is the usual dosage?** The initial dose is usually 75 mg daily in divided doses. This can be increased gradually to 150 mg daily. Some people may require 200 mg to 300 mg daily. Initial doses are lower for patients with medical illnesses and the elderly.

**What are the instructions for taking the drug?** Take this medicine with food, unless your doctor has instructed you otherwise. Taking the medicine on an empty stomach may cause your stomach to become upset. To benefit from the drug, it is important to take the correct dosage each day.

**How quickly will I feel the effect of the drug?** You will probably experience some unpleasant side effects (dry mouth, blurry vision, constipation) right away. It may take days or weeks for the benefits to appear. It usually takes two to four weeks at full dose for a person to feel a positive response. By the third week of treatment, the side effects are usually less severe.

**What if I miss a dose or several doses?** If you are taking one dose at bedtime and miss your dose, do not take the drug in the morning. Check with your doctor. If you are taking more than one dose a day and remember within an hour or so that you have missed a dose, take the dose. However, if it is almost time for your next dose, skip the missed dose. Do not take double doses.

**What if I stop taking the drug?** Do not discontinue this drug abruptly. Your dosage should be gradually reduced. Stopping the drug abruptly may cause flulike symptoms, headache, restlessness, and/or a worsening of your condition. Inform your physician if you notice these side effects, or any others, after stopping the drug. The effects of this drug may last for up to seven days after you have stopped taking it.

**How should I store the drug?** Keep out of reach of children. Store in a dry, tightly closed, light-resistant container. Heat and moisture may cause this drug to break down.

## INTERACTIONS

**Alcohol:** Do not drink alcohol. Amitriptyline *increases* the effect of alcohol, while alcohol *increases* the side effects of the drug. In addition, alcohol use can contribute to depression.

**Food/Beverages:** No restrictions.

**Smoking:** Smoking lowers the blood level of amitriptyline. If you do smoke, blood samples should be taken to test whether the drug is in the therapeutic range.

**Other drugs:** Amitriptyline will increase the effect of medicines known as CNS (central nervous system) depressants. Examples include antihistamines, hay fever medicines, sedatives, narcotics, muscle relaxants, barbiturates, and anesthetics. Check with your physician before taking any of these drugs.

## HABIT-FORMING POTENTIAL

None.

## LONG-TERM USE

Most people who have a beneficial response do not need to take this drug longer than about six months. A few people may need to take the drug for a year or longer because their depression recurs if they attempt to discontinue the drug.

## PLEASE NOTE

Help with side effects: Drinking water and sucking on hard candy can help if you are experiencing dry mouth. To prevent constipation, eat high-fiber foods and take a daily dose of a natural bulk laxative. And you can avoid episodes of light-headedness by making sure you get up slowly from a sitting or prone position. These side effects generally get better or go away after you have been on the drug several weeks.

**DRUG NAME:**    Amytriptyline (*continued*)

| Symptom/Effect | Frequency | | Discuss with Physician | | | Stop Taking Drug Now | Call Physician Now |
|---|---|---|---|---|---|---|---|
| | Common | Rare | Not Necessary | In All Cases | Only If Severe | | |
| drowsiness | X | | | | X | | |
| dry mouth | X | | | | X | | |
| constipation | X | | | | X | | |
| blurred vision | X | | | | X | | |
| low blood pressure | X | | | X | | | |
| racing heartbeat/ palpitations | | X | | | X | | |
| confusion | | X | | X | | | X |
| skin rashes/allergies | | X | | X | | | X |
| insomnia | | X | | | X | | |
| sexual problems | | X | | X | | | |
| increased appetite | | X | | | X | | |
| seizures | | X | | X | | X | X |

DRUG NAME: **Amoxapine**

**BRAND NAME:** Asendin
**For more information:** See Chapter 3, Antidepressant Drugs.

**FAST FACTS**  **Drug group:** Antidepressants.  **Available as generic?** No.
**Prescription needed?** Yes.  **Habit-forming?** No.

 **Overdose:** The danger of an overdose, which can be lethal, is extremely high. The most likely symptoms are grand mal convulsions (which can occur precipitously, most often about twelve hours after the overdose) and coma. Seek immediate emergency medical treatment.

## PRECAUTIONS
### Do not take this drug if:
- You have ever had an allergic or negative reaction to any drug in this group.

### Inform your physician if:
- You have ever had an allergic reaction to any drug.
- You have epilepsy.
- You are taking any other drug—prescription or nonprescription—or vitamins.
- You will be under anesthesia or undergoing surgery or medical testing in the next few months.

 ### Pregnancy/Breast-feeding
If you are pregnant or planning a pregnancy, you should, if possible, use non-drug alternatives for treating your depression. This drug has not been demonstrated to be safe during pregnancy. Nursing mothers should not take this drug since it is passed on to the baby in the mother's milk.

 ### Infants/Children
Safety and effectiveness for children under age sixteen has not been established. Its use in the treatment of depression in children and adolescents must be under the guidance of a child psychiatrist.

 ### Over Sixty
In general, lower doses are required. Side effects may be worse and some older patients may experience confusion. Elderly people may fall after standing up because of the drug's hypotensive (blood pressure lowering) side effects.

 ### Driving/Operating Machinery
Extreme caution is advised. This medicine can impair mental alertness and coordination. If you do drive or operate machinery, this medicine should be taken at bedtime when its sedating effects are less likely to interfere with daytime activities.

**DRUG NAME:**    Amoxapine (*continued*)

## GENERAL INFORMATION

Amoxapine is one of the heterocyclic drugs used to treat depression. It works by inhibiting the nerve cell's ability to reabsorb the neurotransmitters norepinephrine and serotonin (see Chapter 3). Amoxapine is among the less sedating heterocyclic drugs. Some studies have shown that it produces beneficial effects more quickly than other heterocyclic drugs—sometimes within four to seven days and usually within two weeks. The brand Asendin is made by Lederle.

## BENEFITS

- Helps 75 percent to 80 percent of people with major depression.

## RISKS

- Produces annoying side effects.
- Potential for use in suicide attempts.
- Tardive dyskinesia syndrome (see Glossary).

## GUIDELINES FOR USERS

**How is the drug taken?** Tablets (25, 50, 100, 150 mg).

**What is the usual dosage?** The initial dose is usually 75 mg daily in divided doses. This can be increased gradually to 150 mg daily. Some people may require 200 mg to 300 mg daily.

**What are the instructions for taking the drug?** Take this medicine with food, unless your doctor has instructed you otherwise. Taking the medicine on an empty stomach may cause your stomach to become upset. To benefit from the drug, it is important to take the correct dosage each day.

**How quickly will I feel the effect of the drug?** You will probably experience some unpleasant side effects (dry mouth, blurry vision, constipation) right away. It may take days or weeks for the benefits to appear. It usually takes two to four weeks at full dose for a person to feel a positive response. By the third week of treatment, the side effects are usually less severe.

**What if I miss a dose or several doses?** If you are taking one dose at bedtime and miss your dose, do not take the drug in the morning. Check with your doctor. If you are taking more than one dose a day and remember within an hour or so that you have missed a dose, take the dose. However, if it is almost time for your next dose, skip the missed dose. Do not take double doses.

**What if I stop taking the drug?** Do not discontinue this drug abruptly. Your dosage should be gradually reduced. Stopping the drug abruptly may cause flulike symptoms, headache, restlessness, and/or a worsening of your condition. Inform your physician if you notice these side effects, or any others, after stopping the drug. The effects of this drug may last for up to seven days after you have stopped taking it.

**How should I store the drug?** Keep out of reach of children. Store in a dry, tightly closed, light-resistant container. Heat and moisture may cause this drug to break down.

## INTERACTIONS

**Alcohol:** Do not drink alcohol. Amoxapine may *increase* the effect of alcohol, while alcohol may *increase* the side effects of the drug. In addition, alcohol use can contribute to depression.

**Food/Beverages:** No restrictions.

**Smoking:** Smoking lowers the blood level of amoxapine. If you must smoke, blood samples should be taken to test whether the drug is in the therapeutic range.

**Other drugs:** Amoxapine may increase the effect of medicines known as CNS (central nervous system) depressants. Examples include antihistamines, hay fever medicines, sedatives, narcotics, muscle relaxants, barbiturates, and anesthetics. Check with your physician before taking any of these drugs.

## HABIT-FORMING POTENTIAL

None.

## LONG-TERM USE

Most people who have a beneficial response do not need to take this drug longer than about six months. A few people may need to take the drug for a year or longer because their depression recurs if they attempt to discontinue the drug.

## PLEASE NOTE

Tardive dyskinesia: Some patients who use this drug will develop tardive dyskinesia, a syndrome consisting of irreversible, involuntary dyskinetic movements. The risk of developing the syndrome increases with the length of treatment and the cumulative dosage. The syndrome is most common among the elderly, and specifically elderly women, although other age groups may also be affected. You may wish to discuss the risks of tardive dyskinesia with your physician.

Help with side effects: Drinking water and sucking on hard candy can help if you are experiencing dry mouth. To prevent constipation, eat high-fiber foods and take a daily dose of a natural bulk laxative. And you can avoid episodes of light-headedness by making sure you get up slowly from a sitting or prone position. These side effects generally get better or go away after you have been on the drug several weeks.

**Drug Name:**    Amoxapine (*continued*)

| Symptom/Effect | Frequency | | Discuss with Physician | | | Stop Taking Drug Now | Call Physician Now |
|---|---|---|---|---|---|---|---|
| | Common | Rare | Not Necessary | In All Cases | Only If Severe | | |
| drowsiness | X | | | | X | | |
| dry mouth | X | | | | X | | |
| constipation | X | | | | X | | |
| blurred vision | X | | | | X | | |
| low blood pressure | X | | | X | | | |
| racing heartbeat/ palpitations | | X | | | X | | |
| confusion | | X | | X | | | |
| skin rashes/allergies | | X | | X | | | |
| insomnia | | X | | | X | | |
| sexual problems | | X | | X | | | |
| increased appetite | | X | | | X | | |
| seizures | | X | | X | | X | X |
| involuntary facial or tongue movements | | X | | X | | | X |

DRUG NAME: **Benztropine**

**BRAND NAME:** Cogentin
**For more information:** See Chapter 7, Antipsychotic Drugs.

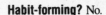

**FAST FACTS**    **Drug group:** Antiparkinsonian medications.

**Available as generic?** Yes.

**Prescription needed?** Yes.

**Habit-forming?** No.

 **Overdose:** Symptoms include severe drowsiness, mental confusion, disorientation, convulsions, trouble breathing, loss of coordination, hallucinations. If any of these symptoms are present, seek immediate emergency medical treatment.

## PRECAUTIONS

### Do not take this drug if:

- You have ever had an allergic reaction to this drug or any drug that treats movement disorders (antidyskinetic drug).

### Inform your physician if:

- You have ever had an allergic reaction to any drug.
- You have asthma, glaucoma, urinary problems, or an enlarged prostate.
- You have epilepsy.
- You have heart problems, kidney, or liver disease.
- You are taking any other drug—prescription or nonprescription—or vitamins.
- You will be under anesthesia or undergoing surgery or medical testing in the next few months.

 **Pregnancy/Breast-feeding**

Except in unusual cases where the mother's life or the pregnancy is endangered, this drug should not be taken by pregnant women. To be safe, women taking benztropine should not breast-feed, although benztropine has not been shown to cause problems in nursing babies.

 **Infants/Children**

May be used in children in lower doses. Child psychiatrists frequently prescribe this to children with parkinsonian side effects of other psychiatric drugs, with careful monitoring for side effects.

 **Over Sixty**

Side effects, some serious, can be worse. In men, this drug may cause problems with urinating. If you experience confusion, memory loss, changes in vision, or eye pain, check immediately with your doctor.

 **Driving/Operating Machinery**

This drug may impair mental alertness and coordination. Do not drive or operate machinery until you are certain this drug will not affect your performance.

**DRUG NAME:**    Benztropine (*continued*)

## GENERAL INFORMATION

Benztropine is in a class of drugs referred to as *antidyskinetics*. It is used to treat Parkinson's disease and to control movement side effects that occur fairly commonly with antipsychotic drugs. Benztropine improves muscle control and decreases stiffness and tremors.

## BENEFITS

- Generally effective in controlling the symptoms of Parkinson's disease and movement side effects of antipsychotic drugs.

## RISKS

- In some cases, this drug does not alleviate movement symptoms and may even aggravate them.
- In some patients, particularly the elderly or brain injured, this drug can cause confusion or memory problems.
- This drug can aggravate glaucoma.

## GUIDELINES FOR USERS

**How is the drug taken?** Tablets (0.5, 1, 2 mg).

**What is the usual dosage?** The initial dose should be a 1 mg or 2 mg injection in healthy young people. The usual maximum daily dose is 6 mg.

**What are the instructions for taking the drug?** Your dose should be taken with meals to prevent stomach upset. The syrup may be mixed with water or juice to improve the taste and prevent stomach upset. If dry mouth is a problem, it is often better to take before meals.

**How quickly will I feel the effect of the drug and how long does it last?** If you have stiffness or other movement side effects of psychiatric medications, you should experience an improvement in your symptoms with the first several days of treatment. Certain other, more rare, movement disorders respond much more rapidly to intramuscular doses.

**What if I miss a dose or several doses?** If you miss a dose and remember within an hour or so, take the missed dose. Otherwise, skip the missed dose and continue on your regular dosing schedule. Do not take double doses.

**What if I stop taking the drug?** Do not stop taking this drug without consulting your physician. Your medication should be tapered slowly to prevent a reemergence of your symptoms.

**How should I store the drug?** Keep out of reach of children. Store in a dry, tightly closed, light-resistant container. Heat and moisture may cause this drug to break down. The liquid form does not require refrigeration.

## INTERACTIONS

**Alcohol:** Do not drink alcohol. Benztropine may increase some of the effects of alcohol.

**Food/Beverages:** No restrictions.

**Smoking:** No restrictions.

**Other drugs:** Benztropine will *increase* the effect of other CNS (central nervous system) depressants. Examples include hay fever medicines, sedatives, narcotics, muscle relaxants, barbiturates, and anesthetics. Check with your physician before taking any of these drugs.

Antacids with aluminum or magnesium (Maalox, for example) and diarrhea medicines should not be taken for one hour before or after taking benztropine because they may interfere with the absorption of this drug.

## HABIT-FORMING POTENTIAL

None.

## LONG-TERM USE

Poses no danger.

| | Benztropine | | | | | | |
|---|---|---|---|---|---|---|---|
| | Frequency | | Discuss with Physician | | | | |
| Symptom/Effect | Common | Rare | Not Necessary | In All Cases | Only If Severe | Stop Taking Drug Now | Call Physician Now |
| blurred vision | X | | | | X | | |
| constipation | X | | | | X | | |
| decreased sweating | X | | | | X | | |
| drowsiness | X | | | | X | | |
| nausea/vomiting | X | | | X | | | |
| sensitivity to light | X | | | | X | | |
| dry mouth | X | | | | X | | |
| severe headache | | X | | X | | | |
| dizziness/ light-headedness | | X | | X | | | |
| anxiety | | X | | X | | | |
| numbness or tingling in hands or feet | | X | | X | | | |
| muscle cramps | | X | | X | | | |
| eye pain | | X | | X | | X | X |
| skin rash | | X | | X | | X | X |
| memory loss | | X | | X | | | |
| confusion | | X | | X | | | |
| problems urinating | | X | | X | | X | X |

DRUG NAME: **Bupropion**

**BRAND NAME:** Wellbutrin
**For more information:** See Chapter 3, Antidepressant Drugs.

---

**FAST FACTS**  **Drug group:** Antidepressants.  **Available as generic?** No.

 **Prescription needed?** Yes.  **Habit-forming?** No.

**Overdose:** Symptoms include confusion, convulsions, and coma. Seek emergency medical treatment.

---

## PRECAUTIONS

### Do not take this drug if:

- You have epilepsy or a history of seizures.
- You have bulimia or anorexia nervosa.

### Inform your physician if:

- You have ever had an allergic reaction to any drug.
- You have heart, kidney, or liver disease.
- You are taking any other drug— prescription or nonprescription —or vitamins.
- You will be under anesthesia or undergoing surgery or medical testing in the next few months.

 ### Pregnancy/Breast-feeding

Do not take this drug if you are pregnant, are planning a pregnancy, or are breast-feeding. There is a potential for serious adverse reactions in nursing infants from this drug.

 ### Infants/Children

Do not give to children. The safety and effectiveness of this drug for those under age eighteen have not been proven.

 ### Over Sixty

No research is available.

 ### Driving/Operating Machinery

This drug may impair mental alertness and coordination. Do not drive or operate machinery until you are certain this drug will not affect your performance.

---

## GENERAL INFORMATION

Bupropion was introduced in 1986 for the treatment of depression in patients who did not tolerate well or benefit from usual antidepressant therapy. A short time later, the manufacturer withdrew the drug because of reports of seizures in patients with bulimia. In 1989, the drug was reintroduced with a cautionary note that seizures occur in approximately 4 out of every 1,000 patients. Bupropion is chemically unrelated to the heterocyclics and other antidepressant drugs. Early research has shown it may be as effective as other antidepression drugs, but more will be learned about bupropion as its use becomes more common. Exactly how bupropion works is not known.

## BENEFITS

- Effective antidepressant.
- Produces little or no drowsiness.
- Has few effects on the cardiovascular system.
- Does not significantly reduce blood pressure.
- Is not associated with weight gain.
- Has fewer anticholinergic (dry mouth, blurred vision, confusion) side effects than do heterocyclics.

## RISKS

- Greater risk of seizures than with other antidepressant drugs.
- Cannot be used in combination with monoamine oxidase inhibitor.

## GUIDELINES FOR USERS

**How is the drug taken?** Tablets (75, 100 mg).

**What is the usual dosage?** The initial dose is 200 mg daily in divided doses. This can be increased gradually to 300 mg, as needed. Some people may require up to 450 mg daily. No *single* dose should exceed 150 mg.

**What are the instructions for taking the drug?** You should take this drug in equally divided doses during the day. In order to minimize the risk of seizures, you should never take more than 150 mg of bupropion in a single dose.

**How quickly will I feel the effect of the drug?** Usually a person will begin to experience relief from depression by the third week after a treatment dose is achieved.

**What if I miss a dose or several doses?** If you miss a dose and remember within an hour or so, take the dose. However, if it is almost time for your next dose, skip the missed dose. Do not take double doses.

**What if I stop taking the drug?** Do not discontinue this drug abruptly. Your dosage should be gradually reduced.

**How should I store the drug?** Keep out of reach of children. Store in a dry, tightly closed, light-resistant container. Heat and moisture may cause this drug to break down.

## INTERACTIONS

**Alcohol:** Do not drink alcohol. Using alcohol with this drug can increase the danger of seizures. In addition, alcohol use can contribute to depression.

**Food/Beverages:** No restrictions.

**Smoking:** Smoking can lower the blood level of this drug. If you do smoke, blood samples should be taken to test whether the drug is in the therapeutic range.

**Other drugs:** Care should be used if combined with carbamazepine, cimetidine, phenobarbital, phenytoin, and other drugs that affect liver metabolic activity. Blood levels of bupropion and the other drug may be affected when used in combination.

Do not combine with L-dopa without careful discussion with your physician.

**DRUG NAME:**    Bupropion (*continued*)

## HABIT-FORMING POTENTIAL
None.

## LONG-TERM USE
Poses no danger.

| Bupropion | | | | | | | |
|---|---|---|---|---|---|---|---|
| | Frequency | | Discuss with Physician | | | | |
| Symptom/Effect | Common | Rare | Not Necessary | In All Cases | Only If Severe | Stop Taking Drug Now | Call Physician Now |
| dizziness | | X | | | X | | |
| racing heartbeat/ palpitations | | X | | X | | | |
| agitation | | X | | X | | | |
| nausea/vomiting | | X | | X | | | |
| headaches | | X | | X | | | |
| skin rashes | | X | | X | | | X |
| constipation | | X | | | X | | |
| change in appetite | | X | | X | | | |
| diarrhea | | X | | | X | | |
| weight gain or loss | | X | | | X | | |
| sexual problems | | X | | X | | | |
| seizures | | X | | X | | X | X |
| insomnia | | X | | | X | | |

# DRUG NAME: **Buspirone**

**BRAND NAME:** BuSpar
**For more information:** See Chapter 4, Antianxiety Drugs.

**FAST FACTS**
**Drug group:** Antianxiety agents. •
**Prescription needed?** Yes.

**Available as generic?** No.
**Habit-forming?** No.

**Overdose:** There is usually little danger of overdosing. However, signs of an overdose include dizziness, confusion, nausea, and sleepiness. If these symptoms are present, seek emergency medical treatment.

## PRECAUTIONS

**Do not take this drug if:**

- You have ever had an allergic reaction to this drug.

**Inform your physician if:**

- You have ever had an allergic reaction to any drug.
- You have epilepsy.
- You are taking any other drugs—prescription or nonprescription—or vitamins.
- You will be under anesthesia or undergoing surgery or medical testing in the next few months.

### Pregnancy/Breast-feeding

Do not take this drug if you are pregnant, planning a pregnancy, or breast-feeding.

### Infants/Children

Not recommended for treatment of infants and children.

### Over Sixty

This medicine has not been tested specifically in older people. However, clinical experience indicates that it is safe and effective in this age group.

### Driving/Operating Machinery

Buspirone normally does not impair coordination and is safe for people who need to drive.

## GENERAL INFORMATION

Buspirone is a relatively new antianxiety drug with a chemical structure different from the benzodiazepines. Recent research suggests that it may be as effective as the benzodiazepines in treating most kinds of anxiety. It produces fewer side effects than do the benzodiazepines and has little potential for addiction. However, more studies are needed on the drug's safety and effectiveness. The only brand, BuSpar, is manufactured by Mead Johnson.

**DRUG NAME:** Buspirone (*continued*)

## BENEFITS

- No sedation.
- Does not cause memory loss.
- Does not impair coordination.
- No withdrawal syndrome.
- No alcohol interaction.
- May be beneficial in the treatment of agitation and aggression.
- Is helpful in treating anxiety with depressive symptoms.
- Few subjective side effects.

## RISKS

- Takes two or three weeks to produce antianxiety effects.
- No muscle relaxant properties.
- Requires multiple daily dosing.
- Less acceptance by recent benzodiazepine users.

## GUIDELINES FOR USERS

**How is the drug taken?** Tablets (5 and 10 mg).

**What is the usual dosage?** The initial dose should be 5 mg three times per day, with increases as needed to control symptoms. A maximum daily dose of up to 60 mg may be used, if necessary.

**What are the instructions for taking the drug?** Buspirone must be taken at least three times a day. Follow your dosage instructions carefully. The tablets may be taken before, during, or after meals and can be crushed and dissolved in water before taking, if you prefer. Your physician may request that you drink extra fluids while taking this drug to prevent kidney problems.

**How quickly will I feel the effect of the drug and how long does it last?** It may take as long as three weeks before you feel the effects of the drug. There is thought to be less "rebound anxiety" between doses of buspirone than with many benzodiazepines.

**What if I miss a dose or several doses?** If you miss a dose, skip the missed dose and go back to your regular dosing schedule. Do not take double doses.

**What if I stop taking the drug?** Do not stop taking this drug without consulting your physician.

**How should I store the drug?** Keep out of reach of children. Store in a dry, tightly closed, light-resistant container. Heat and moisture may cause buspirone to break down.

## INTERACTIONS

**Alcohol:** Buspirone does not interact dangerously with alcohol.

**Food/Beverages:** No restrictions on food. Control caffeine intake, as caffeine makes anxiety worse.

**Smoking:** Smoking may reduce the blood levels of this drug.

**Other drugs:** Buspirone may cause drowsiness when taken with antihistamines or hay fever medicines. Sedatives, tranquilizers, muscle relaxants, and prescription pain medicine also may increase drowsiness. Consult your doctor before taking any of these drugs.

## HABIT-FORMING POTENTIAL

None.

## LONG-TERM USE

Buspirone can be used for periods longer than four weeks.

## PLEASE NOTE

If you are taking a benzodiazepine, your doctor may gradually switch you to buspirone. He would first add buspirone to your current benzodiazepine dose and after several weeks on buspirone, gradually taper you off the benzodiazepine.

Immunizations: While you are taking this drug, do not have any immunizations without consulting your doctor. Buspirone may lower your body's resistance, and it is possible you could get the infection the vaccination is designed to prevent.

| Buspirone | | | | | | | |
|---|---|---|---|---|---|---|---|
| | Frequency | | Discuss with Physician | | | | |
| Symptom/Effect | Common | Rare | Not Necessary | In All Cases | Only If Severe | Stop Taking Drug Now | Call Physician Now |
| nervousness | | X | | | X | | |
| insomnia | | X | | | X | | |
| dizziness/light-headedness | | X | | X | | | |
| nausea/diarrhea | | X | | | X | | |
| headaches | | X | | X | | | |
| chest pain | | X | | X | | | |
| racing heartbeat/palpitations | | X | | X | | | |
| numbness/tingling | | X | | X | | | |
| confusion | | X | | X | | | X |
| depression | | X | | X | | | |

# DRUG NAME: Carbamazepine

**BRAND NAMES:** Epitol, Tegretol
**For more information:** See Chapter 6, Antimanic Drugs.

**FAST FACTS**
**Drug groups:** Antimanic agents; anticonvulsants.

**Available as generic?** Yes.

**Prescription needed?** Yes.

**Habit-forming?** No.

 **Overdose:** The first symptoms may appear one to three hours after taking a toxic dose. Symptoms include difficulty breathing, muscle twitching, restlessness, drowsiness, dizziness, and coma. Seek immediate emergency medical treatment.

## PRECAUTIONS

**Do not take this drug if:**

- You have ever had an allergic reaction to this drug or to a heterocyclic antidepressant.
- You have a blood-related disorder.

**Inform your physician if:**

- You have ever had an allergic reaction to any drug.
- You are taking any other drug— prescription or nonprescription —or vitamins.
- You have epilepsy.
- You are taking an MAO inhibitor or have taken one within the last two weeks.
- You will be under anesthesia or undergoing surgery or medical testing in the next few months.

 **Pregnancy/Breast-feeding**

Except in unusual cases where the mother or the baby's life is endangered, this drug should not be taken by pregnant women. Women taking antipsychotics should not breast-feed.

 **Infants/Children**

Safety and effectiveness of this drug have not been proved in children under age six.

 **Over Sixty**

Lower doses are generally required and side effects may be worse.

 **Driving/Operating Machinery**

This drug may impair mental alertness and coordination. Do not drive or operate machinery until you are certain this drug will not affect your performance.

## GENERAL INFORMATION

Carbamazepine is prescribed to treat some types of seizures (epilepsy) and is the second most frequently prescribed drug for people experiencing mania. It is usually prescribed to treat manic-depressive patients who have not responded to lithium or who develop serious side effects with lithium. In some cases, a physician may prescribe both carbamazepine and lithium. While carbamazepine is effective in treating mania, it probably does not treat depression. Other treatments are required when a manic person becomes depressed. Carbamazepine may be more effective than lithium for people who experience frequent episodes of mania ("rapid cyclers"). Frequent blood tests are required when taking this drug because of a potentially serious—and sometimes fatal—side effect involving abnormalities of blood cells (aplastic anemia, agranulocytosis, thrombocytopenia, and leukopenia).

| BENEFITS | RISKS |
|---|---|
| • Effective in treating manic illness. | • Blood-related side effects including aplastic anemia, which, though rare, can be fatal. |
| • Particularly effective in cases where people experience "cycling," or frequent episodes of mania. | • Low white blood cell count may increase risk of infection. |
| • Fewer drug interactions than with lithium. | • Can cause hypersensitivity hepatitis, a disorder of the liver. |
| • Useful in patients who suffer severe side effects with lithium. | |

## GUIDELINES FOR USERS

**How is the drug taken?** Tablets (100 and 200 mg); suspension.

**What is the usual dosage?** Initial dose should be 100 mg twice a day in healthy young people, with increases as needed to control symptoms. The dose is usually increased by 200 mg every five to seven days until the therapeutic levels are obtained. The maximum daily dose is 1,600 mg, but this is rarely required. Your carbamazepine blood levels should be measured every week until your therapeutic dose is determined. Periodic monitoring of your blood levels should continue while you are taking this drug.

**What are the instructions for taking the drug?** Take carbamazepine with meals to reduce gastrointestinal side effects such as nausea and vomiting. Follow your physician's instructions carefully to maintain the correct blood level of this drug.

**How quickly will I feel the effect of the drug?** Manic behavior usually diminishes after seven to ten days of treatment. Carbamazepine should even out the intense ups and downs of your moods and, after several weeks of treatment, you should feel reasonably normal. At the same time, you may experience some side effects from the drug such as dry mouth, a slight tremor in your hands, and a frequent need to urinate. These side effects usually peak about one to two hours after taking your dose.

**What if I miss a dose or several doses?** If you miss a dose and remember within an hour or so, take the dose. Otherwise, skip the missed dose and continue on your regular dosing schedule. Do not take double doses. Notify your physician if you are missing doses regularly. To obtain the full benefit of this drug and lessen the chance of side effects, it is important to take doses regularly.

**What if I stop taking the drug?** Do not stop taking this drug without consulting your physician. When discontinuing carbamazepine, it should be tapered gradually to monitor for potential recurrence of symptoms of mania or depression.

**How should I store the drug?** Keep out of reach of children. Store in a dry, tightly closed, light-resistant container. Heat and moisture may cause this drug to break down.

**DRUG NAME:**    Carbamazepine (*continued*)

## INTERACTIONS

**Alcohol:** Avoid alcohol. When combined with alcohol, this medicine can cause excessive sedation and dangerously lower blood pressure.

**Food/Beverages:** No restrictions.

**Smoking:** No restrictions.

**Other drugs:** Tagamet and cimetidine, which are used to treat ulcers, may *increase* blood levels of carbamazepine.

The antibiotic erythromycin can *increase* plasma carbamazepine levels.

Isoniazid, a drug used to treat tuberculosis, can *increase* plasma carbamazepine levels.

Barbiturates (e.g., phenobarbital, amobarbital, pentobarbital, and secobarbital) may *decrease* blood levels of carbamazepine by speeding up its breakdown in the liver.

## HABIT-FORMING POTENTIAL

None.

## LONG-TERM USE

Complete laboratory testing of blood is required before starting treatment and at regular intervals—weekly during the first three months of treatment and monthly for two years thereafter. Evaluation of the liver and kidney functions should also be done on a regular basis.

## PLEASE NOTE

In combination with lithium: For people who do not respond to either lithium carbonate or carbamazepine alone, some physicians prescribe a combination of the two drugs. When the combination is used, the side effects are similar to those experienced when each medication is taken alone.

| Carbamazepine | | | | | | |
|---|---|---|---|---|---|---|
| | Frequency | | Discuss with Physician | | | |
| Symptom/Effect | Common | Rare | Not Necessary | In All Cases | Only If Severe | Stop Taking Drug Now | Call Physician Now |
| high fever | | X | | X | | X | X |
| blurred vision | | X | | X | | | |
| pigmentation in eyes | | X | | X | | X | X |
| infection | | X | | X | | | X |
| weakness | | X | | X | | X | X |
| abnormal bleeding | | X | | X | | X | X |
| constipation | | X | | X | | | |
| dry mouth | | X | | X | | | |
| dizziness | X | | | | X | | |
| drowsiness | X | | | | X | | |
| skin changes | | X | | X | | X | X |
| yellowing of skin or eyes | | X | | X | | X | X |
| urinary changes | | X | | X | | X | X |
| poor coordination | | X | | X | | | |
| mental changes | | X | | X | | | X |
| nausea/vomiting | | X | | X | | | |
| aching joints | | X | | X | | | |
| gastric distress | | X | | X | | | |

# DRUG NAME: Chloral hydrate

**BRAND NAME:** Noctec
**For more information:** See Chapter 8, Sedatives and Sleeping Pills.

**FAST FACTS**  **Drug group:** Sedatives.                **Available as generic?** Yes.

**Prescription needed?** Yes.           **Habit-forming?** Yes.

 **Overdose:** The overdose danger is especially high when this drug is combined with alcohol. Signs of toxicity include sedation, trouble breathing, confusion, nausea, loss of coordination, staggering, and slurred speech. If these symptoms are present, seek immediate emergency medical treatment.

## PRECAUTIONS

### Do not take this drug if:

- You have ever had an allergic reaction to this drug.
- You have kidney or liver disease.

### Inform your physician if:

- You have ever had an allergic reaction to any drug.
- You are taking any other drug— prescription or nonprescription —or vitamins.
- You will be under anesthesia or undergoing surgery or medical testing in the next few months.
- You have a history of drug or alcohol dependence.

 **Pregnancy/Breast-feeding**

Do not take this drug if you are pregnant, planning a pregnancy, or are breast-feeding. Using this drug during pregnancy can cause the baby to become dependent and may lead to withdrawal symptoms.

 **Infants/Children**

Do not give this drug to children. Safety and effectiveness for children have not been established.

 **Over Sixty**

People over age sixty should take this drug only under strict medical supervision, such as for a brief time in the hospital setting after surgery.

 **Driving/Operating Machinery**

This drug may impair mental alertness and coordination. Do not drive or operate machinery until you are certain this drug will not affect your performance.

## GENERAL INFORMATION

Chloral hydrate is among the sleeping medications with the longest history of use. It is generally prescribed as a generic. If it is taken on a regular basis, it can be mildly habit-forming. This was more of a problem in the 1800s, when the drug was widely abused, than today. In the 1930s and 1940s, chloral hydrate was frequently an element in movie plots—the supposed knock-out drug slipped into drinks of heroes like Humphrey Bogart's characters. Although this drug does induce sleep, its effect is not so rapid as portrayed in the movies. For most physicians, chloral hydrate is a drug of second choice, and is prescribed as a sleeping pill when a person cannot take benzodiazepines. Some physicians, however, prefer chloral hydrate over benzodiazepines because it may be less addictive and less likely to cause daytime drowsiness.

| BENEFITS | RISKS |
|---|---|
| • More effective and fewer side effects than barbiturates in treating insomnia.<br>• Less addictive and less likely to cause daytime drowsiness for some patients than the benzodiazepines. | • Overdose danger, especially when combined with alcohol.<br>• Physically and psychologically addictive.<br>• Can sometimes worsen original sleep problem.<br>• Potentially harmful to kidneys, liver, and lungs. |

## GUIDELINES FOR USERS

**How is the drug taken?** Tablets (500 mg); capsules; syrup.

**What is the usual dosage?** The initial dose for insomnia should be 500 mg in healthy young people. This may be increased, as needed, to 1,000 mg.

**What are the instructions for taking the drug?** Your dose should be taken at bedtime with a full glass of water to prevent stomach upset. If you are taking the capsule form, swallow the capsule whole. The syrup may be mixed with water or juice to improve the taste and prevent stomach upset.

**How quickly will I feel the effect of the drug and how long does it last?** You should experience the sedative effects within fifteen to thirty minutes, and these effects should not persist beyond six to eight hours.

**What if I miss a dose or several doses?** If you miss a dose, skip the missed dose. Do not take double doses.

**What if I stop taking the drug?** If you take this drug regularly for three weeks or more, you should not stop abruptly. Your dosage should be gradually reduced. Abrupt cessation can cause psychological and physical withdrawal symptoms.

**How should I store the drug?** Keep out of reach of children and in a locked cabinet. This drug has a high potential for abuse. Store in a dry, tightly closed, light-resistant container. Heat and moisture may cause this drug to break down.

## INTERACTIONS

**Alcohol:** Do not drink alcohol. Chloral hydrate is highly dangerous when combined with alcohol. It can dangerously lower blood pressure, decrease the breathing rate, and lead to loss of consciousness.

**Food/Beverages:** No restrictions on food. Control caffeine intake, as caffeine can contribute to insomnia.

**Smoking:** Heavy smoking of tobacco may reduce the sedative effects of this drug. Marijuana smoking may increase many of the drug's side effects and significantly reduce mental alertness.

**DRUG NAME:**   Chloral hydrate (*continued*)

## INTERACTIONS (*continued*)

**Other drugs:** Chloral hydrate may *increase* the action of anticoagulant (blood-thinning) medications. It should be used very cautiously when combined with these drugs.

Do not use narcotics, barbiturates or other sedatives with this drug.

The following drugs may reduce the liver's ability to remove this drug from the body, making the drug more powerful and increasing its side effects:
• ulcer drugs
• birth control pills
• propranolol
• disulfiram (Antabuse)

Chloral hydrate will *increase* the effect of medicines known as CNS (central nervous system) depressants. Examples include antihistamines, hay fever medicines, sedatives, narcotics, muscle relaxants, barbiturates, and anesthetics. Check with your physician before taking any of these drugs.

## HABIT-FORMING POTENTIAL

Moderate to high.

## LONG-TERM USE

Chloral hydrate is habit-forming if taken on a regular basis.

## PLEASE NOTE

For most patients, we advise that no medication for sleep be used on a regular basis. For most individuals, tolerance to the sedative effects occurs with continuous use; and, therefore, doses must be increased regularly to induce sleep. Side effects and dependency often develop under these circumstances.

| Chloral Hydrate | | | | | | | |
|---|---|---|---|---|---|---|---|
| | **Frequency** | | **Discuss with Physician** | | | | |
| **Symptom/Effect** | **Common** | **Rare** | **Not Necessary** | **In All Cases** | **Only If Severe** | **Stop Taking Drug Now** | **Call Physician Now** |
| nausea/vomiting | X | | | | X | | |
| stomach pain | | X | | X | | | |
| drowsiness | X | | | X | | | |
| dizziness/ light-headedness | | X | | X | | | |
| diarrhea | | X | | X | | | |
| rash | | X | | X | | X | |
| confusion | | X | | X | | | |
| anxiety/restlessness | | X | | X | | | |
| memory loss | | X | | X | | | |
| irritability | | X | | X | | | |

DRUG NAME: **Chlordiazepoxide**

**BRAND NAMES:** Libritabs, Librium
**For more information:** See Chapter 4, Antianxiety Drugs, and Chapter 9, Antiaddiction Drugs.

**FAST FACTS**

**Drug group:** Antianxiety agents (benzodiazepines).

**Available as generic?** Yes.

**Prescription needed?** Yes.

**Habit-forming?** Yes.

**Overdose:** It is possible, though not easy, to overdose. Signs of toxicity include sedation, decreased breathing rate, confusion, and loss of coordination. If these symptoms are present, seek immediate emergency medical treatment.

## PRECAUTIONS

**Do not take this drug if:**

- You have had previously negative reactions to benzodiazepines.
- You have a history of drug dependence.
- You have Alzheimer's disease, have had a stroke, or have multiple sclerosis or other brain disorders.
- You are seriously depressed.

**Inform your physician if:**

- You are taking any other drug— prescription or nonprescription —or vitamins.
- You have ever had an allergic reaction to any drug.
- You will be under anesthesia or undergoing surgery or medical testing within the next few months.

**Pregnancy/Breast-feeding**

Do not take this drug if you are pregnant, planning a pregnancy, or are breast-feeding.

**Infants/Children**

This drug should not be used by children under six.

**Over Sixty**

Smaller doses are advised and should be monitored very closely.

**Driving/Operating Machinery**

WARNING: Do not fly, drive, or operate heavy machinery since this drug can impair mental alertness and coordination.

## GENERAL INFORMATION

Chlordiazepoxide was the first antianxiety drug. Introduced in 1960, it virtually revolutionized drug treatment. In addition to being more effective than any drug used previously in the treatment of anxiety, it has proved to be far safer in cases of deliberate or accidental overdose. Other drugs have since been found as effective, or perhaps more effective, and chlordiazepoxide's use has declined somewhat. It is now the seventh most frequently prescribed benzodiazepine. It is sometimes prescribed before surgery to

**DRUG NAME:**    Chlordiazepoxide (*continued*)

## GENERAL INFORMATION (*continued*)

reduce apprehension. It also may be used to treat withdrawal symptoms of acute alcoholism (D.T.'s). Roche Products manufactures two brands, Librium and Libritabs. Generic manufacturers include Barr, Danbury, Geneva, and Lederle. Roche also makes chlordiazepoxide in combination with amitriptyline, clidinium, and estrogen. (The brands, respectively, are Limbitrol, Librax, and Menrium.) However, combination products are not recommended. For an explanation of how this drug works, see Chapter 4.

## BENEFITS

- More effective and fewer side effects than barbiturates.
- Less addictive and safer in overdoses than barbiturates.
- Relieves anxiety in about 65 percent to 70 percent of users.
- Helpful in treating alcohol withdrawal.

## RISKS

- Physically and psychologically addictive if misused.
- Makes some people feel lethargic, less able to concentrate, less alert.
- Can affect physical coordination.

## GUIDELINES FOR USERS

**How is the drug taken?** Tablets and capsules (5, 10, and 25 mg); intramuscular; intravenous.

**What is the usual dosage?** The initial dose should be 15 mg to 75 mg per day, with increases as needed to control symptoms. A maximum daily dose of up to 300 mg may be used, if necessary.

**What are the instructions for taking the drug?** As with all benzodiazepines, if you are taking this drug for the first time, take your first dose at home and during a time when you are not required to work or drive. Your physician should tell you how often to take subsequent doses. Follow these instructions carefully. This drug can be taken before, during, or after meals. The tablets can be crushed and dissolved in water before taking, if you prefer.

**How quickly will I feel the effect of the drug?** Those who benefit from this drug will usually experience a positive response within the first week. Many people feel the drug's effect the first day of treatment.

**What if I miss a dose or several doses?** If you miss a dose and remember within an hour or so, take the missed dose. However, if more than an hour has elapsed, skip the dose and continue on your regular schedule. Do not take double doses.

**What if I stop taking the drug?** If you take this drug regularly for three weeks or more, you should not stop abruptly. Your dosage should be gradually reduced. Abrupt cessation can cause psychological and physical withdrawal symptoms.

**How should I store the drug?** Keep out of reach of children, since all benzodiazepines can be extremely dangerous to children. Store in a dry, tightly closed, light-resistant container. Heat and moisture may cause this drug to break down.

## INTERACTIONS

**Alcohol:** Do not drink alcohol. Chlordiazepoxide is highly dangerous when combined with alcohol. It can dangerously lower blood pressure, decrease the breathing rate, and lead to loss of consciousness.

**Food/Beverages:** No restrictions on food. Control caffeine intake, as caffeine makes anxiety worse.

**Smoking:** Heavy smoking of tobacco may reduce the sedative effects of this drug. Marijuana smoking may increase side effects and significantly reduce mental alertness.

**Other drugs:** Narcotics (e.g., Demerol, Percodan, codeine, morphine, Talwin) may *increase* the sedative effects of this drug. The combination can be fatal. Do not use narcotics with this drug.

Barbiturates and other sedatives (e.g., phenobarbital, pentobarbital, Seconal, Tuinal) may *increase* sedation to dangerous levels. Do not combine sedatives with this drug.

Do not take other benzodiazepines when using this drug, since the combination is both unnecessary and unsafe.

Do not take sleeping pills while taking this drug. If you are having trouble sleeping, your doctor may prescribe larger doses of chlordiazepoxide.

The following drugs may reduce the liver's ability to remove this drug from the body, making the drug more powerful and increasing side effects:

- ulcer drugs
- birth control pills
- propranolol
- disulfiram (Antabuse)

## HABIT-FORMING POTENTIAL

High.

## LONG-TERM USE

Physical and psychological dependence are common problems. A clear treatment plan is important. It is possible to become dependent in as short a time span as two to four weeks. This drug should not be taken longer than four weeks on a regular basis (i.e., daily). Long-term use can also increase the risk of side effects.

## PLEASE NOTE

Nondrug alternatives: See Chapter 4 for a discussion of the value of exercise and a good diet in the treatment of anxiety. One of the best nondrug ways to reduce anxiety is to identify and reduce sources of stress in your life.

Correct diagnosis: You should always consult a physician to be sure that any medical causes of anxiety (such as hyperthyroidism) are diagnosed and treated. Anxiety may be a component of depression, in which case the symptoms of anxiety are treated by treating the underlying depression with antidepressants and/or other therapies for mood disorders.

| Chlordiazepoxide | | | | | | | |
|---|---|---|---|---|---|---|---|
| | Frequency | | Discuss with Physician | | | | |
| Symptom/Effect | Common | Rare | Not Necessary | In All Cases | Only If Severe | Stop Taking Drug Now | Call Physician Now |
| clumsiness/sleepiness | X | | | | X | | |
| abdominal cramps | | X | | X | | | |
| blurred vision | | X | | X | | | |
| dry mouth | | X | | X | | | |
| racing heartbeat/ palpitations | | X | | X | | | |
| shaking/slurred speech | | X | | X | | | |
| urination problems | | X | | X | | | |
| convulsions | | X | | X | | X | X |
| hallucinations | | X | | X | | X | X |
| memory loss | | X | | X | | | X |
| trouble breathing | | X | | X | | X | X |
| staggering/trembling | | X | | X | | | X |
| headache | | X | | X | | | |
| confusion | | X | | X | | | X |

# DRUG NAME: **Chlorpromazine**

**BRAND NAME:** Thorazine
**For more information:** See Chapter 7, Antipsychotic Drugs.

**FAST FACTS**   **Drug group:** Antipsychotics.   **Available as generic?** Yes.
**Prescription needed?** Yes.   **Habit-forming?** No.

 **Overdose:** Symptoms include light-headedness, sedation, confusion, agitation, disorientation, restlessness, convulsions, fever, and coma. Seek immediate emergency medical treatment.

## PRECAUTIONS

### Do not take this drug if:

- You have ever had an allergic reaction to this drug or any phenothiazine.

### Inform your physician if:

- You have ever had an allergic reaction to any drug.
- You have epilepsy or asthma.
- You have cardiovascular or liver disease.
- You are taking any other drug—prescription or nonprescription —or vitamins.
- You are on a low-salt, low-sugar, or any other special diet.
- You will be under anesthesia or undergoing surgery or medical testing in the next few months.

 **Pregnancy/Breast-feeding**

Except in unusual cases where the mother or the baby's life is endangered, this drug should not be taken by pregnant women. Women taking chlorpromazine should not breast-feed.

 **Infants/Children**

This drug should not be given to children under six months of age.

 **Over Sixty**

Side effects, some serious, can be worse. Initial dose should be low, with careful monitoring for side effects. Special care should be taken when sitting up from a lying position, or standing from a sitting position, as blood pressure may be lowered and balance impaired.

 **Driving/Operating Machinery**

Extreme caution is advised. This medicine can impair mental alertness and coordination. If you do drive or operate machinery, this medicine should be taken at bedtime when its sedating effects are less likely to interfere with daytime activities.

## GENERAL INFORMATION

Chlorpromazine is a low-potency antipsychotic used to treat people who are experiencing disorganized, psychotic thinking and perceptions such as delusions and hallucinations. Chlorpromazine is sometimes prescribed to treat severe psychotic problems in children. It is also used to treat severe hiccups or protracted nausea. Introduced in the 1950s, it was the first antipsychotic drug widely used in the United States. This

**DRUG NAME:**     Chlorpromazine (*continued*)

## GENERAL INFORMATION (*continued*)

medication has been proved scientifically to reverse psychotic symptoms (hallucinations, delusions, illogical thoughts, etc.) in people with schizophrenia, manic depression, or as the result of other types of brain and medical disorders. This drug is quite sedating, and often causes lowered blood pressure. However, it also has fewer movement side effects than certain other antipsychotics. The sedating side effects may be beneficial in calming people with acute agitation or violent behavior. For an explanation of how this drug works, see Chapter 7.

## BENEFITS

- Effective in treating hallucinations, delusions, confused thinking, and mania.
- Useful to treat severe hiccups or protracted nausea.
- Sedating effects helpful in calming agitated persons.

## RISKS

- Can dangerously lower white blood cell count.
- Can cause tardive dyskinesia.
- Can cause neuroleptic malignant syndrome.
- Can dangerously lower blood pressure.

## GUIDELINES FOR USERS

**How is the drug taken?** Tablets (10, 25, 50, 100, 200 mg); extended-release capsules (30, 75, 150, 200, 300 mg); concentrate; intramuscular; suppository.

**What is the usual dosage?** The initial dose should be 25 mg to 100 mg in healthy young people, with increases as needed to control symptoms. A maximum daily dose of up to 2,000 mg may be used if necessary, although doses above 800 mg per day are rarely required. Maintenance doses should be as low as possible and still be able to control the psychotic symptoms.

**What are the instructions for taking the drug?** It is best to take this drug on an empty stomach with a full glass of water. Sometimes, it is possible to take a single dose at bedtime. In other cases, several doses a day may be prescribed. If you are taking the extended-release form, do not break open the capsule. Follow your physician's instructions carefully.

**How quickly will I feel the effect of the drug?** It usually takes several weeks for you to experience the full benefit of this drug. However, you may feel more calm and relaxed after the first dose or two. The drug should also help you sleep better, if this is a problem.

**What if I miss a dose or several doses?** If you are taking one dose at night, take the missed dose in the morning. If you do not remember until the afternoon, skip the missed dose. Do not take double doses.

If you are taking several doses a day, and remember within an hour or so, take the missed dose. Otherwise, skip the missed dose and continue on your regular dosing schedule. Do not take double doses.

If you are missing doses on a frequent basis, notify your psychiatrist. An extended-release form of this drug is available and may help with your compliance and help avoid a relapse.

**What if I stop taking the drug?** Do not stop taking this drug without consulting your physician. Abruptly stopping this medication will lead to uncomfortable but not dangerous physical symptoms. Should your physician and you agree that the drug should be discontinued, your medication should be tapered slowly to prevent physical symptoms of withdrawal and a reemergence of your psychotic symptoms.

**How should I store the drug?** Keep out of reach of children. Store in a dry, tightly closed, light-resistant container. Heat and moisture may cause this drug to break down. The liquid form does not require refrigeration.

## INTERACTIONS

**Alcohol:** Avoid alcohol. When combined with alcohol, this medicine can cause excessive sedation and dangerously lower blood pressure.

**Food/Beverages:** No restrictions.

**Smoking:** Smoking lowers the blood level of chlorpromazine. If you do smoke, blood samples should be taken to test whether the drug is in the therapeutic range.

**Other drugs:** Antacids with aluminum or magnesium (Maalox, for example) should not be taken for two hours before or after taking chlorpromazine because they may interfere with the absorption of this drug.

Heterocyclic antidepressants can increase the plasma level of this drug and cause a worsening of side effects. Conversely, this drug can increase the blood level of antidepressants. The concurrent use of these two types of drugs must be carefully monitored.

Blood pressure can be dangerously lowered when antipsychotics are combined with vasodilators (medications that dilate blood vessels). Chlorpromazine, taken with the antihypertensives clonidine or guanethidine, can also cause the blood pressure to be dangerously lowered.

Chlorpromazine will increase the effect of medicines known as CNS (central nervous system) depressants. Examples include antihistamines, hay fever medicines, sedatives, narcotics, muscle relaxants, barbiturates, and anesthetics. Check with your physician before taking any of these drugs.

## HABIT-FORMING POTENTIAL

None.

## LONG-TERM USE

Prolonged use of chlorpromazine is associated with increased risk of developing tardive dyskinesia, a potentially irreversible side effect involving disfiguring movements of the face, tongue, and limbs. For more information on tardive dyskinesia, please see Chapter 7.

**DRUG NAME:**   Chlorpromazine (*continued*)

## PLEASE NOTE

Not a sleeping pill: This drug, which has a sedating effect, is sometimes misused as a sleeping pill. There are much safer medications available as sleeping aids.

Not specifically antiaggressive: Because of the potential serious side effects of the antipsychotic drugs, especially over the long term, this medication should not be used to treat anxiety or chronic aggression and agitation.

Frequent examinations required: While taking this medication, your blood pressure and pulse rate should be monitored frequently. Regular checks should also be made for the early signs of tardive dyskinesia.

Classification: Chlorpromazine is classified as a phenothiazine. Other antipsychotics in the same group include acetophenazine, fluphenazine, mesoridazine, perphenazine, promazine, thioridazine, trifluoperazine, and triflupromazine. In general, if you have a poor response to one drug in this family, you will likely have a similar poor response to other drugs in the family.

| | Chlorpromazine | | | | | | |
|---|---|---|---|---|---|---|---|
| | Frequency | | Discuss with Physician | | | | |
| Symptom/Effect | Common | Rare | Not Necessary | In All Cases | Only If Severe | Stop Taking Drug Now | Call Physician Now |
| lethargy/sleepiness | X | | | | X | | |
| low blood pressure | X | | | X | | | |
| dizziness | | X | | X | | | |
| dry mouth | X | | | | X | | |
| blurred vision | X | | | | X | | |
| constipation | X | | | | X | | |
| difficulty urinating | X | | | X | | | |
| reduced urinary output | | X | | X | | | |
| racing heartbeat/ palpitations | | X | | X | | | |
| weakness | | X | | X | | | |
| sexual problems | | X | | X | | | |
| restlessness | | X | | X | | | |
| skin rash | | X | | X | | | X |
| weight gain | X | | | | X | | |
| seizures | | X | | X | | X | X |
| low white blood cell count | | X | | X | | | |
| tremors | | X | | X | | | |
| stiffness | X | | | X | | | |
| involuntary facial or tongue movements | | X | | X | | | X |

**BRAND NAME:** Taractan
**For more information:** See Chapter 7, Antipsychotic Drugs.

**FAST FACTS**
**Drug group:** Antipsychotics.
**Prescription needed?** Yes.

**Available as generic?** No.
**Habit-forming?** No.

**Overdose:** Symptoms include difficulty breathing, light-headedness, sedation, confusion, muscle twitching, agitation, disorientation, restlessness, shock, and coma. Seek immediate emergency medical treatment.

## PRECAUTIONS

**Do not take this drug if:**

- You have ever had an allergic reaction to this drug.

**Inform your physician if:**

- You have ever had an allergic reaction to any drug.
- You have epilepsy or asthma.
- You have cardiovascular disease.
- You are taking any other drug— prescription or nonprescription —or vitamins.
- You are on a low-salt, low-sugar, or other special diet.
- You will be under anesthesia or undergoing surgery or medical testing in the next few months.

### Pregnancy/Breast-feeding

Safe use in pregnancy has not been established. Except in unusual cases where the mother or the baby's life is endangered, this drug should not be taken by pregnant women. Women taking chlorprothixene should not breast-feed.

### Infants/Children

The safety and effectiveness of this drug has not been determined for children under age six.

### Over Sixty

Side effects, some serious, can be worse. Initial dose should be low, with careful monitoring for side effects. Special care should be taken when sitting up from a lying position, or standing from a sitting position, as blood pressure may be lowered and balance impaired.

### Driving/Operating Machinery

Extreme caution is advised. This medicine can impair mental alertness and coordination. If you do drive or operate machinery, this medicine should be taken at bedtime when its sedating effects are less likely to interfere with daytime activities.

**DRUG NAME:**  Chlorprothixene (*continued*)

## GENERAL INFORMATION

Chlorprothixene is a low-potency antipsychotic in the family of medicines known as thioxanthenes. It is used to treat people who are experiencing disorganized, psychotic thinking and perceptions such as delusions and hallucinations. This drug is quite sedating, and often causes lowered blood pressure. However, it also has fewer movement side effects than certain other antipsychotics. The sedating side effects may be beneficial in calming people with acute agitation or violent behavior. For an explanation of how this drug works, see Chapter 7.

## BENEFITS

- Effective in treating hallucinations, delusions, confused thinking, and mania.
- Sedating effects helpful in calming agitated persons.

## RISKS

- Can dangerously lower white blood cell count.
- Can cause neuroleptic malignant syndrome.
- Can cause tardive dyskinesia.

## GUIDELINES FOR USERS

**How is the drug taken?** Tablets (10, 25, 50, 100 mg); oral concentrate; intramuscular.

**What is the usual dosage?** Initial dose should be 50 mg to 200 mg per day in healthy young people, with increases as needed to control symptoms. A maximum daily dose of up to 600 mg may be used if necessary. Maintenance doses should be as low as possible but still control the psychotic symptoms. Single doses above 150 mg are rarely given.

**What are the instructions for taking the drug?** It is best to take this drug on an empty stomach with a full glass of water. The liquid form can be taken with juice. Follow your physician's instructions carefully.

**How quickly will I feel the effect of the drug?** It usually takes several weeks for you to experience the full benefit of this drug. However, you may feel more calm and relaxed after the first dose or two.

**What if I miss a dose or several doses?** If you miss a dose and remember within an hour or so, take the missed dose. However, if more than an hour has elapsed, skip the dose and continue on your regular schedule. Do not take double doses.

If you are missing doses on a frequent basis, notify your psychiatrist. A slow-release form of an antipsychotic drug may help with your compliance and help avoid a relapse.

**What if I stop taking the drug?** Do not stop taking this drug without consulting your physician. Abruptly stopping this medication will lead to uncomfortable but not dangerous physical symptoms. Should your physician and you agree that the drug should be discontinued, your medication should be tapered slowly to prevent physical symptoms of withdrawal and a reemergence of your psychotic symptoms.

**How should I store the drug?** Keep out of reach of children. Store in a dry, tightly closed, light-resistant container. Heat and moisture may cause this drug to break down. The liquid form does not require refrigeration.

## INTERACTIONS

**Alcohol:** Avoid alcohol. When combined with alcohol, this medicine can cause excessive sedation and dangerously lower blood pressure.

**Food/Beverages:** No restrictions.

**Smoking:** Smoking lowers the blood level of chlorprothixene. If you do smoke, blood samples should be taken to test whether the drug is in the therapeutic range.

**Other drugs:** Antacids with aluminum or magnesium (Maalox, for example) should not be taken for two hours before or after taking chlorprothixene because they may interfere with the absorption of this drug.

Heterocyclic antidepressants can increase the plasma level of this drug and cause a worsening of side effects. Conversely, this drug can increase the blood level of antidepressants. The concurrent use of these two types of drugs must be carefully monitored.

Blood pressure can be dangerously lowered when antipsychotics are combined with vasodilators (medications that dilate blood vessels).

Chlorprothixene will increase the effect of medicines known as CNS (central nervous system) depressants. Examples include antihistamines, hay fever medicines, sedatives, narcotics, muscle relaxants, barbiturates, and anesthetics. Check with your physician before taking any of these drugs.

## HABIT-FORMING POTENTIAL

None.

## LONG-TERM USE

Prolonged use of chlorprothixene is associated with increased risk of developing tardive dyskinesia, a potentially irreversible side effect involving disfiguring movements of the face, tongue, and limbs. For more information on tardive dyskinesia, please see Chapter 7.

## PLEASE NOTE

Not specifically antiaggressive: Because of the potential serious side effects of the antipsychotic drugs, especially over the long term, this medicine should not be used to treat anxiety or chronic aggression and agitation.

Less sweating: Chlorprothixene may cause you to sweat less, which in turn causes your body temperature to rise. When the weather is hot or you are exercising, make sure you do not become too hot or dehydrated, since overheating may result in a heat stroke.

Frequent examinations required: While taking this medication, your blood pressure and pulse rate should be monitored frequently. Regular checks should also be made for the early signs of tardive dyskinesia.

Classification: Chlorprothixene is classified in the family of medicines known as the thioxanthenes. Thiothixene is another antipsychotic in the same group. In general, if you have a poor response to one drug in this family, you will likely have a similar poor response to other drugs in the family.

**DRUG NAME:**    Chlorprothixene (*continued*)

| Symptom/Effect | Frequency | | Discuss with Physician | | | Stop Taking Drug Now | Call Physician Now |
|---|---|---|---|---|---|---|---|
| | Common | Rare | Not Necessary | In All Cases | Only If Severe | | |
| lethargy/sleepiness | X | | | | X | | |
| low blood pressure | X | | | X | | | |
| dizziness | | X | | X | | | |
| dry mouth | X | | | | X | | |
| blurred vision | X | | | | X | | |
| constipation | X | | | | X | | |
| difficulty urinating | X | | | X | | | |
| reduced urinary output | | X | | X | | | X |
| racing heartbeat/ palpitations | | X | | X | | | |
| weakness | | X | | X | | | |
| sexual problems | | X | | X | | | |
| restlessness | | X | | X | | | |
| skin rash | | X | | X | | | X |
| weight gain | X | | | | X | | |
| seizures | | X | | X | | X | X |
| low white blood cell count | | X | | X | | | X |
| tremors | | X | | X | | | |
| stiffness | X | | | X | | | |
| involuntary facial or tongue movements | | X | | X | | | X |

## Drug Name: **Clomipramine**

**Brand Name:** Anafranil
**For more information:** See Chapter 3, Antidepressant Drugs, and Chapter 4, Antianxiety Drugs.

**FAST FACTS**    **Drug group:** Antidepressants.     **Available as generic?** No.
**Prescription needed?** Yes.     **Habit-forming?** No.

 **Overdose:** The danger of an overdose, which can be lethal, is extremely high. Symptoms include difficulty breathing, shock, agitation, delirium, and coma. Seek immediate emergency medical treatment.

## PRECAUTIONS

### Do not take this drug if:

- You have ever had an allergic or negative reaction to any drug in this group.

### Inform your physician if:

- You have ever had an allergic reaction to any drug.
- You have epilepsy.
- You are taking any other drug— prescription or nonprescription —or vitamins.
- You will be under anesthesia or undergoing surgery or medical testing in the next few months.

### Pregnancy/Breast-feeding

If you are pregnant or planning a pregnancy, you should, if possible, use non-drug alternatives for treating your depression. This drug has not been demonstrated to be safe during pregnancy. Nursing mothers should not take this drug since it is passed on to the baby in the mother's milk.

### Infants/Children

Not recommended for children under age ten. Adolescents should be given lower doses. Its use in the treatment of depression in children and adolescents must be under the guidance of a child psychiatrist.

### Over Sixty

In general, lower doses are required. Side effects may be worse and some older patients may experience confusion. Elderly people may fall after standing up because of the drug's hypotensive (blood pressure lowering) side effects.

### Driving/Operating Machinery

Extreme caution is advised. This medicine can impair mental alertness and coordination. If you drive or operate machinery, this medicine should be taken at bedtime when its sedating effects are less likely to interfere with daytime activities.

417

**DRUG NAME:**    Clomipramine (*continued*)

## GENERAL INFORMATION

Clomipramine is in the heterocyclic antidepressant family of drugs. Although this drug has been used widely internationally for more than twenty years to treat depression, it was not available in the United States until February 1990. Clomipramine is the only FDA-approved drug marketed specifically to treat obsessive-compulsive disorder.

| BENEFITS | RISKS |
|---|---|
| • Effective in treating depression and obsessive-compulsive disorder. | • Produces annoying side effects. |
| | • Potential for use in suicide attempts. |

## GUIDELINES FOR USERS

**How is the drug taken?** Tablets (25, 50, 75 mg).

**What is the usual dosage?** The initial dose is usually 25 mg daily in divided doses. This can be increased gradually to 100 mg daily. Some people may require 200 mg to 300 mg daily. Initial doses are lower for patients with medical illnesses, and the elderly.

**What are the instructions for taking the drug?** Take this medicine with food, unless your doctor has instructed you otherwise. Taking the medicine on an empty stomach may cause your stomach to become upset. To benefit from the drug, it is important to take the correct dosage each day.

**How quickly will I feel the effect of the drug?** You will probably experience some unpleasant side effects (dry mouth, blurry vision, constipation) right away. It may take days or weeks for the benefits to appear. It usually takes two to four weeks at full dose for a person to feel a positive response. By the third week of treatment, the side effects are usually less severe.

**What if I miss a dose or several doses?** If you are taking one dose at bedtime and miss your dose, do not take the drug in the morning. Check with your doctor. If you are taking more than one dose a day and remember within an hour or so that you have missed a dose, take the dose. However, if it is almost time for your next dose, skip the missed dose. Do not take double doses.

**What if I stop taking the drug?** Do not discontinue this drug abruptly. Your dosage should be gradually reduced. Stopping the drug abruptly may cause flulike symptoms, headache, restlessness, and/or a worsening of your condition. Inform your physician if you notice these side effects, or any others, after stopping the drug. The effects of this drug may last for up to seven days after you have stopped taking it.

**How should I store the drug?** Keep out of reach of children. Store in a dry, tightly closed, light-resistant container. Heat and moisture may cause this drug to break down.

## INTERACTIONS

**Alcohol:** Do not drink alcohol. Clomipramine *increases* the effect of alcohol, while alcohol *increases* the side effects of the drug. In addition, alcohol use can contribute to depression.

**Food/Beverages:** No restrictions.

**Smoking:** Smoking lowers the blood level of clomipramine. If you do smoke, blood samples should be taken to test whether the drug is in the therapeutic range.

**Other drugs:** Clomipramine will increase the effect of medicines known as CNS (central nervous system) depressants. Examples include antihistamines, hay fever medicines, sedatives, narcotics, muscle relaxants, barbiturates, and anesthetics. Check with your physician before taking any of these drugs.

Clomipramine should not be taken in combination with MAO inhibitors, or within fourteen days of taking an MAO inhibitor.

Clomipramine may block the effects of guanethidine, clonidine, or similar drugs.

Concurrent use of neuroleptics, methylphenidate, carbamazepine, haloperidol, or cimetidine may increase the blood levels of clomipramine.

## HABIT-FORMING POTENTIAL

None.

## LONG-TERM USE

Most people who have a beneficial response do not need to take this drug longer than about six months. A few people may need to take the drug for a year or longer because their depression or obsessive-compulsive symptoms recur if they attempt to discontinue the drug.

## PLEASE NOTE

Help with side effects: Drinking water and sucking on hard candy can help if you are experiencing dry mouth. To prevent constipation, eat high-fiber foods and take a daily dose of a natural bulk laxative. And you can avoid episodes of light-headedness by making sure you get up slowly from a sitting or prone position. These side effects generally get better or go away after you have been on the drug several weeks.

**DRUG NAME:**    Clomipramine (*continued*)

| Symptom/Effect | Frequency | | Discuss with Physician | | | Stop Taking Drug Now | Call Physician Now |
| --- | --- | --- | --- | --- | --- | --- | --- |
| | Common | Rare | Not Necessary | In All Cases | Only If Severe | | |
| drowsiness | X | | | | X | | |
| dry mouth | X | | | | X | | |
| constipation | X | | | | X | | |
| blurred vision | X | | | | X | | |
| low blood pressure | X | | | X | | | |
| racing heartbeat/ palpitations | | X | | | X | | |
| confusion | | X | | X | | | X |
| skin rashes/allergies | | X | | X | | | X |
| insomnia | | X | | | X | | |
| sexual problems | | X | | X | | | |
| increased appetite | | X | | | X | | |
| seizures | | X | | X | | X | X |

DRUG NAME: **Clonazepam**

**BRAND NAME:** Klonopin
**For more information:** See Chapter 4, Antianxiety Drugs.

**FAST FACTS**  **Drug group:** Antianxiety agents (benzodiazepines).

**Available as generic?** No.

**Prescription needed?** Yes.

**Habit-forming?** Yes.

 **Overdose:** It is possible, though not easy, to overdose. Signs of toxicity include sedation, decreased breathing rate, confusion, and loss of coordination. If these symptoms are present, seek immediate emergency medical treatment.

## PRECAUTIONS

**Do not take this drug if:**

- You have had previously negative reactions to benzodiazepines.
- You have a history of drug dependence.
- You have Alzheimer's disease, have had a stroke, or have multiple sclerosis or other brain disorders.
- You are seriously depressed.

**Inform your physician if:**

- You are taking any other drug—prescription or nonprescription —or vitamins.
- You will be under anesthesia or undergoing surgery or medical testing within the next few months.

 **Pregnancy/Breast-feeding**

Do not take this drug if you are pregnant, planning a pregnancy, or are breast-feeding.

 **Infants/Children**

Safety and effectiveness have not been established for children and adolescents under eighteen.

 **Over Sixty**

Smaller doses are advised and should be monitored very closely.

 **Driving/Operating Machinery**

WARNING: Do not fly, drive, or operate heavy machinery, since this drug can impair mental alertness and coordination.

## GENERAL INFORMATION

Clonazepam is used for the short-term treatment of mild to moderate anxiety. It may also be prescribed for certain convulsive disorders such as epilepsy. Some case reports have suggested that this drug may have certain antimanic effects and may treat certain movement disorders like tics and tremors. As with other benzodiazepines, long-term use can lead to dependence. Roche Products manufactures the brand Klonopin. For an explanation of how this drug works, see Chapter 4.

**DRUG NAME:**   Clonazepam (*continued*)

## BENEFITS

- More effective and fewer side effects than barbiturates.
- Less addictive and safer in overdoses than barbiturates.
- Relieves anxiety in about 65 percent to 70 percent of users.

## RISKS

- Physically and psychologically addictive if misused.
- Makes some people feel lethargic, less able to concentrate, less alert.
- Can affect physical coordination.

## GUIDELINES FOR USERS

**How is the drug taken?** Tablets (0.5, 1, 2 mg).

**What is the usual dosage?** The initial dose should be 1.5 mg per day, with increases as needed to control symptoms. A maximum daily dose of up to 20 mg may be used, if necessary.

**What are the instructions for taking the drug?** As with all benzodiazepines, if you are taking this drug for the first time, take your first dose at home and during a time when you are not required to work or drive. Your physician should tell you how often to take subsequent doses. Follow these instructions carefully. This drug can be taken before, during, or after meals. The tablets can be crushed and dissolved in water before taking, if you prefer.

**How quickly will I feel the effect of the drug?** Those who benefit from this drug will usually experience a positive response within the first week. Many people feel the drug's effect the first day of treatment.

**What if I miss a dose or several doses?** If you miss a dose and remember within an hour or so, take the missed dose. However, if more than an hour has elapsed, skip the dose and continue on your regular schedule. Do not take double doses.

**What if I stop taking the drug?** If you take this drug regularly for three weeks or more, you should not stop abruptly. Your dosage should be gradually reduced. Abrupt cessation can cause psychological and physical withdrawal symptoms.

**How should I store the drug?** Keep out of reach of children, since all benzodiazepines can be extremely dangerous to children. Store in a dry, tightly closed, light-resistant container. Heat and moisture may cause this drug to break down.

## INTERACTIONS

**Alcohol:** Do not drink alcohol. Clonazepam is highly dangerous when combined with alcohol. It can dangerously lower blood pressure, decrease the breathing rate, and lead to loss of consciousness.

**Food/Beverages:** No restrictions on food. Control caffeine intake, as caffeine makes anxiety worse.

**Smoking:** Heavy smoking of tobacco may reduce the sedative effects of this drug. Marijuana smoking may increase side effects and significantly reduce mental alertness.

**Other drugs:** Narcotics (e.g., Demerol, Percodan, codeine, morphine, Talwin) may *increase* the sedative effects of this drug. The combination can be fatal. Do not use narcotics with this drug.

Barbiturates and other sedatives (e.g., phenobarbital, pentobarbital, Seconal, Tuinal) may *increase* sedation to dangerous levels. Do not combine sedatives with this drug.

Do not take other benzodiazepines when using this drug, since the combination is both unnecessary and unsafe.

Do not take sleeping pills while taking this drug. If you are having trouble sleeping, your doctor may prescribe larger doses of clonazepam.

The following drugs may reduce the liver's ability to remove this drug from the body, making the drug more powerful and increasing side effects:

- ulcer drugs
- birth control pills
- propranolol
- disulfiram (Antabuse)

## HABIT-FORMING POTENTIAL

High.

## LONG-TERM USE

Physical and psychological dependence are common problems. A clear treatment plan is important. It is possible to become dependent in as short a time span as two to four weeks. This drug should not be taken longer than four weeks on a regular basis (i.e., daily). Long-term use can also increase the risk of side effects.

| | Frequency | | Discuss with Physician | | | | |
|---|---|---|---|---|---|---|---|
| Symptom/Effect | Common | Rare | Not Necessary | In All Cases | Only If Severe | Stop Taking Drug Now | Call Physician Now |
| clumsiness/sleepiness | X | | | | X | | |
| abdominal cramps | | X | | X | | | |
| blurred vision | | X | | X | | | |
| dry mouth | | X | | X | | | |
| racing heartbeat/ palpitations | | X | | X | | | |
| shaking/slurred speech | | X | | X | | | |
| urination problems | | X | | X | | | |
| convulsions | | X | | X | | X | X |
| hallucinations | | X | | X | | X | X |
| memory loss | | X | | X | | X | X |
| trouble breathing | | X | | X | | X | X |
| staggering/trembling | | X | | X | | X | X |
| headache | | X | | X | | | |
| confusion | | X | | X | | | X |

*Table title: Clonazepam*

DRUG NAME: **Clorazepate**

**BRAND NAME:** Tranxene
**For more information:** See Chapter 4, Antianxiety Drugs.

**FAST FACTS** **Drug group:** Antianxiety agents (benzodiazepines).

**Available as generic?** Yes.

**Prescription needed?** Yes.

**Habit-forming?** Yes.

 **Overdose:** It is possible, though not easy, to overdose. Signs of toxicity include sedation, decreased breathing rate, confusion, and loss of coordination. If these symptoms are present, seek immediate emergency medical treatment.

## PRECAUTIONS

**Do not take this drug if:**

- You have had previously negative reactions to benzodiazepines.
- You have a history of drug dependence.
- You have Alzheimer's disease, have had a stroke, or have multiple sclerosis or other brain disorders.
- You are seriously depressed.

**Inform your physician if:**

- You are taking any other drug— prescription or nonprescription —or vitamins.
- You have ever had an allergic reaction to any drug.
- You will be under anesthesia or undergoing surgery or medical testing in the next few months.

 **Pregnancy/Breast-feeding**

Do not take this drug if you are pregnant, planning a pregnancy, or breast-feeding.

 **Infants/Children**

This drug should not be given to children under nine.

 **Over Sixty**

Smaller doses are advised and should be monitored very closely.

 **Driving/Operating Machinery**

WARNING: Do not fly, drive, or operate heavy machinery, since this drug can impair mental alertness and coordination.

## GENERAL INFORMATION

Clorazepate, the third most frequently prescribed benzodiazepine, is used to treat anxiety. It is sometimes prescribed for persons with acute alcohol withdrawal syndrome and for epilepsy and other convulsive disorders. Abbott manufactures the drug under the brand name Tranxene. Generic manufacturers include Alra Laboratories, Lederle, Martec, Mylan, Par, Squibb, and Warner Chilcott. For an explanation of how this drug works, see Chapter 4.

## BENEFITS

- More effective and fewer side effects than barbiturates.
- Less addictive and safer in overdoses than barbiturates.
- Relieves anxiety in about 65 percent to 70 percent of users.

## RISKS

- Physically and psychologically addictive if misused.
- Makes some people feel lethargic, less able to concentrate, less alert.
- Can affect physical coordination.

## GUIDELINES FOR USERS

**How is the drug taken?** Tablets (3.75, 7.5, 11.25, 15, 22.5 mg).

**What is the usual dosage?** The initial dose should be 15 mg per day, with increases as needed to control symptoms. A maximum daily dose of up to 60 mg may be used, if necessary.

**What are the instructions for taking the drug?** As with all benzodiazepines, if you are taking this drug for the first time, take your first dose at home and during a time when you are not required to work or drive. Your physician should tell you how often to take subsequent doses. Follow these instructions carefully. This drug can be taken before, during, or after meals. The tablets can be crushed and dissolved in water before taking, if you prefer.

**How quickly will I feel the effect of the drug?** Those who benefit from this drug will usually experience a positive response within the first week. Many people feel the drug's effect the first day of treatment.

**What if I miss a dose or several doses?** If you miss a dose and remember within an hour or so, take the missed dose. However, if more than an hour has elapsed, skip the dose and continue on your regular schedule. Do not take double doses.

**What if I stop taking the drug?** If you take this drug regularly for three weeks or more, you should not stop abruptly. Your dosage should be gradually reduced. Abrupt cessation can cause psychological and physical withdrawal symptoms.

**How should I store the drug?** Keep out of reach of children, since all benzodiazepines can be extremely dangerous to children. Store in a dry, tightly closed, light-resistant container. Heat and moisture may cause this drug to break down.

## INTERACTIONS

**Alcohol:** Do not drink alcohol. Clorazepate is highly dangerous when combined with alcohol. It can dangerously lower blood pressure, decrease the breathing rate, and lead to loss of consciousness.

**Food/Beverages:** No restrictions on food. Control caffeine intake, as caffeine makes anxiety worse.

**Smoking:** Heavy smoking of tobacco may reduce the sedative effects of this drug. Marijuana smoking may increase side effects and significantly reduce mental alertness.

**Other drugs:** Narcotics (e.g., Demerol, Percodan, codeine, morphine, Talwin) may

**DRUG NAME:**    Clorazepate (*continued*)

---

## INTERACTIONS (*continued*)

*increase* the sedative effects of this drug. The combination can be fatal. Do not use narcotics with this drug.

Barbiturates and other sedatives (e.g., phenobarbital, pentobarbital, Seconal, Tuinal) may *increase* sedation to dangerous levels. Do not combine sedatives with this drug.

Do not take other benzodiazepines when using this drug, since the combination is both unnecessary and unsafe.

Do not take sleeping pills while taking this drug. If you are having trouble sleeping, your doctor may prescribe larger doses of clorazepate.

The following drugs may reduce the liver's ability to remove this drug from the body, making the drug more powerful and increasing side effects:
- ulcer drugs
- birth control pills
- propranolol
- disulfiram (Antabuse)

---

## HABIT-FORMING POTENTIAL

High.

---

## LONG-TERM USE

Physical and psychological dependence are common problems. A clear treatment plan is important. It is possible to become dependent in as short a time span as two to four weeks. This drug should not be taken longer than four weeks on a regular basis (i.e., daily). Long-term use can also increase the risk of side effects.

---

## PLEASE NOTE

Nondrug alternatives: See Chapter 4 for a discussion of the value of exercise and a good diet in the treatment of anxiety. One of the best nondrug ways to reduce anxiety is to identify and reduce sources of stress in your life.

Correct diagnosis: You should always consult a physician to be sure that any medical causes of anxiety (such as hyperthyroidism) are diagnosed and treated. Anxiety may be a component of depression, in which case the symptoms of anxiety are treated by treating the underlying depression with antidepressants and/or other therapies for mood disorders.

## Clorazepate

| Symptom/Effect | Frequency | | Discuss with Physician | | | Stop Taking Drug Now | Call Physician Now |
|---|---|---|---|---|---|---|---|
| | Common | Rare | Not Necessary | In All Cases | Only If Severe | | |
| clumsiness/sleepiness | X | | | | X | | |
| abdominal cramps | | X | | X | | | |
| blurred vision | | X | | X | | | |
| dry mouth | | X | | X | | | |
| racing heartbeat/ palpitations | | X | | X | | | |
| shaking/slurred speech | | X | | X | | | |
| urination problems | | X | | X | | | |
| convulsions | | X | | X | | X | X |
| hallucinations | | X | | X | | X | X |
| memory loss | | X | | X | | X | X |
| trouble breathing | | X | | X | | X | X |
| staggering/trembling | | X | | X | | X | X |
| headache | | X | | X | | | X |
| confusion | | X | | X | | | X |

# DRUG NAME: Clozapine

**BRAND NAME:** Clozaril
**For more information:** See Chapter 7, Antipsychotic Drugs.

**FAST FACTS**    **Drug group:** Antipsychotics.      **Available as generic?** No.

**Prescription needed?** Yes.      **Habit-forming?** No.

 **Overdose:** Symptoms include light-headedness, sedation, confusion, salivation, agitation, restlessness, disorientation, convulsions, fever, and coma. Seek immediate emergency medical treatment.

## PRECAUTIONS

### Do not take this drug if:

- You have ever had an allergic reaction to this drug.
- You have a history of myeloproliferative disease (a disorder of your bone marrow and white blood cells).

### Inform your physician if:

- You have ever had an allergic reaction to any drug.
- You have epilepsy.
- You have anemia or any other blood disorder.
- You are taking any other drug—prescription or nonprescription—or vitamins.
- You are on a low-salt, low-sugar, or any other special diet.
- You will be under anesthesia or undergoing surgery or medical testing in the next few months.

 **Pregnancy/Breast-feeding**

Except in unusual cases where the mother or the baby's life is endangered, this drug should not be taken by pregnant women. Women taking clozapine should not breast-feed. Studies suggest that clozapine is excreted in breast milk and will affect the nursing infant.

 **Infants/Children**

Safety and effectiveness have not been established in children under age sixteen.

 **Over Sixty**

Side effects, some serious, can be worse. Initial dose should be low, with careful monitoring for side effects.

 **Driving/Operating Machinery**

Do not fly, drive, or operate machinery because of the high risks of seizures during clozapine treatment.

## GENERAL INFORMATION

The antipsychotic clozapine has been widely used in Europe, but currently its use in the United States is limited because it has a 1 percent to 2 percent risk of causing agranulocytosis, the cessation of the production of white blood cells. If this condition is detected and the medication stopped, it will usually resolve itself. However, if not detected in time, the person may die. Clozapine also is associated with a high risk of seizures, 1 percent to 2 percent risk at low doses and a 3 percent to 5 percent risk at doses above 600 mg daily. Clozapine must be used with the "clozapine patient management system," in which weekly blood samples are taken to test for blood-related side effects. At the present time, clozapine is mainly used for the treatment of people with schizophrenia. It should not be used to treat insomnia, agitation, anxiety, or violence not associated with psychosis.

## BENEFITS

- Effective in treating hallucinations, delusions, confused thinking, and mania.
- May be effective for patients whose symptoms have not been controlled by other antipsychotics.
- Causes fewer movement side effects than all other antipsychotics.
- Does not cause tardive dyskinesia.

## RISKS

- May dangerously lower white blood cell count.
- Can cause neuroleptic malignant syndrome.
- 1 percent to 2 percent risk of agranulocytosis.
- Can cause seizures.

## GUIDELINES FOR USERS

**How is the drug taken?** Tablets (25, 100 mg).

**What is the usual dosage?** The initial dose should be 25 mg to 50 mg per day, with increases as needed to control symptoms. A maximum daily dose of up to 600 mg may be used if necessary. Maintenance doses should be as low as possible but still be able to control the symptoms.

**What are the instructions for taking the drug?** It is best to take this drug on an empty stomach, with a full glass of water.

**How quickly will I feel the effect of the drug?** It usually takes several weeks for you to experience the full benefit of this drug. However, you may feel more calm and relaxed after the first dose or two. The drug should also help you sleep better, if this is a problem.

**What if I miss a dose or several doses?** If you miss a dose and remember within an hour or so, take the missed dose. Otherwise, skip the missed dose and continue on your regular dosing schedule. Do not take double doses.

If you are missing doses on a frequent basis, notify your psychiatrist. A slow-release form of another antipsychotic drug may help with your compliance and help avoid a relapse.

**What if I stop taking the drug?** Do not stop taking this drug without consulting your physician. Abruptly stopping this medication will lead to uncomfortable but not dangerous physical symptoms. Should your physician and you agree that the drug should be discontinued, your medication should be tapered slowly to prevent physical symptoms of withdrawal and a reemergence of your psychotic symptoms.

**How should I store the drug?** Keep out of reach of children. Store in a dry, tightly closed, light-resistant container. Heat and moisture may cause this drug to break down.

**DRUG NAME:**    Clozapine (*continued*)

## INTERACTIONS

**Alcohol:** Avoid if possible since this medication will add to the effects of alcohol, especially sedation, confusion, and low blood pressure.

**Food/Beverages:** No restrictions.

**Smoking:** Smoking lowers the blood level of clozapine. If you do smoke, blood samples should be taken to test whether the drug is in the therapeutic range.

**Other drugs:** The risks of using clozapine with other drugs have not been fully established. It is important to inform your physician if you are taking any prescription or over-the-counter drug.

Clozapine should not be used with any other drug known to suppress bone marrow function.

Clozapine may interact with medicines known as CNS (central nervous system) depressants. Examples include antihistamines, hay fever medicines, sedatives, narcotics, muscle relaxants, barbiturates, and anesthetics. Check with your physician before taking any of these drugs.

Clozapine may increase the effects of antihypertensive drugs and the anticholinergic effects of atropine-type drugs.

## HABIT-FORMING POTENTIAL

None.

## LONG-TERM USE

The effects and side effects of this drug are still being studied in the United States. However, its use in Europe does not indicate long-term hazards.

## Clozapine

| Symptom/Effect | Frequency | | Discuss with Physician | | | Stop Taking Drug Now | Call Physician Now |
|---|---|---|---|---|---|---|---|
| | Common | Rare | Not Necessary | In All Cases | Only If Severe | | |
| drowsiness/sedation | X | | | | X | | |
| dizziness/light-headedness | X | | | | X | | |
| low blood pressure | X | | | | X | | |
| headache | | X | | | X | | |
| agitation/restlessness | | X | | X | | | |
| sleep disturbances/nightmares | | X | | X | | | |
| seizures | | X | | X | | X | X |
| increased salivation | X | | | X | | | |
| sweating | | X | | | X | | |
| dry mouth | | X | | | X | | |
| visual changes | | X | | X | | | |
| racing heartbeat/palpitations | X | | | X | | | |
| constipation | X | | | X | | | |
| abdominal discomfort | | X | | | X | | |
| nausea/vomiting | | X | | X | | | |
| fever | | X | | X | | | X |
| weight gain | | X | | X | | | |
| sore throat | | X | | X | | | X |
| reduced urinary output | | X | | X | | | X |

**BRAND NAMES:** Norpramine, Pertofrane
**For more information:** See Chapter 3, Antidepressant Drugs.

**FAST FACTS**

| | |
|---|---|
| **Drug group:** Antidepressants. | **Available as generic?** Yes. |
| **Prescription needed?** Yes. | **Habit-forming?** No. |

 **Overdose:** The danger of an overdose, which can be lethal, is extremely high. Symptoms include difficulty breathing, shock, agitation, delirium, convulsions, and coma. Seek immediate emergency medical treatment.

## PRECAUTIONS

### Do not take this drug if:

- You have ever had an allergic or negative reaction to any drug in this group.

### Inform your physician if:

- You have ever had an allergic reaction to any drug.
- You have epilepsy, glaucoma, cardiovascular disease, or thyroid disease.
- You are taking any other drug—prescription or nonprescription—or vitamins.
- You will be under anesthesia or undergoing surgery or medical testing in the next few months.

 ### Pregnancy/Breast-feeding

If you are pregnant or planning a pregnancy, you should, if possible, use non-drug alternatives for treating your depression. This drug has not been demonstrated to be safe during pregnancy. Nursing mothers should not take this drug, since it is passed on to the baby in the mother's milk.

 ### Infants/Children

The safety of this drug has not been established for children. Lower doses are recommended for adolescents. Its use in the treatment of depression in children and adolescents must be under the guidance of a child psychiatrist.

 ### Over Sixty

In general, lower doses are required. Side effects may be worse and some older patients may experience confusion. Elderly people may fall after standing up because of the drug's hypotensive (blood pressure lowering) side effects.

 ### Driving/Operating Machinery

Extreme caution is advised. This medicine can impair mental alertness and coordination. If you do drive or operate machinery, this medicine should be taken at bedtime, when its sedating effects are less likely to interfere with daytime activities.

## GENERAL INFORMATION

Desipramine is one of the heterocyclic drugs used to treat depression. It is sometimes prescribed when a person is withdrawing from cocaine to reduce the craving for cocaine and to treat the associated depression. It works by inhibiting the nerve cell's ability to reabsorb the neurotransmitters norepinephrine and serotonin (see Chapter 3). Desipramine is among the less sedating heterocyclic drugs.

| BENEFITS | RISKS |
|---|---|
| • Helps 75 percent to 80 percent of people with major depression. | • Produces annoying side effects.<br>• Potential for use in suicide attempts. |

## GUIDELINES FOR USERS

**How is the drug taken?** Tablets (10, 25, 50, 75, 100, 150 mg); capsules (25, 50 mg).

**What is the usual dosage?** The initial dose is usually 75 mg daily in divided doses. This can be increased gradually to 150 mg daily. Some people may require 200 mg to 300 mg daily.

**What are the instructions for taking the drug?** Take this medicine with food, unless your doctor has instructed you otherwise. Taking the medicine on an empty stomach may cause your stomach to become upset. To benefit from the drug, it is important to take the correct dosage each day.

**How quickly will I feel the effect of the drug?** You will probably experience some unpleasant side effects (dry mouth, blurry vision, constipation) right away. It may take days or weeks for the benefits to appear. It usually takes two to four weeks at full dose for a person to feel a positive response. By the third week of treatment, the side effects are usually less severe.

**What if I miss a dose or several doses?** If you are taking one dose at bedtime and miss your dose, do not take the drug in the morning. Check with your doctor. If you are taking more than one dose a day and remember within an hour or so that you have missed a dose, take the dose. However, if it is almost time for your next dose, skip the missed dose. Do not take double doses.

**What if I stop taking the drug?** Do not discontinue this drug abruptly. Your dosage should be gradually reduced. Stopping the drug abruptly may cause flulike symptoms, headache, restlessness, and/or a worsening of your condition. Inform your physician if you notice these side effects, or any others, after stopping the drug. The effects of this drug may last for up to seven days after you have stopped taking it.

**How should I store the drug?** Keep out of reach of children. Store in a dry, tightly closed, light-resistant container. Heat and moisture may cause this drug to break down.

## INTERACTIONS

**Alcohol:** Do not drink alcohol. Desipramine *increases* the effect of alcohol, while alcohol *increases* the side effects of the drug. In addition, alcohol use can contribute to depression.

**Food/Beverages:** No restrictions.

**DRUG NAME:**    Desipramine (*continued*)

## INTERACTIONS (*continued*)

**Smoking:** Smoking lowers the blood level of desipramine. If you do smoke, blood samples should be taken to test whether the drug is in the therapeutic range.

**Other drugs:** Desipramine will increase the effect of medicines known as CNS (central nervous system) depressants. Examples include antihistamines, hay fever medicines, sedatives, narcotics, muscle relaxants, barbiturates, and anesthetics. Check with your physician before taking any of these drugs.

## HABIT-FORMING POTENTIAL

None.

## LONG-TERM USE

Most people who have a beneficial response do not need to take this drug longer than about six months. A few people may need to take the drug for a year or longer because their depression recurs if they attempt to discontinue the drug.

## PLEASE NOTE

Help with side effects: Drinking water and sucking on hard candy can help if you are experiencing dry mouth. To prevent constipation, eat high-fiber foods and take a daily dose of a natural bulk laxative. And you can avoid episodes of light-headedness by making sure you get up slowly from a sitting or prone position. These side effects generally get better or go away after you have been on the drug several weeks.

| Desipramine | | | | | | | |
|---|---|---|---|---|---|---|---|
| | Frequency | | Discuss with Physician | | | | |
| Symptom/Effect | Common | Rare | Not Necessary | In All Cases | Only If Severe | Stop Taking Drug Now | Call Physician Now |
| drowsiness | X | | | | X | | |
| dry mouth | X | | | | X | | |
| constipation | X | | | | X | | |
| blurred vision | X | | | | X | | |
| low blood pressure | X | | | X | | | |
| racing heartbeat/ palpitations | | X | | | X | | |
| confusion | | X | | X | | | X |
| skin rashes/allergies | | X | | X | | | X |
| insomnia | | X | | | X | | |
| sexual problems | | X | | X | | | |
| increased appetite | | X | | | X | | |
| seizures | | X | | X | | X | X |

**DRUG NAME: Dextroamphetamine**

**BRAND NAME:** Dexedrine

**For more information:** See Chapter 10, Drugs for Attention-Deficit Hyperactivity Disorder.

---

**FAST FACTS**  **Drug group:** Stimulants.  **Available as generic?** Yes.

**Prescription needed?** Yes.  **Habit-forming?** Yes.

 **Overdose:** Symptoms include restlessness, tremors, insomnia, trouble breathing, confusion, hallucinations, and panic. These symptoms may be followed by lethargy, and in acute poisoning, convulsions and coma. Seek emergency medical treatment.

---

## PRECAUTIONS

### Do not take this drug if:

- You have ever had an allergic reaction to this drug or another amphetamine.
- You have a history of drug or alcohol abuse.

### Inform your physician if:

- You have ever had an allergic reaction to any drug.
- You have epilepsy or a history of Tourette's syndrome.
- You have glaucoma, or heart or blood vessel disease.
- You have high blood pressure.
- You are taking any other drug—prescription or nonprescription—or vitamins.
- You are now taking or have taken within two weeks a monoamine oxidase (MAO) inhibitor.
- You will be under anesthesia or undergoing surgery or medical testing in the next few months.

 **Pregnancy/Breast-feeding**

Do not take this drug if you are pregnant, planning a pregnancy, or are breast-feeding.

 **Infants/Children**

Not recommended for children under age three.

 **Over Sixty**

Little research has been done on the effect of amphetamines in the elderly. This drug is prescribed by some psychiatrists to increase mental alertness in the elderly and is known to augment the effects of heterocyclic antidepressants for people with treatment-resistant depression.

 **Driving/Operating Machinery**

This drug may impair mental alertness and coordination. Do not drive or operate machinery until you are certain this drug will not affect your performance. This drug has been abused by those wishing to increase alertness and to combat sleepiness while driving. This is a dangerous practice as tolerance buildup for its mental alertness effects and psychological side effects can impair perception or judgment.

**DRUG NAME:**    Dextroamphetamine (*continued*)

## GENERAL INFORMATION

Dextroamphetamine is an amphetamine in the family of medicines known as *central nervous system stimulants*. This drug is used to treat narcolepsy and attention-deficit disorders in children. In children, amphetamines increase the ability to concentrate and reduce restlessness. When hyperactivity is a problem, dextroamphetamine is often the drug of first choice. Dextroamphetamine's side effects can be bothersome, and in cases where they are serious, methylphenidate is one alternative drug choice with fewer side effects. Children who suffer from schizophrenia or other psychotic disorders that may produce symptoms similar to attention-deficit disorders should not be given stimulants. In rare cases, dextroamphetamine may be used to treat depression. Amphetamines, which produce feelings of euphoria and excitation when taken in large doses by adults, have been widely abused. Street names for this drug include *brownies, Christmas trees, dexies, hearts,* and *wakeups*. Dextroamphetamine is available in combination with amphetamine; however, combination drugs are not recommended. For an explanation of how this drug works, see Chapter 10.

## BENEFITS

- Effective in treating attention-deficit hyperactivity disorder in children and adolescents.
- Augments the antidepressant effects of heterocyclic antidepressants.

## RISKS

- Stimulants sometimes induce Tourette's syndrome.
- Increases vulnerability to seizure disorders.
- Can be abused by people prone to drug dependence.

## GUIDELINES FOR USERS

**How is the drug taken?** Tablets (5, 10, 20 mg); long-acting capsules; syrup.

**What is the usual dosage?** Initial doses are 5 mg two or three times per day. Dosages must be increased and adjusted to the individual in response to therapeutic benefits and side effects.

**What are the instructions for taking the drug?** If you are taking the short-acting form of dextroamphetamine (three to six hours), take your last dose at least six hours before bedtime to prevent trouble sleeping. If you are taking the long-acting capsules (eight to sixteen hours), take your dose in the morning. Do not break, crush, or chew the tablets or capsules before swallowing them. For some children, the long-acting form of this drug may cause uneven blood levels that may not be acceptable.

**How quickly will I feel the effect of the drug and how long does it last?** When this drug is effective, adults will usually notice some improvement in the child from almost the first day the medication is taken. The effects of dextroamphetamine last about three to four hours, and it must be given several times a day. The sustained-release form of the drug can be taken once a day. However, this form does not work for all children.

**What if I miss a dose or several doses?** If you are taking several doses a day and remember the missed dose within an hour or so, take the dose. However, if it is almost time for your next dose, skip the missed dose and continue on your regular schedule. Do not take a dose within six hours of sleeping and do not take double doses.

If you are taking the long-acting capsule, take the missed dose only if you remember within an hour or so and if it is at least twelve hours before bedtime. Otherwise, skip the missed dose. Do not take double doses.

**What if I stop taking the drug?** Do not stop taking this drug without consulting your physician. Your physician may wish to taper off your doses to prevent withdrawal symptoms.

**How should I store the drug?** Keep out of reach of children. Store in a dry, tightly closed, light-resistant container. Heat and moisture may cause this drug to break down. As this drug has a high potential for abuse, we recommend that it be kept in a locked cabinet and that careful records be maintained to check for missing tablets.

## INTERACTIONS

**Alcohol:** Alcohol may aggravate the symptoms of attention-deficit hyperactivity disorder and react dangerously with central nervous system effects of dextroamphetamine.

**Food/Beverages:** No restrictions; however, caffeine may increase nervousness, anxiety, and other emotional side effects.

**Smoking:** No restrictions.

**Other drugs:** The danger of overdose is high when dextroamphetamine is combined with heterocyclic antidepressants.

Monoamine oxidase (MAO) inhibitors slow the absorption of amphetamines and can cause toxic blood levels. This drug should not be used with MAO inhibitors.

Antihistamines have a sedative effect that may counteract the effect of dextroamphetamine.

Take special care to consult your physician before taking any drug but especially the following drugs in combination with dextroamphetamine: chlorpromazine, ethosuximide, haloperidol, antihypertensive medications, meperidine, norepinephrine, phenytoin, propoxyphene, any beta blocker, digitalis, and thyroid hormones.

## HABIT-FORMING POTENTIAL

High.

## LONG-TERM USE

Addiction is primarily a problem with adults. It is extremely rare for children with attention-deficit hyperactivity disorder to become addicted. Because this drug has been widely abused by adults, its use is tightly regulated by the Food and Drug Administration. When high doses are taken for a long time, a person may experience severe side effects, including paranoia, delusions, and other psychoses. Children who take this drug on a long-term basis should be examined every four to six months. The physician should monitor height and weight, look for the presence of tics, measure blood pressure and pulse, and ask about side effects.

**DRUG NAME:**    Dextramphetamine (*continued*)

## PLEASE NOTE

Signs of amphetamine abuse: When abused, dextroamphetamine can cause an increase in the heart rate, elevated blood pressure, dilation of the pupils, and agitation. As dosages increase, more severe side effects—including irritability, confusion, hostility, and sleep disturbances—may be noticed. At the highest doses, a person's symptoms (bizarre thoughts, delusions, and agitation) may resemble common symptoms of schizophrenia.

Treatment for withdrawal: In most cases, a person who has abused dextroamphetamine and who is suffering withdrawal symptoms can be treated on an outpatient basis. Symptoms of withdrawal include fatigue, insomnia, or hypersomnia. An antipsychotic medication may be prescribed if a person is experiencing delusions, hallucinations, agitation, or confusion. Inpatient treatment may be required when the drug was taken intravenously, when a person is depressed or suicidal, or when a person has lost touch with reality.

Effects on growth in children: Stimulants may suppress the production of growth hormones and can reduce weight and height gain in growing children. In most cases, this lag is temporary. However, the effects on growth caused by long-term use of stimulants with children has lead some clinicians to believe that the drug should never be prescribed for children.

| Dextroamphetamine | | | | | | | |
|---|---|---|---|---|---|---|---|
| | Frequency | | Discuss with Physician | | | | |
| Symptom/Effect | Common | Rare | Not Necessary | In All Cases | Only If Severe | Stop Taking Drug Now | Call Physician Now |
| loss of appetite | X | | | | X | | |
| difficulty sleeping | X | | | | X | | |
| weight loss | X | | | X | | | |
| abdominal pain | | X | | X | | X | X |
| headache | | X | | X | | X | X |
| drowsiness | | X | | | X | | |
| dizziness | | X | | | X | | |
| mood changes | | X | | X | | | |
| lack of coordination | | X | | X | | X | |
| tics or unusual movements | | X | | X | | X | |
| irritability/nervousness | | X | | X | | | |
| skin rash or hives | | X | | X | | X | |
| blurred vision | | X | | X | | | |
| diarrhea | X | | | | X | | |
| nausea | X | | | | X | | |
| sexual problems | | X | | X | | | |
| paranoia | | X | | X | | X | X |

DRUG NAME: **Diazepam**

**BRAND NAMES:** T-Quil, Valium, Valrelease,
**For more information:** See Chapter 4, Antianxiety Drugs, and Chapter 9, Antiaddiction Drugs.

**FAST FACTS** **Drug group:** Antianxiety agents (benzodiazepines).
**Available as generic?** Yes.

**Prescription needed?** Yes. **Habit-forming?** Yes.

 **Overdose:** It is possible, though not easy, to overdose. Signs of toxicity include sedation, decreased breathing rate, confusion, and loss of coordination. If these symptoms are present, seek immediate emergency medical treatment.

## PRECAUTIONS

### Do not take this drug if:

- You have had previously negative reactions to benzodiazepines.
- You have had a history of drug dependence.
- You have Alzheimer's disease, have had a stroke, or have multiple sclerosis or other brain disorders.
- You are seriously depressed.

### Inform your physician if:

- You are taking any other drug—prescription or nonprescription—or vitamins.
- You have ever had an allergic reaction to any drug.
- You will be under anesthesia or undergoing surgery or medical testing in the next few months.

 **Pregnancy/Breast-feeding**

Do not take this drug if you are pregnant, planning a pregnancy, or breast-feeding.

 **Infants/Children**

Never give this drug to a child under six months. Never use with hyperactive or psychotic children. Watch carefully for excessive sedation and lack of coordination.

 **Over Sixty**

Smaller doses are advised and should be monitored very closely.

 **Driving/Operating Machinery**

WARNING: Do not fly, drive, or operate heavy machinery since this drug can impair mental alertness and coordination.

## GENERAL INFORMATION

Diazepam is most familiar as Valium, the trade name for tablets manufactured by the Hoffmann-La Roche pharmaceutical company. The drug also has several common street names: tranks, yellows, and downs. It is currently available under its generic name from seven drug companies. Diazepam is used primarily to provide short-term relief for mild to moderate anxiety; to treat symptoms of acute alcohol withdrawal (D.T.'s); to relieve muscle spasms; and to control epilepsy. As has been widely reported in the media, diazepam (Valium) is addictive. For an explanation of how this drug works, see Chapter 4.

**DRUG NAME:** Diazepam (*continued*)

| BENEFITS | RISKS |
|---|---|

**BENEFITS**
- More effective and fewer side effects than barbiturates.
- Less addictive and safer in overdoses than barbiturates.
- Relieves anxiety in about 65 percent to 70 percent of users.

**RISKS**
- Physically and psychologically addictive if misused.
- Makes some people feel lethargic, less able to concentrate, less alert.
- Can affect physical coordination.
- Highly dangerous when combined with alcohoi and certain other drugs.

## GUIDELINES FOR USERS

**How is the drug taken?** Tablets (2, 5, 10 mg); capsules; intramuscular; intravenous.

**What is the usual dosage?** The initial dose should be 2 mg to 5 mg per day in healthy young people, with increases as needed to control symptoms. Most experts advise beginning with a low, divided dose, (e.g., for a healthy adult male, three 2 mg tablets at eight-hour intervals during the day). The maximum daily dose usually does not exceed 40 mg.

**What are the instructions for taking the drug?** As with all benzodiazepines, if you are taking this drug for the first time, take your first dose at home and during a time when you are not required to work or drive. Your physician should tell you how often to take subsequent doses. Follow these instructions carefully. This drug can be taken before, during, or after meals. The capsules should not be opened. The tablets can be crushed and dissolved in water before taking, if you prefer.

**How quickly will I feel the effect of the drug and how long does it last?** Those who benefit from this drug will usually experience a positive response within the first week. Many people feel the drug's effect the first day of treatment.

**What if I miss a dose or several doses?** If you miss a dose and remember within an hour or so, take the missed dose. However, if more than an hour has elapsed, skip the dose and continue on your regular schedule. Do not take double doses.

**What if I stop taking the drug?** If you take this drug regularly for three weeks or more, you should not stop abruptly. Your dosage should be gradually reduced. Abrupt cessation can cause psychological and physical withdrawal symptoms.

**How should I store the drug?** Keep out of reach of children, since all benzodiazepines can be extremely dangerous to children. Store in a dry, tightly closed, light-resistant container. Heat and moisture may cause this drug to break down.

## INTERACTIONS

**Alcohol:** Do not drink alcohol. Diazepam is highly dangerous when combined with alcohol. It can dangerously lower blood pressure, decrease the breathing rate, and lead to loss of consciousness.

**Food/Beverages:** No restrictions on food. Control caffeine intake, as caffeine makes anxiety worse.

**Smoking:** Heavy smoking of tobacco may reduce the sedative effects of the drug. Marijuana smoking may increase many of the drug's side effects and significantly reduce mental alertness.

**Other drugs:** Narcotics (e.g., Demerol, Percodan, codeine, morphine, Talwin) may *increase* the sedative effects of this drug. The combination can be fatal. Do not use narcotics with this drug.

Barbiturates and other sedatives (e.g., phenobarbital, pentobarbital, Seconal, Tuinal) may *increase* sedation to dangerous levels. Do not combine sedatives with this drug.

Do not take other benzodiazepines when using this drug, since the combination is both unnecessary and unsafe.

Do not take sleeping pills while taking this drug. If you are having trouble sleeping, your doctor may prescribe larger doses of diazepam.

The following drugs may reduce the liver's ability to remove this drug from the body, making the drug more powerful and increasing side effects:

- ulcer drugs
- birth control pills
- propranolol
- disulfiram (Antabuse)

Diazepam may *decrease* the effects of levodopa (Sinemet, etc.) and reduce its effectiveness in treating Parkinson's disease.

## HABIT-FORMING POTENTIAL

High.

## LONG-TERM USE

Physical and psychological dependence are common problems. A clear treatment plan is important. It is possible to become dependent in as short a time span as two to four weeks. This drug should not be taken longer than four weeks on a regular basis (i.e., daily). Long-term use can also increase the risk of side effects.

## PLEASE NOTE

Use as a sleeping pill: Diazepam has strong sedative effects and may be used as a sleeping pill on an occasional basis. But this drug is excreted from the body rather slowly, and consequently can build up in the system and produce daytime sleepiness. Thus, shorter-acting benzodiazepines are generally more effective as sleeping pills.

Nondrug alternatives: See Chapter 4 for a discussion of the value of exercise and a good diet in the treatment of anxiety. One of the best nondrug ways to reduce anxiety is to identify and reduce sources of stress in your life.

Correct diagnosis: You should always consult a physician to be sure that any medical causes of anxiety (such as hyperthyroidism) are diagnosed and treated. Anxiety may be a component of depression, in which case the symptoms of anxiety are treated by treating the underlying depression with antidepressants and/or other therapies for mood disorders.

DRUG NAME:   Diazepam (*continued*)

**PLEASE NOTE** (*continued*)

Pregnancy studies: Research on the effects of diazepam on pregnant women is conflicting and inconclusive. It is important to note, however, that some studies have found an increase in serious birth defects when this drug is used. Frequent use in late pregnancy is a suspected cause of "floppy infant" syndrome.

| Diazepam | | | | | | | |
|---|---|---|---|---|---|---|---|
| | **Frequency** | | **Discuss with Physician** | | | | |
| **Symptom/Effect** | **Common** | **Rare** | **Not Necessary** | **In All Cases** | **Only If Severe** | **Stop Taking Drug Now** | **Call Physician Now** |
| clumsiness/sleepiness | X | | | | X | | |
| abdominal cramps | | X | | X | | | |
| blurred vision | | X | | X | | | |
| dry mouth | | X | | X | | | |
| racing heartbeat/ palpitations | | X | | X | | | |
| shaking/slurred speech | | X | | X | | | |
| urination problems | | X | | X | | | |
| convulsions | | X | | X | | X | X |
| hallucinations | | X | | X | | X | X |
| memory loss | | X | | X | | X | X |
| trouble breathing | | X | | X | | X | X |
| staggering/trembling | | X | | X | | X | X |
| headache | | X | | X | | | |
| confusion | | X | | X | | | X |

# DRUG NAME: **Diphenhydramine**

**BRAND NAMES:** Allerdryl, Benadryl, Dytuss
**For more information:** See Chapter 8, Sedatives and Sleeping Pills.

**FAST FACTS** **Drug groups:** Sedatives; antihistamines. **Available as generic?** Yes.
**Prescription needed?** No. **Habit-forming?** No.

 **Overdose:** Symptoms include severe drowsiness, convulsions, confusion, trouble breathing, and loss of coordination. If these symptoms are present, seek immediate emergency medical treatment.

## PRECAUTIONS

### Do not take this drug if:

- You have ever had an allergic reaction to this drug.

### Inform your physician if:

- You have ever had an allergic reaction to any drug.
- You have asthma, glaucoma, urinary problems, or an enlarged prostate.
- You are taking any other drug—prescription or nonprescription—or vitamins.
- You will be under anesthesia or undergoing surgery or medical testing in the next few months.
- You are now taking or have taken in the last two weeks an MAO inhibitor.

 **Pregnancy/Breast-feeding**

Do not take this drug if you are pregnant, planning a pregnancy, or are breast-feeding.

 **Infants/Children**

Children may take the drug, but only under the direction of a pediatrician and/or children's psychiatrist.

 **Over Sixty**

Elderly people are more sensitive to antihistamines. People over age sixty-five should not take this medication.

 **Driving/Operating Machinery**

WARNING: Do not fly, drive, or operate heavy machinery since this drug can impair mental alertness and coordination.

## GENERAL INFORMATION

Diphenhydramine is an antihistamine frequently used as a sleeping pill. It is also prescribed for people with Parkinson's disease to decrease stiffness and tremors. Antihistamines are sold over the counter and by prescription and are used primarily to treat allergies, motion sickness, nausea, vomiting, and dizziness. Because they cause drowsiness, they are also effective sleeping pills. Some physicians feel diphenhydramine is safer as a sleeping pill than benzodiazepines or barbiturates. Other physicians say there is inadequate research on the safety of antihistamines used as sleeping pills. Antihistamines are often prescribed for minor or short-term sleeping problems and for patients who have trouble falling asleep in the hospital. Diphenhydramine is rapidly absorbed by the body and quickly induces sleep. A combination product with acetaminophen is available. However, combination products are not recommended.

**DRUG NAME:**  Diphenhydramine (*continued*)

## BENEFITS

- No risk of addiction.
- Little daytime drowsiness.

## RISKS

- Generally not so effective as the benzodiazepines in inducing sleep.

## GUIDELINES FOR USERS

**How is the drug taken?** Capsules (25, 50 mg); syrup.

**What is the usual dosage?** The initial dose for insomnia should be 25 mg in healthy young people. Occasionally, 50 mg to 70 mg may be used to induce sleep.

**What are the instructions for taking the drug?** Your dose should be taken at bedtime with a full glass of water to prevent stomach upset. The syrup may be mixed with water or juice to improve the taste and prevent stomach upset.

**How quickly will I feel the effect of the drug and how long does it last?** This drug is rapidly absorbed by the body and when taken for insomnia should rapidly induce sleep.

**What if I miss a dose or several doses?** If you miss a dose, skip the missed dose. Do not take double doses.

**What if I stop taking the drug?** If your physician has prescribed this drug for a sleeping problem, do not stop taking it without consulting your physician.

**How should I store the drug?** Keep out of reach of children. Store in a dry, tightly closed, light-resistant container. Heat and moisture may cause this drug to break down.

## INTERACTIONS

**Alcohol:** Do not drink alcohol. Diphenhydramine increases the effect of alcohol. In addition, alcohol can contribute to insomnia.

**Food/Beverages:** No restrictions on food. Control caffeine intake, as caffeine can contribute to insomnia.

**Smoking:** Heavy smoking of tobacco may reduce the sedative effects of this drug. Marijuana smoking may increase many of the drug's side effects and significantly reduce mental alertness.

**Other drugs:** Do not use narcotics, barbiturates, or other sedatives with this drug.

Diphenhydramine will *increase* the effect of other CNS (central nervous system) depressants. Examples include hay fever medicines, sedatives, narcotics, muscle relaxants, barbiturates, and anesthetics. Check with your physician before taking any of these drugs.

## HABIT-FORMING POTENTIAL

None.

## LONG-TERM USE

Poses no danger.

## Diphenhydramine

| Symptom/Effect | Frequency | | Discuss with Physician | | | Stop Taking Drug Now | Call Physician Now |
|---|---|---|---|---|---|---|---|
| | Common | Rare | Not Necessary | In All Cases | Only If Severe | | |
| nausea/vomiting | | X | | X | | | |
| headache | | X | | X | | | |
| dizziness | X | | | | X | | |
| coordination problems | | X | | X | | | |
| blurred vision | | X | | X | | | |
| tightness of the chest | | X | | X | | X | X |
| wheezing | | X | | X | | | |
| abnormal heartbeat | | X | | X | | | |
| dry mouth, nose | X | | | | X | | |
| nervous/restless | | X | | X | | | |
| drowsy/sedated | X | | | | X | | |
| confusion | | X | | X | | X | X |
| insomnia | | X | | X | | | |
| flushing | | X | | X | | X | X |
| seizures | | X | | X | | X | X |
| hallucinations | | X | | X | | X | X |
| problems urinating | | X | | X | | X | X |
| nightmares | | X | | X | | X | X |
| skin rash | | X | | X | | X | X |

DRUG NAME: **Disulfiram**

**BRAND NAME:** Antabuse
**For more information:** See Chapter 9, Antiaddiction Drugs.

FAST FACTS  **Drug group:** Antiaddiction agents.     **Available as generic?** Yes.
**Prescription needed?** Yes.     **Habit-forming?** No.

 **Overdose:** This drug is most dangerous when used with alcohol. Serious elevations of blood pressure may result. Seek emergency medical treatment.

## PRECAUTIONS

**Do not take this drug if:**

- You have ever had an allergic reaction to this drug.

**Inform your physician if:**

- You have ever had an allergic reaction to any drug.
- You have epilepsy.
- You have had a stroke.
- You have heart, kidney, or liver disease.
- You have skin allergies.
- You are taking any other drug—prescription or nonprescription —or vitamins.
- You will be under anesthesia or undergoing surgery or medical testing in the next few months.

 **Pregnancy/Breast-feeding**

If you are pregnant or planning a pregnancy, you should, if possible, use non-drug alternatives. This drug has not been demonstrated to be safe during pregnancy. Women who are breast-feeding should not take this drug.

 **Infants/Children**

Do not give to children.

 **Over Sixty**

No research is available.

**Driving/Operating Machinery**

 This medicine can cause drowsiness. Do not drive or operate machinery until you are certain this drug will not affect your performance.

## GENERAL INFORMATION

Disulfiram is an aversive drug that combines with alcohol to make the user sick. The reaction—which can include weakness, vomiting, throbbing in the head, dizziness, blurred vision, and confusion—discourages the person from drinking. This drug is normally prescribed only after other methods to treat alcoholism have failed. Because of the potential for a serious reaction if combined with alcohol, it is used only as part of an inpatient treatment program or under careful medical monitoring.

## BENEFITS

- Used in combination with other treatments, it can aid an alcohol-dependent person in resisting the temptation to drink.

## RISKS

- Severe reaction, and even death, if combined with alcohol.

## GUIDELINES FOR USERS

**How is the drug taken?** Tablets (250, 500 mg).

**What is the usual dosage?** The initial dose is usually 500 mg, which is reduced to a maintenance dose of 250 mg. However, daily doses can vary from 125 mg to 500 mg depending on the person. Before taking the first dose, it is very important that the person not have consumed alcohol for at least twelve hours.

**What are the instructions for taking the drug?** Patients are normally instructed to take their dose in the morning, unless drowsiness occurs.

**How quickly will I feel the effect of the drug and how long does it last?** Within twelve hours of taking the drug, it can produce an alcohol-drug reaction. The drug will continue to react with alcohol for two weeks. If you consume any alcohol during that time, you will become violently ill.

**What if I miss a dose or several doses?** If you realize you have missed a dose, take your regular dose, then continue the following day as prescribed. If you have missed several doses, do not drink alcohol, since the drug remains in your system and you will become violently ill.

**What if I stop taking the drug?** Contact your physician or alcohol treatment center to discuss your decision to discontinue the drug. Do not drink any alcohol for at least two weeks.

**How should I store the drug?** Keep out of reach of children. Store in a dry, tightly closed, light-resistant container. Heat and moisture may cause this drug to break down.

## INTERACTIONS

**Alcohol:** Do not drink alcohol. Drinking even a small amount of alcohol with this drug may result in breathing problems, nausea, chest pain, heart palpitations, dizziness, and confusion. A severe reaction can lead to heart failure, coma, seizures, and death. Also avoid alcohol in sauces, desserts, and cough medicines. Do not breathe vapors from substances that may contain alcohol, such as perfume and some paints. Do not use any alcohol products on the skin.

**Food/Beverages:** No restrictions.

**Smoking:** No restrictions.

**Other drugs:** Disulfiram should be used cautiously by people taking Dilantin (phenytoin) for seizures, since the metabolism of Dilantin by the liver may be considerably decreased and Dilantin may build up in your body to dangerous levels.

## HABIT-FORMING POTENTIAL

None.

## LONG-TERM USE

Poses no danger.

**DRUG NAME:**    Disulfiram (*continued*)

| | Frequency | | Discuss with Physician | | | | |
|---|---|---|---|---|---|---|---|
| **Symptom/Effect** | **Common** | **Rare** | **Not Necessary** | **In All Cases** | **Only If Severe** | **Stop Taking Drug Now** | **Call Physician Now** |
| drowsiness | X | | | | X | | |
| decreased sexual ability | | X | | X | | | |
| headache | | X | | X | | | |
| skin rash | | X | | | X | X | X |
| upset stomach | | X | | | X | | |
| eye problems | | X | | X | | | |
| numbness/tingling | | X | | X | | | |
| jaundice | | X | | X | | X | X |

DRUG NAME: **Doxepin**

**BRAND NAMES:** Adapin, Sinequan
**For more information:** See Chapter 3, Antidepressant Drugs.

**FAST FACTS**   **Drug group:** Antidepressants.     **Available as generic?** Yes.
**Prescription needed?** Yes.     **Habit-forming?** No.

**Overdose:** The danger of an overdose, which can be lethal, is extremely high. Symptoms include difficulty breathing, shock, agitation, delirium, and coma. Seek immediate emergency medical treatment.

## PRECAUTIONS

### Do not take this drug if:

- You have ever had an allergic or negative reaction to any drug in this group.

### Inform your physician if:

- You have ever had an allergic reaction to any drug.
- You have epilepsy or glaucoma.
- You are taking any other drug— prescription or nonprescription —or vitamins.
- You will be under anesthesia or undergoing surgery or medical testing in the next few months.

### Pregnancy/Breast-feeding

If you are pregnant or planning a pregnancy, you should, if possible, use non-drug alternatives for treating your depression. This drug has not been demonstrated to be safe during pregnancy. Nursing mothers should not take this drug since it is passed on to the baby in the mother's milk.

### Infants/Children

The safety of this drug has not been established for children under age twelve. Its use in the treatment of depression in children and adolescents must be under the guidance of a child psychiatrist.

### Over Sixty

In general, lower doses are required. Side effects may be worse and some older patients may experience confusion. Elderly people may fall after standing up because of the drug's hypotensive (blood pressure lowering) side effects.

### Driving/Operating Machinery

Extreme caution is advised. This medicine can impair mental alertness and coordination. If you do drive or operate machinery, this medicine should be taken at bedtime when its sedating effects are less likely to interfere with daytime activities.

**DRUG NAME:**    Doxepin (*continued*)

## GENERAL INFORMATION

Doxepin is one of the heterocyclic drugs used to treat depression. It works by inhibiting the nerve cell's ability to reabsorb the neurotransmitters norepinephrine and serotonin (see Chapter 3). Doxepin is among the more sedating heterocyclic drugs. Brands include Adapin manufactured by Pennwalt and Sinequan made by Roerig. Generic manufacturers include Barr, Danbury, Geneva, Lederle, Martec, Mylan, and Par.

## BENEFITS

- Helps 75 percent to 80 percent of people with major depression.

## RISKS

- Produces annoying side effects.
- Potential for use in suicide attempts.

## GUIDELINES FOR USERS

**How is the drug taken?** Capsules (10, 25, 75, 100, 150 mg); oral concentrate.

**What is the usual dosage?** The initial dose is usually 75 mg daily in divided doses. This can be increased gradually to 150 mg daily. Some people may require 200 mg to 300 mg daily. Initial doses are lower for patients with medical illnesses and the elderly.

**What are the instructions for taking the drug?** Take this medicine with food, unless your doctor has instructed you otherwise. Taking the medicine on an empty stomach may cause your stomach to become upset. To benefit from the drug, it is important to take the correct dosage each day.

**How quickly will I feel the effect of the drug?** You will probably experience some unpleasant side effects (dry mouth, blurry vision, constipation) right away. It may take days or weeks for the benefits to appear. It usually takes two to four weeks at full dose for a person to feel a positive response. By the third week of treatment, the side effects are usually less severe.

**What if I miss a dose or several doses?** If you are taking one dose at bedtime and miss your dose, do not take the drug in the morning. Check with your doctor. If you are taking more than one dose a day and remember within an hour or so that you have missed a dose, take the dose. However, if it is almost time for your next dose, skip the missed dose. Do not take double doses.

**What if I stop taking the drug?** Do not discontinue this drug abruptly. Your dosage should be gradually reduced. Stopping the drug abruptly may cause flulike symptoms, headache, restlessness, and/or a worsening of your condition. Inform your physician if you notice these side effects, or any others, after stopping the drug. The effects of this drug may last for up to seven days after you have stopped taking it.

**How should I store the drug?** Keep out of reach of children. Store in a dry, tightly closed, light-resistant container. Heat and moisture may cause this drug to break down.

## INTERACTIONS

**Alcohol:** Do not drink alcohol. Doxepin *increases* the effect of alcohol, while alcohol *increases* the side effects of the drug. In addition, alcohol use can contribute to depression.

**Food/Beverages:** No restrictions.

**Smoking:** Smoking lowers the blood level of doxepin. If you do smoke, blood samples should be taken to test whether the drug is in the therapeutic range.

**Other drugs:** Doxepin will increase the effect of medicines known as CNS (central nervous system) depressants. Examples include antihistamines, hay fever medicines, sedatives, narcotics, muscle relaxants, barbiturates, and anesthetics. Check with your physician before taking any of these drugs.

## HABIT-FORMING POTENTIAL

None.

## LONG-TERM USE

Most people who have a beneficial response do not need to take this drug longer than about six months. A few people may need to take the drug for a year or longer because their depression recurs if they attempt to discontinue the drug.

## PLEASE NOTE

Help with side effects: Drinking water and sucking on hard candy can help if you are experiencing dry mouth. To prevent constipation, eat high-fiber foods and take a daily dose of a natural bulk laxative. And you can avoid episodes of light-headedness by making sure you get up slowly from a sitting or prone position. These side effects generally get better or go away after you have been on the drug several weeks.

| Doxepin | | | | | | | |
|---|---|---|---|---|---|---|---|
| | **Frequency** | | **Discuss with Physician** | | | | |
| **Symptom/Effect** | **Common** | **Rare** | **Not Necessary** | **In All Cases** | **Only If Severe** | **Stop Taking Drug Now** | **Call Physician Now** |
| drowsiness | X | | | | X | | |
| dry mouth | X | | | | X | | |
| constipation | X | | | | X | | |
| blurred vision | X | | | | X | | |
| low blood pressure | X | | | X | | | |
| racing heartbeat/ palpitations | | X | | | X | | |
| confusion | | X | | X | | | |
| skin rashes/allergies | | X | | X | | X | X |
| insomnia | | X | | | X | | |
| sexual problems | | X | | X | | | |
| increased appetite | | X | | | X | | |
| seizures | | X | | X | | X | X |

DRUG NAME: **Fluoxetine**

**BRAND NAME:** Prozac
**For more information:** See Chapter 3, Antidepressant Drugs.

**FAST FACTS**  **Drug group:** Antidepressants.   **Available as generic?** No.
**Prescription needed?** Yes.   **Habit-forming?** No.

 **Overdose:** Symptoms of overdose include agitation, convulsions, and nausea. Seek immediate emergency medical treatment. Although it appears that overdoses with this drug are rarely fatal, more data are required to assess fully its safety in situations of overdose.

## PRECAUTIONS

**Do not take this drug if:**

• You have ever had an allergic or negative reaction to this drug.

**Inform your physician if:**

• You have ever had an allergic reaction to any drug.
• You have epilepsy, kidney disease, or liver disease.
• You are taking any other drug— prescription or nonprescription —or vitamins.
• You will be under anesthesia or undergoing surgery or medical testing in the next few months.

 **Pregnancy/Breast-feeding**

If you are pregnant or planning a pregnancy, you should, if possible, use non-drug alternatives for treating your depression. This drug has not been demonstrated to be safe during pregnancy. Nursing mothers should not take this drug since it is passed on to the baby in the mother's milk.

 **Infants/Children**

This drug has not been tested in children and is not recommended for use in infants or children.

 **Over Sixty**

Lower doses may be required and side effects may be worse.

 **Driving/Operating Machinery**

This drug causes drowsiness in some people. It is best to avoid driving for the first several days of treatment—until you are certain that your alertness and coordination are not affected by the drug.

## GENERAL INFORMATION

Fluoxetine is a serotonin-specific drug used to treat depression and several other psychological problems. At one time, fluoxetine was prescribed for depression only if a patient failed to respond to the heterocyclic antidepressants. However, more and more physicians are prescribing this drug as a "first-line" treatment for depression. Fluoxetine is also used to treat obsessive-compulsive disorder and may have some antipanic, antiphobic effects. For an explanation of how this drug works, see Chapter 3.

## BENEFITS

- Fewer cardiovascular side effects and less sedating than heterocyclic drugs.
- Better tolerated by people with heart disease, stroke, Alzheimer's disease.
- Higher margin of overdose safety than heterocyclics.
- Not associated with weight gain.

## RISKS

- Some people become highly anxious when taking this drug.
- Some people have difficulty sleeping.

## GUIDELINES FOR USERS

**How is drug taken?** Capsules (20 mg); liquid (20 mg per 5 cc).

**What is the usual dosage?** The initial dose is 20 mg daily. If no improvement is seen after three weeks, the dose may be gradually increased to a maximum 60 mg daily. Some people may be maintained on 20 mg of the drug every other day. People being treated for obsessive-compulsive disorder generally require higher doses (80 mg to 100 mg daily).

**What are the instructions for taking the drug?** This drug should be taken in the morning following your physician's instructions. The capsules can be opened and dissolved in water before taking, if you prefer. Be sure to wash your hands after breaking the capsule, as the powder may be irritating to your eyes. For long-term use at doses below 20 mg, the liquid may be preferred.

**How quickly will I feel the effect of the drug?** It could take as long as three or four weeks before you experience a positive response to this drug.

**What if I miss a dose or several doses?** If you miss a dose, skip the missed dose and continue on your regular dosing schedule. Do not take double doses.

**What if I stop taking the drug?** Do not discontinue this drug abruptly. Your dosage should be gradually reduced. With gradual tapering of this medication, you should experience very few, if any, withdrawal symptoms.

**How should I store the drug?** Keep out of reach of children. Store in a dry, tightly closed, light-resistant container. Heat and moisture may cause this drug to break down.

## INTERACTIONS

**Alcohol:** Do not drink alcohol since fluoxetine can increase its effects. In addition, alcohol use can contribute to depression.

**Food/Beverages:** No restrictions.

**Smoking:** Smoking may lower the blood level of fluoxetine and this may reduce the drug's efficiency in treating depression.

**Other drugs:** Fluoxetine may increase the effect of medicines known as CNS (central nervous system) depressants. Examples include antihistamines, hay fever medicines, sedatives, narcotics, muscle relaxants, barbiturates, and anesthetics. Check with your physician before taking any of these drugs.

DRUG NAME: Fluoxetine (*continued*)

## HABIT-FORMING POTENTIAL

None.

## LONG-TERM USE

Most people may be tapered safely from the medication six months after their depression has responded to treatment. A small percentage of patients have symptoms of depression return after their dosage is reduced. These individuals may benefit from remaining on fluoxetine for a year or longer.

| Fluoxetine | | | | | | | |
|---|---|---|---|---|---|---|---|
| | Frequency | | Discuss with Physician | | | | |
| Symptom/Effect | Common | Rare | Not Necessary | In All Cases | Only If Severe | Stop Taking Drug Now | Call Physician Now |
| anxiety/nervousness | X | | | X | | | |
| nausea | | X | | X | | | |
| trouble sleeping | | X | | X | | | |
| headache | | X | | X | | | |
| sedation | | X | | | X | | |
| diarrhea | | X | | | X | | |
| abnormal sweating | | X | | X | | | |
| constipation | | X | | | X | | |
| change in appetite | | X | | X | | | |
| seizure | | X | | X | | X | X |
| skin rash | | X | | X | | X | X |
| stomach cramps | | X | | X | | | |

## PLEASE NOTE

The controversy about Prozac: In 1991 there were highly publicized charges that fluoxetine induced suicidality and violent behavior among patients who were neither violent nor suicidal prior to their taking the antidepressant. The FDA, the American Psychiatric Association, the Alcohol, Drug Abuse, and Mental Health Adminstration, and the National Mental Health Association subsequently spoke in favor of Prozac, when properly prescribed and used. The experience of the authors is that fluoxetine is a highly safe and unusually effective drug. As we have stated elsewhere in this book, with regard to the treatment of depression the greatest danger lies for those who do *not* receive, when warranted, appropriate treatment with antidepressant drugs.

# DRUG NAME: Fluphenazine

**BRAND NAMES:** Permitil, Prolixin, Prolixin Decanoate, Prolixin Enanthate
**For more information:** See Chapter 7, Antipsychotic Drugs.

**FAST FACTS**   **Drug group:** Antipsychotics.    **Available as generic?** Yes.
**Prescription needed?** Yes.    **Habit-forming?** No.

 **Overdose:** Symptoms include light-headedness, sedation, agitation, confusion, restlessness, disorientation, convulsions, fever, and coma. Seek immediate emergency medical treatment.

## PRECAUTIONS

### Do not take this drug if:

- You have ever had an allergic reaction to this drug or any other phenothiazine.

### Inform your physician if:

- You have ever had an allergic reaction to any drug.
- You have epilepsy or asthma.
- You are taking any other drug— prescription or nonprescription —or vitamins.
- You are on a low-salt, low-sugar, or any other special diet.
- You will be under anesthesia or undergoing surgery or medical testing in the next few months.

 **Pregnancy/Breast-feeding**

Except in unusual cases where the mother or the baby's life is endangered, this drug should not be taken by pregnant women. Women taking fluphenazine should not breast-feed.

 **Infants/Children**

Safety and effectiveness have not been established.

 **Over Sixty**

Side effects, some serious, can be worse. Initial dose should be low, with careful monitoring for side effects. Special care should be taken when sitting up from a lying position, or standing from a sitting position, as blood pressure may be lowered and balance impaired.

 **Driving/Operating Machinery**

Extreme caution is advised. This medicine can impair mental alertness and coordination. If you do drive or operate machinery, this medicine should be taken at bedtime when its sedating effects are less likely to interfere with daytime activities.

## GENERAL INFORMATION

Fluphenazine is a high-potency antipsychotic used to treat people who are experiencing disorganized, psychotic thinking and perceptions, such as delusions and hallucinations. High-potency antipsychotics are more likely to cause movement side effects such as dystonic reactions, parkinsonian features, and akathisia, but they are less sedating and

**DRUG NAME:**  Fluphenazine (*continued*)

## GENERAL INFORMATION (*continued*)

cause fewer problems with low blood pressure. The choice of which antipsychotic drug to use is often determined by side effects. For an explanation of how this drug works, see Chapter 7.

| BENEFITS | RISKS |
|---|---|
| • Effective in treating hallucinations, delusions, confused thinking, and mania.<br>• Less sedating than many other phenothiazines.<br>• Long-acting injectable form is useful for patients who may forget to take doses or who are not compliant with their treatment plan. | • May dangerously lower white blood cell count.<br>• Can cause tardive dyskinesia.<br>• Can cause neuroleptic malignant syndrome. |

## GUIDELINES FOR USERS

**How is the drug taken?** Tablets (1, 2.5, 5, 10 mg); oral concentrate; intramuscular; long-acting injectable (decanoate and enanthate forms).

**What is the usual dosage?** The initial dose should be 2.5 mg to 10 mg per day in healthy young people, with increases as needed to control symptoms. A maximum daily dose of up to 40 mg may be used if necessary. Maintenance doses should be as low as possible, ideally in the range of 1 mg to 5 mg per day, and still be able to control the psychotic symptoms.

**What are the instructions for taking the drug?** It is best to take this drug on an empty stomach, with a full glass of water.

**How quickly will I feel the effect of the drug?** It usually takes several weeks for you to experience the full benefit of this drug. However, you may feel more calm and relaxed after the first dose or two. The drug should also help you sleep better, if this is a problem.

**What if I miss a dose or several doses?** If you miss a dose and remember within an hour or so, take the missed dose. Otherwise, skip the missed dose and continue on your regular dosing schedule. Do not take double doses.

If you are missing doses on a frequent basis, notify your psychiatrist. A slow-release form of this drug or another antipsychotic drug may help with your compliance and help avoid a relapse.

**What if I stop taking the drug?** Do not stop taking this drug without consulting your physician. Abruptly stopping this medication will lead to uncomfortable but not dangerous physical symptoms. Should your physician and you agree that the drug should be discontinued, your medication should be tapered slowly to prevent physical symptoms of withdrawal and a reemergence of your psychotic symptoms.

**How should I store the drug?** Keep out of reach of children. Store in a dry, tightly closed, light-resistant container. Heat and moisture may cause this drug to break down. The liquid form does not require refrigeration.

## INTERACTIONS

**Alcohol:** Avoid alcohol. When combined with alcohol, this medicine can cause excessive sedation and dangerously lower blood pressure.

**Food/Beverages:** No restrictions.

**Smoking:** Smoking lowers the blood level of fluphenazine. If you do smoke, blood samples should be taken to test whether the drug is in the therapeutic range.

**Other drugs:** Antacids with aluminum or magnesium (Maalox, for example) should not be taken for two hours before or after taking fluphenazine because they may interfere with the absorption of this drug.

Heterocyclic antidepressants can increase the plasma level of this drug and cause a worsening of side effects. Conversely, this drug can increase the blood level of antidepressants. The concurrent use of these two types of drugs must be carefully monitored.

Blood pressure can be dangerously lowered when antipsychotics are combined with vasodilators (medications that dilate blood vessels.)

Fluphenazine will increase the effect of medicines known as CNS (central nervous system) depressants. Examples include antihistamines, hay fever medicines, sedatives, narcotics, muscle relaxants, barbiturates, and anesthetics. Check with your physician before taking any of these drugs.

## HABIT-FORMING POTENTIAL

None.

## LONG-TERM USE

Prolonged use of fluphenazine is associated with increased risk of developing tardive dyskinesia, a potentially irreversible side effect involving disfiguring movements of the face, tongue, and limbs. For more information on tardive dyskinesia, please see Chapter 7.

## PLEASE NOTE

Not a sleeping pill: This drug, which has a sedating effect, is sometimes misused as a sleeping pill. There are much safer medications available as sleeping aids.

Not specifically antiaggressive: Because of the potential serious side effects of the antipsychotic drugs, especially over the long term, this medication should not be used to treat anxiety or chronic aggression and agitation.

Frequent examinations required: While taking this medication, your blood pressure and pulse rate should be monitored frequently. Regular checks should also be made for the early signs of tardive dyskinesia.

**DRUG NAME:**  Fluphenazine (*continued*)

**PLEASE NOTE** (*continued*)

Classification: Fluphenazine is classified as a phenothiazine. Other antipsychotics in the same group include acetophenazine, chlorpromazine, mesoridazine, perphenazine, promazine, thioridazine, trifluoperazine, and triflupromazine. In general, if you have a poor response to one drug in this family, you will likely have a similar poor response to other drugs in the family.

| Fluphenazine | | | | | | | |
|---|---|---|---|---|---|---|---|
| | Frequency | | Discuss with Physician | | | | |
| Symptom/Effect | Common | Rare | Not Necessary | In All Cases | Only If Severe | Stop Taking Drug Now | Call Physician Now |
| lethargy/sleepiness | X | | | | X | | |
| low blood pressure | X | | | X | | | |
| dizziness | | X | | X | | | |
| dry mouth | X | | | | X | | |
| blurred vision | X | | | | X | | |
| constipation | X | | | | X | | |
| difficulty urinating | X | | | X | | | |
| reduced urinary output | | X | | X | | | X |
| racing heartbeat/ palpitations | | X | | X | | | |
| weakness | | X | | X | | | |
| sexual problems | | X | | X | | | |
| restlessness | | X | | X | | | |
| skin rash | | X | | X | | | |
| weight gain | X | | | | X | | |
| seizures | | X | | X | | X | X |
| low white blood cell count | | X | | X | | | X |
| tremors | | X | | X | | | |
| stiffness | X | | | X | | | |
| involuntary facial or tongue movements | | X | | X | | | |

# DRUG NAME: Flurazepam

**BRAND NAME:** Dalmane
**For more information:** See Chapter 8, Sedatives and Sleeping Pills, and Chapter 4, Antianxiety Drugs.

**FAST FACTS**   **Drug group:** Sedatives (benzodiazepines).

**Available as generic?** Yes.

**Prescription needed?** Yes.

**Habit-forming?** Yes.

 **Overdose:** The overdose danger is especially high when this drug is combined with alcohol. Signs of toxicity include sedation, a decreased breathing rate, confusion, and loss of coordination. If these symptoms are present, seek immediate emergency medical treatment.

## PRECAUTIONS

### Do not take this drug if:

- You have ever had an allergic reaction to this drug or any other benzodiazepine.
- You have a chronic breathing problem.
- You have kidney or liver disease.

### Inform your physician if:

- You have ever had an allergic reaction to any drug.
- You are taking any other drug—prescription or nonprescription—or vitamins.
- You have a history of alcohol or drug dependency.
- You have epilepsy.
- You will be under anesthesia or undergoing surgery or medical testing in the next few months.

 **Pregnancy/Breast-feeding**

Do not take this drug if you are pregnant, planning a pregnancy, or are breast-feeding. Some benzodiazepines are associated with birth defects.

 **Infants/Children**

Do not give this drug to children. Safety and effectiveness for children have not been established.

 **Over Sixty**

People over age sixty should take this medication only under strict medical supervision.

 **Driving/Operating Machinery**

This drug may impair mental alertness and coordination. Do not drive or operate machinery until you are certain this drug will not affect your performance.

## GENERAL INFORMATION

Flurazepam was the first benzodiazepine to be approved for use principally as a sleeping pill. It has a half-life of between two to four days, meaning half the drug will still be in your body two to four days after you take it. With daily use, it builds up in the body rapidly, and daytime drowsiness can become a problem, particularly in older people.

**DRUG NAME:**    Flurazepam (*continued*)

## BENEFITS

- More effective and fewer side effects than barbiturates in treating insomnia.
- Safer than barbiturates when taken in overdose.

## RISKS

- Overdose danger, especially when combined with alcohol.
- Can interfere with breathing and be dangerous in people with chronic respiratory problems.
- Physically and psychologically addictive if misused.
- Can sometimes worsen original sleep problem.
- Potentially harmful to kidneys, liver, and lungs.
- Birth defects are possible if this drug is taken during pregnancy; central nervous system depression of the newborn occurs if the drug is taken during the last weeks of pregnancy.

## GUIDELINES FOR USERS

**How is the drug taken?** Tablets (15 and 30 mg).

**What is the usual dosage?** The initial dose should be 15 mg in healthy young people. The dose may be increased to 30 mg per evening if required.

**What are the instructions for taking the drug?** As with all benzodiazepines, if you are taking this drug for the first time, take your first dose at home and during a time when you are not required to work or drive. Your physician should tell you how often to take subsequent doses. Follow these instructions carefully. This drug can be taken before, during, or after meals. The tablets can be crushed and dissolved in water before taking, if you prefer.

**How quickly will I feel the effect of the drug and how long does it last?** If you are taking this drug for insomnia, you should sleep better the first night. However, the full effect of the drug may not be felt for two or three nights.

**What if I miss a dose or several doses?** If you miss a dose and remember within an hour or so, take the missed dose. However, if more than an hour has elapsed, skip the dose and continue on your regular schedule. Do not take double doses.

**What if I stop taking the drug?** If you take this drug regularly for three weeks or more, you should not stop abruptly. Your dosage should be gradually reduced. Abrupt cessation can cause psychological and physical withdrawal symptoms.

**How should I store the drug?** Keep out of reach of children and in a locked cabinet. This drug has a high potential for abuse. Store in a dry, tightly closed, light-resistant container. Heat and moisture may cause this drug to break down.

## INTERACTIONS

**Alcohol:** Do not drink alcohol. Flurazepam is highly dangerous when combined with alcohol. It can dangerously lower blood pressure, decrease the breathing rate, and lead to loss of consciousness.

**Food/Beverages:** No restrictions on food. Control caffeine intake, as caffeine can contribute to insomnia.

**Smoking:** Heavy smoking of tobacco may reduce the sedative effects of the drug. Marijuana smoking may increase many of the drug's side effects and significantly reduce mental alertness.

**Other drugs:** Narcotics (e.g., Demerol, Percodan, codeine, morphine, Talwin) may *increase* the sedative effects of this drug. The combination can be fatal. Do not use narcotics with this drug.

Barbiturates and other sedatives (e.g., phenobarbital, pentobarbital, Seconal, Tuinal) may *increase* sedation to dangerous levels. Do not combine other sedatives or sleeping pills with this drug.

Do not take other benzodiazepines when using this drug, since the combination is both unnecessary and unsafe.

The following drugs may reduce the liver's ability to remove this drug from the body, making the drug more powerful and increasing its side effects:
- ulcer drugs
- birth control pills
- propranolol
- disulfiram (Antabuse)

## HABIT-FORMING POTENTIAL

High.

## LONG-TERM USE

With continued use, people taking flurazepam will have as much of the drug in their system during the day as during the night. Physical and psychological dependence are common problems. It is possible to become dependent in as short a time span as two to four weeks. This drug should not be taken longer than four weeks. Long-term use increases the risk of side effects and dependency.

## PLEASE NOTE

If you use this drug for a week or more, you may find that when you stop taking the drug, your insomnia is worse than before. This is called *rebound insomnia*. Taking flurazepam again will not solve the problem. Nondrug treatments or a gradual tapering of the benzodiazepine will be required.

**DRUG NAME:**    Flurazepam (*continued*)

| Symptom/Effect | Frequency | | Discuss with Physician | | | Stop Taking Drug Now | Call Physician Now |
|---|---|---|---|---|---|---|---|
| | Common | Rare | Not Necessary | In All Cases | Only If Severe | | |
| clumsiness/sleepiness | X | | | | X | | |
| abdominal cramps | | X | | X | | | |
| blurred vision | | X | | X | | | |
| dry mouth | | X | | X | | | |
| fast heartbeat | | X | | X | | | |
| shaking/slurred speech | | X | | X | | | |
| urination problems | | X | | X | | | |
| convulsions | | X | | X | | X | X |
| hallucinations | | X | | X | | X | X |
| memory loss | | X | | X | | | |
| trouble breathing | | X | | X | | X | X |
| staggering/trembling | | X | | X | | X | X |
| headache | | X | | X | | | |
| confusion | | X | | X | | | |

# DRUG NAME: Haloperidol

**BRAND NAMES:** Haldol, Haldol Decanoate
**For more information:** See Chapter 7, Antipsychotic Drugs.

## FAST FACTS

**Drug group:** Antipsychotics.
**Prescription needed?** Yes.

**Available as generic?** Yes.
**Habit-forming?** No.

 **Overdose:** Symptoms include light-headedness, sedation, confusion, agitation, disorientation, restlessness, shock, muscle tremors, and coma. Seek immediate emergency medical treatment.

## PRECAUTIONS

### Do not take this drug if:

- You have ever had an allergic reaction to this drug.

### Inform your physician if:

- You have ever had an allergic reaction to any drug.
- You have epilepsy or asthma.
- You are taking any other drug—prescription or nonprescription—or vitamins.
- You are on a low-salt, low-sugar, or other special diet.
- You will be under anesthesia or undergoing surgery or medical testing in the next few months.

 ### Pregnancy/Breast-feeding

Except in unusual cases where the mother or the baby's life is endangered, this drug should not be taken by pregnant women. Women taking haloperidol should not breast-feed.

 ### Infants/Children

Children may take the drug, but only under the direction of a pediatrician and/or children's psychiatrist.

 ### Over Sixty

Side effects, some serious, can be worse in the elderly. Initial dose should be low, with careful monitoring for side effects. Special care should be taken when sitting up from a lying position, or standing from a sitting position, as blood pressure may be lowered and balance impaired.

 ### Driving/Operating Machinery

Extreme caution is advised. This medicine can impair mental alertness and co-ordination. If you do drive or operate machinery, this medicine should be taken at bedtime when its sedating effects are less likely to interfere with daytime activities.

## GENERAL INFORMATION

Haloperidol is a high-potency antipsychotic used to treat people who are experiencing disorganized, psychotic thinking such as paranoia and delusions and impaired perceptions such as auditory hallucinations. In addition, haloperidol is frequently prescribed

**DRUG NAME:** Haloperidol (*continued*)

## GENERAL INFORMATION (*continued*)

to treat the neurologic disorder Gilles de la Tourette syndrome. High-potency antipsychotics are more likely to cause movement side effects such as dystonic reactions, parkinsonian features, and agitated restlessness (akathisia), but they are less sedating than the low-potency antipsychotics and cause fewer problems with low blood pressure and the cardiovascular system. Many psychiatrists prescribe an anticholinergic medication with haloperidol to reduce its movement side effects. Haloperidol is also available in a long-acting, injectable form. For an explanation of how this drug works, see Chapter 7.

## BENEFITS

- Effective in treating hallucinations, delusions, confused thinking, and mania.
- Effective in treating Gilles de la Tourette syndrome.
- Injectable form helpful for people who forget to take doses prescribed or may be noncompliant with their treatment plans.

## RISKS

- May dangerously lower white blood cell count.
- Can cause neuroleptic malignant syndrome.
- Can cause tardive dyskinesia.

## GUIDELINES FOR USERS

**How is the drug taken?** Tablets (0.5, 1, 2, 5, 10, 20 mg); oral concentrate; injectable—short- or long-acting (Haldol Decanoate).

**What is the usual dosage?** Initial dose should be 1 mg to 10 mg per day in healthy young people, with increases as needed to control symptoms. A maximum daily dose of up to 100 mg may be used if necessary. Maintenance doses should be as low as possible and still be able to control the psychotic symptoms. Maintenance doses rarely exceed 20 mg per day. Doses of the decanoate (long-acting) form of this drug are larger (e.g., 100 mg to 200 mg) and the interval between doses is usually four weeks.

**What are the instructions for taking the drug?** It is best to take the tablet form of this drug on an empty stomach and drink a full glass of water. The liquid form may be mixed with juice. Follow your physician's instructions carefully.

**How quickly will I feel the effect of the drug?** It usually takes several weeks for you to experience the full antipsychotic benefit of this drug. However, you may feel more calm and relaxed after the first dose or two.

**What if I miss a dose or several doses?** If you miss a dose and remember within an hour or so, take the missed dose. However, if more than an hour has elapsed, skip the dose and continue on your regular schedule. Do not take double doses.

If you are missing doses on a frequent basis, notify your psychiatrist. A slow-release form of haloperidol is available.

**What if I stop taking the drug?** Do not stop taking this drug without consulting your physician. Abruptly stopping this medication will lead to uncomfortable but not dangerous physical symptoms. Should your physician and you agree that the drug should be discontinued, your medication should be tapered slowly to prevent physical symptoms of withdrawal and a reemergence of your psychotic symptoms.

**How should I store the drug?** Keep out of reach of children. Store in a dry, tightly closed, light-resistant container. Heat and moisture may cause this drug to break down. The liquid form does not require refrigeration.

## INTERACTIONS

**Alcohol:** Avoid alcohol. When combined with alcohol, this medicine can cause excessive sedation and dangerously lower blood pressure.

**Food/Beverages:** No restrictions.

**Smoking:** Smoking lowers the blood level of haloperidol. If you do smoke, blood samples should be taken to test whether the drug is in the therapeutic range.

**Other drugs:** Antacids with aluminum or magnesium (Maalox, for example) should not be taken for two hours before or after taking haloperidol because they may interfere with the absorption of this drug.

Heterocyclic antidepressants can increase the plasma level of this drug and cause a worsening of side effects. Conversely, this drug can increase the blood level of antidepressants. The concurrent use of these two types of drugs must be carefully monitored.

Blood pressure can be dangerously lowered when antipsychotics are combined with vasodilators (medications that dilate blood vessels.)

Haloperidol will increase the effect of medicines known as CNS (central nervous system) depressants. Examples include antihistamines, hay fever medicines, sedatives, narcotics, muscle relaxants, barbiturates, and anesthetics. Check with your physician before taking any of these drugs.

## HABIT-FORMING POTENTIAL

None.

## LONG-TERM USE

Prolonged use of haloperidol is associated with increased risk of developing tardive dyskinesia, a potentially irreversible side effect involving disfiguring movements of the face, tongue, and limbs. For more information on tardive dyskinesia, please see Chapter 7.

## PLEASE NOTE

Not specifically antiaggressive: Because of the potential serious side effects of the antipsychotic drugs, especially over the long term, this medication should not be used to treat anxiety or chronic aggression and agitation.

Frequent examinations required: While taking this medication, your blood pressure and pulse rate should be monitored frequently. Regular checks should also be made for the early signs of tardive dyskinesia.

**DRUG NAME:**    Haloperidol (*continued*)

**PLEASE NOTE** (*continued*)

Less sweating: Haloperidol may cause you to sweat less, which in turn causes your body temperature to rise. When the weather is hot or you are exercising, make sure you do not become too hot or dehydrated, since overheating may result in a heat stroke.

Extended-release form: Haldol Decanoate, manufactured by McNeil Pharmaceutical, is the extended-release form of haloperidol. This long-acting form is called a "depot" injection. The drug is contained in sesame oil, which is injected into a muscle and then slowly released into the body over a period of weeks. Except for its long-acting nature, the decanoate is no different from other forms of haloperidol.

| Haloperidol | | | | | | | |
|---|---|---|---|---|---|---|---|
| | **Frequency** | | **Discuss with Physician** | | | | |
| **Symptom/Effect** | **Common** | **Rare** | **Not Necessary** | **In All Cases** | **Only If Severe** | **Stop Taking Drug Now** | **Call Physician Now** |
| lethargy/sleepiness | X | | | | X | | |
| low blood pressure | X | | | X | | | |
| dizziness | | X | | X | | | |
| dry mouth | X | | | | X | | |
| blurred vision | X | | | | X | | |
| constipation | X | | | | X | | |
| difficulty urinating | X | | | X | | | |
| reduced urinary output | | X | | X | | | X |
| racing heartbeat/ palpitations | | X | | X | | | |
| weakness | | X | | X | | | |
| sexual problems | | X | | X | | | |
| restlessness | | X | | X | | | |
| skin rash | | X | | X | | | |
| weight gain | X | | | | X | | |
| seizures | | X | | X | | X | X |
| low white blood cell count | | X | | X | | | |
| tremors | | X | | X | | | |
| stiffness | X | | | X | | | |
| involuntary facial or tongue movements | | X | | X | | | |

DRUG NAME: **Imipramine**

**BRAND NAMES:** Janimine, Tofranil
**For more information:** See Chapter 3, Antidepressant Drugs, and Chapter 5, Antipanic and Antiphobic Drugs.

---

**FAST FACTS**  **Drug group:** Antidepressants.

**Prescription needed?** Yes.

**Available as generic?** Yes.

**Habit-forming?** No.

 **Overdose:** The danger of an overdose, which can be lethal, is extremely high. Symptoms include difficulty breathing, shock, agitation, delirium, and coma. Seek immediate emergency medical treatment.

---

## PRECAUTIONS

### Do not take this drug if:

- You have ever had an allergic or negative reaction to any drug in this group.

### Inform your physician if:

- You have ever had an allergic reaction to any drug.
- You have epilepsy.
- You are taking any other drug— prescription or nonprescription —or vitamins.
- You will be under anesthesia or undergoing surgery or medical testing in the next few months.

 **Pregnancy/Breast-feeding**

If you are pregnant or planning a pregnancy, you should, if possible, use non-drug alternatives for treating your depression. This drug has not been demonstrated to be safe during pregnancy. Nursing mothers should not take this drug.

 **Infants/Children**

This drug may be prescribed to children for short-term treatment of bedwetting, but only to children age six and above. Its use in the treatment of depression in children and adolescents must be under the guidance of a child psychiatrist.

 **Over Sixty**

In general, lower doses are required. Side effects may be worse and some older patients may experience confusion. Elderly people may fall after standing up because of the drug's hypotensive (blood pressure lowering) side effects.

 **Driving/Operating Machinery**

Extreme caution is advised. This medicine can impair mental alertness and coordination. If you do drive or operate machinery, this medicine should be taken at bedtime, when its sedating effects are less likely to interfere with daytime activities.

**DRUG NAME:**    Imipramine (*continued*)

## GENERAL INFORMATION

Imipramine is one of the heterocyclic drugs used to treat depression. It is sometimes prescribed when a person is withdrawing from cocaine to reduce the craving for cocaine and to treat the associated depression. In addition, it is the most commonly used antidepressant to treat panic attacks. Imipramine has been shown effective in treating panic disorder in 50 percent to 90 percent of all patients treated. The drug works by inhibiting the nerve cell's ability to reabsorb the neurotransmitters norepinephrine and serotonin (see Chapter 3). Imipramine is sometimes prescribed to treat chronic bedwetting in children age six and older, although this use is controversial.

## BENEFITS

- Helps 75 percent to 80 percent of people with major depression.
- Effective in treating panic attacks.

## RISKS

- Produces annoying side effects.
- Highly dangerous in overdose.

## GUIDELINES FOR USERS

**How is the drug taken?** Tablets (10, 25, 50 mg); capsules (75, 100, 125, 150 mg); injection.

**What is the usual dosage?** The initial dose for treating depression is usually 75 mg daily in divided doses. This can be increased gradually to 150 mg daily. Some people may require 200 mg to 300 mg daily. Antipanic dosages are generally smaller to begin with, though they may also be increased to 300 mg or even higher. Initial doses are lower for patients with medical illnesses and the elderly.

**What are the instructions for taking the drug?** Take this medicine with food, unless your doctor has instructed you otherwise. Taking the medicine on an empty stomach may cause your stomach to become upset. To benefit from the drug, it is important to take the correct dosage each day.

**How quickly will I feel the effect of the drug?** You will probably experience some unpleasant side effects (dry mouth, blurry vision, constipation) right away. It may take days or weeks for the antidepressant benefits to appear. It usually takes two to four weeks at full dose for a person to feel a positive response. By the third week of treatment, the side effects are usually less severe.

**What if I miss a dose or several doses?** If you are taking one dose at bedtime and miss your dose, do not take the drug in the morning. Check with your physician. If you are taking more than one dose a day and remember within an hour or so that you have missed a dose, take the dose. However, if it is almost time for your next dose, skip the missed dose. Do not take double doses.

**What if I stop taking the drug?** Do not discontinue this drug abruptly. Your dosage should be gradually reduced. Stopping the drug abruptly may cause flulike symptoms, headache, restlessness, and/or a worsening of your condition. Inform your physician if you notice these side effects, or any others, after stopping the drug. The effects of this drug may last for up to seven days after you have stopped taking it.

**How should I store the drug?** Keep out of reach of children. Store in a dry, tightly closed, light-resistant container. Heat and moisture may cause this drug to break down.

## INTERACTIONS

**Alcohol:** Do not drink alcohol. Imipramine *increases* the effect of alcohol, while alcohol *increases* the side effects of the drug. In addition, alcohol use can contribute to depression.

**Food/Beverages:** No restrictions.

**Smoking:** Smoking lowers the blood level of imipramine. If you do smoke, blood samples should be taken to test whether the drug is in the therapeutic range.

**Other drugs:** Imipramine will increase the effect of medicines known as CNS (central nervous system) depressants. Examples include antihistamines, hay fever medicines, sedatives, narcotics, muscle relaxants, barbiturates, and anesthetics. Check with your physician before taking any of these drugs.

## HABIT-FORMING POTENTIAL

None.

## LONG-TERM USE

Most people who have a beneficial response do not need to take this drug longer than about six months. A few people may need to take the drug for a year or longer, because their depression recurs if they attempt to discontinue the drug.

## PLEASE NOTE

Help with side effects: Drinking water and sucking on hard candy can help if you are experiencing dry mouth. To prevent constipation, eat high-fiber foods and take a daily dose of a natural bulk laxative. And you can avoid episodes of light-headedness by making sure you get up slowly from a sitting or prone position. These side effects generally get better or go away after you have been on the drug several weeks.

Antipanic use: Roughly two-thirds of the patients who take imipramine to control panic attacks will not experience another attack after discontinuing the medicine.

| Imipramine | | | | | | | |
|---|---|---|---|---|---|---|---|
| | Frequency | | Discuss with Physician | | | | |
| Symptom/Effect | Common | Rare | Not Necessary | In All Cases | Only If Severe | Stop Taking Drug Now | Call Physician Now |
| drowsiness | X | | | | X | | |
| dry mouth | X | | | | X | | |
| constipation | X | | | | X | | |
| blurred vision | X | | | | X | | |
| low blood pressure | X | | | X | | | |
| racing heartbeat/ palpitations | | X | | | X | | |
| confusion | | X | | X | | | X |
| skin rashes/allergies | | X | | X | | | X |
| insomnia | | X | | | X | | |
| sexual problems | | X | | X | | | |
| increased appetite | | X | | | X | | |
| seizures | | X | | X | | X | X |

DRUG NAME: **Isocarboxazid**

**BRAND NAME:** Marplan
**For more information:** See Chapter 3, Antidepressant Drugs.

**FAST FACTS**  **Drug group:** Antidepressants (monoamine oxidase inhibitors).

**Available as generic?** No.

**Prescription needed?** Yes.

**Habit-forming?** No.

 **Overdose:** Symptoms include drowsiness, hypotension, breathing problems, convulsions, and coma. If you suspect an overdose or experience these symptoms, seek immediate emergency medical treatment.

## PRECAUTIONS

### Do not take this drug if:

- You have ever had an allergic or negative reaction to this or any other MAO inhibitor.

### Inform your physician if:

- You have ever had an allergic reaction to any drug.
- You have epilepsy.
- You have high blood pressure or heart problems.
- You are taking any other drug—prescription or nonprescription—or vitamins.
- You will be under anesthesia or undergoing surgery or medical testing in the next few months.
- You have severe or frequent headaches.

 **Pregnancy/Breast-feeding**

If you are pregnant, planning a pregnancy, or breast-feeding, you should not take this drug.

 **Infants/Children**

Should not be given to anyone under age sixteen since safety and effectiveness have not been proved.

 **Over Sixty**

Side effects may be worse.

 **Driving/Operating Machinery**

This drug may cause drowsiness. You should not drive a car during the initial phase of treatment. When you are confident that you are alert and have full motor coordination, ask your doctor if you can resume driving. We suggest having a passenger present on your initial trips to help ascertain safety.

## GENERAL INFORMATION

Isocarboxazid is a monoamine oxidase inhibitor used in the treatment of depression and panic. In most cases, isocarboxazid should not be the first treatment choice for depression. Rather, this drug is prescribed for people whose symptoms have failed to respond to other common antidepression drugs. This drug is just as effective in treating depression as the heterocyclic drugs; however, it poses a potential problem because of possible toxic food-drug interactions. If you are on this drug, it is extremely important to follow the dietary guidelines given to you by your physician. (For an explanation of how this drug works and a discussion of food-drug interactions, see Chapter 3.)

**DRUG NAME:**    Isocarboxazid (*continued*)

## BENEFITS

- As effective as heterocyclics in treating depression.
- May be effective in treating depression in patients who have not responded to other medications.
- May have special benefits in treating atypical depression.
- Effective in treating panic and phobic symptoms.

## RISKS

- Possible toxic interaction with some foods, beverages, and drugs.

## GUIDELINES FOR USERS

**How is the drug taken?** Tablets (10 mg).

**What is the usual dosage?** The initial dose for the treatment of depression is 10 mg to 20 mg daily. This can be increased to 50 mg as needed. Because this drug has a cumulative effect, the dosage is normally reduced after a benefit is noticed.

**What are the instructions for taking the drug?** Follow your physician's instructions carefully. This drug can be taken before, during, or after meals. The tablets can be crushed and dissolved in water before taking, if you prefer.

**How quickly will I feel the effect of the drug?** You may experience a benefit within the first week. However, some people do not feel the effects of this drug until the third or fourth week.

**What if I miss a dose or several doses?** If you miss a dose and remember within an hour or so, take the dose. However, if it is within two hours of your next dose, skip the missed dose. Do not take double doses.

**What if I stop taking the drug?** Do not stop taking isocarboxazid without consulting your physician. If this drug has been taken regularly, withdrawal symptoms may appear unless it is discontinued gradually. After stopping this medicine, you must continue following the dietary guidelines for at least three weeks to avoid a toxic food-drug interaction.

**How should I store the drug?** Keep out of reach of children. Store in a dry, tightly closed, light-resistant container. Heat and moisture may cause this drug to break down.

## INTERACTIONS

**Alcohol:** Do not drink alcohol since this drug can increase the effects of alcohol and alcohol can increase isocarboxazid's side effects. In addition, alcohol use can contribute to depression.

**Food/Beverages:** Do not eat foods or drink beverages with tyramine. Tyramine can interact with this drug and cause severe or fatal increases in blood pressure. Among the food and beverages to be avoided are:

    *Meat and fish:* lox, pickled herring, liver, dry sausage;

    *Fruits and vegetables:* broad (fava) beans, raisins, figs, avocado;

*Dairy products:* Cheese (cottage cheese and cream cheese are allowed), yogurt;

*Beverages:* beer, wine, hard liquor, sherry, large amounts of caffeine (coffee, cocoa, or chocolate);

*Miscellaneous:* Yeast products (including brewer's yeast in large quantities), pickles, sauerkraut, soy sauce, sour cream, snails, licorice.

**Smoking:** Smoking may lower the blood level of isocarboxazid and this may reduce the drug's efficiency in treating depression.

**Other drugs:** All "recreational" or illegal drugs should be avoided by people with depression and may be highly dangerous when combined with isocarboxazid.

Do not take any other medicine without consulting your physician. This includes over-the-counter medicines (nonprescription) such as decongestants, other cold tablets or formulas, nasal drops or sprays, hay fever medications, sinus medications, appetite suppressants, weight-reducing preparations, or "pep" pills.

Do not take procaine (Novocain and others) while on this drug.

Notify your surgeon and anesthesiologist that you take this medication prior to any surgical procedure, as this MAO inhibitor reacts with certain anesthetics.

## HABIT-FORMING POTENTIAL

None.

## LONG-TERM USE

Most people may be tapered safely from the medication six months after their depression has responded to treatment. A small percentage of patients have symptoms of depression return after their dosage is reduced. These individuals may benefit from remaining on isocarboxazid for a year or longer.

## PLEASE NOTE

Cocaine use: Cocaine, when combined with an MAO inhibitor such as isocarboxazid, can dangerously increase blood pressure.

Surgery: If you are taking this drug, you should notify the anesthesiologist before undergoing surgery requiring general anesthesia. Dental procedures requiring Novocain (procaine) are dangerous. Isocarboxazid must be discontinued at least ten days prior to surgery.

ID card: Your physician may suggest you carry an identification card that states you are taking this medicine. In addition, it's a good idea to carry with you at all times a wallet-sized list of foods high in tyramine content.

**DRUG NAME:** Isocarboxazid (*continued*)

| | Frequency | | Discuss with Physician | | | | |
|---|---|---|---|---|---|---|---|
| **Isocarboxazid** | | | | | | | |
| **Symptom/Effect** | **Common** | **Rare** | **Not Necessary** | **In All Cases** | **Only If Severe** | **Stop Taking Drug Now** | **Call Physician Now** |
| blurred vision | X | | | | X | | |
| dizziness/light-headedness | X | | | X | | | |
| drowsiness/weakness | X | | | | X | | |
| decreased sexual ability | X | | | X | | | |
| constipation | | X | | | X | | |
| diarrhea | | X | | | X | | |
| allergies/rashes | | X | | X | | X | X |
| chest pain | | X | | X | | X | X |
| fast or slow heartbeat | X | | | X | | | |
| severe headache | | X | | | | X | X |
| chills/shivering | | X | | | X | | |
| dry mouth | X | | | | X | | |
| jaundice | | X | | X | | X | X |

DRUG NAME: **Lithium**

**BRAND NAMES:** Cibalith-S, Eskalith, Eskalith CR, Lithane, Lithobid, Lithonate, Lithotabs
**For more information:** See Chapter 6, Antimanic Drugs.

**FAST FACTS**   **Drug group:** Antimanic agents.     **Available as generic?** Yes.
**Prescription needed?** Yes.     **Habit-forming?** No.

 **Overdose:** Symptoms include diarrhea, drowsiness, muscle weakness, vomiting or nausea, slurred speech, blurred confusion, convulsions, and severe trembling. Seek immediate emergency medical treatment.

## PRECAUTIONS

### Do not take this drug if:

- You have ever had an allergic reaction to this drug.

### Inform your physician if:

- You have ever had an allergic reaction to any drug.
- You are taking any other drug—prescription or nonprescription—or vitamins. In particular, it is important to tell your physician if you are taking antipsychotics, antithyroid pills, diuretics (water pills), or any medication for asthma, bronchitis, emphysema, sinusitis, or cystic fibrosis.
- You have epilepsy.
- You have kidney, thyroid, or cardiovascular disease.
- You will be under anesthesia or undergoing surgery or medical testing in the next few months.
- You are on a low-salt, low-sugar, or any other special diet.

 **Pregnancy/Breast-feeding**

Do not take this drug if you are pregnant, planning a pregnancy, or breast-feeding. Lithium, when taken during pregnancy, appears to increase the risk of certain types of birth defects, including heart malformations.

 **Infants/Children**

Safety and effectiveness of this drug have not been proved for children under age twelve.

 **Over Sixty**

Lower doses are generally required and side effects may be worse.

 **Driving/Operating Machinery**

This drug may impair mental alertness and coordination. Do not drive or operate machinery until you are certain this drug will not affect your performance.

## GENERAL INFORMATION

Lithium is the most commonly prescribed drug for people experiencing mania. It is effective in treating both the manic and depressive phases of manic-depressive disorder. People with milder forms of mania may also benefit from lithium. In some cases, lithium may be prescribed in combination with carbamazepine and with heterocyclic antidepressants. Lithium is thought to augment the antidepressant effects of the hetero-

**DRUG NAME:**   Lithium (*continued*)

## GENERAL INFORMATION (*continued*)

cyclics. It is sometimes given to people after electroconvulsive therapy to prevent a reoccurrence of depression. Toxic levels of this drug may be close to the therapeutic levels, so it is important to monitor blood levels periodically, take doses regularly, and watch for signs of overdose. For children, a flavored preparation is available. For a list of the medical tests you should have before taking lithium, see Chapter 6.

## BENEFITS

- Effective in treating both mania and depression.
- Augments antidepressant effects of heterocyclics.

## RISKS

- Can damage the kidney and thyroid and parathyroid glands.
- Poses some risk in people with cardiovascular problems.
- Overdose danger is relatively high.

## GUIDELINES FOR USERS

**How is the drug taken?** Tablets (300 mg); time-release capsules (300 and 450 mg).

**What is the usual dosage?** Initial dose should be 300 mg to 600 mg in healthy young people, with increases as needed to control symptoms. The usual maximum daily dose is up to 1,800 mg. The tablets usually are taken either two or three times a day. The time-release capsules, which produce fewer gastrointestinal side effects, are usually taken twice a day. Your lithium blood levels should be measured twice a week until your therapeutic dose is determined. Periodic monitoring of your blood levels should continue while you are taking this drug.

**What are the instructions for taking the drug?** Take lithium with meals to reduce gastrointestinal side effects such as nausea, diarrhea, and stomach cramps. Follow your physician's instructions carefully to maintain the correct blood level of this drug. If you are taking the time-release form of this drug, swallow the tablet or capsule whole.

**How quickly will I feel the effect of the drug?** Manic behavior usually diminishes after seven to ten days of treatment. Lithium should even out the intense ups and downs of your moods, and after several weeks of treatment, you should feel reasonably normal. At the same time, you may experience some side effects from the drug such as dry mouth, a slight tremor in your hands, and a frequent need to urinate. These side effects usually peak about one to two hours after taking your dose.

**What if I miss a dose or several doses?** If you miss a dose and remember within an hour or so, take the missed dose. If it is within two hours of your next dose (or six hours of a time-release dose), skip the missed dose. Do not take double doses.

**What if I stop taking the drug?** Do not stop taking this drug without consulting your physician. When discontinuing lithium, taper gradually to monitor for potential recurrence of symptoms of mania or depression.

**How should I store the drug?** Keep out of reach of children. Store in a dry, tightly closed, light-resistant container. Heat and moisture may cause this drug to break down.

## INTERACTIONS

**Alcohol:** Do not drink alcohol. Lithium *increases* the effect of alcohol, while alcohol *increases* the side effects of the drug. In addition, alcohol use can contribute to depression.

**Food/Beverages:** Drinking large amounts of coffee, tea, or a caffeine beverage may increase your nervousness and reduce the effect of this drug.

**Smoking:** Smoking does not appear to alter blood levels of treatment efficacy of lithium.

**Other drugs:** Diuretics can alter the kidney's ability to remove lithium from the blood, *increase* lithium blood levels, and cause potentially severe side effects. Hydrochlorothiazide diuretics, which are used to treat high blood pressure, can have the same effect. Common brands are Maxzide, Hydropres, and HydroDIURIL.

The antibiotic tetracycline, commonly used to treat infections and acne, may *increase* lithium blood levels.

Theophylline and theophylline-containing compounds *decrease* lithium blood levels. Examples of brand names are Bronkaid, Constant-T, Marax, Mudrane, Primatene, Quibron, Respbid, Slo-Phyllin, Sustaire, Theo-Dur, and Theospan-SR.

Nonsteroidal anti-inflammatory drugs (e.g., indomethacin and ibuprofen) may *decrease* lithium blood levels. Examples of brand names are Indocin, Midol, Motrin, and Nuprin.

Antipsychotic drugs are frequently used in conjunction with lithium and may increase the risk of toxicity.

## HABIT-FORMING POTENTIAL

None.

## LONG-TERM USE

Long-term use is associated with irreversible changes in thyroid and kidney tissue. Your thyroid and renal functions should be monitored at least every six months while you are taking lithium.

## PLEASE NOTE

Avoid dehydration: While you are taking lithium, be careful not to become dehydrated. About 60 percent of people taking this drug experience frequent urination. Drinking plenty of water—ten to twelve glasses a day—will help avoid dehydration. In addition, do not go on a diet without checking with your doctor, since improper dieting can cause dehydration.

Treatment for a resting tremor: About 50 percent of people taking this drug experience a tremor in their hands. The tremor often becomes less noticeable after the person has taken lithium for several weeks. In some cases, the beta-adrenergic blocking drug propranolol may be used to treat the problem.

**DRUG NAME:**   Lithium (*continued*)

**PLEASE NOTE** (*continued*)

In combination with carbamazepine: For people who do not respond to either lithium or carbamazepine alone, some physicians prescribe a combination of the two drugs. When the combination is used, the side effects are similar to those experienced when each medication is taken alone.

| | Frequency | | Discuss with Physician | | | | |
|---|---|---|---|---|---|---|---|
| Symptom/Effect | Common | Rare | Not Necessary | In All Cases | Only If Severe | Stop Taking Drug Now | Call Physician Now |
| tremor | X | | | X | | | |
| weight gain | X | | | X | | | |
| nausea | X | | | X | | | |
| diarrhea | X | | | X | | | |
| skin rashes | X | | | X | | | X |
| frequent urination | X | | | | X | | |
| heat or cold intolerance | | X | | X | | | |
| lethargy/muscle weakness | | X | | X | | | |
| mood changes | | X | | X | | | |
| anxiety | | X | | X | | | |
| aggressiveness | | X | | X | | | |
| sleep disturbances | | X | | | X | | |
| memory or concentration problems | | X | | X | | | |
| convulsions | | X | | X | | X | X |
| delirium/stupor | | X | | X | | X | X |
| blurred vision | | X | | X | | X | X |
| acne | | X | | X | | | |

# DRUG NAME: **Lorazepam**

**BRAND NAME:** Ativan
**For more information:** See Chapter 4, Antianxiety Drugs.

**FAST FACTS**   **Drug group:** Antianxiety agents (benzodiazepines).

**Available as generic?** Yes.

**Prescription needed?** Yes.

**Habit-forming?** Yes.

 **Overdose:** It is possible, though not easy, to overdose. Signs of toxicity include sedation, decreased breathing rate, confusion, and loss of coordination. If these symptoms are present, seek immediate emergency medical treatment.

## PRECAUTIONS

### Do not take this drug if:

- You have had previously negative reactions to benzodiazepines.
- You have a history of drug dependence.
- You have Alzheimer's disease, have had a stroke, or have multiple sclerosis or other brain disorders.
- You are seriously depressed.

### Inform your physician if:

- You are taking any other drug—prescription or nonprescription—or vitamins.
- You will be under anesthesia or undergoing surgery or medical testing in the next few months.
- You have epilepsy.

 ### Pregnancy/Breast-feeding

Do not take this drug if you are pregnant, planning a pregnancy, or breast-feeding.

 ### Infants/Children

This drug should not be taken by children under twelve.

 ### Over Sixty

Smaller doses are advised and should be monitored very closely.

### Driving/Operating Machinery

WARNING: Do not fly, drive, or operate heavy machinery since this drug can impair mental alertness and coordination.

## GENERAL INFORMATION

Lorazepam, the fourth most frequently prescribed benzodiazepine, is used to treat anxiety. It is sometimes administered via injection prior to surgery to relieve anxiety. The drug has less effect on the liver than other benzodiazepines. Thus, it is better suited for those taking ulcer medications, birth control pills, propranolol, Antabuse, or other drugs that affect liver function. Lorazepam is one of the benzodiazepines that is eliminated from the body quickly and can produce withdrawal symptoms unless it is discontinued very gradually. The advantage is that this drug is less likely to build up in the body over time. Generic manufacturers of the drug include Barr, Danbury, Geneva, Lederle, Martec, Mylan, Par, Squibb, and Warner Chilcott. Wyeth-Ayerst markets the drug under the name Ativan. For an explanation of how this drug works, see Chapter 4.

**DRUG NAME:**    Lorazepam (*continued*)

## BENEFITS

- More effective and fewer side effects than barbiturates.
- Less addictive and safer in overdoses than barbiturates.
- Relieves anxiety in about 65 percent to 70 percent of users.
- Less effect on the liver than other benzodiazepines.
- Injectable forms useful in management of acute agitation in the hospital setting.

## RISKS

- Physically and psychologically addictive if misused.
- Makes some people feel lethargic, less able to concentrate, less alert.
- Can affect physical coordination.

## GUIDELINES FOR USERS

**How is the drug taken?** Tablets (0.5, 1, 2 mg); intramuscular; intravenous.

**What is the usual dosage?** The initial dose should be 2 mg to 3 mg per day, with increases as needed to control symptoms. A maximum daily dose of up to 10 mg may be used, if necessary.

**What are the instructions for taking the drug?** As with all benzodiazepines, if you are taking this drug for the first time, take your first dose at home and during a time when you are not required to work or drive. This drug can be taken before, during, or after meals. The tablets can be crushed and dissolved in water before taking, if you prefer.

**How quickly will I feel the effect of the drug?** Those who benefit from this drug will usually experience a positive response within the first week. Many people feel the drug's effect the first day of treatment.

**What if I miss a dose or several doses?** If you miss a dose and remember within an hour or so, take the missed dose. However, if more than an hour has elapsed, skip the dose and continue on your regular schedule. Do not take double doses.

**What if I stop taking the drug?** If you take this drug regularly for three weeks or more, you should not stop abruptly. Your dosage should be gradually reduced. Abrupt cessation can cause psychological and physical withdrawal symptoms.

**How should I store the drug?** Keep out of reach of children, since all benzodiazepines can be extremely dangerous to children. Store in a dry, tightly closed, light-resistant container. Heat and moisture may cause this drug to break down.

## INTERACTIONS

**Alcohol:** Do not drink alcohol. Lorazepam is highly dangerous when combined with alcohol. It can dangerously lower blood pressure, decrease the breathing rate, and lead to loss of consciousness.

**Food/Beverages:** No restrictions on food. Control caffeine intake, as caffeine makes anxiety worse.

**Smoking:** Heavy smoking of tobacco may reduce the sedative effects of this drug. Marijuana smoking may increase side effects and significantly reduce mental alertness.

**Other drugs:** Narcotics (e.g., Demerol, Percodan, codeine, morphine, Talwin) may *increase* the sedative effects of this drug. The combination can be fatal. Do not use narcotics with this drug.

Barbiturates and other sedatives (e.g., phenobarbital, pentobarbital, Seconal, Tuinal) may *increase* sedation to dangerous levels. Do not combine sedatives with this drug.

Do not take other benzodiazepines when using this drug, since the combination is both unnecessary and unsafe.

Do not take sleeping pills while taking this drug. If you are having trouble sleeping, your doctor may prescribe larger doses of lorazepam.

The following drugs may reduce the liver's ability to remove this drug from the body, making the drug more powerful and increasing side effects:

- ulcer drugs
- birth control pills
- propranolol
- disulfiram (Antabuse)

## HABIT-FORMING POTENTIAL

High.

## LONG-TERM USE

Physical and psychological dependence are common problems. A clear treatment plan is important. It is possible to become dependent in as short a time span as two to four weeks. This drug should not be taken longer than four weeks on a regular basis (i.e., daily). Long-term use can also increase the risk of side effects.

## PLEASE NOTE

Nondrug alternatives: See Chapter 4 for a discussion of the value of exercise and a good diet in the treatment of anxiety. One of the best nondrug ways to reduce anxiety is to identify and reduce sources of stress in your life.

Correct diagnosis: You should always consult a physician to be sure that any medical causes of anxiety (such as hyperthyroidism) are diagnosed and treated. Anxiety may be a component of depression, in which case the symptoms of anxiety are treated by treating the underlying depression with antidepressants and/or other therapies for mood disorders.

**DRUG NAME:**    Lorazepam (*continued*)

| | Frequency | | Discuss with Physician | | | | |
|---|---|---|---|---|---|---|---|
| Symptom/Effect | Common | Rare | Not Necessary | In All Cases | Only If Severe | Stop Taking Drug Now | Call Physician Now |
| clumsiness/sleepiness | X | | | | X | | |
| abdominal cramps | | X | | X | | | |
| blurred vision | | X | | X | | | |
| dry mouth | | X | | X | | | |
| racing heartbeat/ palpitations | | X | | X | | | |
| shaking/slurred speech | | X | | X | | | |
| urination problems | | X | | X | | | |
| convulsions | | X | | X | | X | X |
| hallucinations | | X | | X | | X | X |
| memory loss | | X | | X | | X | X |
| trouble breathing | | X | | X | | X | X |
| staggering/trembling | | X | | X | | X | X |
| headache | | X | | X | | | |
| confusion | | X | | X | | | |

*Table title: Lorazepam*

## DRUG NAME: **Loxapine**

**BRAND NAME:** Loxitane
**For more information:** See Chapter 7, Antipsychotic Drugs.

**FAST FACTS**

**Drug group:** Antipsychotics.
**Prescription needed?** Yes.

**Available as generic?** Yes.
**Habit-forming?** No.

 **Overdose:** Symptoms include light-headedness, sedation, confusion, agitation, disorientation, restlessness, convulsions, fever, and coma. Seek immediate emergency medical treatment.

## PRECAUTIONS

### Do not take this drug if:

- You have ever had an allergic reaction to this drug or amoxapine.

### Inform your physician if:

- You have ever had an allergic reaction to any drug.
- You have cardiovascular disease
- You have epilepsy or asthma.
- You are taking any other drug— prescription or nonprescription —or vitamins.
- You are on a low-salt, low-sugar, or any other special diet.
- You will be under anesthesia or undergoing surgery or medical testing in the next few months.

 ### Pregnancy/Breast-feeding

Safe use of this drug during pregnancy has not been established. Except in unusual cases where the mother or the baby's life is endangered, this drug should not be taken by pregnant women. Women taking loxapine should not breast-feed.

 ### Infants/Children

This drug has not been proved safe or effective for children under the age of sixteen.

 ### Over Sixty

Side effects, some serious, can be worse. Initial dose should be low, with careful monitoring for side effects. Special care should be taken when sitting up from a lying position, or standing from a sitting position, as blood pressure may be lowered and balance impaired.

 ### Driving/Operating Machinery

Extreme caution is advised. This medicine can impair mental alertness and coordination. If you do drive or operate machinery, this medicine should be taken at bedtime when its sedating effects are less likely to interfere with daytime activities.

**DRUG NAME:** Loxapine (*continued*)

## GENERAL INFORMATION

Loxapine is an intermediate-potency antipsychotic belonging to the dibenzoxapine class of antipsychotics. It is used to treat people who are experiencing disorganized, psychotic thinking and who may be having delusions or hallucinations. For an explanation of how this drug works, see Chapter 7.

| BENEFITS | RISKS |
|---|---|
| • Effective in treating hallucinations, delusions, confused thinking, and mania. | • May dangerously lower white blood cell count. |
| • Sedating effects helpful in calming agitated persons. | • Can cause tardive dyskinesia. |
| | • Can cause neuroleptic malignant syndrome. |

## GUIDELINES FOR USERS

**How is the drug taken?** Capsules (5, 10, 25, 50 mg); oral concentrate; intramuscular.

**What is the usual dosage?** Initial dose should be 10 mg to 50 mg per day in healthy young people, with increases as needed to control symptoms. A maximum daily dose of up to 250 mg may be used, if necessary. Maintenance doses should be as low as possible and still be able to control the psychotic symptoms.

**What are the instructions for taking the drug?** It is best to take this drug on an empty stomach and drink a full glass of water. The liquid form of loxapine can be taken with juice to make it easier to take. Follow your physician's instructions carefully.

**How quickly will I feel the effect of the drug?** It usually takes several weeks for you to experience the full benefit of this drug. However, you may feel more calm and relaxed after the first dose or two. The drug should also help you sleep better, if this is a problem.

**What if I miss a dose or several doses?** If you miss a dose and remember within an hour or so, take the missed dose. Otherwise, skip the missed dose and continue on your regular dosing schedule. Do not take double doses.

If you are missing doses on a frequent basis, notify your psychiatrist. A slow-release form of an antipsychotic drug may help with your compliance and help avoid a relapse.

**What if I stop taking the drug?** Do not stop taking this drug without consulting your physician. Abruptly stopping this medication will lead to uncomfortable, but not dangerous, physical symptoms. Should your physician and you agree that the drug should be discontinued, your medication should be tapered slowly to prevent physical symptoms of withdrawal and a reemergence of your psychotic symptoms.

**How should I store the drug?** Keep out of reach of children. Store in a dry, tightly closed, light-resistant container. Heat and moisture may cause this drug to break down. The liquid form does not require refrigeration.

## INTERACTIONS

**Alcohol:** Avoid alcohol. When combined with alcohol, this medicine can cause excessive sedation and dangerously lower blood pressure.

**Food/Beverages:** No restrictions.

**Smoking:** Smoking lowers the blood level of loxapine. If you do smoke, blood samples should be taken to test whether the drug is in the therapeutic range.

**Other drugs:** Antacids with aluminum or magnesium (Maalox, for example) should not be taken for two hours before or after taking loxapine because they may interfere with the absorption of this drug.

Heterocyclic antidepressants can increase the plasma level of this drug and cause a worsening of side effects. Conversely, this drug can increase the blood level of antidepressants. The concurrent use of these two types of drugs must be carefully monitored.

Blood pressure can be dangerously lowered when antipsychotics are combined with vasodilators (medications that dilate blood vessels).

Loxapine will increase the effect of medicines known as CNS (central nervous system) depressants. Examples include antihistamines, hay fever medicines, sedatives, narcotics, muscle relaxants, barbiturates, and anesthetics. Check with your physician before taking any of these drugs.

## HABIT-FORMING POTENTIAL

None.

## LONG-TERM USE

Prolonged use of loxapine is associated with increased risk of developing tardive dyskinesia, a potentially irreversible side effect involving disfiguring movements of the face, tongue, and limbs. For more information on tardive dyskinesia, please see Chapter 7.

## PLEASE NOTE

Not a sleeping pill: This drug, which has a sedating effect, is sometimes misused as a sleeping pill. There are much safer medications available as sleeping aids.

Not specifically antiaggressive: Because of the potential serious side effects of the antipsychotic drugs, especially over the long term, this medication should not be used to treat anxiety or chronic aggression and agitation.

Frequent examinations required: While taking this medication, your blood pressure and pulse rate should be monitored frequently. Regular checks should also be made for the early signs of tardive dyskinesia.

**DRUG NAME:**  Loxapine (*continued*)

| Symptom/Effect | Frequency | | Discuss with Physician | | | Stop Taking Drug Now | Call Physician Now |
| | Common | Rare | Not Necessary | In All Cases | Only If Severe | | |
|---|---|---|---|---|---|---|---|
| lethargy/sleepiness | X | | | | X | | |
| low blood pressure | X | | | X | | | |
| dizziness | | X | | X | | | |
| dry mouth | X | | | | X | | |
| blurred vision | | X | | | X | | |
| constipation | X | | | | X | | |
| difficulty urinating | | X | | X | | | X |
| reduced urinary output | | X | | X | | | X |
| racing heartbeat/ palpitations | | X | | X | | | |
| weakness | | X | | X | | | |
| sexual problems | | X | | X | | | |
| restlessness | | X | | X | | | |
| skin rash | | X | | X | | | X |
| weight gain | X | | | | X | | |
| seizures | | X | | X | | X | X |
| low white blood cell count | | X | | X | | | X |
| tremors | | X | | X | | | |
| stiffness | X | | | X | | | |
| involuntary facial or tongue movements | | X | | X | | | |

DRUG NAME: **Maprotiline**

**BRAND NAME:** Ludiomil
**For more information:** See Chapter 3, Antidepressant Drugs.

FAST FACTS  **Drug group:** Antidepressants.  **Available as generic?** Yes.
**Prescription needed?** Yes.  **Habit-forming?** No.

 **Overdose:** The danger of an overdose, which can be lethal, is extremely high. Symptoms include difficulty breathing, shock, agitation, delirium, convulsions, and coma. Seek immediate emergency medical treatment.

## PRECAUTIONS
### Do not take this drug if:
- You have ever had an allergic or negative reaction to any drug in this group.

### Inform your physician if:
- You have ever had an allergic reaction to any drug.
- You have epilepsy or any seizures.
- You are taking any other drug— prescription or nonprescription —or vitamins.
- You will be under anesthesia or undergoing surgery or medical testing in the next few months.

 **Pregnancy/Breast-feeding**

If you are pregnant or planning a pregnancy, you should, if possible, use non-drug alternatives for treating your depression. This drug has not been demonstrated to be safe during pregnancy. Nursing mothers should not take this drug since it is passed on to the baby in the mother's milk.

 **Infants/Children**

Safety and effectiveness have not been determined for those under age eighteen. Its use in the treatment of depression in children and adolescents must be under the guidance of a child psychiatrist.

 **Over Sixty**

In general, lower doses are required. Side effects may be worse and some older patients may experience confusion. Elderly people may fall after standing up because of the drug's hypotensive (blood pressure lowering) side effects.

 **Driving/Operating Machinery**

Extreme caution is advised. This medicine can impair mental alertness and co-ordination. If you do drive or operate machinery, this medicine should be taken at bedtime, when its sedating effect will not interfere with daytime activities.

DRUG NAME:    Maprotiline (*continued*)

## GENERAL INFORMATION

Maprotiline is one of the heterocyclic drugs used to treat depression. It works by inhibiting the nerve cell's ability to reabsorb the neurotransmitters norepinephrine and serotonin (see Chapter 3). Although the risk is small, your physician should advise you that seizures have been associated with maprotiline. Most of the seizures have occurred in cases where the dosage was rapidly escalated, other medicines interacted with maprotiline, or the dosage exceeded the recommended range.

## BENEFITS

• Helps 75 percent to 80 percent of people with major depression.

## RISKS

• Produces annoying side effects.
• Potential for use in suicide attempts.

## GUIDELINES FOR USERS

**How is the drug taken?** Tablets (25, 50, 75 mg).

**What is the usual dosage?** The initial dose is usually 75 mg daily in divided doses. This can be increased gradually to 150 mg daily. Daily dosage of 225 mg should not be exceeded. Initial doses are lower for patients with medical illnesses, and the elderly.

**What are the instructions for taking the drug?** Take this medicine with food, unless your doctor has instructed you otherwise. Taking the medicine on an empty stomach may cause your stomach to become upset. To benefit from the drug, it is important to take the correct dosage each day.

**How quickly will I feel the effect of the drug?** You will probably experience some unpleasant side effects (dry mouth, blurry vision, constipation) right away. It may take days or weeks for the benefits to appear. It usually takes two to four weeks at full dose for a person to feel a positive response. By the third week of treatment, the side effects are usually less severe.

**What if I miss a dose or several doses?** If you are taking one dose at bedtime and miss your dose, do not take the drug in the morning. Check with your physician. If you are taking more than one dose a day and remember within an hour or so that you have missed a dose, take the dose. However, if it is almost time for your next dose, skip the missed dose. Do not take double doses.

**What if I stop taking the drug?** Do not discontinue this drug abruptly. Your dosage should be gradually reduced. Stopping the drug abruptly may cause flulike symptoms, headache, restlessness, and/or a worsening of your condition. Inform your physician if you notice these side effects, or any others, after stopping the drug. The effects of this drug may last for up to seven days after you have stopped taking it.

**How should I store the drug?** Keep out of reach of children. Store in a dry, tightly closed, light-resistant container. Heat and moisture may cause this drug to break down.

## INTERACTIONS

**Alcohol:** Do not drink alcohol. Maprotiline *increases* the effect of alcohol, while alcohol *increases* the side effects of the drug. In addition, alcohol use can contribute to depression.

**Food/Beverages:** No restrictions.

**Smoking:** Smoking lowers the blood level of maprotiline. If you do smoke, blood samples should be taken to test whether the drug is in the therapeutic range.

**Other drugs:** Maprotiline will increase the effect of medicines known as CNS (central nervous system) depressants. Examples include antihistamines, hay fever medicines, sedatives, narcotics, muscle relaxants, barbiturates, and anesthetics. Check with your physician before taking any of these drugs.

## HABIT-FORMING POTENTIAL

None.

## LONG-TERM USE

Most people who have a beneficial response do not need to take this drug longer than about six months. A few people may need to take the drug for a year or longer because their depression recurs if they attempt to discontinue the drug.

## PLEASE NOTE

Help with side effects: Drinking water and sucking on hard candy can help if you are experiencing dry mouth. To prevent constipation, eat high-fiber foods and take a daily dose of a natural bulk laxative. And you can avoid episodes of light-headedness by making sure you get up slowly from a sitting or prone position. These side effects generally get better or go away after you have been on the drug several weeks.

**DRUG NAME:**    Maprotiline (*continued*)

| | Frequency | | Discuss with Physician | | | | |
|---|---|---|---|---|---|---|---|
| Symptom/Effect | Common | Rare | Not Necessary | In All Cases | Only If Severe | Stop Taking Drug Now | Call Physician Now |
| drowsiness | X | | | | X | | |
| dry mouth | X | | | | X | | |
| constipation | X | | | | X | | |
| blurred vision | X | | | | X | | |
| low blood pressure | X | | | X | | | |
| racing heartbeat/ palpitations | | X | | | X | | |
| confusion | | X | | X | | | X |
| skin rashes/allergies | | X | | X | | | X |
| insomnia | | X | | | X | | |
| sexual problems | | X | | X | | | |
| increased appetite | | X | | | X | | |
| seizures | | X | | X | | X | X |

DRUG NAME: **Meprobamate**

**BRAND NAMES:** Equanil, Meprospan, Miltown
**For more information:** See Chapter 4, Antianxiety Drugs.

**FAST FACTS** **Drug group:** Antianxiety agents. **Available as generic?** Yes.
**Prescription needed?** Yes. **Habit-forming?** Yes.

**Overdose:** Signs of an overdose include severe confusion, drowsiness, trouble breathing, slurred speech, and staggering. If these symptoms are present, seek immediate emergency medical treatment.

## PRECAUTIONS

**Do not take this drug if:**

- You have ever had an allergic reaction to this drug.

**Inform your physician if:**

- You have ever had an allergic reaction to any drug.
- You are taking any other drug—prescription or nonprescription—or vitamins.
- You will be under anesthesia or undergoing surgery or medical testing in the next few months.
- You have epilepsy, kidney disease, liver disease, or porphyria.

**Pregnancy/Breast-feeding**

Do not take this drug if you are pregnant, planning a pregnancy, or breast-feeding.

**Infants/Children**

Meprobamate should not be given to children under age six since there is a lack of evidence of safety and effectiveness with this age group.

**Over Sixty**

Side effects may be more likely to occur.

**Driving/Operating Machinery**

Do not drive. This drug can impair mental alertness and coordination.

## GENERAL INFORMATION

Meprobamate is used to relieve anxiety and nervousness on a short-term basis. Generic manufacturers include Barr, Danbury, Geneva, Martec, Par, and Pharmafair. Meprobamate is also marketed in combination with aspirin, benactyzine, and estrogen; however, these combinations are not recommended. In general, this drug is less effective and poses more overdose danger than the benzodiazepines or buspirone used in the treatment of anxiety.

## BENEFITS

- Few benefits that cannot be obtained with other drugs.

## RISKS

- High danger of oversedation.
- Can cause mental confusion and loss of coordination.
- Highly addictive if used longer than three weeks.

**DRUG NAME:**    Meprobamate (*continued*)

## GUIDELINES FOR USERS

**How is the drug taken?** Tablets (200, 400, 600 mg).

**What is the usual dosage?** The initial dose is 1,200 mg to 1,600 mg daily in divided doses. The dosage may be gradually increased to 2,400 mg a day, if necessary.

**What are the instructions for taking the drug?** Take as low a dose as possible to treat anxiety symptoms. Do not remain on continuous doses for longer than three weeks.

**How quickly will I feel the effect of the drug?** Most people experience the antianxiety effects of this drug shortly after it is initiated.

**What if I miss a dose or several doses?** If you miss a dose and remember within an hour or so, take the missed dose. However, if more than an hour has elapsed, skip the dose and continue on your regular schedule. Do not take double doses.

**What if I stop taking the drug?** Do not stop taking this medicine without consulting your physician. If you took meprobamate for a long time, your body may need several days to adjust when you stop taking the drug. Meprobamate should be gradually tapered off over several days to avoid withdrawal symptoms, including restlessness, irritability, insomnia, poor concentration, and headache.

**How should I store the drug?** Keep out of reach of children. Store in a dry, tightly closed, light-resistant container. Heat and moisture may cause this drug to break down.

## INTERACTIONS

**Alcohol:** Do not drink alcohol. Meprobamate is highly dangerous when combined with alcohol. It can dangerously lower blood pressure, decrease the breathing rate, and lead to loss of consciousness.

**Food/Beverages:** No restrictions on food. Control caffeine intake, as caffeine makes anxiety worse.

**Smoking:** Poses no danger.

**Other drugs:** Meprobamate will increase the effect of medicines known as CNS (central nervous system) depressants. Examples include antihistamines, hay fever medicines, sedatives, narcotics, muscle relaxants, barbiturates, and anesthetics. Check with your physician before taking any of these drugs.

## HABIT-FORMING POTENTIAL

Very high.

## LONG-TERM USE

In most cases, this drug should not be used for longer than three weeks.

## Meprobamate

| Symptom/Effect | Frequency | | Discuss with Physician | | | Stop Taking Drug Now | Call Physician Now |
|---|---|---|---|---|---|---|---|
| | Common | Rare | Not Necessary | In All Cases | Only If Severe | | |
| skin rash/itching | | X | | X | | | |
| confusion | | X | | X | | | X |
| racing heartbeat/ palpitations | | X | | X | | | X |
| unusual bleeding/bruising | | X | | X | | | X |
| clumsiness/unsteadiness | X | | | X | | | |
| drowsiness | X | | | | X | | |
| blurred vision | | X | | X | | | |
| diarrhea | | X | | X | | | |
| headache | | X | | X | | | |
| nausea/vomiting | | X | | X | | | |
| dry mouth | X | | | | X | | |
| dependency | X | | | X | | | X |

DRUG NAME: **Mesoridazine**

**BRAND NAME:** Serentil
**For more information:** See Chapter 7, Antipsychotic Drugs.

**FAST FACTS** **Drug group:** Antipsychotics.     **Available as generic?** No.
**Prescription needed?** Yes.     **Habit-forming?** No.

 **Overdose:** Symptoms include light-headedness, sedation, agitation, confusion, restlessness, disorientation, convulsions, fever, and coma. Seek immediate emergency medical treatment.

## PRECAUTIONS

### Do not take this drug if:

- You have ever had an allergic reaction to this drug or any phenothiazine.

### Inform your physician if:

- You have ever had an allergic reaction to any drug.
- You have epilepsy or asthma.
- You are taking any other drug— prescription or nonprescription —or vitamins.
- You are on a low-salt, low-sugar, or any other special diet.
- You will be under anesthesia or undergoing surgery or medical testing in the next few months.

 **Pregnancy/Breast-feeding**

Except in unusual cases where the mother or the baby's life is endangered, this drug should not be taken by pregnant women. Women taking mesoridazine should not breast-feed.

 **Infants/Children**

Not recommended for children under age twelve.

 **Over Sixty**

Side effects, some serious, can be worse. Initial dose should be low, with careful monitoring for side effects. Special care should be taken when sitting up from a lying position, or standing from a sitting position, as blood pressure may be lowered and balance impaired.

 **Driving/Operating Machinery**

Extreme caution is advised. This medicine can impair mental alertness and coordination. If you do drive or operate machinery, this medicine should be taken at bedtime when its sedating effects are less likely to interfere with daytime activities.

## GENERAL INFORMATION

Mesoridazine is a low-potency antipsychotic used to treat people who are experiencing disorganized, psychotic thinking and who may be having delusions or hallucinations. It is sometimes prescribed to treat schizophrenia. This drug is quite sedating, and often causes lowered blood pressure. It should be used carefully by people taking antihypertensive (high blood pressure) medications. The sedating side effects may be beneficial in calming people with acute agitation or violent behavior. Mesoridazine has fewer movement side effects than certain other antipsychotics. The choice of which antipsychotic drug to use is often determined by the side effects. For an explanation of how this drug works, see Chapter 7.

## BENEFITS

- Effective in treating hallucinations, delusions, confused thinking, and mania.
- Sedating effects helpful in calming agitated persons.

## RISKS

- Can dangerously lower white blood cell count.
- Can dangerously lower blood pressure.
- Can cause tardive dyskinesia.
- Can cause neuroleptic malignant syndrome.

## GUIDELINES FOR USERS

**How is the drug taken?** Tablets (10, 25, 50, 100 mg); oral concentrate; intramuscular.

**What is the usual dosage?** The initial dose should be between 25 mg and 50 mg per day in healthy young people, with increases as needed to control symptoms. Maintenance doses should be as low as possible and still be able to control the psychotic symptoms.

**What are the instructions for taking the drug?** It is best to take this drug on an empty stomach and drink a full glass of water. The oral concentrate may be diluted with water, orange juice, or grape juice. However, this should be done just prior to taking the dose.

**How quickly will I feel the effect of the drug?** It usually takes several weeks for you to experience the full benefit of this drug. However, you may feel more calm and relaxed after the first dose or two. The drug should also help you sleep better, if this is a problem.

**What if I miss a dose or several doses?** If you miss a dose and remember within an hour or so, take the missed dose. Otherwise, skip the missed dose and continue on your regular dosing schedule. Do not take double doses.

If you are missing doses on a frequent basis, notify your psychiatrist. A slow-release form of an antipsychotic drug may help with your compliance and help avoid a relapse.

**What if I stop taking the drug?** Do not stop taking this drug without consulting your physician. Abruptly stopping this medication will lead to uncomfortable but not dangerous physical symptoms. Should your physician and you agree that the drug should be discontinued, your medication should be tapered slowly to prevent physical symptoms of withdrawal and a reemergence of your psychotic symptoms.

**How should I store the drug?** Keep out of reach of children. Store in a dry, tightly closed, light-resistant container. Heat and moisture may cause this drug to break down. The liquid form does not require refrigeration.

## INTERACTIONS

**Alcohol:** Avoid alcohol. When combined with alcohol, this medicine can cause excessive sedation and dangerously lower blood pressure.

**DRUG NAME:**   Mesoridazine (*continued*)

## INTERACTIONS (*continued*)

**Food/Beverages:** No restrictions.

**Smoking:** Smoking lowers the blood level of mesoridazine. If you do smoke, blood samples should be taken to test whether the drug is in the therapeutic range.

**Other drugs:** Antacids with aluminum or magnesium (Maalox, for example) should not be taken for two hours before or after taking mesoridazine because they may interfere with the absorption of this drug.

Heterocyclic antidepressants can increase the plasma level of this drug and cause a worsening of side effects. Conversely, this drug can increase the blood level of antidepressants. The concurrent use of these two types of drugs must be carefully monitored.

Blood pressure can be dangerously lowered when antipsychotics are combined with vasodilators (medications that dilate blood vessels).

Mesoridazine will increase the effect of medicines known as CNS (central nervous system) depressants. Examples include antihistamines, hay fever medicines, sedatives, narcotics, muscle relaxants, barbiturates, and anesthetics. Check with your physician before taking any of these drugs.

## HABIT-FORMING POTENTIAL

None.

## LONG-TERM USE

Prolonged use of mesoridazine is associated with increased risk of developing tardive dyskinesia, a potentially irreversible side effect involving disfiguring movements of the face, tongue, and limbs. For more information on tardive dyskinesia, please see Chapter 7.

## PLEASE NOTE

Not a sleeping pill: This drug, which has a sedating effect, is sometimes misused as a sleeping pill. There are much safer medications available as sleeping aids.

Not specifically antiaggressive: Because of the potential serious side effects of the antipsychotic drugs, especially over the long term, this medication should not be used to treat anxiety or chronic aggression and agitation.

Frequent examinations required: While taking this medication, your blood pressure and pulse rate should be monitored frequently. Regular checks should also be made for the early signs of tardive dyskinesia.

Classification: Mesoridazine is classified as a phenothiazine. Other antipsychotics in the same group include acetophenazine, chlorpromazine, fluphenazine, perphenazine, promazine, thioridazine, trifluoperazine, and triflupromazine. In general, if you have a poor response to one drug in this family, you will likely have a similar poor response to other drugs in the family.

## Mesoridazine

| Symptom/Effect | Frequency | | Discuss with Physician | | | Stop Taking Drug Now | Call Physician Now |
| --- | --- | --- | --- | --- | --- | --- | --- |
| | Common | Rare | Not Necessary | In All Cases | Only If Severe | | |
| lethargy/sleepiness | X | | | | X | | |
| low blood pressure | X | | | X | | | |
| dizziness | | X | | X | | | |
| dry mouth | X | | | | X | | |
| blurred vision | X | | | | X | | |
| constipation | X | | | | X | | |
| difficulty urinating | X | | | X | | | |
| reduced urinary output | | X | | X | | | X |
| racing heartbeat/ palpitations | | X | | X | | | |
| weakness | | X | | X | | | |
| sexual problems | | X | | X | | | |
| restlessness | | X | | X | | | |
| skin rash | | X | | X | | | X |
| weight gain | X | | | | X | | |
| seizures | | X | | X | | X | X |
| low white blood cell count | | X | | X | | | X |
| tremors | | X | | X | | | |
| stiffness | X | | | X | | | |
| involuntary facial or tongue movements | | X | | X | | | |

## DRUG NAME: **Methamphetamine**

**BRAND NAME:** Desoxyn
**For more information:** See Chapter 10, Drugs for Attention-Deficit Hyperactivity Disorder.

**FAST FACTS**  **Drug group:** Stimulants.  **Available as generic?** Yes.

**Prescription needed?** Yes.  **Habit-forming?** Yes.

 **Overdose:** Symptoms include restlessness, tremors, insomnia, trouble breathing, confusion, hallucinations, and panic. These symptoms may be followed by lethargy, and in acute poisoning, convulsions and coma. Seek emergency medical treatment.

## PRECAUTIONS

**Do not take this drug if:**

- You have ever had an allergic reaction to this drug or another amphetamine.
- You have a history of drug or alcohol abuse.

**Inform your physician if:**

- You have ever had an allergic reaction to any drug.
- You have epilepsy or a history of Tourette's syndrome.
- You have glaucoma, or heart or blood vessel disease.
- You have high blood pressure.
- You are taking any other drug— prescription or nonprescription —or vitamins.
- You are now taking or have taken within two weeks a monoamine oxidase (MAO) inhibitor.
- You will be under anesthesia or undergoing surgery or medical testing in the next few months.

 **Pregnancy/Breast-feeding**

Do not take this drug if you are pregnant, planning a pregnancy, or are breast-feeding.

 **Infants/Children**

Not recommended for children under age six.

 **Over Sixty**

Little research has been done on the effect of amphetamines in the elderly. This drug is prescribed by some psychiatrists to increase mental alertness in the elderly and is known to augment the effects of heterocylic antidepressants for people with treatment-resistant depression.

 **Driving/Operating Machinery**

This drug may impair mental alertness and coordination. Do not drive or operate machinery until you are certain this drug will not affect your performance. This drug has been abused by those wishing to increase alertness and to combat sleepiness while driving. This is a dangerous practice as tolerance builds up for its mental alertness effects, and its psychological side effects can impair perception or judgment.

498

## GENERAL INFORMATION

Methamphetamine is an amphetamine in the family of medicines known as *central nervous system stimulants*. This drug is used to treat narcolepsy and attention-deficit disorders in children. In rare cases, methamphetamine may be used to treat depression. In children, amphetamines increase the ability to concentrate and reduce restlessness. Children who suffer from schizophrenia or other psychotic disorders that may produce symptoms similar to attention-deficit disorders should not be given stimulants. Amphetamines, which produce feelings of euphoria and excitation when taken in large doses by adults, have been widely abused. Street names for this drug include *bombit, crank, crystal, meth,* and *speed*. For more information on how this drug works, see Chapter 10.

## BENEFITS

- Effective in treating attention-deficit hyperactivity disorder in children and adolescents.
- Augments the antidepressant effects of heterocyclic antidepressants.

## RISKS

- Stimulants sometimes induce Tourette's syndrome.
- Increases vulnerability to seizure disorders.
- Can be abused by people prone to drug dependence.

## GUIDELINES FOR USERS

**How is the drug taken?** Tablets (5, 10, 20 mg).

**What is the usual dosage?** Initial doses are 5 mg two or three times per day. Dosages must be increased and adjusted to the individual in response to therapeutic benefits and side effects.

**What are the instructions for taking the drug?** Take your last dose at least six hours before bedtime to prevent trouble sleeping. Do not break, crush, or chew the tablets.

**How quickly will I feel the effect of the drug and how long does it last?** When this drug is effective, adults will usually notice some improvement in the child from almost the first day the medication is taken. The effects of methamphetamine last about three to four hours, and the drug must be given several times a day.

**What if I miss a dose or several doses?** If you remember the missed dose within an hour or so, take the dose. However, if it is almost time for your next dose, skip the missed dose and continue on your regular schedule. Do not take a dose within six hours of sleeping and do not take double doses.

**What if I stop taking the drug?** Do not stop taking this drug without consulting your physician. Your physician may wish to taper off your doses to prevent withdrawal symptoms.

**How should I store the drug?** Keep out of reach of children. Store in a dry, tightly closed, light-resistant container. Heat and moisture may cause this drug to break down. As this drug has a high potential for abuse, we recommend that it be kept in a locked cabinet and that careful records be maintained to check for missing tablets.

DRUG NAME:    Methamphetamine (*continued*)

## INTERACTIONS

**Alcohol:** Alcohol may aggravate the symptoms of attention-deficit hyperactivity disorder and react dangerously with central nervous system effects of methamphetamine.

**Food/Beverages:** No restrictions; however, caffeine may increase nervousness, anxiety, and other emotional side effects.

**Smoking:** No restrictions.

**Other drugs:** The danger of overdose is high when methamphetamine is combined with heterocyclic antidepressants.

Monoamine oxidase (MAO) inhibitors slow the absorption of amphetamines and can cause toxic blood levels. This drug should not be used with MAO inhibitors.

Antihistamines have a sedative effect that may counteract the effect of methamphetamine.

Take special care to consult your physician before taking any drug but especially the following drugs in combination with methamphetamine: chlorpromazine, ethosuximide, haloperidol, antihypertensive medications, meperidine, norepinephrine, phenytoin, propoxyphene, any beta blocker, digitalis, and thyroid hormones.

## HABIT-FORMING POTENTIAL

High.

## LONG-TERM USE

Addiction is a problem primarily with adults. It is extremely rare for children with attention-deficit hyperactivity disorder to become addicted. Because this drug has been widely abused by adults, its use is tightly regulated by the Food and Drug Administration. When high doses are taken for a long time, a person may experience severe side effects, including paranoia, delusions, and other psychoses. Children who take this drug on a long-term basis should be examined every four to six months. The physician should monitor height and weight, look for the presence of tics, measure blood pressure and pulse, and ask about side effects.

## PLEASE NOTE

Signs of amphetamine abuse: When abused, methamphetamine can cause an increase in the heart rate, elevated blood pressure, dilation of the pupils, and agitation. As dosages increase, more severe side effects—including irritability, confusion, hostility, and sleep disturbances—may be noticed. At the highest doses, a person's symptoms (bizarre thoughts, delusions, and agitation) may resemble common symptoms of schizophrenia.

Treatment for withdrawal: In most cases, a person who has abused methamphetamine and who is suffering withdrawal symptoms can be treated on an outpatient basis. Symptoms of withdrawal include fatigue, insomnia, or hypersomnia. An antipsychotic medication may be prescribed if a person is experiencing delusions, hallucinations, agitation, or confusion. Inpatient treatment may be required when the drug was taken intravenously, when a person is depressed or suicidal, or when a person has lost touch with reality.

Effects on growth in children: Stimulants may suppress the production of growth hormones and can reduce weight and height gain in growing children. In most cases, this lag is temporary. However, the effects on growth that the long-term use of stimulants has on children lead some physicians to believe that this drug should never be prescribed for children.

| | Methamphetamine | | | | | | |
|---|---|---|---|---|---|---|---|
| | Frequency | | Discuss with Physician | | | | |
| Symptom/Effect | Common | Rare | Not Necessary | In All Cases | Only If Severe | Stop Taking Drug Now | Call Physician Now |
| loss of appetite | X | | | | X | | |
| difficulty sleeping | X | | | | X | | |
| weight loss | X | | | X | | | |
| abdominal pain | | X | | X | | X | X |
| headache | | X | | X | | X | X |
| drowsiness | | X | | | X | | |
| dizziness | | X | | | X | | |
| mood changes | | X | | X | | | |
| lack of coordination | | X | | X | | X | |
| tics or unusual movements | | X | | X | | X | |
| irritability/nervousness | | X | | X | | | |
| skin rash or hives | | X | | X | | X | |
| blurred vision | | X | | X | | | |
| diarrhea | X | | | | X | | |
| nausea | X | | | | X | | |
| sexual problems | | X | | X | | | |
| paranoia | | X | | X | | X | X |

# Drug Name: **Methylphenidate**

**BRAND NAME:** Ritalin

**For more information:** See Chapter 10, Drugs for Attention-Deficit Hyperactivity Disorder.

---

**FAST FACTS** **Drug group:** Stimulants. **Available as generic?** Yes.

**Prescription needed?** Yes. **Habit-forming?** Yes.

 **Overdose:** Symptoms of overdose include extreme anxiety, insomnia, confusion, muscle tremors or twitching, nausea, convulsions, a severe headache, fever and sweating, and hallucinations. Seek emergency medical treatment.

---

## PRECAUTIONS

### Do not take this drug if:

- You have ever had an allergic reaction to this drug.
- You have glaucoma.
- You have a history of alcohol or drug dependence.

### Inform your physician if:

- You have ever had an allergic reaction to any drug.
- You have epilepsy or a family history of seizures.
- You have a family history of tics or Tourette's syndrome.
- You are taking any other drug— prescription or nonprescription —or vitamins.
- You are now taking or have taken in the past two weeks a monoamine oxidase (MAO) inhibitor.
- You have used or are now using cocaine.
- You will be under anesthesia or undergoing surgery or medical testing in the next few months.

 **Pregnancy/Breast-feeding**

Do not take this drug if you are pregnant, planning a pregnancy, or are breast-feeding.

 **Infants/Children**

This drug should not be given to children under age six. Long-term use may affect growth.

 **Over Sixty**

Little research is available on the effect of methylphenidate on elderly people. This drug is prescribed by some psychiatrists to increase mental alertness in the elderly and is known to augment the effects of heterocyclic antidepressants for people with treatment-resistant depression.

 **Driving/Operating Machinery**

This drug may impair mental alertness and coordination. Do not drive or operate machinery until you are certain this drug will not affect your performance. This drug has been abused by those wishing to increase alertness and to combat sleepiness while driving. This is a dangerous practice as tolerance builds up for its mental alertness effects, and its psychological side effects can impair perception or judgment.

## GENERAL INFORMATION

Methylphenidate belongs to a group of medicines known as *central nervous system stimulants*. This drug is, by far, the most commonly prescribed medication for attention-deficit hyperactivity disorder in children. In particular, it is often the drug of first choice for children who have problems with attention and concentration, but show few signs of hyperactivity. Methylphenidate causes fewer side effects than the amphetamines. Children who suffer from schizophrenia or other psychotic disorders that may produce symptoms similar to attention-deficit disorders should not be given stimulants. A sustained-release form of methylphenidate is available, although it is not effective with all children. For an explanation of how this drug works, see Chapter 10.

## BENEFITS

- Effective in treating attention deficit hyperactivity disorder in children and adolescents.
- Augments the antidepressant effects of heterocyclic antidepressants.

## RISKS

- Stimulants sometimes induce Tourette's syndrome.
- Increases vulnerability to seizure disorders.
- Can be abused in people prone to drug dependence.

## GUIDELINES FOR USERS

**How is the drug taken?** Tablets (5, 10, 20 mg); sustained-release form.

**What is the usual dosage?** The initial dose for a child with attention-deficit hyperactivity disorder may range from 5 mg to 15 mg per day. Dosages must be increased and adjusted to the individual in response to therapeutic benefits and side effects.

**What are the instructions for taking the drug?** Take methylphenidate about a half-hour before meals. Your last dose should be taken before 6:00 P.M. to prevent trouble sleeping. Do not crush, break, or chew the tablets before swallowing.

**How quickly will I feel the effect of the drug and how long does it last?** When this drug is effective, adults will usually notice some improvement in the child from almost the first day the medication is taken. The effects of methylphenidate last about three to four hours, and it must be given several times a day. The sustained-release form of the drug can be taken once a day. However, this form does not work for all children.

**What if I miss a dose or several doses?** If you are taking several doses a day and remember the missed dose within an hour or so, take the dose. However, if it is almost time for your next dose, skip the missed dose and continue on your regular schedule. Do not take a dose after 6:00 P.M. Do not take double doses.

If you are taking the long-acting capsule, take the missed dose only if you remember within an hour or so. Otherwise, skip the missed dose. Do not take double doses.

**What if I stop taking the drug?** Do not stop taking this drug without consulting your physician. Your physician may wish to taper off your doses to prevent withdrawal symptoms.

**How should I store the drug?** Keep out of reach of children. Store in a dry, tightly closed, light-resistant container. Heat and moisture may cause this drug to break down.

**DRUG NAME:**    Methylphenidate (*continued*)

## GUIDELINES FOR USERS (*continued*)

As this drug has a high potential for abuse, we recommend that it be kept in a locked cabinet and that careful records be maintained to check for missing tablets.

## INTERACTIONS

**Alcohol:** Alcohol may aggravate the symptoms of attention-deficit hyperactivity disorder and react dangerously with central nervous system effects of methylphenidate.

**Food/Beverages:** No restrictions; however, caffeine may increase nervousness, anxiety, and other emotional side effects.

**Smoking:** No restrictions.

**Other drugs:** Cocaine in combination with methylphenidate can be extremely dangerous. The combination can produce severe anxiety, disturbed sleeping, irregular heartbeat, and seizures.

The danger of overdose is high when methylphenidate is combined with heterocyclic antidepressants. This drug should not be combined with monoamine oxidase inhibitors.

Antihistamines have a sedative effect that may counteract the effect of methylphenidate.

Methylphenidate may decrease the hypotensive effect of guanethidine.

Methylphenidate may increase the effects of the anticoagulants and anticonvulsants (phenobarbital, diphenylhydantoin, primidone, phenylbutazone).

## HABIT-FORMING POTENTIAL

High.

## LONG-TERM USE

Addiction is primarily a problem with adults. It is extremely rare for children with attention-deficit hyperactivity disorder to become addicted. Because this drug has been widely abused by adults, its use is tightly regulated by the Food and Drug Administration. When high doses are taken for a long time, a person may experience severe side effects, including paranoia, delusions, and other psychoses. Children who take this drug on a long-term basis should be examined every four to six months. The physician should monitor height and weight, look for the presence of tics, measure blood pressure and pulse, and ask about side effects.

## PLEASE NOTE

Signs of methylphenidate abuse: When abused, this drug can cause an increase in the heart rate, elevated blood pressure, dilation of the pupils, and agitation. As dosages increase, more severe side effects—including irritability, confusion, hostility, and sleep disturbances—may be noticed. At the highest doses, a person's symptoms (bizarre thoughts, delusions, and agitation) may resemble common symptoms of schizophrenia.

Treatment for withdrawal: In most cases, a person who has abused methylphenidate and who is suffering withdrawal symptoms can be treated on an outpatient basis. Symptoms of withdrawal include fatigue, insomnia, or hypersomnia. An antipsychotic medication may be prescribed if a person is experiencing delusions, hallucinations, agitation, or confusion. Inpatient treatment may be required when the drug was taken intravenously, when a person is depressed or suicidal, or when a person has lost touch with reality.

Effects on growth in children: Stimulants may suppress the production of growth hormone and can reduce weight and height gain in growing children. In most cases, this lag is temporary. However, the effects on growth that the long-term use of stimulants has on children lead some physicians to believe that this drug should never be prescribed for children.

| Methylphenidate | | | | | | | |
|---|---|---|---|---|---|---|---|
| | Frequency | | Discuss with Physician | | | | |
| Symptom/Effect | Common | Rare | Not Necessary | In All Cases | Only If Severe | Stop Taking Drug Now | Call Physician Now |
| loss of appetite | X | | | X | | | |
| difficulty sleeping | X | | | X | | | |
| weight loss | X | | | X | | | |
| abdominal pain | | X | | X | | X | X |
| headache | | X | | X | | | |
| drowsiness | | X | | X | | | |
| dizziness | | X | | X | | | |
| mood changes | | X | | X | | | |
| lack of coordination | | X | | X | | | |
| tics or unusual movements | | X | | X | | | |
| fast heartbeat | | X | | X | | | |
| blurred vision | | X | | X | | | |
| nausea | X | | | | X | | |
| joint pain | | X | | X | | | |
| chest pain | | X | | X | | X | X |
| skin rash or hives | | X | | X | | X | X |

DRUG NAME: **Molindone**

**BRAND NAMES:** Lidone, Moban
**For more information:** See Chapter 7, Antipsychotic Drugs.

FAST FACTS   **Drug group:** Antipsychotics.     **Available as generic?** No.
**Prescription needed?** Yes.     **Habit-forming?** No.

 **Overdose:** Symptoms include light-headedness, sedation, confusion, agitation, disorientation, restlessness, convulsions, fever, and coma. Seek immediate emergency medical treatment.

## PRECAUTIONS

### Do not take this drug if:

- You have ever had an allergic reaction to this drug or any other antipsychotic drug.

### Inform your physician if:

- You have ever had an allergic reaction to any drug.
- You have kidney, thyroid, or liver problems.
- You have epilepsy, asthma, liver disease, or glaucoma.
- You are taking any other drug— prescription or nonprescription —or vitamins.
- You are on a low-salt, low-sugar, or any other special diet.
- You will be under anesthesia or undergoing surgery or medical testing in the next few months.

 ### Pregnancy/Breast-feeding

Safe use of this drug during pregnancy has not been established. Except in unusual cases where the mother or the baby's life is endangered, this drug should not be taken by pregnant women. Women taking molindone should not breast-feed.

 ### Infants/Children

This drug has not been proved safe or effective for children under the age of twelve.

 ### Over Sixty

Side effects, some serious, can be worse. Initial dose should be low, with careful monitoring for side effects. Special care should be taken when sitting up from a lying position, or standing from a sitting position, as blood pressure may be lowered and balance impaired.

 ### Driving/Operating Machinery

Extreme caution is advised. This medicine can impair mental alertness and co-ordination. If you do drive or operate machinery, this medicine should be taken at bedtime when its sedating effects are less likely to interfere with day-time activities.

## GENERAL INFORMATION

Molindone is an intermediate-potency antipsychotic in the dihydroindolone class. It is used to treat people who are experiencing disorganized, psychotic thinking and who may be having delusions or hallucinations. Molindone is less likely to cause seizures than most other antipsychotics. Of all the antipsychotic drugs, it is least likely to cause weight gain. For an explanation of how this drug works, see Chapter 7.

| BENEFITS | RISKS |
|---|---|
| • Effective in treating hallucinations, delusions, confused thinking, and mania. | • Can dangerously lower white blood cell count. |
| • Sedating effects helpful in calming agitated persons. | • Can cause tardive dyskinesia. |
| • Less likely to cause seizures than most other antipsychotics. | • Can cause neuroleptic malignant syndrome. |
| • Less likely to cause weight gain. | |

## GUIDELINES FOR USERS

**How is the drug taken?** Tablets (5, 10, 25, 50, 100 mg); oral concentrate; intramuscular.

**What is the usual dosage?** Initial dose should be 50 mg to 75 mg per day in healthy young people, with increases as needed to control symptoms. A maximum daily dose of up to 225 mg may be used, if necessary. Rarely is more than 75 mg given as a single dose. Maintenance doses should be as low as possible and still be able to control the psychotic symptoms.

**What are the instructions for taking the drug?** It is best to take this drug on an empty stomach and drink a full glass of water. The liquid form of molindone can be taken with juice or milk to make it easier to take. Follow your physician's instructions carefully.

**How quickly will I feel the effect of the drug?** It usually takes several weeks for you to experience the full benefit of this drug. However, you may feel more calm and relaxed after the first dose or two. The drug should also help you sleep better, if this is a problem.

**What if I miss a dose or several doses?** If you miss a dose and remember within an hour or so, take the missed dose. Otherwise, skip the missed dose and continue on your regular dosing schedule. Do not take double doses.

If you are missing doses on a frequent basis, notify your psychiatrist. A slow-release form of an antipsychotic drug may help with your compliance and help avoid a relapse.

**What if I stop taking the drug?** Do not stop taking this drug without consulting your physician. Abruptly stopping this medication will lead to uncomfortable but not dangerous physical symptoms. Should your physician and you agree that the drug should be discontinued, your medication should be tapered slowly to prevent physical symptoms of withdrawal and a reemergence of your psychotic symptoms.

**How should I store the drug?** Keep out of reach of children. Store in a dry, tightly closed, light-resistant container. Heat and moisture may cause this drug to break down. The liquid form does not require refrigeration.

**DRUG NAME:**    Molindone (*continued*)

## INTERACTIONS

**Alcohol:** Avoid alcohol. When combined with alcohol, this medicine can cause excessive sedation and dangerously lower blood pressure.

**Food/Beverages:** No restrictions.

**Smoking:** Smoking lowers the blood level of molindone. If you do smoke, blood samples should be taken to test whether the drug is in the therapeutic range.

**Other drugs:** Antacids with aluminum or magnesium (Maalox, for example) should not be taken for two hours before or after taking molindone because they may interfere with the absorption of this drug.

Heterocyclic antidepressants can increase the plasma level of this drug and cause a worsening of side effects. Conversely, this drug can increase the blood level of antidepressants. The concurrent use of these two types of drugs must be carefully monitored.

Blood pressure can be dangerously lowered when antipsychotics are combined with vasodilators (medications that dilate blood vessels).

Molindone will increase the effect of medicines known as CNS (central nervous system) depressants. Examples include antihistamines, hay fever medicines, sedatives, narcotics, muscle relaxants, barbiturates, and anesthetics. Check with your physician before taking any of these drugs.

## HABIT-FORMING POTENTIAL

None.

## LONG-TERM USE

Prolonged use of molindone is associated with increased risk of developing tardive dyskinesia, a potentially irreversible side effect involving disfiguring movements of the face, tongue, and limbs. For more information on tardive dyskinesia, please see Chapter 7.

## PLEASE NOTE

Not a sleeping pill: This drug, which has a sedating effect, is sometimes misused as a sleeping pill. There are much safer medications available as sleeping aids.

Not specifically antiaggressive: Because of the potential serious side effects of the antipsychotic drugs, especially over the long term, this medication should not be used to treat anxiety or chronic aggression and agitation.

Frequent examinations required: While taking this medication, your blood pressure and pulse rate should be monitored frequently. Regular checks should also be made for the early signs of tardive dyskinesia.

| Molindone | | | | | | | |
|---|---|---|---|---|---|---|---|
| | Frequency | | Discuss with Physician | | | | |
| Symptom/Effect | Common | Rare | Not Necessary | In All Cases | Only If Severe | Stop Taking Drug Now | Call Physician Now |
| lethargy/sleepiness | X | | | | X | | |
| low blood pressure | X | | | X | | | |
| dizziness | | X | | X | | | |
| dry mouth | X | | | | X | | |
| blurred vision | X | | | | X | | |
| constipation | X | | | | X | | |
| difficulty urinating | X | | | X | | | |
| reduced urinary output | | X | | X | | | X |
| racing heartbeat/ palpitations | | X | | X | | | |
| weakness | | X | | X | | | |
| sexual problems | | X | | X | | | |
| restlessness | | X | | X | | | |
| skin rash | | X | | X | | | X |
| weight gain | X | | | | X | | |
| seizures | | X | | X | | X | X |
| low white blood cell count | | X | | X | | | X |
| tremors | | X | | X | | | |
| stiffness | X | | | X | | | |
| involuntary facial or tongue movements | | X | | X | | | |

## DRUG NAME: **Nortriptyline**

**BRAND NAMES:** Aventyl, Pamelor
**For more information:** See Chapter 3, Antidepressant Drugs.

**FAST FACTS**   **Drug group:** Antidepressants.    **Available as generic?** Yes.
**Prescription needed?** Yes.    **Habit-forming?** No.

 **Overdose:** The danger of an overdose, which can be lethal, is extremely high. Symptoms include difficulty breathing, shock, vomiting, agitation, delirium, convulsions, and coma. Seek immediate emergency medical treatment.

## PRECAUTIONS

### Do not take this drug if:

- You have ever had an allergic or negative reaction to any drug in this group.

### Inform your physician if:

- You have ever had an allergic reaction to any drug.
- You have epilepsy or glaucoma.
- You have kidney, liver, or cardiovascular disease.
- You are taking any other drug— prescription or nonprescription —or vitamins.
- You will be under anesthesia or undergoing surgery or medical testing in the next few months.

 ### Pregnancy/Breast-feeding

If you are pregnant or planning a pregnancy, you should, if possible, use non-drug alternatives for treating your depression. This drug has not been demonstrated to be safe during pregnancy. Nursing mothers should not take this drug since it is passed on to the baby in the mother's milk.

 ### Infants/Children

Do not give this drug to children. This drug has not been proved safe or effective for children. Its use in the treatment of depression in children and adolescents must be under the guidance of a child psychiatrist.

 ### Over Sixty

Lower doses are recommended. Side effects may be worse and some older patients may experience confusion. Elderly people may fall after standing up because of the drug's hypotensive (blood pressure lowering) side effects.

 ### Driving/Operating Machinery

Extreme caution is advised. This medicine can impair mental alertness and coordination. If you do drive or operate machinery, this medicine should be taken at bedtime, when its sedating effects are less likely to interfere with daytime activities.

## GENERAL INFORMATION

Nortriptyline is one of the heterocyclic drugs used to treat depression. It works by inhibiting the nerve cell's ability to reabsorb the neurotransmitters norepinephrine and serotonin (see Chapter 3).

## BENEFITS

- Helps 75 percent to 80 percent of people with major depression.

## RISKS

- Produces annoying side effects.
- Potential for use in suicide attempts.

## GUIDELINES FOR USERS

**How is the drug taken?** Capsules (10, 25, 50, 75 mg); oral concentrate.

**What is the usual dosage?** The initial dose is usually 25 mg to 50 mg daily, with increases as needed to control symptoms. The maximum daily dose is 150 mg. Initial doses are lower for patients with medical illnesses, and the elderly.

**What are the instructions for taking the drug?** Take this medicine with food, unless your doctor has instructed you otherwise. Taking the medicine on an empty stomach may cause your stomach to become upset. To benefit from the drug, it is important to take the correct dosage each day.

**How quickly will I feel the effect of the drug?** You will probably experience some unpleasant side effects (dry mouth, blurry vision, constipation) right away. It may take days or weeks for the benefits to appear. It usually takes two to four weeks at full dose for a person to feel a positive response. By the third week of treatment, the side effects are usually less severe.

**What if I miss a dose or several doses?** If you are taking one dose at bedtime and miss your dose, do not take the drug in the morning. Check with your doctor. If you are taking more than one dose a day and remember within an hour or so that you have missed a dose, take the dose. However, if it is almost time for your next dose, skip the missed dose. Do not take double doses.

**What if I stop taking the drug?** Do not discontinue this drug abruptly. Your dosage should be gradually reduced. Stopping the drug abruptly may cause flulike symptoms, headache, restlessness, and/or a worsening of your condition. Inform your physician if you notice these side effects, or any others, after stopping the drug. The effects of this drug may last for up to seven days after you have stopped taking it.

**How should I store the drug?** Keep out of reach of children. Store in a dry, tightly closed, light-resistant container. Heat and moisture may cause this drug to break down.

## INTERACTIONS

**Alcohol:** Do not drink alcohol. Nortriptyline *increases* the effect of alcohol, while alcohol *increases* the side effects of the drug. In addition, alcohol use can contribute to depression.

**Food/Beverages:** No restrictions.

**DRUG NAME:**   Nortriptyline (*continued*)

## INTERACTIONS (*continued*)

**Smoking:** Smoking lowers the blood level of nortriptyline. If you do smoke, blood samples should be taken to test whether the drug is in the therapeutic range.

**Other drugs:** Nortriptyline will increase the effect of medicines known as CNS (central nervous system) depressants. Examples include antihistamines, hay fever medicines, sedatives, narcotics, muscle relaxants, barbiturates, and anesthetics. Check with your physician before taking any of these drugs.

## HABIT-FORMING POTENTIAL

None.

## LONG-TERM USE

Most people who have a beneficial response do not need to take this drug longer than about six months. A few people may need to take the drug for a year or longer because their depression recurs if they attempt to discontinue the drug.

## PLEASE NOTE

Help with side effects: Drinking water and sucking on hard candy can help if you are experiencing dry mouth. To prevent constipation, eat high-fiber foods and take a daily dose of a natural bulk laxative. And you can avoid episodes of light-headedness by making sure you get up slowly from a sitting or prone position. These side effects generally get better or go away after you have been on the drug several weeks.

| Nortriptyline | | | | | | | |
|---|---|---|---|---|---|---|---|
| | **Frequency** | | **Discuss with Physician** | | | | |
| **Symptom/Effect** | **Common** | **Rare** | **Not Necessary** | **In All Cases** | **Only If Severe** | **Stop Taking Drug Now** | **Call Physician Now** |
| drowsiness | X | | | | X | | |
| dry mouth | X | | | | X | | |
| constipation | X | | | | X | | |
| blurred vision | X | | | | X | | |
| low blood pressure | X | | | X | | | |
| racing heartbeat/ palpitations | | X | | | X | | |
| confusion | | X | | X | | | X |
| skin rashes/allergies | | X | | X | | | |
| insomnia | | X | | | X | | |
| sexual problems | | X | | X | | | |
| increased appetite | | X | | | X | | |
| seizures | | X | | X | | X | X |

DRUG NAME: **Oxazepam**

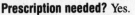

**BRAND NAME:** Serax
**For more information:** See Chapter 4, Antianxiety Drugs.

**FAST FACTS**   **Drug group:** Antianxiety agents (benzodiazepines).

**Available as generic?** Yes.

**Prescription needed?** Yes.

**Habit-forming?** Yes.

 **Overdose:** It is possible, though not easy, to overdose. Signs of toxicity include sedation, decreased breathing rate, confusion, and loss of coordination. If these symptoms are present, seek immediate emergency medical treatment.

## PRECAUTIONS

### Do not take this drug if:

- You have had previously negative reactions to benzodiazepines.
- You have a history of drug dependence.
- You have Alzheimer's disease, have had a stroke, or have multiple sclerosis or other brain disorders.
- You are seriously depressed.

### Inform your physician if:

- You are taking any other drug—prescription or nonprescription—or vitamins.
- You have ever had an allergic reaction to any drug.
- You will be under anesthesia or undergoing surgery or medical testing in the next few months.

 **Pregnancy/Breast-feeding**

Do not take this drug if you are pregnant, planning a pregnancy, or breast-feeding.

 **Infants/Children**

Should not be used by children under six; optimum dosage for children six to twelve has not been established.

 **Over Sixty**

Smaller doses are advised and should be monitored very closely.

 **Driving/Operating Machinery**

WARNING: Do not fly, drive, or operate heavy machinery since this drug can impair mental alertness and coordination.

## GENERAL INFORMATION

Oxazepam is the fifth most frequently prescribed benzodiazepine. Like other drugs in the family, it is used to treat mild to moderate anxiety. It is sometimes prescribed to treat alcohol addiction or alcohol withdrawal symptoms. Serax is the brand name for Wyeth-Ayerst's product. Generics are made by Barr, Danbury, Geneva, Martec, Squibb, and Warner Chilcott. Oxazepam is eliminated from the body quickly after it is discontinued. Thus, it can cause withdrawal symptoms within one to two days after discontinuation. The advantage is that it is less likely than other benzodiazepines to build up in

**DRUG NAME:**    Oxazepam (*continued*)

## GENERAL INFORMATION (*continued*)

the body over time and to produce side effects such as sedation, loss of coordination and memory, and muscle weakness. For an explanation of how this drug works, see Chapter 4.

## BENEFITS

- More effective and fewer side effects than barbiturates.
- Less addictive and safer in overdoses than barbiturates.
- Relieves anxiety in about 65 percent to 70 percent of users.
- Fewer side effects than some benzodiazepines.

## RISKS

- Physically and psychologically addictive if misused.
- Makes some people feel lethargic, less able to concentrate, less alert.
- Can affect physical coordination.

## GUIDELINES FOR USERS

**How is the drug taken?** Tablets (15 mg); capsules (10, 15, 30 mg).

**What is the usual dosage?** The initial dose should be 30 mg to 60 mg per day, with increases as needed to control symptoms. A maximum daily dose of up to 120 mg may be used, if necessary.

**What are the instructions for taking the drug?** As with all benzodiazepines, if you are taking this drug for the first time, take your first dose at home and during a time when you are not required to work or drive. Your physician should tell you how often to take subsequent doses. Follow these instructions carefully. This drug can be taken before, during, or after meals. The capsules should not be opened. The tablets can be crushed and dissolved in water before taking, if you prefer.

**How quickly will I feel the effect of the drug?** Those who benefit from this drug will usually experience a positive response within the first week. Many people feel the drug's effect the first day of treatment.

**What if I miss a dose or several doses?** If you miss a dose and remember within an hour or so, take the missed dose. However, if more than an hour has elapsed, skip the dose and continue on your regular schedule. Do not take double doses.

**What if I stop taking the drug?** If you take this drug regularly for three weeks or more, you should not stop abruptly. Your dosage should be gradually reduced. Abrupt cessation can cause psychological and physical withdrawal symptoms.

**How should I store the drug?** Keep out of reach of children, since all benzodiazepines can be extremely dangerous to children. Store in a dry, tightly closed, light-resistant container. Heat and moisture may cause this drug to break down.

## INTERACTIONS

**Alcohol:** Do not drink alcohol. Oxazepam is highly dangerous when combined with alcohol. It can dangerously lower blood pressure, decrease the breathing rate, and lead to loss of consciousness.

**Food/Beverages:** No restrictions on food. Control caffeine intake, as caffeine makes anxiety worse.

**Smoking:** Heavy smoking of tobacco may reduce the sedative effects of this drug. Marijuana smoking may increase side effects and significantly reduce mental alertness.

**Other drugs:** Narcotics (e.g., Demerol, Percodan, codeine, morphine, Talwin) may *increase* the sedative effects of this drug. The combination can be fatal. Do not use narcotics with this drug.

Barbiturates and other sedatives (e.g., phenobarbital, pentobarbital, Seconal, Tuinal) may *increase* sedation to dangerous levels. Do not combine sedatives with this drug.

Do not take other benzodiazepines when using this drug, since the combination is both unnecessary and unsafe.

Do not take sleeping pills while taking this drug. If you are having trouble sleeping, your doctor may prescribe larger doses of oxazepam.

The following drugs may reduce the liver's ability to remove this drug from the body, making the drug more powerful and increasing side effects:

- ulcer drugs
- birth control pills
- propranolol
- disulfiram (Antabuse)

## HABIT-FORMING POTENTIAL

High.

## LONG-TERM USE

Physical and psychological dependence are common problems. A clear treatment plan is important. It is possible to become dependent in as short a time span as two to four weeks. This drug should not be taken longer than four weeks on a regular basis (i.e., daily). Long-term use can also increase the risk of side effects.

## PLEASE NOTE

Nondrug alternatives: See Chapter 4 for a discussion of the value of exercise and a good diet in the treatment of anxiety. One of the best nondrug ways to reduce anxiety is to identify and reduce sources of stress in your life.

Correct diagnosis: You should always consult a physician to be sure that any medical causes of anxiety (such as hyperthyroidism) are diagnosed and treated. Anxiety may be a component of depression, in which case the symptoms of anxiety are treated by treating the underlying depression with antidepressants and/or other therapies for mood disorders.

**DRUG NAME:**   Oxazepam (*continued*)

| Symptom/Effect | Frequency | | Discuss with Physician | | | Stop Taking Drug Now | Call Physician Now |
|---|---|---|---|---|---|---|---|
| | Common | Rare | Not Necessary | In All Cases | Only If Severe | | |
| clumsiness/sleepiness | X | | | | X | | |
| abdominal cramps | | X | | X | | | |
| blurred vision | | X | | X | | | |
| dry mouth | | X | | X | | | |
| racing heartbeat/ palpitations | | X | | X | | | |
| shaking/slurred speech | | X | | X | | | |
| urination problems | | X | | X | | | X |
| seizures | | X | | X | | X | X |
| hallucinations | | X | | X | | X | X |
| memory loss | | X | | X | | X | X |
| trouble breathing | | X | | X | | X | X |
| staggering/trembling | | X | | X | | X | X |
| headache | | X | | X | | | |
| confusion | | X | | X | | | X |

# DRUG NAME: **Pemoline**

**BRAND NAME:** Cylert

**For more information:** See Chapter 10, Drugs for Attention-Deficit Hyperactivity Disorder.

**FAST FACTS**

**Drug group:** Stimulants.
**Prescription needed?** Yes.

**Available as generic?** No.
**Habit-forming?** Yes.

 **Overdose:** Symptoms of overdose include extreme agitation, confusion, hallucinations, a severe headache, fever, sweating, convulsions, a fast heartbeat, and coma. Seek immediate emergency medical treatment.

## PRECAUTIONS

### Do not take this drug if:

- You have ever had an allergic reaction to this drug.

### Inform your physician if:

- You have ever had an allergic reaction to any drug.
- You have epilepsy or a family history of seizures.
- You have liver, kidney, or heart disease.
- You are taking any other drug—prescription or nonprescription—or vitamins.
- You are now taking or have taken within two weeks a monoamine oxidase (MAO) inhibitor.
- You will be under anesthesia or undergoing surgery or medical testing in the next few months.

 **Pregnancy/Breast-feeding**

Do not take this drug if you are pregnant, planning a pregnancy, or are breast-feeding.

 **Infants/Children**

Safety and effectiveness have not been established for children under age six.

 **Over Sixty**

This drug is prescribed by some psychiatrists to increase mental alertness in the elderly and is known to augment the effects of heterocyclic antidepressants for people with treatment-resistant depression.

 **Driving/Operating Machinery**

This drug may impair mental alertness and coordination. Do not drive or operate machinery until you are certain this drug will not affect your performance. This drug has been abused by those wishing to increase alertness and to combat sleepiness while driving. This is a dangerous practice as tolerance builds up for its mental alertness effects, and its psychological side effects can impair perception or judgment.

## GENERAL INFORMATION

Pemoline is one of the medicines known as *central nervous system stimulants*. Originally, it was prescribed to improve cognitive functioning in older persons. Today, the drug is primarily used to treat attention-deficit hyperactivity disorder in children. Some

**DRUG NAME:**    Pemoline (*continued*)

## GENERAL INFORMATION (*continued*)

psychiatrists prefer pemoline over other stimulants because it produces fewer side effects. However, it is slower to show results, and improvement may not be noticeable for as long as three or four weeks. Children who suffer from schizophrenia or other psychotic disorders that may produce symptoms similar to attention-deficit disorders should not be given stimulants. For an explanation of how this drug works, see Chapter 10.

## BENEFITS

- Effective in treating attention-deficit hyperactivity disorder in children and adolescents.
- Augments the antidepressant effects of heterocyclic antidepressants.

## RISKS

- Stimulants sometimes induce Tourette's syndrome.
- Increases vulnerability to seizure disorders.
- Can be abused in people prone to drug dependence.
- May affect growth in some children.

## GUIDELINES FOR USERS

**How is the drug taken?** Tablets (18.75, 37.5, 75 mg).

**What is the usual dosage?** The initial dose ranges from 18.75 mg to 37.5 mg per day. A few children may require lower doses at first. Dosages must be increased and adjusted to the individual in response to therapeutic benefits and side effects.

**What are the instructions for taking the drug?** Pemoline is usually taken in a single dose in the morning. If you are taking the chewable tablet form of pemoline, the tablet must be chewed before swallowing.

**How quickly will I feel the effect of the drug and how long does it last?** In children who suffer from attention-deficit hyperactivity disorder, improvement may not be noticed for three or four weeks. Usually, it is parents and teachers who notice beneficial effects; children usually do not acknowledge change.

**What if I miss a dose or several doses?** If you miss a dose and remember within an hour or so, take the missed dose. However, if it is almost time for your next dose, skip the missed dose. Do not take double doses.

**What if I stop taking the drug?** Do not stop taking pemoline without consulting your physician. Your medication should be tapered slowly to prevent a reemergence of your symptoms.

**How should I store the drug?** Keep out of reach of children. Store in a dry, tightly closed, light-resistant container. Heat and moisture may cause this drug to break down. As this drug has a high potential for abuse, we recommend that it be kept in a locked cabinet and that careful records be maintained to check for missing tablets.

## INTERACTIONS

**Alcohol:** Alcohol may aggravate the symptoms of attention-deficit hyperactivity disorder and react dangerously with central nervous system effects of pemoline.

**Food/Beverages:** No restrictions; however, caffeine may increase nervousness, anxiety, and other emotional side effects.

**Smoking:** No restrictions.

**Other drugs:** The danger of overdose is high when pemoline is combined with heterocyclic antidepressants. This drug should not be used with monoamine oxidase inhibitors.

Antihistamines have a sedative effect that may counteract the effect of pemoline.

## HABIT-FORMING POTENTIAL

High.

## LONG-TERM USE

Addiction is a problem primarily with adults. It is extremely rare for children with attention-deficit hyperactivity disorder to become addicted. Because this drug has been widely abused by adults, its use is tightly regulated by the Food and Drug Administration. When high doses are taken for a long time, a person may experience severe side effects, including paranoia, delusions, and other psychoses. Children who take this drug on a long-term basis should be examined every four to six months. The physician should monitor height and weight, look for the presence of tics, measure blood pressure and pulse, and ask about side effects.

## PLEASE NOTE

Signs of pemoline abuse: When abused, this drug can cause an increase in the heart rate, elevated blood pressure, dilation of the pupils, and agitation. As dosages increase, more severe side effects—including irritability, confusion, hostility, and sleep disturbances—may be noticed. At the highest doses, a person's symptoms (bizarre thoughts, delusions, and agitation) may resemble common symptoms of schizophrenia.

Treatment for withdrawal: In most cases, a person who has abused pemoline and who is suffering withdrawal symptoms can be treated on an outpatient basis. Symptoms of withdrawal include fatigue, insomnia, or hypersomnia. An antipsychotic medication may be prescribed if a person is experiencing delusions, hallucinations, agitation, or confusion. Inpatient treatment may be required when the drug was taken intravenously, when a person is depressed or suicidal, or when a person has lost touch with reality.

Effects on growth in children: Stimulants may suppress the production of growth hormones and can reduce weight and height gain in growing children. In most cases, this lag is temporary. However, the effects on growth that the long-term use of stimulants has on children lead some physicians to believe that these drugs should never be prescribed for children.

**DRUG NAME:** Pemoline (*continued*)

| | Frequency | | Discuss with Physician | | | | |
|---|---|---|---|---|---|---|---|
| Symptom/Effect | Common | Rare | Not Necessary | In All Cases | Only If Severe | Stop Taking Drug Now | Call Physician Now |
| loss of appetite | X | | | | X | | |
| difficulty sleeping | X | | | X | | | |
| weight loss | X | | | X | | | |
| abdominal pain | | X | | X | | X | X |
| headache | | X | | | X | | |
| drowsiness | | X | | X | | | |
| dizziness | | X | | X | | | |
| mood changes | | X | | X | | | |
| lack of coordination | | X | | X | | | |
| tics or unusual movements | | X | | X | | X | X |
| nausea | X | | | | X | | |
| skin rash | | X | | X | | X | |
| yellow eyes or skin | | X | | X | | X | X |
| chest pain | | X | | X | | X | X |

The table is titled **Pemoline**.

DRUG NAME: **Perphenazine**

**BRAND NAMES:** Etrafon, Trilafon
**For more information:** See Chapter 7, Antipsychotic Drugs.

**FAST FACTS** **Drug group:** Antipsychotics.    **Available as generic?** Yes.
**Prescription needed?** Yes.    **Habit-forming?** No.

 **Overdose:** Symptoms include light-headedness, sedation, agitation, confusion, restlessness, disorientation, convulsions, fever, and coma. Seek immediate emergency medical treatment.

## PRECAUTIONS
### Do not take this drug if:

- You have ever had an allergic reaction to this drug or any phenothiazine.

### Inform your physician if:

- You have ever had an allergic reaction to any drug.
- You have epilepsy or asthma.
- You are taking any other drug—prescription or nonprescription —or vitamins.
- You are on a low-salt, low-sugar, or any other special diet.
- You will be under anesthesia or undergoing surgery or medical testing in the next few months.

 **Pregnancy/Breast-feeding**

Except in unusual cases where the mother or the baby's life is endangered, this drug should not be taken by pregnant women. Women taking perphenazine should not breast-feed.

 **Infants/Children**

Not recommended for children under age twelve.

 **Over Sixty**

Side effects, some serious, can be worse. Initial dose should be low, with careful monitoring for side effects. Special care should be taken when sitting up from a lying position, or standing from a sitting position, as blood pressure may be lowered and balance impaired.

 **Driving/Operating Machinery**

Extreme caution is advised. This medicine can impair mental alertness and co-ordination. If you do drive or operate machinery, this medicine should be taken at bedtime when its sedating effects are less likely to interfere with day-time activities.

## GENERAL INFORMATION

Perphenazine is an intermediate-potency antipsychotic used to treat people who are experiencing disorganized, psychotic thinking and who may be having delusions or hallucinations. The choice of which antipsychotic drug to use is often determined by the side effects. Perphenazine is available in combination with amitriptyline. However, combination products are not recommended. For an explanation of how this drug works, see Chapter 7.

**DRUG NAME:**   Perphenazine (*continued*)

| BENEFITS | RISKS |
|---|---|
| • Effective in treating hallucinations, delusions, confused thinking, and mania. <br> • Sedating effects helpful in calming agitated persons. | • Can dangerously lower white blood cell count. <br> • Can cause tardive dyskinesia. <br> • Can cause neuroleptic malignant syndrome. |

## GUIDELINES FOR USERS

**How is the drug taken?** Tablets (2, 4, 8, 16 mg); oral concentrate; intramuscular.

**What is the usual dosage?** The initial dose should be 4 mg to 12 mg per day in a healthy young person, with increases as needed to control symptoms. Maintenance doses should be as low as possible and still be able to control the psychotic symptoms.

**What are the instructions for taking the drug?** It is best to take this drug on an empty stomach and drink a full glass of water. The oral concentrate may be diluted with water, orange juice, or grape juice. However, this should be done just prior to taking the dose.

**How quickly will I feel the effect of the drug?** It usually takes several weeks for you to experience the full benefit of this drug. However, you may feel more calm and relaxed after the first dose or two. The drug should also help you sleep better, if this is a problem.

**What if I miss a dose or several doses?** If you miss a dose and remember within an hour or so, take the missed dose. Otherwise, skip the missed dose and continue on your regular dosing schedule. Do not take double doses.

If you are missing doses on a frequent basis, notify your psychiatrist. A slow-release form of an antipsychotic drug may help with your compliance and help avoid a relapse.

**What if I stop taking the drug?** Do not stop taking this drug without consulting your physician. Abruptly stopping this medication will lead to uncomfortable but not dangerous physical symptoms. Should your physician and you agree that the drug should be discontinued, your medication should be tapered slowly to prevent physical symptoms of withdrawal and a reemergence of your psychotic symptoms.

**How should I store the drug?** Keep out of reach of children. Store in a dry, tightly closed, light-resistant container. Heat and moisture may cause this drug to break down. The liquid form does not require refrigeration.

## INTERACTIONS

**Alcohol:** Avoid alcohol. When combined with alcohol, this medicine can cause excessive sedation and dangerously lower blood pressure.

**Food/Beverages:** No restrictions.

**Smoking:** Smoking lowers the blood level of perphenazine. If you do smoke, blood samples should be taken to test whether the drug is in the therapeutic range.

**Other drugs:** Antacids with aluminum or magnesium (Maalox, for example) should not be taken for two hours before or after taking perphenazine because they may interfere with the absorption of this drug.

Heterocyclic antidepressants can increase the plasma level of this drug and cause a worsening of side effects. Conversely, this drug can increase the blood level of antidepressants. The concurrent use of these two types of drugs must be carefully monitored.

Blood pressure can be dangerously lowered when antipsychotics are combined with vasodilators (medications that dilate blood vessels).

Perphenazine will increase the effect of medicines known as CNS (central nervous system) depressants. Examples include antihistamines, hay fever medicines, sedatives, narcotics, muscle relaxants, barbiturates, and anesthetics. Check with your physician before taking any of these drugs.

## HABIT-FORMING POTENTIAL

None.

## LONG-TERM USE

Prolonged use of perphenazine is associated with increased risk of developing tardive dyskinesia, a potentially irreversible side effect involving disfiguring movements of the face, tongue, and limbs. For more information on tardive dyskinesia, please see Chapter 7.

## PLEASE NOTE

Not a sleeping pill: This drug, which has a sedating effect, is sometimes misused as a sleeping pill. There are much safer medications available as sleeping aids.

Not specifically antiaggressive: Because of the potential serious side effects of the antipsychotic drugs, especially over the long term, this medication should not be used to treat anxiety or chronic aggression and agitation.

Frequent examinations required: While taking this medication, your blood pressure and pulse rate should be monitored frequently. Regular checks should also be made for the early signs of tardive dyskinesia.

Classification: Perphenazine is classified as a phenothiazine. Other antipsychotics in the same group include acetophenazine, chlorpromazine, fluphenazine, mesoridazine, promazine, thioridazine, trifluoperazine, and triflupromazine. In general, if you have a poor response to one drug in this family, you will likely have a similar poor response to other drugs in the family.

**DRUG NAME:**    Perphenazine (*continued*)

| Perphenazine | | | | | | | |
|---|---|---|---|---|---|---|---|
| | Frequency | | Discuss with Physician | | | | |
| Symptom/Effect | Common | Rare | Not Necessary | In All Cases | Only If Severe | Stop Taking Drug Now | Call Physician Now |
| lethargy/sleepiness | X | | | | X | | |
| low blood pressure | X | | | X | | | |
| dizziness | | X | | X | | | |
| dry mouth | X | | | | X | | |
| blurred vision | X | | | | X | | |
| constipation | X | | | | X | | |
| difficulty urinating | X | | | X | | | |
| reduced urinary output | | X | | X | | | X |
| racing heartbeat/ palpitations | | X | | X | | | |
| weakness | | X | | X | | | |
| sexual problems | | X | | X | | | |
| restlessness | | X | | X | | | |
| skin rash | | X | | X | | | |
| weight gain | X | | | | X | | |
| seizures | | X | | X | | X | X |
| low white blood cell count | | X | | X | | | |
| tremors | | X | | X | | | |
| stiffness | X | | | X | | | |
| involuntary facial or tongue movements | | X | | X | | | |

DRUG NAME: **Phenelzine**

**BRAND NAME:** Nardil
**For more information:** See Chapter 3, Antidepressant Drugs, and Chapter 5, Antipanic and Antiphobic Drugs.

**FAST FACTS**

**Drug group:** Antidepressants (monoamine oxidase inhibitors).

**Available as generic?** No.

**Prescription needed?** Yes.

**Habit-forming?** No.

 **Overdose:** Symptoms include drowsiness, dizziness, hypertension, agitation, hallucinations, convulsions, and coma. These symptoms may not develop until twelve hours after ingestion, reaching a peak twenty-four to forty-eight hours later. If you suspect an overdose or experience these symptoms, seek immediate emergency medical treatment.

## PRECAUTIONS

**Do not take this drug if:**

- You have ever had an allergic or negative reaction to this or any other MAO inhibitor.

**Inform your physician if:**

- You have ever had an allergic reaction to any drug.
- You have high blood pressure or heart problems.
- You have epilepsy.
- You are taking any other drug— prescription or nonprescription —or vitamins.
- You will be under anesthesia or undergoing surgery or medical testing in the next few months.

 **Pregnancy/Breast-feeding**

If you are pregnant, planning a pregnancy, or breast-feeding, you should not take this drug.

 **Infants/Children**

This drug should not be given to anyone under age sixteen since safety and effectiveness have not been proved.

 **Over Sixty**

Side effects may be worse.

 **Driving/Operating Machinery**

This drug may cause drowsiness. You should not drive a car during the initial phase of treatment. When you are confident that you are alert and have full motor coordination, ask your doctor if you can resume driving. We suggest having a passenger present on your initial trips to help ascertain safety.

## GENERAL INFORMATION

Phenelzine is a monoamine oxidase inhibitor used in the treatment of depression and panic. In most cases, phenelzine should not be the first treatment choice for depression. Rather, this drug is prescribed for people whose symptoms have failed to respond to other common antidepression drugs. This drug is just as effective in treating depression as the heterocyclic drugs; however, it poses a potential problem because of possible toxic food-drug interactions. If you are on this drug, it is extremely important to follow the dietary guidelines given to you by your physician. (For an explanation of how this drug works and a discussion of food-drug interactions, see Chapter 3.)

**DRUG NAME:**   Phenelzine (*continued*)

## BENEFITS

- As effective as heterocyclics in treating depression.
- May be effective in treating depression in patients who have not responded to other medications.
- May have special benefits in treating atypical depression.
- Effective in treating panic and phobic symptoms.

## RISKS

- Possible toxic interaction with some foods, beverages, and drugs.

## GUIDELINES FOR USERS

**How is the drug taken?** Tablets (15 mg).

**What is the usual dosage?** The initial dose for the treatment of depression is 15 mg to 30 mg daily. This may be increased gradually to 45 mg to 75 mg daily in divided doses. In rare cases, doses of 90 mg may be prescribed. After the maximum benefit has been achieved, the dosage is normally reduced. When used to treat panic attacks, the initial dose is usually 15 mg per day for three days with increases to 45 mg. If panic symptoms persist, the dosage may be increased to 90 mg.

**What are the instructions for taking the drug?** Follow your physician's instructions carefully. This drug can be taken before, during, or after meals. The tablets can be crushed and dissolved in water before taking, if you prefer.

**How quickly will I feel the effect of the drug?** A few people experience the benefit of this drug during the first week, but it usually takes three or more weeks for a positive effect.

**What if I miss a dose or several doses?** If you miss a dose and remember within an hour or so, take the dose. However, if it is within two hours of your next dose, skip the missed dose. Do not take double doses.

**What if I stop taking the drug?** Do not stop taking phenelzine without consulting your doctor. If this drug has been taken regularly, withdrawal symptoms may appear unless it is discontinued gradually. After stopping this medicine, you must continue following the dietary guidelines for at least three weeks to avoid a toxic food-drug interaction.

**How should I store the drug?** Keep out of reach of children. Store in a dry, tightly closed, light-resistant container. Heat and moisture may cause this drug to break down.

## INTERACTIONS

**Alcohol:** Do not drink alcohol since this drug can *increase* the effects of alcohol and alcohol can *increase* phenelzine's side effects. In addition, alcohol use can contribute to depression.

**Food/Beverages:** Do not eat foods or drink beverages with tyramine. Tyramine can interact with this drug and cause *severe or fatal increases in blood pressure*. Among the food and beverages to be avoided are:

*Meat and fish:* lox, pickled herring, liver, dry sausage;

*Fruits and vegetables:* broad (fava) beans, raisins, figs, avocado;

*Dairy products:* Cheese (cottage cheese and cream cheese are allowed), yogurt;

*Beverages:* beer, wine, hard liquor, sherry, large amounts of caffeine (coffee, cocoa, or chocolate);

*Miscellaneous:* Yeast products (including brewer's yeast in large quantities), pickles, sauerkraut, soy sauce, sour cream, snails, licorice.

**Smoking:** Smoking may lower the blood level of phenelzine and this may reduce the drug's efficiency in treating depression.

**Other drugs:** All "recreational" or illegal drugs should be avoided by people with depression and may be *highly dangerous* when combined with phenelzine.

Do not take any other medicine without consulting your physician. This includes over-the-counter medicines (nonprescription) such as decongestants, other cold tablets or formulas, nasal drops or sprays, hay fever medications, sinus medications, appetite suppressants, weight-reducing preparations, or "pep" pills.

Do not take procaine (Novocain and others) while on this drug.

Notify your surgeon and anesthesiologist that you take this medication prior to any surgical procedure, as this MAO inhibitor reacts with certain anesthetics.

## HABIT-FORMING POTENTIAL

None.

## LONG-TERM USE

Most people may be tapered safely from the medication six months after their depression has responded to treatment. A small percentage of patients have symptoms of depression return after their dosage is reduced. These individuals may benefit from remaining on phenelzine for a year or longer.

## PLEASE NOTE

Cocaine use: Cocaine, when combined with an MAO inhibitor such as phenelzine, can dangerously increase blood pressure.

Surgery: If you are taking this drug, you should not undergo surgery requiring certain types of general anesthesia or a dental procedure requiring Novocain (procaine).

ID card: Your physician may suggest you carry an identification card that states you are taking this medicine. In addition, it's a good idea to carry with you at all times a wallet-sized list of foods high in tyramine content.

**DRUG NAME:**   Phenelzine (*continued*)

| | Frequency | | Discuss with Physician | | | Stop Taking Drug Now | Call Physician Now |
|---|---|---|---|---|---|---|---|
| Symptom/Effect | Common | Rare | Not Necessary | In All Cases | Only If Severe | | |
| blurred vision | X | | | | X | | |
| dizziness/light-headedness | X | | | X | | | |
| drowsiness/weakness | X | | | | X | | |
| decreased sexual ability | X | | | X | | | |
| constipation | | X | | | X | | |
| diarrhea | | X | | | X | | |
| allergies or rashes | | X | | X | | X | X |
| chest pain | | X | | X | | X | X |
| fast or slow heartbeat | X | | | X | | | |
| headache (severe) | | X | | X | | | X |
| chills/shivering | | X | | | X | | |
| dry mouth | X | | | | X | | |

(Table title: **Phenelzine**)

DRUG NAME: **Pimozide**

**BRAND NAME:** Orap
**For more information:** See Chapter 7, Antipsychotic Drugs.

**FAST FACTS**   **Drug group:** Antipsychotics.   **Available as generic?** No.

**Prescription needed?** Yes.   **Habit-forming?** No.

 **Overdose:** Symptoms include light-headedness, sedation, confusion, agitation, disorientation, restlessness, shock, muscle tremors, and coma. Seek immediate emergency medical treatment.

## PRECAUTIONS

**Do not take this drug if:**

- You have ever had an allergic reaction to this drug.

**Inform your physician if:**

- You have ever had an allergic reaction to any drug.
- You have epilepsy or asthma.
- You have kidney, heart, or liver disease.
- You are taking any other drug—prescription or nonprescription —or vitamins.
- You are on a low-salt, low-sugar, or other special diet.
- You will be under anesthesia or undergoing surgery or medical testing in the next few months.

 **Pregnancy/Breast-feeding**

Except in unusual cases where the mother or the baby's life is endangered, this drug should not be taken by pregnant women. Women taking pimozide should not breast-feed.

 **Infants/Children**

Safety and effectiveness have not been proved for children under age twelve.

 **Over Sixty**

Side effects, some serious, can be worse. Initial dose should be low, with careful monitoring for side effects. Special care should be taken when sitting up from a lying position, or standing from a sitting position, as blood pressure may be lowered and balance impaired.

 **Driving/Operating Machinery**

Extreme caution is advised. This medicine can impair mental alertness and coordination. If you do drive or operate machinery, this medicine should be taken at bedtime when its sedating effects are less likely to interfere with daytime activities.

## GENERAL INFORMATION

Pimozide is a high-potency antipsychotic used to treat the neuropsychiatric disorder Gilles de la Tourette syndrome and also to treat people who are experiencing psychotic thinking and hallucinations. Pimozide poses some serious risks and is not intended for treatment of tics that are merely annoying or cosmetically troublesome. Pimozide is usually not the drug of first choice, and is prescribed only if a person has failed to

**DRUG NAME:**    Pimozide (*continued*)

## GENERAL INFORMATION (*continued*)

respond to other medicines. This drug may be less likely to cause tardive dyskinesia than certain other antipsychotics, with the exception of clozapine. For an explanation of how this drug works, see Chapter 7.

## BENEFITS

- Effective in treating hallucinations, delusions, confused thinking, and mania.
- Effective in treating Gilles de la Tourette syndrome.
- Less likely to cause tardive dyskinesia than are certain other antipsychotics.

## RISKS

- Can dangerously lower white blood cell count.
- Can cause neuroleptic malignant syndrome.
- Can cause tardive dyskinesia.

## GUIDELINES FOR USERS

**How is the drug taken?** Tablets (2 mg).

**What is the usual dosage?** Initial dose should be 1 mg to 2 mg per day in healthy young people, with increases as needed to control symptoms. A maximum daily dose of up to 10 mg may be used if necessary. Maintenance doses should be as low as possible and still be able to control the psychotic symptoms or symptoms of Gilles de la Tourette syndrome.

**What are the instructions for taking the drug?** It is best to take this drug on an empty stomach and drink a full glass of water. Follow your physician's instructions carefully.

**How quickly will I feel the effect of the drug?** It usually takes several weeks for you to experience the full benefit of this drug. However, you may feel more calm and relaxed after the first dose or two.

**What if I miss a dose or several doses?** If you miss a dose and remember within an hour or so, take the missed dose. However, if more than an hour has elapsed, skip the dose and continue on your regular schedule. Do not take double doses.

If you are missing doses on a frequent basis, notify your psychiatrist. A slow-release form of another antipsychotic is available.

**What if I stop taking the drug?** Do not stop taking this drug without consulting your physician. Abruptly stopping this medication will lead to uncomfortable but not dangerous physical symptoms. Should your physician and you agree that the drug should be discontinued, your medication should be tapered slowly to prevent physical symptoms of withdrawal and a reemergence of your psychotic symptoms.

**How should I store the drug?** Keep out of reach of children. Store in a dry, tightly closed, light-resistant container. Heat and moisture may cause this drug to break down.

## INTERACTIONS

**Alcohol:** Avoid alcohol. When combined with alcohol, this medicine can cause excessive sedation and dangerously lower blood pressure.

**Food/Beverages:** No restrictions.

**Smoking:** Smoking lowers the blood level of pimozide. If you do smoke, blood samples should be taken to test whether the drug is in the therapeutic range.

**Other drugs:** Antacids with aluminum or magnesium (Maalox, for example) should not be taken for two hours before or after taking pimozide because they may interfere with the absorption of this drug.

Heterocyclic antidepressants can increase the plasma level of this drug and cause a worsening of side effects. Conversely, this drug can increase the blood level of antidepressants. The concurrent use of these two types of drugs must be carefully monitored.

Blood pressure can be dangerously lowered when antipsychotics are combined with vasodilators (medications that dilate blood vessels).

Pimozide may increase the effect of medicines known as CNS (central nervous system) depressants. Examples include antihistamines, hay fever medicines, sedatives, narcotics, muscle relaxants, barbiturates, and anesthetics. Check with your physician before taking any of these drugs.

## HABIT-FORMING POTENTIAL

None.

## LONG-TERM USE

Prolonged use of pimozide is associated with increased risk of developing tardive dyskinesia, a potentially irreversible side effect involving disfiguring movements of the face, tongue, and limbs. For more information on tardive dyskinesia, please see Chapter 7.

## PLEASE NOTE

Frequent examinations required: While taking this medication, your blood pressure and pulse rate should be monitored frequently. Regular checks should also be made for the early signs of tardive dyskinesia.

Use in children: Gilles de la Tourette syndrome often has its onset between the ages of two and fifteen years. However, there is very little information available on the use of this drug in children under the age of twelve.

**DRUG NAME:**  Pimozide (*continued*)

| | Frequency | | Discuss with Physician | | | | |
|---|---|---|---|---|---|---|---|
| **Symptom/Effect** | **Common** | **Rare** | **Not Necessary** | **In All Cases** | **Only If Severe** | **Stop Taking Drug Now** | **Call Physician Now** |
| difficulty speaking, swallowing | | X | | X | | X | X |
| coordination problems | | X | | | X | | |
| muscle spasms | | X | | X | | | |
| trembling/shaking | | X | | X | | | |
| vision problems | X | | | | X | | |
| constipation | X | | | | X | | |
| dizziness/light-headedness | X | | | | X | | |
| dry mouth | X | | | | X | | |
| skin rash | | X | | X | | | X |
| sore breasts/milk secretion | X | | | X | | | |
| diarrhea | | X | | | X | | |
| headache | | X | | | X | | |
| change of appetite | | X | | | X | | |
| nausea/vomiting | | X | | | X | | |
| swelling or puffiness in face | | X | | X | | | X |
| high or low blood pressure | X | | | X | | | |
| seizures | | X | | X | | X | X |
| fever | | X | | X | | | X |
| muscle stiffness | | X | | X | | | |
| sedation | X | | | | X | | |
| restlessness | | X | | X | | | |
| sexual problems | | X | | X | | | |
| reduced urinary output | | X | | X | | | X |

DRUG NAME: **Prazepam**

**BRAND NAME:** Centrax
**For more information:** See Chapter 4, Antianxiety Drugs.

**FAST FACTS**    **Drug group:** Antianxiety agents (benzodiazepines).          **Available as generic?** Yes.

**Prescription needed?** Yes.          **Habit-forming?** Yes.

 **Overdose:** It is possible, though not easy, to overdose. Signs of toxicity include sedation, decreased breathing rate, confusion, and loss of coordination. If these symptoms are present, seek immediate emergency medical treatment.

## PRECAUTIONS

### Do not take this drug if:

- You have had previously negative reactions to benzodiazepines.
- You have a history of drug dependence.
- You have Alzheimer's disease, have had a stroke, or have multiple sclerosis or other brain disorders.
- You are seriously depressed.

### Inform your physician if:

- You are taking any other drug—prescription or nonprescription—or vitamins.
- You have epilepsy.
- You will be under anesthesia or undergoing surgery or medical testing in the next few months.

 ### Pregnancy/Breast-feeding

Do not take this drug if you are pregnant, planning a pregnancy, or breast-feeding.

 ### Infants/Children

Safety and effectiveness have not been established for children and adolescents under eighteen.

 ### Over Sixty

Smaller doses are advised and should be monitored very closely.

 ### Driving/Operating Machinery

WARNING: Do not fly, drive, or operate heavy machinery since this drug can impair mental alertness and coordination.

## GENERAL INFORMATION

Prazepam is the sixth most frequently prescribed benzodiazepine. It is manufactured by Parke-Davis under the brand name Centrax and is available as a generic. Like the other benzodiazepines, it is used to treat anxiety. For an explanation of how this drug works, see Chapter 4.

**DRUG NAME:**    Prazepam (*continued*)

---

| BENEFITS | RISKS |
|---|---|
| • More effective and fewer side effects than barbiturates.<br>• Less addictive and safer in overdoses than barbiturates.<br>• Relieves anxiety in about 65 percent to 70 percent of users. | • Physically and psychologically addictive if misused.<br>• Makes some people feel lethargic, less able to concentrate, less alert.<br>• Can affect physical coordination. |

### GUIDELINES FOR USERS

**How is the drug taken?** Tablets (10 mg); capsules (5, 10, 20 mg).

**What is the usual dosage?** The initial dose should be 20 mg per day, with increases as needed to control symptoms. A maximum daily dose of up to 60 mg may be used, if necessary.

**What are the instructions for taking the drug?** As with all benzodiazepines, if you are taking this drug for the first time, take your first dose at home and during a time when you are not required to work or drive. Your physician should tell you how often to take subsequent doses. Follow these instructions carefully. This drug can be taken before, during, or after meals. The tablets can be crushed and dissolved in water before taking, if you prefer.

**How quickly will I feel the effect of the drug?** Those who benefit from this drug will usually experience a positive response within the first week. Many people feel the drug's effect the first day of treatment.

**What if I miss a dose or several doses?** If you miss a dose and remember within an hour or so, take the missed dose. However, if more than an hour has elapsed, skip the dose and continue on your regular schedule. Do not take double doses.

**What if I stop taking the drug?** If you take this drug regularly for three weeks or more, you should not stop abruptly. Your dosage should be gradually reduced. Abrupt cessation can cause psychological and physical withdrawal symptoms.

**How should I store the drug?** Keep out of reach of children, since all benzodiazepines can be extremely dangerous to children. Store in a dry, tightly closed, light-resistant container. Heat and moisture may cause this drug to break down.

---

### INTERACTIONS

**Alcohol:** Do not drink alcohol. Prazepam is highly dangerous when combined with alcohol. It can dangerously lower blood pressure, decrease the breathing rate, and lead to loss of consciousness.

**Food/Beverages:** No restrictions on food. Control caffeine intake, as caffeine makes anxiety worse.

**Smoking:** Heavy smoking of tobacco may reduce the sedative effects of the drug. Marijuana smoking may increase side effects and significantly reduce mental alertness.

**Other drugs:** Narcotics (e.g., Demerol, Percodan, codeine, morphine, Talwin) may

---

*increase* the sedative effects of this drug. The combination can be fatal. Do not use narcotics with this drug.

Barbiturates and other sedatives (e.g., phenobarbital, pentobarbital, Seconal, Tuinal) may *increase* sedation to dangerous levels. Do not combine sedatives with this drug.

Do not take other benzodiazepines when using this drug, since the combination is both unnecessary and unsafe.

Do not take sleeping pills while taking this drug. If you are having trouble sleeping, your doctor may prescribe larger doses of prazepam.

The following drugs may reduce the liver's ability to remove this drug from the body, making the drug more powerful and increasing side effects:
- ulcer drugs
- birth control pills
- propranolol
- disulfiram (Antabuse)

## HABIT-FORMING POTENTIAL

High.

## LONG-TERM USE

Physical and psychological dependence are common problems. A clear treatment plan is important. It is possible to become dependent in as short a time span as two to four weeks. This drug should not be taken longer than four weeks on a regular basis (i.e., daily). Long-term use can also increase the risk of side effects.

## PLEASE NOTE

Nondrug alternatives: See Chapter 4 for a discussion of the value of exercise and a good diet in the treatment of anxiety. One of the best nondrug ways to reduce anxiety is to identify and reduce sources of stress in your life.

Correct diagnosis: You should always consult a physician to be sure that any medical causes of anxiety (such as hyperthyroidism) are diagnosed and treated. Anxiety may be a component of depression, in which case the symptoms of anxiety are treated by treating the underlying depression with antidepressants and/or other therapies for mood disorders.

**Drug Name:**    Prazepam (*continued*)

| Symptom/Effect | Frequency | | Discuss with Physician | | | Stop Taking Drug Now | Call Physician Now |
|---|---|---|---|---|---|---|---|
| | Common | Rare | Not Necessary | In All Cases | Only If Severe | | |
| clumsiness/sleepiness | X | | | | X | | |
| abdominal cramps | | X | | X | | | |
| blurred vision | | X | | X | | | |
| dry mouth | | X | | X | | | |
| racing heartbeat/ palpitations | | X | | X | | | |
| shaking/slurred speech | | X | | X | | | |
| urination problems | | X | | X | | | |
| convulsions | | X | | X | | X | X |
| hallucinations | | X | | X | | X | X |
| memory loss | | X | | X | | X | X |
| trouble breathing | | X | | X | | X | X |
| staggering/trembling | | X | | X | | X | X |
| headache | | X | | X | | | |
| confusion | | X | | X | | X | X |

# DRUG NAME: **Promazine**

**BRAND NAME:** Sparine
**For more information:** See Chapter 7, Antipsychotic Drugs.

**FAST FACTS**

**Drug group:** Antipsychotics.
**Prescription needed?** Yes.

**Available as generic?** No.
**Habit-forming?** No.

**Overdose:** Symptoms include light-headedness, sedation, agitation, confusion, restlessness, disorientation, convulsions, fever, and coma. Seek immediate emergency medical treatment.

## PRECAUTIONS

### Do not take this drug if:

- You have ever had an allergic reaction to this drug or any phenothiazine.

### Inform your physician if:

- You have ever had an allergic reaction to any drug.
- You have epilepsy or asthma.
- You are taking any other drug—prescription or nonprescription—or vitamins.
- You are on a low-salt, low-sugar, or any other special diet.
- You will be under anesthesia or undergoing surgery or medical testing in the next few months.

### Pregnancy/Breast-feeding

Except in unusual cases where the mother or the baby's life is endangered, this drug should not be taken by pregnant women. Women taking promazine should not breast-feed.

### Infants/Children

Children may take this drug, but only under the direction of a pediatrician and/or children's psychiatrist.

### Over Sixty

Side effects, some serious, can be worse. Initial dose should be low, with careful monitoring for side effects. Special care should be taken when sitting up from a lying position, or standing from a sitting position, as blood pressure may be lowered and balance impaired.

### Driving/Operating Machinery

Extreme caution is advised. This medicine can impair mental alertness and coordination. If you do drive or operate machinery, this medicine should be taken at bedtime when its sedating effects are less likely to interfere with daytime activities.

## GENERAL INFORMATION

Promazine is a low-potency antipsychotic used to treat people who are experiencing disorganized, psychotic thinking, and perceptions such as delusions or hallucinations. Promazine can be quite sedating and often causes lowered blood pressure. However, it

**DRUG NAME:**   Promazine (*continued*)

## GENERAL INFORMATION (*continued*)

also has fewer movement side effects than certain other antipsychotics. The choice of which antipsychotic drug to use is often determined by the side effects. For an explanation of how this drug works, see Chapter 7.

## BENEFITS

- Effective in treating hallucinations, delusions, confused thinking, and mania.
- Sedating effects helpful in calming agitated persons.

## RISKS

- May dangerously lower white blood cell count.
- Can cause tardive dyskinesia.
- Can cause neuroleptic malignant syndrome.
- Can dangerously lower blood pressure.

## GUIDELINES FOR USERS

**How is the drug taken?** Tablets (25, 50, 100 mg).

**What is the usual dosage?** The initial dose should be 25 mg to 50 mg per day in healthy young people, with increases as needed to control symptoms. A maximum daily dose of up to 400 mg may be used, if necessary. Maintenance doses should be as low as possible and still be able to control the psychotic symptoms.

**What are the instructions for taking the drug?** It is best to take this drug on an empty stomach and drink a full glass of water.

**How quickly will I feel the effect of the drug?** It usually takes several weeks for you to experience the full benefit of this drug. However, you may feel more calm and relaxed after the first dose or two. The drug should also help you sleep better, if this is a problem.

**What if I miss a dose or several doses?** If you miss a dose and remember within an hour or so, take the missed dose. Otherwise, skip the missed dose and continue on your regular dosing schedule. Do not take double doses.

If you are missing doses on a frequent basis, notify your psychiatrist. A slow-release form of an antipsychotic drug may help with your compliance and help avoid a relapse.

**What if I stop taking the drug?** Do not stop taking this drug without consulting your physician. Abruptly stopping this medication will lead to uncomfortable but not dangerous physical symptoms. Should your physician and you agree that the drug should be discontinued, your medication should be tapered slowly to prevent physical symptoms of withdrawal and a reemergence of your psychotic symptoms.

**How should I store the drug?** Keep out of reach of children. Store in a dry, tightly closed, light-resistant container. Heat and moisture may cause this drug to break down.

## INTERACTIONS

**Alcohol:** Avoid alcohol. When combined with alcohol, this medicine can cause excessive sedation and dangerously lower blood pressure.

**Food/Beverages:** No restrictions.

**Smoking:** Smoking lowers the blood level of promazine. If you do smoke, blood samples should be taken to test whether the drug is in the therapeutic range.

**Other drugs:** Antacids with aluminum or magnesium (Maalox, for example) should not be taken for two hours before or after taking promazine because they may interfere with the absorption of this drug.

Heterocyclic antidepressants can increase the plasma level of this drug and cause a worsening of side effects. Conversely, this drug can increase the blood level of antidepressants. The concurrent use of these two types of drugs must be carefully monitored.

Blood pressure can be dangerously lowered when antipsychotics are combined with vasodilators (medications that dilate blood vessels).

Promazine will increase the effect of medicines known as CNS (central nervous system) depressants. Examples include antihistamines, hay fever medicines, sedatives, narcotics, muscle relaxants, barbiturates, and anesthetics. Check with your physician before taking any of these drugs.

## HABIT-FORMING POTENTIAL

None.

## LONG-TERM USE

Prolonged use of promazine is associated with increased risk of developing tardive dyskinesia, a potentially irreversible side effect involving disfiguring movements of the face, tongue, and limbs. For more information on tardive dyskinesia, please see Chapter 7.

## PLEASE NOTE

Not a sleeping pill: This drug, which has a sedating effect, is sometimes misused as a sleeping pill. There are much safer medications available as sleeping aids.

Not specifically antiaggressive: Because of the potential serious side effects of the antipsychotic drugs, especially over the long term, this medication should not be used to treat anxiety or chronic aggression and agitation.

Frequent examinations required: While taking this medication, your blood pressure and pulse rate should be monitored frequently. Regular checks should also be made for the early signs of tardive dyskinesia.

Classification: Promazine is classified as a phenothiazine. Other antipsychotics in the same group include acetophenazine, chlorpromazine, fluphenazine, mesoridazine, perphenazine, thioridazine, trifluoperazine, and triflupromazine. In general, if you have a poor response to one drug in this family, you will likely have a similar poor response to other drugs in the family.

**DRUG NAME:**  Promazine (*continued*)

| Symptom/Effect | Frequency | | Discuss with Physician | | | Stop Taking Drug Now | Call Physician Now |
|---|---|---|---|---|---|---|---|
| | Common | Rare | Not Necessary | In All Cases | Only If Severe | | |
| lethargy/sleepiness | X | | | | X | | |
| low blood pressure | X | | | X | | | |
| dizziness | | X | | X | | | |
| dry mouth | X | | | | X | | |
| blurred vision | X | | | | X | | |
| constipation | X | | | | X | | |
| difficulty urinating | X | | | X | | | |
| reduced urinary output | | X | | X | | | X |
| racing heartbeat/ palpitations | | X | | X | | | |
| weakness | | X | | X | | | |
| sexual problems | | X | | X | | | |
| restlessness | | X | | X | | | |
| skin rash | | X | | X | | | X |
| weight gain | X | | | | X | | |
| seizures | | X | | X | | X | X |
| low white blood cell count | | X | | X | | | X |
| tremors | | X | | X | | | |
| stiffness | X | | | X | | | |
| involuntary facial or tongue movements | | X | | X | | | |

# DRUG NAME: **Propranolol**

**BRAND NAME:** Inderal
**For more information:** See Chapter 4, Antianxiety Drugs, and Chapter 5, Antipanic and Antiphobic Drugs.

---

**FAST FACTS**    **Drug group:** Antianxiety agents (beta blockers).

**Available as generic?** Yes.

**Prescription needed?** Yes.

**Habit-forming?** No.

 **Overdose:** It is possible, though not easy, to overdose. Signs of toxicity include a slow heartbeat, dizziness, difficulty breathing, and convulsions. If these symptoms are present, seek immediate emergency medical treatment.

---

## PRECAUTIONS

### Do not take this drug if:

- You have ever had an allergic reaction to a beta-blocker medicine.
- You have asthma, chronic pulmonary disease, severe heart disease, severe allergies, diabetes, or low blood pressure.

### Inform your physician if:

- You have ever had an allergic reaction to any drug.
- You are taking any other drug—prescription or nonprescription—or vitamins.
- You are on a low-salt, low-sugar, or other special diet, or you are diabetic.
- You have liver or kidney problems or a history of heart failure.
- You will be under anesthesia or undergoing surgery or medical testing in the next few months.

 **Pregnancy/Breast-feeding**

Research on the use of beta blockers by pregnant women is inconclusive, although some studies have shown that beta blockers can cause breathing problems in newborns. To be safe, avoid taking this drug if you are pregnant or planning a pregnancy. If you are breast-feeding, propranolol will pass into the breast milk, and you should exercise caution before taking this drug.

 **Infants/Children**

Research has not yet shown if this drug is safe or effective for children.

 **Over Sixty**

Side effects may be more pronounced. Special care must be taken because this drug can lower blood pressure, causing a person to fall after standing up.

 **Driving/Operating Machinery**

This drug can impair mental alertness and coordination. Do not drive or operate machinery until you are certain this drug will not affect your performance.

**DRUG NAME:**   Propranolol (*continued*)

## GENERAL INFORMATION

Propranolol belongs to a group of medicines known as beta blockers, which, in addition to their antianxiety effects, are sometimes used to treat high blood pressure, angina (chest pain), migraine headaches, and a number of other conditions. It should be noted that beta blockers are not FDA-approved for the treatment of any anxiety disorder. Nonetheless, when prescribed to treat anxiety, beta blockers help relieve sweating, hand tremors, nervousness, "stomach butterflies," and other physical symptoms. They are particularly effective in treating performance anxiety, although this use is controversial. Propranolol is the beta blocker most frequently prescribed for this purpose. Some researchers believe that beta blockers can cause or intensify depression, although the evidence for this is controversial at this time. Propranolol is sometimes prescribed to treat manic episodes, aggressive disorders, and hand tremors caused by lithium.

## BENEFITS

- Has few side effects.
- Is not addictive.
- Effective in reducing performance anxiety.
- May reduce agitation, irritability, and aggression without causing sedation.

## RISKS

- Should not be used with certain pre-existing medical conditions.

## GUIDELINES FOR USERS

**How is the drug taken?** Tablets (10, 20, 40, 60, 80, 90 mg); capsules (long-acting 60, 80, 120, 160 mg); injection; intravenous.

**What is the usual dosage?** Effective doses vary from person to person, but the initial dose for treatment of anxiety usually ranges from 80 mg to 320 mg per day in divided doses. For performance anxiety, smaller doses are usually prescribed.

**What are the instructions for taking the drug?** If you are taking this drug for the first time, take your first dose at home and during a time when you are not required to work or drive, since this medicine causes some people to become dizzy and less alert. Propranolol is available in an extended-release form. If you are taking an extended-release capsule or tablet, swallow it whole. Do not crush, break, or chew the extended-release capsule or tablet.

**How quickly will I feel the effect of the drug and how long does it last?** The effect of the drug peaks about one to one and a half hours after taking a dose and lasts for several hours. For some people with performance anxiety, the effect start shortly after the drug is taken. For people with chronic anxiety, several weeks may be required before any benefit is experienced.

**What if I miss a dose or several doses?** It is important not to miss any doses if you are taking this drug on a regular basis. If you miss a dose and several hours have elapsed, skip the missed dose and go back to your regular dosing schedule. Do not take double doses.

**What if I stop taking the drug?** Do not stop the drug without checking with your physician. When discontinuing propranolol after being on the drug for an extended period, the dose must be gradually reduced to avoid withdrawal symptoms. Some people have vivid dreams or nightmares as the drug is being discontinued.

**How should I store the drug?** Keep out of reach of children. Store in a dry, tightly closed, light-resistant container. Heat and moisture may cause this drug to break down.

## INTERACTIONS

**Alcohol:** Control alcohol intake since propranolol and alcohol interact dangerously. The brain-depressing effects of alcohol and propranolol are additive.

**Food/Beverages:** No restrictions on food. Control caffeine intake since caffeine makes anxiety worse.

**Smoking:** No restrictions.

## HABIT-FORMING POTENTIAL

None.

## LONG-TERM USE

Beta blockers may be used safely over months or years. However, regular monitoring of your cardiovascular status is required.

## PLEASE NOTE

Cold temperatures: Beta blockers, which tend to decrease circulation in your hands and feet, can make you more sensitive to cold or hot weather. Dress warmly in winter, and if you exercise in hot weather, watch for symptoms of dizziness and light-headedness.

Word of caution: Beta blockers are more likely to produce highly dangerous side effects in persons with preexisting asthma and other pulmonary disorders, congestive heart failure, insulin-dependent diabetes mellitus, significant vascular disease, hyperthyroidism, and angina pectoris.

Musical note: Several studies have shown that certain musicians perform better when using beta blockers. Both the musicians and panels of "musical experts" rated the beta-blocker performances as superior.

FDA approval: At the present time, although beta blockers are extensively prescribed for the treatment of performance anxiety, general anxiety, irritability, and aggression associated with brain injury, there is no FDA-approved indication for using them in the treatment of any psychiatric disorder.

**DRUG NAME:**  Propranolol (*continued*)

| Symptom/Effect | Frequency | | Discuss with Physician | | | Stop Taking Drug Now | Call Physician Now |
|---|---|---|---|---|---|---|---|
| | Common | Rare | Not Necessary | In All Cases | Only If Severe | | |
| decreased sexual ability | | X | | X | | | |
| dizziness/slight drowsiness | X | | | | X | | |
| trouble sleeping | | X | | | X | | |
| difficulty breathing | | X | | X | | X | X |
| cold hands and feet | | X | | X | | X | |
| hallucinations | | X | | X | | X | X |
| irregular heartbeat | | X | | X | | X | |
| skin rash | | X | | X | | X | X |
| swelling of ankles, feet | | X | | X | | X | X |
| back or joint pain | | X | | X | | | |
| chest pain | | X | | X | | X | X |
| depression | | X | | X | | | X |
| confusion | | X | | X | | X | X |
| nausea | | X | | X | | | |
| fever | | X | | X | | | X |
| Abdominal cramps | | X | | X | | | |

DRUG NAME: **Protriptyline**

**BRAND NAME:** Vivactil
**For more information:** See Chapter 3, Antidepressant Drugs.

**FAST FACTS**  **Drug group:** Antidepressants.   **Available as generic?** No.
**Prescription needed?** Yes.   **Habit-forming?** No.

 **Overdose:** The danger of an overdose, which can be lethal, is extremely high. Symptoms include difficulty breathing, stupor, vomiting, agitation, convulsions, delirium, and coma. Seek immediate emergency medical treatment.

## PRECAUTIONS
### Do not take this drug if:

- You have ever had an allergic or negative reaction to any drug in this group.

### Inform your physician if:

- You have ever had an allergic reaction to any drug.
- You have epilepsy.
- You are taking any other drug—prescription or nonprescription—or vitamins.
- You will be under anesthesia or undergoing surgery or medical testing in the next few months.

 **Pregnancy/Breast-feeding**

If you are pregnant or planning a pregnancy, you should, if possible, use non-drug alternatives for treating your depression. This drug has not been demonstrated to be safe during pregnancy. Nursing mothers should not take this drug since it is passed on to the baby in the mother's milk.

 **Infants/Children**

The safety and effectiveness of this drug for children have not been determined. Lower dosages recommended for adolescents. Its use in the treatment of depression in children and adolescents must be under the guidance of a child psychiatrist.

 **Over Sixty**

In general, lower doses are required. Side effects may be worse and some older patients may experience confusion. Elderly people may fall after standing up because of the drug's hypotensive (blood pressure lowering) side effects.

 **Driving/Operating Machinery**

Extreme caution is advised. This medicine can impair mental alertness and coordination. If you do drive or operate machinery, this medicine should be taken at bedtime, when its sedating effects are less likely to interfere with daytime activities.

**DRUG NAME:**   Protriptyline (*continued*)

## GENERAL INFORMATION

Protriptyline is one of the heterocyclic drugs used to treat depression. It works by inhibiting the nerve cell's ability to reabsorb the neurotransmitters norepinephrine and serotonin (see Chapter 3). Protriptyline is among the less sedating heterocyclic drugs. Some studies have shown that it produces benefits more rapidly than the heterocyclics imipramine or amitriptyline.

## BENEFITS

- Helps 75 percent to 80 percent of people with major depression.

## RISKS

- Produces annoying side effects.
- Potential for use in suicide attempts.

## GUIDELINES FOR USERS

**How is the drug taken?** Tablets (5, 10 mg).

**What is the usual dosage?** The initial dose is usually 15 mg to 40 mg daily in divided doses, with increases as required. The maximum daily dosage is 60 mg. Initial doses are lower for patients with medical illnesses, and the elderly.

**What are the instructions for taking the drug?** Take this medicine with food, unless your physician has instructed you otherwise. Taking the medicine on an empty stomach may cause your stomach to become upset. To benefit from the drug, it is important to take the correct dosage each day.

**How quickly will I feel the effect of the drug?** You will probably experience some unpleasant side effects (dry mouth, blurry vision, constipation) right away. Some people feel a positive response within a week, though it could take up to four weeks at full dose. By the third week of treatment, the side effects are usually less severe.

**What if I miss a dose or several doses?** If you are taking one dose at bedtime and miss your dose, do not take the drug in the morning. Check with your physician. If you are taking more than one dose a day and remember within an hour or so that you have missed a dose, take the dose. However, if it is almost time for your next dose, skip the missed dose. Do not take double doses.

**What if I stop taking the drug?** Do not discontinue this drug abruptly. Your dosage should be gradually reduced. Stopping the drug abruptly may cause flulike symptoms, headache, restlessness, and/or a worsening of your condition. Inform your physician if you notice these side effects, or any others, after stopping the drug. The effects of this drug may last for up to seven days after you have stopped taking it.

**How should I store the drug?** Keep out of reach of children. Store in a dry, tightly closed, light-resistant container. Heat and moisture may cause this drug to break down.

## INTERACTIONS

**Alcohol:** Do not drink alcohol. Protriptyline *increases* the effect of alcohol, while alcohol *increases* the side effects of the drug. In addition, alcohol use can contribute to depression.

**Food/Beverages:** No restrictions.

**Smoking:** Smoking lowers the blood level of protriptyline. If you do smoke, blood samples should be taken to test whether the drug is in the therapeutic range.

**Other drugs:** Protriptyline will increase the effect of medicines known as CNS (central nervous system) depressants. Examples include antihistamines, hay fever medicines, sedatives, narcotics, muscle relaxants, barbiturates, and anesthetics. Check with your physician before taking any of these drugs.

## HABIT-FORMING POTENTIAL

None.

## LONG-TERM USE

Most people who have a beneficial response do not need to take this drug longer than about six months. A few people may need to take the drug for a year or longer because their depression recurs if they attempt to discontinue the drug.

## PLEASE NOTE

Help with side effects: Drinking water and sucking on hard candy can help if you are experiencing dry mouth. To prevent constipation, eat high-fiber foods and take a daily dose of a natural bulk laxative. And you can avoid episodes of light-headedness by making sure you get up slowly from a sitting or prone position. These side effects generally get better or go away after you have been on the drug several weeks.

**DRUG NAME:**    Protriptyline (*continued*)

| | Frequency | | Discuss with Physician | | | | |
|---|---|---|---|---|---|---|---|
| Symptom/Effect | Common | Rare | Not Necessary | In All Cases | Only If Severe | Stop Taking Drug Now | Call Physician Now |
| drowsiness | X | | | | X | | |
| dry mouth | X | | | | X | | |
| constipation | X | | | | X | | |
| blurred vision | X | | | | X | | |
| low blood pressure | X | | | X | | | |
| racing heartbeat/ palpitations | | X | | | X | | |
| confusion | | X | | X | | | X |
| skin rashes/allergies | | X | | X | | | X |
| insomnia | | X | | | X | | |
| sexual problems | | X | | X | | | |
| increased appetite | | X | | | X | | |
| seizures | | X | | X | | X | X |

# Drug Name: **Temazepam**

**Brand Name:** Restoril

**For more information:** See Chapter 8, Sedatives and Sleeping Pills, and Chapter 4, Antianxiety Drugs.

**FAST FACTS** **Drug group:** Sedatives (benzodiazepines).      **Available as generic?** Yes.

**Prescription needed?** Yes.      **Habit-forming?** Yes.

 **Overdose:** The overdose danger is especially high when this drug is combined with alcohol. Signs of toxicity include sedation, a decreased breathing rate, confusion, and loss of coordination. If these symptoms are present, seek immediate emergency medical treatment.

## PRECAUTIONS

### Do not take this drug if:

- You have ever had an allergic reaction to this drug or any other benzodiazepine.
- You have a chronic breathing problem.
- You have kidney or liver disease.

### Inform your physician if:

- You have ever had an allergic reaction to any drug.
- You are taking any other drug— prescription or nonprescription —or vitamins.
- You have a history of drug or alcohol dependence.
- You have epilepsy.
- You will be under anesthesia or undergoing surgery or medical testing in the next few months.

 **Pregnancy/Breast-feeding**

Do not take this drug if you are pregnant, planning a pregnancy, or are breast-feeding. Some benzodiazepines are associated with birth defects.

 **Infants/Children**

Do not give this drug to children. Safety and effectiveness for children have not been established.

 **Over Sixty**

People over age sixty should take this medication only under strict medical supervision.

 **Driving/Operating Machinery**

This drug may impair mental alertness and coordination. Do not drive or operate machinery until you are certain this drug will not affect your performance.

## GENERAL INFORMATION

Temazepam is a benzodiazepine used principally as a sleeping pill. It is absorbed by the body slowly and you may not feel sleepy immediately after taking the drug. It is excreted from the body very quickly. It has a half-life of about twelve hours, meaning half the drug will still be in your body twelve hours after you take it. Temazepam causes less daytime drowsiness than flurazepam, a benzodiazepine with a half-life of two to four days.

**DRUG NAME:**    Temazepam (*continued*)

## BENEFITS

- More effective and fewer side effects than barbiturates in treating insomnia.
- Safer than barbiturates when taken in overdose.

## RISKS

- Overdose danger, especially when combined with alcohol.
- Can interfere with breathing and be dangerous in people with chronic respiratory problems.
- Physically and psychologically addictive if misused.
- Can sometimes worsen original sleep problem.
- Potentially harmful to kidneys, liver, and lungs.
- Birth defects are possible if this drug is taken during pregnancy; central nervous system depression of the newborn occurs if the drug is taken during the last weeks of pregnancy.

## GUIDELINES FOR USERS

**How is the drug taken?** Tablets (15, 30 mg).

**What is the usual dosage?** The initial dose should be 15 mg in healthy young people. This may be increased to 30 mg per evening if required.

**What are the instructions for taking the drug?** As with all benzodiazepines, if you are taking this drug for the first time, take your first dose at home during a time when you are not required to work or drive. Your physician should tell you how often to take subsequent doses. Follow these instructions carefully. This drug can be taken before, during, or after meals. The tablets can be crushed and dissolved in water before taking, if you prefer.

**How quickly will I feel the effect of the drug and how long does it last?** Because this drug is absorbed by the body very slowly, you may not fall asleep rapidly after taking your dose. However, you should sleep better the first night. The full effect of the drug may not be felt for two or three nights.

**What if I miss a dose or several doses?** If you miss a dose and remember within an hour or so, take the missed dose. However, if more than an hour has elapsed, skip the dose and continue on your regular schedule. Do not take double doses.

**What if I stop taking the drug?** If you take this drug regularly for three weeks or more, you should not stop abruptly. Your dosage should be gradually reduced. Abrupt cessation can cause psychological and physical withdrawal symptoms and perhaps rebound insomnia.

**How should I store the drug?** Keep out of reach of children, since all benzodiazepines can be extremely dangerous to children. Store in a dry, tightly closed, light-resistant container. Heat and moisture may cause this drug to break down.

## INTERACTIONS

**Alcohol:** Do not drink alcohol. Temazepam is highly dangerous when combined with alcohol. It can dangerously lower blood pressure, decrease the breathing rate, and lead to loss of consciousness.

**Food/Beverages:** No restrictions on food. Control caffeine intake, as caffeine can contribute to insomnia.

**Smoking:** Heavy smoking of tobacco may reduce the sedative effects of the drug. Marijuana smoking may increase many of the drug's side effects and significantly reduce mental alertness.

**Other drugs:** Narcotics (e.g., Demerol, Percodan, codeine, morphine, Talwin) may *increase* the sedative effects of this drug. The combination can be fatal. Do not use narcotics with this drug.

Barbiturates and other sedatives (e.g., phenobarbital, pentobarbital, Seconal, Tuinal) may *increase* sedation to dangerous levels. Do not combine other sedatives or sleeping pills with this drug.

Do not take other benzodiazepines when using this drug, since the combination is both unnecessary and unsafe.

The following drugs may reduce the liver's ability to remove this drug from the body, making the drug more powerful and increasing side effects:
- ulcer drugs
- birth control pills
- propranolol
- disulfiram (Antabuse)

## HABIT-FORMING POTENTIAL

High.

## LONG-TERM USE

With continued use, people taking temazepam will have as much of the drug in their system during the day as during the night. Physical and psychological dependence are common problems. It is possible to become dependent in as short a time span as two to four weeks. The drug should not be taken longer than four weeks. Long-term use increases the risk of side effects and dependency.

## PLEASE NOTE

If you use this drug for a week or more, you may find that when you stop taking the drug your insomnia is worse than before. This is called *rebound insomnia*. Taking temazepam again will not solve the problem. Nondrug treatments or a gradual tapering of the benzodiazepine will be required.

**DRUG NAME:**  Temazepam (*continued*)

| Temazepam | | | | | | | |
|---|---|---|---|---|---|---|---|
| | **Frequency** | | **Discuss with Physician** | | | | |
| **Symptom/Effect** | **Common** | **Rare** | **Not Necessary** | **In All Cases** | **Only If Severe** | **Stop Taking Drug Now** | **Call Physician Now** |
| clumsiness/sleepiness | X | | | | X | | |
| abdominal cramps | | X | | X | | | |
| blurred vision | | X | | X | | | |
| dry mouth | | X | | X | | | |
| fast heartbeat | | X | | X | | | |
| shaking/slurred speech | | X | | X | | | |
| urination problems | | X | | X | | | |
| convulsions | | X | | X | | X | X |
| hallucinations | | X | | X | | X | X |
| memory loss | | X | | X | | | |
| trouble breathing | | X | | X | | X | X |
| staggering/trembling | | X | | X | | X | X |
| headache | | X | | X | | | |
| confusion | | X | | X | | | |
| memory loss | | X | | X | | | |

DRUG NAME: **Thioridazine**

**BRAND NAME:** Mellaril
**For more information:** See Chapter 7, Antipsychotic Drugs.

**FAST FACTS**  **Drug group:** Antipsychotics.   **Available as generic?** Yes.
**Prescription needed?** Yes.   **Habit-forming?** No.

 **Overdose:** Symptoms include light-headedness, sedation, agitation, confusion, restlessness, disorientation, convulsions, fever, and coma. Seek immediate emergency medical treatment.

## PRECAUTIONS

### Do not take this drug if:

- You have ever had an allergic reaction to this drug or any other phenothiazine.

### Inform your physician if:

- You have ever had an allergic reaction to any drug.
- You have epilepsy, asthma, or heart disease.
- You are taking any other drug—prescription or nonprescription —or vitamins.
- You are on a low-salt, low-sugar, or any other special diet.
- You will be under anesthesia or undergoing surgery or medical testing in the next few months.

 **Pregnancy/Breast-feeding**

Except in unusual cases where the mother or the baby's life is endangered, this drug should not be taken by pregnant women. Women taking thioridazine should not breast-feed.

 **Infants/Children**

Children may take this drug, but only under the direction of a pediatrician and/or children's psychiatrist.

 **Over Sixty**

Side effects, some serious, can be worse. Initial dose should be low, with careful monitoring for side effects. Special care should be taken when sitting up from a lying position, or standing from a sitting position, as blood pressure may be lowered and balance impaired.

 **Driving/Operating Machinery**

Extreme caution is advised. This medicine can impair mental alertness and coordination. If you do drive or operate machinery, this medicine should be taken at bedtime when its sedating effects are less likely to interfere with daytime activities.

## GENERAL INFORMATION

Thioridazine is a low-potency antipsychotic used to treat people who are experiencing disorganized, psychotic thinking, and who may be having delusions or hallucinations. This drug is quite sedating, and often causes lowered blood pressure. Thioridazine is associated with a harmful side effect called retinitis pigmentosa (deposits of pigment in

**DRUG NAME:**    Thioridazine (*continued*)

## GENERAL INFORMATION (*continued*)

the retina), which can lead to blindness. For this reason, it may not be prescribed in doses higher than 800 mg per day. It is also associated with sexual dysfunction and painful priapism (sustained erections). It also may cause dangerous heart rhythms in people with preexisting heart disease. The choice of which antipsychotic drug to use is often determined by the side effects. For an explanation of how this drug works, see Chapter 7.

## BENEFITS

- Effective in treating hallucinations, delusions, confused thinking, and mania.
- Sedating effects helpful in calming agitated persons.

## RISKS

- Can cause retinitis pigmentosa leading to blindness.
- Can dangerously lower blood pressure.
- Can cause tardive dyskinesia.
- Can cause neuroleptic malignant syndrome.
- A few men experience painful priapism (sustained erection).

## GUIDELINES FOR USERS

**How is the drug taken?** Tablets (10, 15, 25, 50, 100, 150, 200 mg); oral concentrate.

**What is the usual dosage?** The initial dose should be 25 mg to 75 mg per day in healthy young people, with increases as needed to control symptoms. Maintenance doses should be as low as possible and still be able to control the psychotic symptoms.

**What are the instructions for taking the drug?** It is best to take this drug on an empty stomach and drink a full glass of water.

**How quickly will I feel the effect of the drug?** It usually takes several weeks for you to experience the full benefit of this drug. However, you may feel more calm and relaxed after the first dose or two. The drug should also help you sleep better, if this is a problem.

**What if I miss a dose or several doses?** If you miss a dose and remember within an hour or so, take the missed dose. Otherwise, skip the missed dose and continue on your regular dosing schedule. Do not take double doses.

If you are missing doses on a frequent basis, notify your psychiatrist. A slow-release form of an antipsychotic drug may help with your compliance and help avoid a relapse.

**What if I stop taking the drug?** Do not stop taking this drug without consulting your physician. Abruptly stopping this medication will lead to uncomfortable but not dangerous physical symptoms. Should your physician and you agree that the drug should be discontinued, your medication should be tapered slowly to prevent physical symptoms of withdrawal and a reemergence of your psychotic symptoms.

**How should I store the drug?** Keep out of reach of children. Store in a dry, tightly closed, light-resistant container. Heat and moisture may cause this drug to break down. The liquid form does not require refrigeration.

## INTERACTIONS

**Alcohol:** Avoid alcohol. When combined with alcohol, this medicine can cause excessive sedation and dangerously lower blood pressure.

**Food/Beverages:** No restrictions.

**Smoking:** Smoking lowers the blood level of thioridazine. If you do smoke, blood samples should be taken to test whether the drug is in the therapeutic range.

**Other drugs:** Antacids with aluminum or magnesium (Maalox, for example) should not be taken for two hours before or after taking thioridazine because they may interfere with the absorption of this drug.

Thioridazine, when combined with the heart medication quinidine, can cause irregular heart rhythms.

Heterocyclic antidepressants can increase the plasma level of this drug and cause a worsening of side effects. Conversely, this drug can increase the blood level of antidepressants. The concurrent use of these two types of drugs must be carefully monitored.

Blood pressure can be dangerously lowered when antipsychotics are combined with vasodilators (medications that dilate blood vessels).

Thioridazine will increase the effects and side effects of medicines known as CNS (central nervous system) depressants. Examples include antihistamines, hay fever medicines, sedatives, narcotics, muscle relaxants, barbiturates, and anesthetics. Check with your physician before taking any of these drugs.

## HABIT-FORMING POTENTIAL

None.

## LONG-TERM USE

Prolonged use of thioridazine is associated with increased risk of developing tardive dyskinesia, a potentially irreversible side effect involving disfiguring movements of the face, tongue, and limbs. For more information on tardive dyskinesia, please see Chapter 7.

## PLEASE NOTE

Not a sleeping pill: This drug, which has a sedating effect, is sometimes misused as a sleeping pill. There are much safer medications available as sleeping aids.

Not specifically antiaggressive: Because of the potential serious side effects of the antipsychotic drugs, especially over the long term, they should not be used to treat anxiety or chronic aggression and agitation.

Frequent examinations required: While you are taking this medication, your blood pressure and pulse rate should be monitored frequently. In addition, you should have periodic eye examinations in order to detect any changes in your retina.

Classification: Thioridazine is classified as a phenothiazine. Other antipsychotics in the same group include acetophenazine, chlorpromazine, fluphenazine, mesoridazine,

**DRUG NAME:**    Thioridazine (*continued*)

**PLEASE NOTE** (*continued*)

perphenazine, promazine, trifluoperazine, and triflupromazine. In general, if you have a poor response to one drug in this family, you will likely have a similar poor response to other drugs in the family.

| Thioridazine | | | | | | | |
|---|---|---|---|---|---|---|---|
| | Frequency | | Discuss with Physician | | | | |
| Symptom/Effect | Common | Rare | Not Necessary | In All Cases | Only If Severe | Stop Taking Drug Now | Call Physician Now |
| lethargy/sleepiness | X | | | | X | | |
| low blood pressure | X | | | X | | | |
| dizziness | | X | | X | | | |
| dry mouth | X | | | | X | | |
| blurred vision | X | | | | X | | |
| constipation | X | | | | X | | |
| difficulty urinating | X | | | X | | | |
| reduced urinary output | | X | | X | | | X |
| racing heartbeat/ palpitations | | X | | X | | | |
| weakness | | X | | X | | | |
| sexual problems | | X | | X | | | |
| restlessness | | X | | X | | | |
| skin rash | | X | | X | | | X |
| weight gain | X | | | | X | | |
| seizures | | X | | X | | X | X |
| low white blood cell count | | X | | X | | | X |
| tremors | | X | | X | | | |
| stiffness | X | | | X | | | |
| involuntary facial or tongue movements | | X | | X | | | |
| chest pain | | X | | X | | X | X |
| breathlessness | | X | | X | | X | X |

**BRAND NAME:** Navane
**For more information:** See Chapter 7, Antipsychotic Drugs.

**FAST FACTS** **Drug group:** Antipsychotics. **Available as generic?** Yes.
**Prescription needed?** Yes. **Habit-forming?** No.

 **Overdose:** Symptoms include difficulty breathing, light-headedness, sedation, confusion, muscle twitching, agitation, disorientation, restlessness, shock, and coma. Seek immediate emergency medical treatment.

## PRECAUTIONS

### Do not take this drug if:

- You have ever had an allergic reaction to this drug.

### Inform your physician if:

- You have ever had an allergic reaction to any drug.
- You have epilepsy or asthma.
- You have cardiovascular disease.
- You are taking any other drug— prescription or nonprescription —or vitamins.
- You are on a low-salt, low-sugar, or other special diet.
- You will be under anesthesia or undergoing surgery or medical testing in the next few months.

 ### Pregnancy/Breast-feeding

Safe use in pregnancy has not been established. Except in unusual cases where the mother or the baby's life is endangered, this drug should not be taken by pregnant women. Women taking thiothixene should not breast-feed.

 ### Infants/Children

The safety and effectiveness of this drug have not been determined for children under age twelve.

 ### Over Sixty

Side effects, some serious, can be worse. Initial dose should be low, with careful monitoring for side effects. Special care should be taken when sitting up from a lying position, or standing from a sitting position, as blood pressure may be lowered and balance impaired.

 ### Driving/Operating Machinery

Extreme caution is advised. This medicine can impair mental alertness and coordination. If you do drive or operate machinery, this medicine should be taken at bedtime when its sedating effects are less likely to interfere with daytime activities.

**DRUG NAME:**    Thiothixene (*continued*)

## GENERAL INFORMATION

Thiothixene is a high-potency antipsychotic in the family of medicines known as thioxanthenes. It is used to treat people who are experiencing disorganized, psychotic thinking and perceptions such as delusions and hallucinations. High-potency antipsychotics are more likely to cause movement side effects such as dystonic reactions, parkinsonian features, and agitated restlessness (akathisia), but they are less sedating than the low-potency antipsychotics and cause fewer problems with low blood pressure and the cardiovascular system. Many psychiatrists prescribe an anticholinergic medication with thiothixene to reduce its movement side effects. For an explanation of how this drug works, see Chapter 7.

## BENEFITS

- Effective in treating hallucinations, delusions, confused thinking, and mania.
- Sedating effects helpful in calming agitated persons.

## RISKS

- Can dangerously lower white blood cell count.
- Can cause neuroleptic malignant syndrome.
- Can cause tardive dyskinesia.

## GUIDELINES FOR USERS

**How is the drug taken?** Tablets (1, 2, 5, 10, 20 mg); oral concentrate; intramuscular.

**What is the usual dosage?** Initial dose should be 4 mg to 10 mg per day in healthy young people, with increases as needed to control symptoms. A maximum daily dose of up to 60 mg may be used if necessary. Maintenance doses should be as low as possible and still be able to control the psychotic symptoms.

**What are the instructions for taking the drug?** It is best to take this drug on an empty stomach and drink a full glass of water. The liquid form must be diluted before you take it. You can mix it with water, milk, juice, soup, or a carbonated beverage. Follow your physician's instructions carefully.

**How quickly will I feel the effect of the drug?** It usually takes several weeks for you to experience the full benefit of this drug. However, you may feel more calm and relaxed after the first dose or two.

**What if I miss a dose or several doses?** If you miss a dose and remember within an hour or so, take the missed dose. However, if more than an hour has elapsed, skip the dose and continue on your regular schedule. Do not take double doses.

If you are missing doses on a frequent basis, notify your psychiatrist. A slow-release form of an antipsychotic drug may help with your compliance and help avoid a relapse.

**What if I stop taking the drug?** Do not stop taking this drug without consulting your physician. Abruptly stopping this medication will lead to uncomfortable but not dangerous physical symptoms. Should your physician and you agree that the drug should be discontinued, your medication should be tapered slowly to prevent physical symptoms of withdrawal and a reemergence of your psychotic symptoms.

**How should I store the drug?** Keep out of reach of children. Store in a dry, tightly closed, light-resistant container. Heat and moisture may cause this drug to break down. The liquid form does not require refrigeration.

## INTERACTIONS

**Alcohol:** Avoid alcohol. When combined with alcohol, this medicine can cause excessive sedation and dangerously lower blood pressure.

**Food/Beverages:** No restrictions.

**Smoking:** Smoking lowers the blood level of thiothixene. If you do smoke, blood samples should be taken to test whether the drug is in the therapeutic range.

**Other drugs:** Antacids with aluminum or magnesium (Maalox, for example) should not be taken for two hours before or after taking thiothixene because they may interfere with the absorption of this drug.

Heterocyclic antidepressants can increase the plasma level of this drug and cause a worsening of side effects. Conversely, this drug can increase the blood level of antidepressants. The concurrent use of these two types of drugs must be carefully monitored.

Blood pressure can be dangerously lowered when antipsychotics are combined with vasodilators (medications that dilate blood vessels.)

Thiothixene will increase the effect of medicines known as CNS (central nervous system) depressants. Examples include antihistamines, hay fever medicines, sedatives, narcotics, muscle relaxants, barbiturates, and anesthetics. Check with your physician before taking any of these drugs.

## HABIT-FORMING POTENTIAL

None.

## LONG-TERM USE

Prolonged use of thiothixene is associated with increased risk of developing tardive dyskinesia, a potentially irreversible side effect involving disfiguring movements of the face, tongue, and limbs. For more information on tardive dyskinesia, please see Chapter 7.

## PLEASE NOTE

Less sweating: Thiothixene may cause you to sweat less, which in turn causes your body temperature to rise. When the weather is hot or you are exercising, make sure you do not become too hot or dehydrated, since overheating may result in a heat stroke.

Not specifically antiaggressive: Because of the potential serious side effects of the antipsychotic drugs, especially over the long term, this medication should not be used to treat anxiety or chronic aggression and agitation.

Frequent examinations required: While taking this medication, your blood pressure and pulse rate should be monitored frequently. Regular checks should also be made for the early signs of tardive dyskinesia.

**DRUG NAME:**    Thiothixene (*continued*)

**PLEASE NOTE** (*continued*)

Classification: Thiothixene is classified in the family of medicines known as the thioxanthenes. Chlorprothixene is another antipsychotic in the same group. In general, if you have a poor response to one drug in this family, you will likely have a similar poor response to other drugs in the family.

| | Frequency | | Discuss with Physician | | | | |
|---|---|---|---|---|---|---|---|
| **Symptom/Effect** | **Common** | **Rare** | **Not Necessary** | **In All Cases** | **Only If Severe** | **Stop Taking Drug Now** | **Call Physician Now** |
| lethargy/sleepiness | X | | | | X | | |
| low blood pressure | X | | | X | | | |
| dizziness | | X | | X | | | |
| dry mouth | X | | | | X | | |
| blurred vision | X | | | | X | | |
| constipation | X | | | | X | | |
| difficulty urinating | X | | | X | | | |
| reduced urinary output | | X | | X | | | X |
| racing heartbeat/ palpitations | | X | | X | | | |
| weakness | | X | | X | | | |
| sexual problems | | X | | X | | | |
| restlessness | | X | | X | | | |
| skin rash | | X | | X | | | X |
| weight gain | X | | | | X | | |
| seizures | | X | | X | | X | X |
| low white blood cell count | | X | | X | | | X |
| tremors | | X | | X | | | |
| stiffness | X | | | X | | | |
| involuntary facial or tongue movements | | X | | X | | | |

# Tranylcypromine

**BRAND NAME:** Parnate

**For more information:** See Chapter 3, Antidepressant Drugs, and Chapter 5, Antipanic and Antiphobic Drugs.

**FAST FACTS**   **Drug group:** Antidepressants (monoamine oxidase inhibitors).

**Available as generic?** Yes.

**Prescription needed?** Yes.

**Habit-forming?** No.

 **Overdose:** Symptoms of an overdose or a dangerous hypertensive reaction include a severe headache, neck stiffness, nausea or vomiting, chest pain, dizziness, and shock.

## PRECAUTIONS

### Do not take this drug if:

- You have ever had an allergic or negative reaction to this or any other MAO inhibitor.
- You have a confirmed or suspected cerebrovascular defect, cardiovascular disease, hypertension, or a history of headaches.

### Inform your physician if:

- You have ever had an allergic reaction to any drug.
- You have epilepsy.
- You have high blood pressure or a history of stroke.
- You are taking any other drug—prescription or nonprescription—or vitamins.
- You will be under anesthesia or undergoing surgery or medical testing in the next few months.

 **Pregnancy/Breast-feeding**

If you are pregnant, planning a pregnancy, or breast-feeding, you should not take this drug.

 **Infants/Children**

The safety and effectiveness of tranylcypromine have not been established for children under age sixteen.

 **Over Sixty**

Side effects may be pronounced in the elderly. Initial dose should be low, with careful monitoring for side effects. Special care should be taken when sitting up from a lying position, or standing from a sitting position, as blood pressure may be lowered and balance impaired.

 **Driving/Operating Machinery**

This drug may cause drowsiness. You should not drive a car during the initial phase of treatment. When you are confident that you are alert and have full motor coordination, ask your doctor if you can resume driving. We suggest having a passenger present on your initial trips to help ascertain safety.

## GENERAL INFORMATION

Tranylcypromine is a monoamine oxidase inhibitor used in the treatment of depression and panic. In most cases, tranylcypromine should not be the first treatment choice for depression. Rather, this drug is prescribed for people whose symptoms have failed to respond to other common antidepression drugs. This drug is just as effective in treating

**DRUG NAME:**   Tranylcypromine (*continued*)

## GENERAL INFORMATION (*continued*)

depression as the heterocyclic drugs; however, it poses a potential problem because of possible toxic food-drug interactions. If you are on this drug, it is extremely important to follow the dietary guidelines given to you by your physician. (For an explanation of how this drug works and a discussion of food-drug interactions, see Chapter 3.)

## BENEFITS

- As effective as heterocyclics in treating depression.
- May be effective in treating depression in patients who have not responded to other classes of antidepressants.
- May have special benefits in treating atypical depression (including special sensitivity to rejection, oversleeping, overeating, and prominent anxiety).
- Effective in treating panic and phobic symptoms.

## RISKS

- Possible toxic interaction with some foods, beverages, and drugs.

## GUIDELINES FOR USERS

**How is the drug taken?** Tablets (10 mg).

**What is the usual dosage?** The initial dose for the treatment of depression is 10 mg twice a day in the healthy adult. The dose is raised gradually, but rarely higher than 50 mg per day.

**What are the instructions for taking the drug?** Follow your physician's instructions carefully. This drug can be taken before, during, or after meals. The tablets can be crushed and dissolved in water before taking, if you prefer.

**How quickly will I feel the effect of the drug?** A few people experience the benefit of this drug during the first week, but it usually takes three or more weeks for a positive effect.

**What if I miss a dose or several doses?** If you miss a dose and remember within an hour or so, take the dose. However, if it is within two hours of your next dose, skip the missed dose. Do not take double doses.

**What if I stop taking the drug?** Do not stop taking tranylcypromine without consulting your doctor. If this drug has been taken regularly, withdrawal symptoms may appear unless it is discontinued gradually. Some people experience disturbances including vivid dreams or nightmares during the withdrawal period. After stopping this medicine, you must continue following the dietary guidelines for at least three weeks to avoid a toxic food-drug interaction.

**How should I store the drug?** Keep out of reach of children. Store in a dry, tightly closed, light-resistant container. Heat and moisture may cause this drug to break down.

## INTERACTIONS

**Alcohol:** Do not drink alcohol since this drug can increase the effects of alcohol and alcohol can increase tranylcypromine's side effects. In addition, alcohol use can contribute to depression.

**Food/Beverages:** Do not eat foods or drink beverages with tyramine. Tyramine can interact with this drug and cause severe or fatal increases in blood pressure. Among the food and beverages to be avoided are:

*Meat and fish:* lox, pickled herring, liver, dry sausage;

*Fruits and vegetables:* broad (fava) beans, raisins, figs, avocado;

*Dairy products:* Cheese (cottage cheese and cream cheese are allowed), yogurt;

*Beverages:* beer, wine, hard liquor, sherry, large amounts of caffeine (coffee, tea, cocoa, or chocolate);

*Miscellaneous:* Yeast products (including brewer's yeast in large quantities), pickles, sauerkraut, soy sauce, sour cream, snails, licorice.

**Smoking:** Smoking may lower the blood level of tranylcypromine and this may reduce the drug's efficiency in treating depression.

**Other drugs:** All "recreational" or illegal drugs should be avoided by people with depression and may be highly dangerous when combined with tranylcypromine.

Do not take any other medicine without consulting your physician. This includes over-the-counter medicines such as decongestants, other cold tablets or formulas, nasal drops or sprays, hay fever medications, sinus medications, appetite suppressants, weight-reducing preparations, or "pep" pills.

Do not take procaine (Novocain and others) while on this drug.

Notify your surgeon and anesthesiologist that you take this medication prior to any surgical procedure, as this MAO inhibitor reacts with certain anesthetics.

## HABIT-FORMING POTENTIAL

None.

## LONG-TERM USE

Poses no danger.

## PLEASE NOTE

Cocaine use: Cocaine, when combined with an MAO inhibitor such as tranylcypromine, can dangerously increase blood pressure. Certain over-the-counter drugs may also be highly dangerous.

Surgery: If you are taking this drug, you should not undergo surgery requiring certain general anesthetics or a dental procedure requiring Novocain (procaine).

ID card: Your physician may suggest you carry an identification card that states you are taking this medicine. In addition, it's a good idea to carry with you at all times a wallet-sized list of foods high in tyramine content.

**DRUG NAME:** Tranylcypromine (*continued*)

| Symptom/Effect | Frequency Common | Frequency Rare | Not Necessary | In All Cases | Only If Severe | Stop Taking Drug Now | Call Physician Now |
|---|---|---|---|---|---|---|---|
| | **Frequency** | | **Discuss with Physician** | | | | |
| blurred vision | X | | | | X | | |
| dizziness/light-headedness | X | | | X | | | |
| drowsiness/weakness | X | | | | X | | |
| decreased sexual ability | X | | | X | | | |
| constipation | | X | | | X | | |
| diarrhea | | X | | | X | | |
| allergies or rashes | | X | | X | | | |
| chest pain | | X | | X | | X | X |
| fast or slow heartbeat | X | | | X | | | |
| headache (severe) | | X | | | X | X | X |
| chills/shivering | | X | | | X | | |
| dry mouth | X | | | | X | | |
| agitation/restlessness | | X | | X | | | X |
| reduced urinary output | | X | | X | | | X |

## DRUG NAME: Trazodone

**BRAND NAME:** Desyrel
**For more information:** See Chapter 3, Antidepressant Drugs.

**FAST FACTS**

**Drug group:** Antidepressants.
**Prescription needed?** Yes.
**Available as generic?** Yes.
**Habit-forming?** No.
**Overdose:** Symptoms include drowsiness, vomiting, difficulty breathing, and convulsions. Seek immediate emergency medical treatment.

## PRECAUTIONS

### Do not take this drug if:

- You have ever had an allergic or negative reaction to this drug.

### Inform your physician if:

- You have ever had an allergic reaction to any drug.
- You have epilepsy.
- You have heart, kidney, or liver disease.
- You are taking any other drug— prescription or nonprescription —or vitamins.
- You will be under anesthesia or undergoing surgery or medical testing in the next few months.

### Pregnancy/Breast-feeding

If you are pregnant or planning a pregnancy, you should, if possible, use nondrug alternatives for treating your depression. This drug has not been demonstrated to be safe during pregnancy. Nursing mothers should not take this drug since it is passed on to the baby in the mother's milk.

### Infants/Children

Do not give this drug to children. Safety and effectiveness have not been established for those under the age of eighteen.

### Over Sixty

Lower doses are required. Side effects may be worse.

### Driving/Operating Machinery

This drug may cause drowsiness. You should not drive a car during the initial phase of treatment. When you are confident that you are alert and have full motor coordination, ask your doctor if you can resume driving. We suggest having a passenger present on your initial trips to help ascertain safety.

## GENERAL INFORMATION

Trazodone is a serotonin-specific drug used to treat depression and several other psychological problems. At one time, trazodone was prescribed for depression only if a patient failed to respond to the heterocyclic antidepressants. However, more and more physicians are prescribing this drug as a "first-line" treatment for depression. Mead Johnson manufactures the brand Desyrel. Seven companies market a generic. For an explanation of how this drug works, see Chapter 3.

**DRUG NAME:**    Trazodone (*continued*)

## BENEFITS

- Fewer side effects than heterocyclic drugs.
- Better tolerated by people with heart disease, stroke, Alzheimer's disease.
- Sedating effects can be helpful for people whose symptoms of depression include insomnia.
- High margin of overdose safety.

## RISKS

- A few men develop serious penile erection problems that require emergency medical intervention.

## GUIDELINES FOR USERS

**How is the drug taken?** Tablets (50, 100, 150 mg).

**What is the usual dosage?** The initial dose is 50 mg daily in divided doses, then increased gradually to 300 mg daily. Some people may require up to 400 mg or more daily.

**What are the instructions for taking the drug?** Take your dose shortly after a meal or a light snack to decrease the risk of feeling dizzy or light-headed.

**How quickly will I feel the effect of the drug?** A few people experience the benefit of this drug during the first week, but it usually takes three or more weeks for a positive effect.

**What if I miss a dose or several doses?** If you miss a dose and an hour or so has elapsed, take the dose. If it is within four hours of your next dose, skip the missed dose. Do not take double doses.

**What if I stop taking the drug?** Do not stop taking this medicine without consulting your physician. Your dosage may need to be gradually reduced to prevent a recurrence of your condition.

**How should I store the drug?** Keep out of reach of children. Store in a dry, tightly closed, light-resistant container. Heat and moisture may cause this drug to break down.

## INTERACTIONS

**Alcohol:** Do not drink alcohol, since this drug can increase its effects. In addition, alcohol use can contribute to depression.

**Food/Beverages:** No restrictions.

**Smoking:** Smoking lowers the blood level of trazodone and this may reduce the drug's efficiency in treating depression.

**Other drugs:** Trazodone may increase the effect of medicines known as CNS (central nervous system) depressants. Examples include antihistamines, hay fever medicines, sedatives, narcotics, muscle relaxants, barbiturates, and anesthetics. Check with your physician before taking any of these drugs.

## HABIT-FORMING POTENTIAL

None.

## LONG-TERM USE

Most people may be tapered safely from the medication six months after their depression has responded to treatment. A small percentage of patients have symptoms of depression return after their dosage is reduced. These individuals may benefit from remaining on trazodone for a year or longer.

| Trazodone | | | | | | | |
|---|---|---|---|---|---|---|---|
| | **Frequency** | | **Discuss with Physician** | | | | |
| **Symptom/Effect** | **Common** | **Rare** | **Not Necessary** | **In All Cases** | **Only If Severe** | **Stop Taking Drug Now** | **Call Physician Now** |
| dizziness/light-headedness | X | | | | X | | |
| drowsiness | X | | | | X | | |
| dry mouth | | X | | | X | | |
| headache | | X | | | X | | |
| anxiousness/nervousness | | X | | | X | | |
| blurred vision | | X | | | X | | |
| constipation | | X | | | X | | |
| skin rash | | X | | X | | X | X |
| inappropriate or painful erection | | X | | X | | X | X |
| shortness of breath | | X | | X | | | X |
| confusion | | X | | X | | X | X |
| nausea/vomiting | | X | | | X | | |
| decreased concentration | | X | | X | | | |
| muscle pain | | X | | X | | | |

# DRUG NAME: **Triazolam**

**BRAND NAME:** Halcion
**For more information:** See Chapter 8, Sedatives and Sleeping Pills, and Chapter 4, Antianxiety Drugs.

**FAST FACTS**  **Drug group:** Sedatives (benzodiaze-pines).   **Available as generic?** No.

**Prescription needed?** Yes.   **Habit-forming?** Yes.

 **Overdose:** The overdose danger is especially high when this drug is combined with alcohol. Signs of toxicity include sedation, a decreased breathing rate, confusion, and loss of coordination. If these symptoms are present, seek immediate emergency medical treatment.

## PRECAUTIONS

### Do not take this drug if:

- You have ever had an allergic reaction to this drug or any other benzodiazepine.
- You have a chronic breathing problem.
- You have kidney or liver disease.

### Inform your physician if:

- You have ever had an allergic reaction to any drug.
- You are taking any other drug—prescription or nonprescription—or vitamins.
- You have epilepsy.
- You will be under anesthesia or undergoing surgery or medical testing in the next few months.

 **Pregnancy/Breast-feeding**

Do not take this drug if you are pregnant, planning a pregnancy, or are breast-feeding.

 **Infants/Children**

Do not give this drug to children. Safety and effectiveness for children have not been established.

 **Over Sixty**

People over age sixty should take this medication only under strict medical supervision.

 **Driving/Operating Machinery**

This drug may impair mental alertness and coordination. Do not drive or operate machinery until you are certain this drug will not affect your performance.

## GENERAL INFORMATION

Triazolam is one of the more recently developed benzodiazepines used principally as a sleeping pill. It is rapidly absorbed, produces a rapid onset of sleep, and is rapidly eliminated by the body. It has a half-life of about three to six hours, which means half the drug will still be in your body three to six hours after you take it. Triazolam causes less daytime drowsiness than flurazepam, a benzodiazepine with a half-life of two to four days. Some physicians recommend triazolam to prevent jet lag. However, one problem with this use is that travelers may experience memory problems the next morning.

## BENEFITS

- More effective and fewer side effects than barbiturates in treating insomnia.
- Safer than barbiturates when taken in overdose.

## RISKS

- Overdose danger, especially when combined with alcohol.
- Can interfere with breathing and be dangerous in people with chronic respiratory problems.
- Physically and psychologically addictive if misused.
- Can sometimes worsen original sleep problem.
- Birth defects are possible if this drug is taken during pregnancy; central nervous system depression of the newborn occurs if the drug is taken during the last weeks of pregnancy.

## GUIDELINES FOR USERS

**How is the drug taken?** Tablets (0.125, 0.25 mg).

**What is the usual dosage?** The initial dose should be 0.125 mg to 0.25 mg in healthy young people, with increases as needed to control symptoms. A maximum daily dose of up to 0.5 mg per night may be used, if necessary. See also pages 570–71.

**What are the instructions for taking the drug?** As with all benzodiazepines, if you are taking this drug for the first time, take your first dose at home during a time when you are not required to work or drive. Your physician should tell you how often to take subsequent doses. Follow these instructions carefully. This drug can be taken before, during, or after meals.

**How quickly will I feel the effect of the drug and how long does it last?** This drug reaches the brain more rapidly than certain other benzodiazepines, so you may fall asleep fairly rapidly after taking your dose. You should sleep better the first night.

**What if I stop taking the drug?** If you take this drug regularly for three weeks or more, you should not stop abruptly. Your dosage should be gradually reduced. Abrupt cessation can cause psychological and physical withdrawal symptoms, and, perhaps, rebound insomnia.

**How should I store the drug?** Keep out of reach of children and store in a locked cabinet. This drug has high potential for abuse. Store in a dry, tightly closed, light-resistant container. Heat and moisture may cause this drug to break down.

**DRUG NAME:**    Triazolam (*continued*)

## INTERACTIONS

**Alcohol:** Do not drink alcohol. Triazolam is highly dangerous when combined with alcohol. It can dangerously lower blood pressure, decrease the breathing rate, interfere with normal sleep patterns, and lead to loss of consciousness.

**Food/Beverages:** No restrictions on food. Control caffeine intake, as caffeine can contribute to insomnia.

**Smoking:** Heavy smoking of tobacco may reduce the sedative effects of the drug. Marijuana smoking may increase many of the drug's side effects and significantly reduce mental alertness.

**Other drugs:** Narcotics (e.g., Demerol, Percodan, codeine, morphine, Talwin) may *increase* the sedative effects of this drug. The combination can be fatal. Do not use narcotics with this drug.

Barbiturates and other sedatives (e.g., phenobarbital, pentobarbital, Seconal, Tuinal) may *increase* sedation to dangerous levels. Do not combine other sedatives or sleeping pills with this drug.

Do not take other benzodiazepines when using this drug, since the combination is both unnecessary and unsafe.

The following drugs may reduce the liver's ability to remove this drug from the body, making the drug more powerful and increasing side effects:
• ulcer drugs
• birth control pills
• propranolol
• disulfiram (Antabuse)

## HABIT-FORMING POTENTIAL

High.

## LONG-TERM USE

Physical and psychological dependence are common problems. It is possible to become dependent in as short a time span as two to four weeks. This drug should not be taken longer than four weeks. Long-term use can also increase the risk of side effects.

## PLEASE NOTE

Rebound insomnia: If you use this drug for a week or more, you may find that when you stop taking the drug, your insomnia is worse than before. This is called *rebound insomnia*. Taking triazolam again will not solve the problem. Nondrug treatments or a gradual tapering of the benzodiazepine will be required.

Memory gaps: Triazolam has been associated in some people with discrete memory losses ranging from minutes to hours. Memory loss is more likely to occur if the dose is too high or if the medication is taken with alcohol.

The controversy about Halcion: Halcion is the most widely prescribed sleep medication in the world, largely because its brief half life does not permit buildup of the drug during daytime hours. Because of its extraordinary potency and the many side effects associated with Halcion at high doses, the manufacturer, Upjohn, reduced the recommended dose to between 0.25 mg., and 0.125 mg. In addition to the side effects reported in Chapter 4, there have been claims that Halcion causes extraordinarily violent behavior. Although most physicians and scientists who specialize in the assessment and treatment of sleep disorders do not believe that Halcion has any more dangerous side effects than the other benzodiazepines marketed as hypnotics or as antianxiety agents, other highly-prominent research scientists disagree. At the time of this writing, Halcion's safety and efficacy are currently under review by the FDA. We continue to prescribe Halcion at very low doses (usually 0.125 mg.) for specific indications and for brief periods of time as described in Chapters 4 and 8.

| Triazolam | | | | | | | |
|---|---|---|---|---|---|---|---|
| | Frequency | | Discuss with Physician | | | | |
| Symptom/Effect | Common | Rare | Not Necessary | In All Cases | Only If Severe | Stop Taking Drug Now | Call Physician Now |
| sleepiness | X | | | | X | | |
| abdominal cramps | | X | | X | | | |
| blurred vision | | X | | X | | | |
| dry mouth | | X | | X | | | |
| fast heartbeat | | X | | X | | | |
| shaking/slurred speech | | X | | X | | | |
| urination problems | | X | | X | | | |
| convulsions | | | | X | | X | X |
| hallucinations | | X | | X | | X | X |
| memory loss | | X | | X | | | |
| trouble breathing | | X | | X | | X | X |
| staggering/trembling | | X | | X | | X | X |
| headache | | X | | X | | | |
| confusion | | X | | X | | | |
| clumsiness | | X | | X | | | |

DRUG NAME: **Trifluoperazine**

**BRAND NAME:** Stelazine
**For more information:** See Chapter 7, Antipsychotic Drugs.

**FAST FACTS**  **Drug group:** Antipsychotics.     **Available as generic?** Yes.
**Prescription needed?** Yes.     **Habit-forming?** No.

 **Overdose:** Symptoms include light-headedness, sedation, agitation, confusion, restlessness, disorientation, convulsions, fever, and coma. Seek immediate emergency medical treatment.

## PRECAUTIONS
### Do not take this drug if:

- You have ever had an allergic reaction to this drug or any other phenothiazine.

### Inform your physician if:

- You have ever had an allergic reaction to any drug.
- You have epilepsy or asthma.
- You are taking any other drug— prescription or nonprescription —or vitamins.
- You are on a low-salt, low-sugar, or any other special diet.
- You will be under anesthesia or undergoing surgery or medical testing in the next few months.

 **Pregnancy/Breast-feeding**

Except in unusual cases where the mother or the baby's life is endangered, this drug should not be taken by pregnant women. Women taking trifluoperazine should not breast-feed.

 **Infants/Children**

Children may take this drug, but only under the direction of a pediatrician and/or children's psychiatrist.

 **Over Sixty**

Side effects, some serious, can be worse among the elderly. Initial dose should be low, with careful monitoring for side effects. Special care should be taken when sitting up from a lying position, or standing from a sitting position, as blood pressure may be lowered and balance impaired.

 **Driving/Operating Machinery**

Extreme caution is advised. This medicine can impair mental alertness and coordination. If you do drive or operate machinery, this medicine should be taken at bedtime when its sedating effects are less likely to interfere with daytime activities.

## GENERAL INFORMATION
Trifluoperazine is a high-potency antipsychotic used to treat people who are experiencing disorganized, psychotic thinking and who may be having delusions or hallucinations. High-potency antipsychotics are more likely to cause movement side effects such as dystonic reactions, parkinsonian features, and akathisia, but they are less sedating

and cause fewer problems with low blood pressure. The choice of which antipsychotic drug to use is often determined by the side effects. For an explanation of how this drug works, see Chapter 7.

## BENEFITS

- Effective in treating hallucinations, delusions, confused thinking, and mania.
- Less likely to lower blood pressure than certain other phenothiazines.
- Less sedating than some other phenothiazines.

## RISKS

- Can dangerously lower white blood cell count.
- Can cause tardive dyskinesia.
- Can cause neuroleptic malignant syndrome.

## GUIDELINES FOR USERS

**How is the drug taken?** Tablets (1, 2, 5, 10 mg); oral concentrate; intramuscular.

**What is the usual dosage?** The initial dose should be 2 mg to 6 mg per day in healthy young people, with increases as needed to control symptoms. Maintenance doses should be as low as possible and still be able to control the psychotic symptoms.

**What are the instructions for taking the drug?** It is best to take this drug on an empty stomach and drink a full glass of water.

**How quickly will I feel the effect of the drug?** It usually takes several weeks for you to experience the full benefit of this drug. However, you may feel more calm and relaxed after the first dose or two. The drug should also help you sleep better, if this is a problem.

**What if I miss a dose or several doses?** If you miss a dose and remember within an hour or so, take the missed dose. Otherwise, skip the missed dose and continue on your regular dosing schedule. Do not take double doses.

If you are missing doses on a frequent basis, notify your psychiatrist. A slow-release form of an antipsychotic drug may help with your compliance and help avoid a relapse.

**What if I stop taking the drug?** Do not stop taking this drug without consulting your physician. Abruptly stopping this medication will lead to uncomfortable but not dangerous physical symptoms. Should your physician and you agree that the drug should be discontinued, your medication should be tapered slowly to prevent physical symptoms of withdrawal and a reemergence of your psychotic symptoms.

**How should I store the drug?** Keep out of reach of children. Store in a dry, tightly closed, light-resistant container. Heat and moisture may cause this drug to break down. The liquid form does not require refrigeration.

## INTERACTIONS

**Alcohol:** Avoid alcohol. When combined with alcohol, this medicine can cause excessive sedation and dangerously lower blood pressure.

**Food/Beverages:** No restrictions.

**Smoking:** Smoking lowers the blood level of trifluoperazine. If you do smoke, blood samples should be taken to test whether the drug is in the therapeutic range.

DRUG NAME:    Trifluoperazine (*continued*)

## INTERACTIONS (*continued*)

**Other drugs:** Antacids with aluminum or magnesium (Maalox, for example) should not be taken for two hours before or after taking trifluoperazine because they may interfere with the absorption of this drug.

Heterocyclic antidepressants can increase the plasma level of this drug and cause a worsening of side effects. Conversely, this drug can increase the blood level of antidepressants. The concurrent use of these two types of drugs must be carefully monitored.

Blood pressure can be dangerously lowered when antipsychotics are combined with vasodilators (medications that dilate blood vessels).

Trifluoperazine will increase the effect of medicines known as CNS (central nervous system) depressants. Examples include antihistamines, hay fever medicines, sedatives, narcotics, muscle relaxants, barbiturates, and anesthetics. Check with your physician before taking any of these drugs.

## HABIT-FORMING POTENTIAL

None.

## LONG-TERM USE

Prolonged use of trifluoperazine is associated with increased risk of developing tardive dyskinesia, a potentially irreversible side effect involving disfiguring movements of the face, tongue, and limbs. For more information on tardive dyskinesia, please see Chapter 7.

## PLEASE NOTE

Not a sleeping pill: This drug, which has a sedating effect, is sometimes misused as a sleeping pill. There are much safer medications available as sleeping aids.

Not specifically antiaggressive: Because of the potential serious side effects of the antipsychotic drugs, especially over the long term, this medication should not be used to treat anxiety or chronic aggression and agitation.

Frequent examinations required: While taking this medication, your blood pressure and pulse rate should be monitored frequently. Regular checks should also be made for the early signs of tardive dyskinesia.

Classification: Trifluoperazine is classified as a phenothiazine. Other antipsychotics in the same group include acetophenazine, chlorpromazine, fluphenazine, mesoridazine, perphenazine, promazine, thioridazine, and triflupromazine. In general, if you have a poor response to one drug in this family, you will likely have a similar poor response to other drugs in the family.

| Trifluoperazine | | | | | | | |
|---|---|---|---|---|---|---|---|
| | Frequency | | Discuss with Physician | | | | |
| Symptom/Effect | Common | Rare | Not Necessary | In All Cases | Only If Severe | Stop Taking Drug Now | Call Physician Now |
| lethargy/sleepiness | X | | | | X | | |
| low blood pressure | X | | | X | | | |
| dizziness | | X | | X | | | |
| dry mouth | X | | | | X | | |
| blurred vision | X | | | | X | | |
| constipation | X | | | | X | | |
| difficulty urinating | X | | | X | | | |
| reduced urinary output | | X | | X | | | X |
| racing heartbeat/ palpitations | | X | | X | | | |
| weakness | | X | | X | | | |
| sexual problems | | X | | X | | | |
| restlessness | | X | | X | | | |
| skin rash | | X | | X | | X | X |
| weight gain | X | | | | X | | |
| seizures | | X | | X | | X | X |
| low white blood cell count | | X | | X | | | X |
| tremors | | X | | X | | | |
| stiffness | X | | | X | | | |
| involuntary facial or tongue movements | | X | | X | | | |

DRUG NAME: **Triflupromazine**

**BRAND NAME:** Vesprin
**For more information:** See Chapter 7, Antipsychotic Drugs.

**FAST FACTS**　**Drug group:** Antipsychotics.　　**Available as generic?** No.

**Prescription needed?** Yes.　　**Habit-forming?** No.

 **Overdose:** Symptoms include light-headedness, sedation, confusion, agitation, disorientation, restlessness, convulsions, fever, and coma. Seek immediate emergency medical treatment.

## PRECAUTIONS

### Do not take this drug if:

- You have ever had an allergic reaction to this drug or any phenothiazine.

### Inform your physician if:

- You have ever had an allergic reaction to any drug.
- You have epilepsy or asthma.
- You are taking any other drug—prescription or nonprescription—or vitamins.
- You are on a low-salt, low-sugar, or any other special diet.
- You will be under anesthesia or undergoing surgery or medical testing in the next few months.

 **Pregnancy/Breast-feeding**

Except in unusual cases where the mother or the baby's life is endangered, this drug should not be taken by pregnant women. Women taking triflupromazine should not breast-feed.

 **Infants/Children**

Children may take this drug, but only under the direction of a pediatrician and/or children's psychiatrist.

 **Over Sixty**

Side effects, some serious, can be worse. Initial dose should be low, with careful monitoring for side effects. Special care should be taken when sitting up from a lying position, or standing from a sitting position, as blood pressure may be lowered and balance impaired.

 **Driving/Operating Machinery**

Extreme caution is advised. This medicine can impair mental alertness and coordination. If you do drive or operate machinery, this medicine should be taken at bedtime when its sedating effects are less likely to interfere with daytime activities.

## GENERAL INFORMATION

Triflupromazine is an intermediate-potency antipsychotic used to treat people who are experiencing disorganized, psychotic thinking and who may be having delusions or hallucinations. The choice of which antipsychotic drug to use is often determined by the side effects. For an explanation of how this drug works, see Chapter 7.

## BENEFITS

- Effective in treating hallucinations, delusions, confused thinking, and mania.
- Sedating effects helpful in calming agitated persons.

## RISKS

- Can dangerously lower white blood cell count.
- Can cause tardive dyskinesia.
- Can cause neuroleptic malignant syndrome.

## GUIDELINES FOR USERS

**How is the drug taken?** Tablets (10, 25, 50 mg); concentrate; intramuscular.

**What is the usual dosage?** Initial dose should be 50 mg per day in healthy young people, with increases as needed to control symptoms. A maximum daily dose of up to 200 mg may be used, if necessary. Maintenance doses should be as low as possible and still control the psychotic symptoms.

**What are the instructions for taking the drug?** It is best to take this drug on an empty stomach and drink a full glass of water. Sometimes it is possible to take a single dose at bedtime. In other cases, several doses a day may be prescribed. If you are taking the extended-release form, do not break open the capsule. Follow your physician's instructions carefully.

**How quickly will I feel the effect of the drug?** It usually takes several weeks for you to experience the full benefit of this drug. However, you may feel more calm and relaxed after the first dose or two. The drug should also help you sleep better, if this is a problem.

**What if I miss a dose or several doses?** If you are taking one dose at night, take the missed dose in the morning. If you do not remember until the afternoon, skip the missed dose. Do not take double doses.

If you are taking several doses a day, and remember within an hour or so, take the missed dose. Otherwise, skip the missed dose and continue on your regular dosing schedule. Do not take double doses.

If you are missing doses on a frequent basis, notify your psychiatrist. A slow-release form of an antipsychotic drug may help with your compliance and help avoid a relapse.

**What if I stop taking the drug?** Do not stop taking this drug without consulting your physician. Abruptly stopping this medication will lead to uncomfortable but not dangerous physical symptoms. Should your physician and you agree that the drug should be discontinued, your medication should be tapered slowly to prevent physical symptoms of withdrawal and a reemergence of your psychotic symptoms.

**How should I store the drug?** Keep out of reach of children. Store in a dry, tightly closed, light-resistant container. Heat and moisture may cause this drug to break down.

## INTERACTIONS

**Alcohol:** Avoid alcohol. When combined with alcohol, this medicine can cause excessive sedation and dangerously lower blood pressure.

**Food/Beverages:** No restrictions.

DRUG NAME:    Triflupromazine (*continued*)

## INTERACTIONS (*continued*)

**Smoking:** Smoking lowers the blood level of triflupromazine. If you do smoke, blood samples should be taken to test whether the drug is in the therapeutic range.

**Other drugs:** Antacids with aluminum or magnesium (Maalox, for example) should not be taken for two hours before or after taking triflupromazine because they may interfere with the absorption of this drug.

Heterocyclic antidepressants can increase the plasma level of this drug and cause a worsening of side effects. Conversely, this drug can increase the blood level of antidepressants. The concurrent use of these two types of drugs must be carefully monitored.

Blood pressure can be dangerously lowered when antipsychotics are combined with vasodilators (medications that dilate blood vessels).

Triflupromazine will increase the effect of medicines known as CNS (central nervous system) depressants. Examples include antihistamines, hay fever medicines, sedatives, narcotics, muscle relaxants, barbiturates, and anesthetics. Check with your physician before taking any of these drugs.

## HABIT-FORMING POTENTIAL

None.

## LONG-TERM USE

Prolonged use of triflupromazine is associated with increased risk of developing tardive dyskinesia, a potentially irreversible side effect involving disfiguring movements of the face, tongue, and limbs. For more information on tardive dyskinesia, please see Chapter 7.

## PLEASE NOTE

Not a sleeping pill: This drug, which has a sedating effect, is sometimes misused as a sleeping pill. There are much safer medications available as sleeping aids.

Not specifically antiaggressive: Because of the potential serious side effects of the antipsychotic drugs, especially over the long term, this medication should not be used to treat anxiety or chronic aggression and agitation.

Frequent examinations required: While taking this medication, your blood pressure and pulse rate should be monitored frequently. Regular checks should also be made for the early signs of tardive dyskinesia.

Classification: Triflupromazine is classified as a phenothiazine. Other antipsychotics in the same group include acetophenazine, chlorpromazine, fluphenazine, mesoridazine, perphenazine, promazine, thioridazine, trifluoperazine. In general, if you have a poor response to one drug in this family, you will likely have a similar poor response to other drugs in the family.

## Triflupromazine

| Symptom/Effect | Frequency | | Discuss with Physician | | | Stop Taking Drug Now | Call Physician Now |
|---|---|---|---|---|---|---|---|
| | Common | Rare | Not Necessary | In All Cases | Only If Severe | | |
| lethargy/sleepiness | X | | | | X | | |
| low blood pressure | X | | | X | | | |
| dizziness | | X | | X | | | |
| dry mouth | X | | | | X | | |
| blurred vision | X | | | | X | | |
| constipation | X | | | | X | | |
| difficulty urinating | X | | | X | | | |
| reduced urinary output | | X | | X | | | X |
| increased heart rate | | X | | X | | | |
| weakness | | X | | X | | | |
| sexual problems | | X | | X | | | |
| restlessness | | X | | X | | | |
| skin rash | | X | | X | | X | X |
| weight gain | X | | | | X | | |
| seizures | | X | | X | | X | X |
| low white blood cell count | | X | | | | | X |
| tremors | | X | | X | | | |
| stiffness | X | | | X | | | |
| involuntary facial or tongue movements | | X | | X | | | |

# Drug Name: **Trihexyphenidyl**

**Brand Name:** Artane
**For more information:** See Chapter 10, Drugs for Attention-Deficit Hyperactivity Disorder.

**FAST FACTS**   **Drug group:** Antiparkinsonian medications.

**Available as generic?** Yes.

**Prescription needed?** Yes.

**Habit-forming?** No.

 **Overdose:** Symptoms include severe drowsiness, mental confusion, disorientation, convulsions, trouble breathing, loss of coordination, hallucinations. If any of these symptoms are present, seek immediate emergency medical treatment.

## PRECAUTIONS

### Do not take this drug if:

- You have ever had an allergic reaction to this drug or any drug that treats movement disorders (antidyskinetic drug).

### Inform your physician if:

- You have ever had an allergic reaction to any drug.
- You have asthma, glaucoma, urinary problems, or an enlarged prostate.
- You have epilepsy.
- You have heart problems, or kidney or liver disease.
- You are taking any other drug— prescription or nonprescription —or vitamins.
- You will be under anesthesia or undergoing surgery or medical testing in the next few months.

 ### Pregnancy/Breast-feeding

Except in unusual cases where the mother's life or the pregnancy is endangered, this drug should not be taken by pregnant women. To be safe, women taking trihexyphenidyl should not breast-feed, although trihexyphenidyl has not been shown to cause problems in nursing babies.

 ### Infants/Children

May be used in children in lower doses. Child psychiatrists frequently prescribe this to children with parkinsonian side effects of other psychiatric drugs, with careful monitoring for side effects.

 ### Over Sixty

Side effects, some serious, can be worse. In men, this drug may cause problems with urinating. If you experience confusion, a memory loss, changes in vision, or eye pain, check immediately with your doctor.

 ### Driving/Operating Machinery

This drug may impair mental alertness and coordination. Do not drive or operate machinery until you are certain this drug will not affect your performance.

## GENERAL INFORMATION

Trihexyphenidyl is in a class of drugs referred to as *antidyskinetics*. It is used to treat Parkinson's disease and to control movement side effects that occur fairly commonly with antipsychotic drugs. Trihexyphenidyl improves muscle control and decreases stiffness and tremors.

## BENEFITS

- Generally effective in controlling the symptoms of Parkinson's disease and movement side effects of antipsychotic drugs.

## RISKS

- In some cases, this drug does not alleviate movement symptoms and may even aggravate them.
- In some patients, particularly the elderly or brain injured, this drug can cause confusion or memory problems.
- This drug can aggravate glaucoma.

## GUIDELINES FOR USERS

**How is the drug taken?** Tablets (2, 5 mg); syrup.

**What is the usual dosage?** The initial daily dose should be 2 mg or 4 mg in healthy young people. The usual daily dose is 2 mg twice per day, but it may be prescribed in doses up to 15 mg per day in very rare cases.

**What are the instructions for taking the drug?** Your dose should be taken with meals to prevent stomach upset. The syrup may be mixed with water or juice to improve the taste and prevent stomach upset. If dry mouth is a problem, it is often better to take this drug before meals.

**How quickly will I feel the effect of the drug and how long does it last?** If you have stiffness or other movement side effects of psychiatric medications, you should experience an improvement in your symptoms with the first several days of treatment.

**What if I miss a dose or several doses?** If you miss a dose and remember within an hour or so, take the missed dose. Otherwise, skip the missed dose and continue on your regular dosing schedule. Do not take double doses.

**What if I stop taking the drug?** Do not stop taking this drug without consulting your physician. Your medication should be tapered slowly to prevent a reemergence of your symptoms.

**How should I store the drug?** Keep out of reach of children. Store in a dry, tightly closed, light-resistant container. Heat and moisture may cause this drug to break down. The liquid form does not require refrigeration.

## INTERACTIONS

**Alcohol:** Do not drink alcohol. Trihexyphenidyl may increase some of the effects of alcohol.

**Food/Beverages:** No restrictions.

**Smoking:** No restrictions.

**DRUG NAME:** Trihexyphenidyl (*continued*)

## INTERACTIONS (*continued*)

**Other drugs:** Trihexyphenidyl will *increase* the effect of other CNS (central nervous system) depressants. Examples include hay fever medicines, sedatives, narcotics, muscle relaxants, barbiturates, and anesthetics. Check with your physician before taking any of these drugs.

Antacids with aluminum or magnesium (Maalox, for example) and diarrhea medicines should not be taken for one hour before or after taking trihexyphenidyl because they may interfere with the absorption of this drug.

## HABIT-FORMING POTENTIAL

None.

## LONG-TERM USE

Poses no danger.

| Trihexyphenidyl | | | | | | | |
|---|---|---|---|---|---|---|---|
| | **Frequency** | | **Discuss with Physician** | | | | |
| **Symptom/Effect** | **Common** | **Rare** | **Not Necessary** | **In All Cases** | **Only If Severe** | **Stop Taking Drug Now** | **Call Physician Now** |
| blurred vision | X | | | | X | | |
| constipation | X | | | | X | | |
| decreased sweating | X | | | | X | | |
| drowsiness | X | | | | X | | |
| nausea/vomiting | X | | | X | | | |
| sensitivity to light | X | | | | X | | |
| dry mouth | X | | | | X | | |
| severe headache | | X | | X | | | |
| dizziness/ light-headedness | | X | | X | | | |
| anxiety | | X | | X | | | |
| numbness or tingling in hands or feet | | X | | X | | | |
| muscle cramps | | X | | X | | | |
| eye pain | | X | | X | | X | X |
| skin rash | | X | | X | | X | X |
| memory loss | | X | | X | | | |
| confusion | | X | | X | | | |
| problems urinating | | X | | X | | X | X |

DRUG NAME: **Trimipramine**

**BRAND NAME:** Surmontil
**For more information:** See Chapter 3, Antidepressant Drugs.

**FAST FACTS**  **Drug group:** Antidepressants.  **Available as generic?** No.
**Prescription needed?** Yes.  **Habit-forming?** No.

**Overdose:** The danger of an overdose, which can be lethal, is extremely high. Symptoms include difficulty breathing, shock, agitation, delirium, and coma. Seek immediate emergency medical treatment.

## PRECAUTIONS

### Do not take this drug if:

- You have ever had an allergic or negative reaction to any drug in this group.

### Inform your physician if:

- You have ever had an allergic reaction to any drug.
- You have epilepsy.
- You are taking any other drug—prescription or nonprescription—or vitamins.
- You will be under anesthesia or undergoing surgery or medical testing in the next few months.

### Pregnancy/Breast-feeding

If you are pregnant or planning a pregnancy, you should, if possible, use non-drug alternatives for treating your depression. This drug has not been demonstrated to be safe during pregnancy. Nursing mothers should not take this drug since it is passed on to the baby in the mother's milk.

### Infants/Children

The safety of this drug has not been established for children. Lower doses are recommended for adolescents. Its use in the treatment of depression in children and adolescents must be under the guidance of a child psychiatrist.

### Over Sixty

In general, lower doses are required. Side effects may be worse and some older patients may experience confusion. Elderly people may fall after standing up because of the drug's hypotensive (blood pressure lowering) side effects.

### Driving/Operating Machinery

Extreme caution is advised. This medicine can impair mental alertness and coordination. If you do drive or operate machinery, this medicine should be taken at bedtime, when its sedating effects are less likely to interfere with daytime activities.

**DRUG NAME:**    Trimipramine (*continued*)

## GENERAL INFORMATION

Trimipramine is one of the heterocyclic drugs used to treat depression. It works by inhibiting the nerve cell's ability to reabsorb the neurotransmitters norepinephrine and serotonin (see Chapter 3). Trimipramine is among the more sedating heterocyclic drugs. Wyeth-Ayerst manufactures the brand Surmontil.

## BENEFITS

- Helps 75 percent to 80 percent of people with major depression.

## RISKS

- Produces annoying side effects.
- Potential for use in suicide attempts.

## GUIDELINES FOR USERS

**How is the drug taken?** Capsules (25, 50, 100 mg).

**What is the usual dosage?** The initial dose is usually 75 mg daily in divided doses. This can be increased gradually to 150 mg daily. Some people may require 200 mg to 300 mg daily.

**What are the instructions for taking the drug?** Take this medicine with food, unless your physician has instructed you otherwise. Taking the medicine on an empty stomach may cause your stomach to become upset. To benefit from the drug, it is important to take the correct dosage each day.

**How quickly will I feel the effect of the drug?** You will probably experience some unpleasant side effects (dry mouth, blurry vision, constipation) right away. It may take days or weeks for the benefits to appear. It usually takes two to four weeks at full dose for a person to feel a positive response. By the third week of treatment, the side effects are usually less severe.

**What if I miss a dose or several doses?** If you are taking one dose at bedtime and miss your dose, do not take the drug in the morning. Check with your physician. If you are taking more than one dose a day and remember within an hour or so that you have missed a dose, take the dose. However, if it is almost time for your next dose, skip the missed dose. Do not take double doses.

**What if I stop taking the drug?** Do not discontinue this drug abruptly. Your dosage should be gradually reduced. Stopping the drug abruptly may cause flulike symptoms, headache, restlessness, and/or a worsening of your condition. Inform your physician if you notice these side effects, or any others, after stopping the drug. The effects of this drug may last for up to seven days after you have stopped taking it.

**How should I store the drug?** Keep out of reach of children. Store in a dry, tightly closed, light-resistant container. Heat and moisture may cause this drug to break down.

## INTERACTIONS

**Alcohol:** Do not drink alcohol. Trimipramine *increases* the effect of alcohol, while alcohol *increases* the side effects of the drug. In addition, alcohol use can contribute to depression.

**Food/Beverages:** No restrictions.

**Smoking:** Smoking lowers the blood level of trimipramine. If you do smoke, blood samples should be taken to test whether the drug is in the therapeutic range.

**Other drugs:** Trimipramine will increase the effect of medicines known as CNS (central nervous system) depressants. Examples include antihistamines, hay fever medicines, sedatives, narcotics, muscle relaxants, barbiturates, and anesthetics. Check with your physician before taking any of these drugs.

## HABIT-FORMING POTENTIAL

None.

## LONG-TERM USE

Most people who have a beneficial response do not need to take this drug longer than about six months. A few people may need to take the drug for a year or longer because their depression recurs if they attempt to discontinue the drug.

## PLEASE NOTE

Help with side effects: Drinking water and sucking on hard candy can help if you are experiencing dry mouth. To prevent constipation, eat high-fiber foods and take a daily dose of a natural bulk laxative. And you can avoid episodes of light-headedness by making sure you get up slowly from a sitting or prone position. These side effects generally get better or go away after you have been on the drug several weeks.

| Trimipramine | | | | | | | |
|---|---|---|---|---|---|---|---|
| | Frequency | | Discuss with Physician | | | | |
| Symptom/Effect | Common | Rare | Not Necessary | In All Cases | Only If Severe | Stop Taking Drug Now | Call Physician Now |
| drowsiness | X | | | | X | | |
| dry mouth | X | | | | X | | |
| constipation | X | | | | X | | |
| blurred vision | X | | | | X | | |
| low blood pressure | X | | | X | | | |
| racing heartbeat/ palpitations | | X | | | X | | |
| confusion | | X | | X | | | X |
| skin rashes/allergies | | X | | X | | X | X |
| insomnia | | X | | | X | | |
| sexual problems | | X | | X | | | |
| increased appetite | | X | | | X | | |
| seizures | | X | | X | | X | X |

DRUG NAME: **Valproic acid**

**BRAND NAME:** Depakene
**For more information:** See Chapter 6, Antimanic Drugs.

---

**FAST FACTS**  **Drug group:** Antimanic agents.

**Available as generic?** Yes.

**Prescription needed?** Yes.

**Habit-forming?** No.

**Overdose:** Valproic acid is absorbed very rapidly, and overdose may result in a deep coma. Seek immediate emergency medical treatment.

---

## PRECAUTIONS

### Do not take this drug if:

- You have ever had an allergic reaction to this drug or divalproex.
- You have liver disease or dysfunction.
- You are taking phenobarbital or phenytoin (Dilantin).

### Inform your physician if:

- You have ever had an allergic reaction to any drug.
- You have epilepsy.
- You are taking any other drug—prescription or nonprescription—or vitamins.
- You will be under anesthesia or undergoing surgery or medical testing in the next few months.

 **Pregnancy/Breast-feeding**

Birth defects have been reported in babies born to mothers who took this drug during pregnancy. Except in the most unusual cases where the mother or the baby's life is endangered, this drug should not be taken by pregnant women. Women taking valproic acid should not breast-feed.

 **Infants/Children**

Children under age two are at increased risk of developing fatal liver disease. This drug has not been tested systematically as an antimanic agent for children under sixteen years of age.

 **Over Sixty**

Lower doses are generally required and side effects may be worse.

 **Driving/Operating Machinery**

This drug may impair mental alertness and coordination. Do not drive or operate machinery until you are certain this drug will not affect your performance.

---

## GENERAL INFORMATION

Valproic acid is an antiseizure medication prescribed to treat some types of seizures (epilepsy) and sometimes prescribed for people experiencing mania. Valproic acid is not usually the drug of first choice to treat manic depression. Most often, it is prescribed to treat manic-depressive patients who have not responded to lithium or carbamazepine. Liver failure has been reported in some people taking this drug. Children under the age of two appear to be at particular risk. Because of the risk of liver failure, which can be fatal, liver function tests should be performed prior to therapy and at frequent intervals thereafter.

---

## BENEFITS

- Treats mania in people whose symptoms have not responded to or who cannot tolerate the side effects of other antimanic medications.

## RISKS

- Liver failure can occur and is sometimes fatal.
- When used during pregnancy, birth defects have been reported.

## GUIDELINES FOR USERS

**How is the drug taken?** Capsules (250 mg); syrup.

**What is the usual dosage?** Initial daily dose should be 5 mg to 10 mg per kilogram of weight in healthy young people, with increases as needed to control symptoms. The usual maximum daily dose is up to 60 mg per kilogram of weight. If the total daily dose is greater than 250 mg, the drug should be given in divided doses (e.g. 125 mg twice a day).

**What are the instructions for taking the drug?** Take valproic acid with meals to reduce gastrointestinal side effects such as nausea and vomiting. If you are taking the capsule form of this drug, swallow the capsule whole, without chewing. The syrup form of valproic acid may be mixed with liquid or food before taking. Follow your physician's instructions carefully to maintain the correct blood level of this drug and lessen the possibility of side effects.

**How quickly will I feel the effect of the drug?** Manic behavior usually diminishes after seven to ten days of treatment. Valproic acid should even out the intense ups and downs of your moods, and after several weeks of treatment, you should feel reasonably normal. At the same time, you may experience some side effects from the drug such as dry mouth, a slight tremor in your hands, and a frequent need to urinate. These side effects usually peak about one to two hours after taking your dose.

**What if I miss a dose or several doses?** If you miss a dose and remember within an hour or so, take the dose. Otherwise, skip the missed dose and continue on your regular dosing schedule. Do not take double doses. Notify your physician if you are missing doses regularly. To obtain the full benefit of this drug and lessen the chance of side effects, it is important to take doses regularly.

**What if I stop taking the drug?** Do not stop taking this drug without consulting your physician. When discontinuing valproic acid, it should be tapered gradually to monitor for potential recurrence of symptoms of mania or depression.

**How should I store the drug?** Keep out of reach of children. Store in a dry, tightly closed, light-resistant container. Heat and moisture may cause this drug to break down.

## INTERACTIONS

**Alcohol:** Avoid alcohol. When combined with alcohol, this medicine can cause excessive sedation and dangerously lower blood pressure.

**Food/Beverages:** No restrictions.

**Smoking:** No restrictions.

**DRUG NAME:**    Valproic acid (*continued*)

## INTERACTIONS (*continued*)

**Other drugs:** Valproic acid will *increase* the effect of medicines known as CNS (central nervous system) depressants. Examples include antihistamines, hay fever medicines, sedatives, narcotics, muscle relaxants, barbiturates, and anesthetics. Check with your physician before taking any of these drugs.

This drug can dangerously *increase* blood levels of phenobarbital. If your physician prescribes a combination of valproic acid and phenobarbital, you should be closely monitored for toxicity. Primidone is metabolized into a barbiturate and therefore may cause a similar interaction.

When combined with phenytoin (Dilantin), phenytoin concentrations are reduced and seizures can occur.

Consult your physician if you plan on taking aspirin or any drug affecting coagulation.

## HABIT-FORMING POTENTIAL

None.

## LONG-TERM USE

Although liver damage, when it occurs, usually happens in the first six months of treatment, liver functions must be monitored regularly while you are taking this drug. This medicine may also interfere with the clotting mechanism of your blood, so platelet counts and coagulation tests should be taken before beginning treatment and at regular intervals.

| Valproic Acid | | | | | | |
|---|---|---|---|---|---|---|
| | Frequency | | Discuss with Physician | | | |
| Symptom/Effect | Common | Rare | Not Necessary | In All Cases | Only If Severe | Stop Taking Drug Now | Call Physician Now |
| stomach upset or cramps | X | | | X | | | |
| diarrhea | X | | | | X | | |
| indigestion | X | | | | X | | |
| weight gain or loss | | X | | X | | | |
| trembling in hands | | X | | X | | | |
| confusion | | X | | X | | | X |
| drowsiness | X | | | | X | | |
| dizziness | X | | | X | | | |
| headache | | X | | X | | | |
| constipation | | X | | | X | | |
| restlessness/anxiety | | X | | X | | | |
| rash | | X | | X | | X | X |
| yellow eyes or skin | | X | | X | | X | X |
| unusual bruising/ bleeding | | X | | X | | X | X |
| lethargy | X | | | | X | | |
| swelling of face | | X | | X | | | X |
| hair loss | | X | | X | | | |
| depression | | X | | X | | | X |
| psychosis | | X | | X | | X | X |
| painful menstrual cramps | | X | | X | | | |

# Drug Name: **Verapamil**

**Brand Names:** Calan, Isoptin
**For more information:** See Chapter 6, Antimanic Drugs.

---

**FAST FACTS**  **Drug group:** Antimanic agents.  **Available as generic?** Yes.
**Prescription needed?** Yes.  **Habit-forming?** No.

 **Overdose:** Serious lowering of your blood pressure and heart failure may occur. Symptoms include dizziness, nausea, vomiting, headache, lethargy, confusion, and poor equilibrium. Seek immediate emergency medical treatment.

---

## PRECAUTIONS

### Do not take this drug if:

- You have ever had an allergic reaction to this drug or any other calcium channel blocker.

### Inform your physician if:

- You have ever had an allergic reaction to any drug.
- You have epilepsy, low blood pressure, or any heart problems.
- You are taking any other drug—prescription or nonprescription —or vitamins.
- You will be under anesthesia or undergoing surgery or medical testing in the next few months.
- You have liver or kidney disease or dysfunction.
- You have a heart condition.

 ### Pregnancy/Breast-feeding

Except in unusual cases where the mother or the baby's life is endangered, this drug should not be taken by pregnant women. Women taking antipsychotics should not breast-feed.

 ### Infants/Children

Safety and effectiveness have not been established for children under the age of eighteen.

 ### Over Sixty

Lower doses are generally required and side effects may be worse.

### Driving/Operating Machinery

This drug may impair mental alertness and coordination. Do not drive or operate machinery until you are certain this drug will not affect your performance.

---

## GENERAL INFORMATION

Verapamil, a drug used to treat irregular heartbeats and high blood pressure, has been found effective in the treatment of mania, though it is not usually the drug of first choice. Most often, it is prescribed to treat manic-depressive patients who have not responded to lithium or carbamazepine. This drug is classified as a calcium channel blocker because it prevents the movement of calcium into the cells of the heart and blood vessels. This relaxes the blood vessels and increases the flow of blood and oxygen to the heart.

---

## BENEFITS

- Treats mania in people whose symptoms have not responded to or who cannot tolerate the side effects of other antimanic medications.

## RISKS

- May result in severe lowering of blood pressure or heart dysfunction in those with preexisting heart illness.
- May damage the liver in certain patients.

## GUIDELINES FOR USERS

**How is the drug taken?** Tablets (40, 80, 120 mg); extended-release tablets.

**What is the usual dosage?** Initial dose should be 40 mg to 120 mg a day in healthy young people, with increases as needed to control symptoms. The usual maximum daily dose is up to 480 mg in divided doses (three to four times a day).

**What are the instructions for taking the drug?** Take verapamil with food or milk to reduce gastrointestinal side effects such as nausea and vomiting.

**How quickly will I feel the effect of the drug?** Manic behavior usually diminishes after seven to ten days of treatment. Verapamil should even out the intense ups and downs of your moods, and after several weeks of treatment, you should feel reasonably normal. At the same time, you may experience some side effects from the drug such as dry mouth, a slight tremor in your hands, and a frequent need to urinate. These side effects usually peak about one to two hours after taking your dose.

**What if I miss a dose or several doses?** If you miss a dose and remember within an hour or so, take the dose. Otherwise, skip the missed dose and continue on your regular dosing schedule. Do not take double doses. Notify your physician if you are missing doses regularly, since an extended-release form of this medicine is available. To obtain the full benefit of this drug and lessen the chance of side effects, it is important to take doses regularly.

**What if I stop taking the drug?** Do not stop taking this drug without consulting your physician. When discontinuing verapamil, it should be tapered gradually to monitor for potential recurrence of symptoms of mania or depression.

**How should I store the drug?** Keep out of reach of children. Store in a dry, tightly closed, light-resistant container. Heat and moisture may cause this drug to break down.

## INTERACTIONS

**Alcohol:** Avoid alcohol. When combined with alcohol, this medicine can cause excessive sedation and dangerously lower blood pressure.

**Food/Beverages:** No restrictions.

**Smoking:** Smoking does not appear to alter blood levels or efficacy of verapamil.

**Other drugs:** When combined with lithium, verapamil may *decrease* the blood level of lithium. Dosage adjustments may be necessary.

When combined with carbamazepine, verapamil may *increase* the blood level of carbamazepine. Dosage adjustments may be necessary.

Verapamil and antihypertensive drugs (vasodilators, diuretics, and beta blockers)

DRUG NAME:    Verapamil (*continued*)

## INTERACTIONS (*continued*)

can significantly lower blood pressure. Do not take water pills or any other antihypertensive drugs in combination with verapamil without consulting your physician.

The following drugs may have interactions with verapamil: disopyramide, quinidine, nitrates, cimetidine, rifampin, inhalation anesthetics, and neuromuscular blocking agents. Do not take any of these drugs in combination with verapamil without consulting your physician.

## HABIT-FORMING POTENTIAL

None.

## LONG-TERM USE

Renal function, liver function, and cardiovascular status must be monitored regularly while you are taking this medication.

| Symptom/Effect | Frequency | | Discuss with Physician | | | Stop Taking Drug Now | Call Physician Now |
|---|---|---|---|---|---|---|---|
| | Common | Rare | Not Necessary | In All Cases | Only If Severe | | |
| constipation | X | | | | X | | |
| dizziness | | X | | X | | | |
| headache | | X | | X | | | |
| stomach upset | | X | | | X | | |
| anxiety/mood changes | | X | | X | | | |
| weakness | | X | | X | | | |
| tiredness | | X | | X | | | |
| rash | | X | | X | | X | X |
| difficulty breathing | | X | | X | | X | X |
| irregular heartbeat | | X | | X | | | X |
| unusual bruising/ bleeding | | X | | X | | | X |
| swelling of limbs | | X | | X | | | X |
| nausea | | X | | X | | | X |
| confusion | | X | | X | | | |
| problems with equilibrium | | X | | X | | | |
| insomnia | | X | | X | | | |
| sexual problems | | X | | X | | | |
| chest pain | | X | | X | | X | X |
| sweating | | X | | X | | | |
| yellow skin | | X | | X | | X | X |
| yellow in whites of eyes | | X | | X | | X | X |

# DSM-III-R Diagnostic Classification of Mental Disorders

## MULTIAXIAL SYSTEM

Axis I    Clinical Syndromes
          V Codes
Axis II   Developmental Disorders
          Personality Disorders
Axis III  Physical Disorders and Conditions
Axis IV   Severity of Psychosocial Stressors
Axis V    Global Assessment of Functioning

## DISORDERS USUALLY FIRST EVIDENT IN INFANCY, CHILDHOOD, OR ADOLESCENCE

### DEVELOPMENTAL DISORDERS
*Note*: These are coded on Axis II.

*Mental Retardation*

317.00   Mild mental retardation
318.00   Moderate mental retardation
318.10   Severe mental retardation
318.20   Profound mental retardation
319.00   Unspecified mental retardation

*Pervasive Developmental Disorders*

299.00   Autistic disorder
                *Specify* if childhood onset
299.80   Pervasive developmental disorder NOS

*Specific Developmental Disorders*

    Academic skills disorders
315.10   Developmental arithmetic disorder
315.80   Developmental expressive writing disorder
315.00   Developmental reading disorder

    Language and speech disorders
315.39   Developmental articulation disorder
315.31   Developmental expressive language disorder
315.31   Developmental receptive language disorder

    Motor skills disorder
315.40   Developmental coordination disorder
315.90   Specific developmental disorder NOS

*Other Developmental Disorders*

315.90   Developmental disorder NOS

**Source:** Reprinted with permission of the American Psychiatric Association.

### Disruptive Behavior Disorders

314.01    Attention-deficit hyperactivity disorder

312.20    Conduct disorder,
312.20        group type
312.00        solitary aggressive type
312.90        undifferentiated type
313.81    Oppositional defiant disorder

### Anxiety Disorders of Childhood or Adolescence

309.21    Separation anxiety disorder
313.21    Avoidant disorder of childhood or adolescence
313.00    Overanxious disorder

### Eating Disorders

307.10    Anorexia nervosa
307.51    Bulimia nervosa
307.52    Pica
307.53    Rumination disorder of infancy
307.50    Eating disorder NOS

### Gender Identity Disorders

302.60    Gender identity disorder of childhood
302.50    Transsexualism
          *Specify* sexual history: asexual, homosexual, heterosexual,
          unspecified
302.85    Gender identity disorder of adolescence or adulthood, nontranssexual
          type
          *Specify* sexual history: asexual, homosexual, heterosexual,
          unspecified
302.85    Gender identity disorder NOS

### Tic Disorders

307.23    Tourette's disorder
307.22    Chronic motor or vocal tic disorder
307.21    Transient tic disorder
          *Specify*: single episode or recurrent
307.20    Tic disorder NOS

### Elimination Disorders

307.70    Functional encopresis
          *Specify*: primary or secondary type
307.60    Functional enuresis

*Specify*: primary or secondary type
*Specify*: nocturnal only, diurnal only, nocturnal and diurnal

## Speech Disorders Not Elsewhere Classified

307.00   Cluttering
307.00   Stuttering

## Other Disorders of Infancy, Childhood, or Adolescence

313.23   Elective mutism
313.82   Identity disorder
313.89   Reactive attachment disorder of infancy or early childhood
307.30   Stereotypy/habit disorder
314.00   Undifferentiated attention-deficit disorder

## ORGANIC MENTAL DISORDERS

### Dementias Arising in the Senium and Presenium

Primary degenerative dementia of the Alzheimer type, senile onset

290.30        with delirium
290.20        with delusions
290.21        with depression
290.00        uncomplicated
   *Note*: code 331.00 Alzheimer's disease on Axis III

Code in fifth digit: 1 = with delirium, 2 = with delusions, 3 = with depression, 0 = uncomplicated.

290.1x   Primary degenerative dementia of the Alzheimer type, presenile onset,

   ————

   *Note*: code 331.00 Alzheimer's disease on Axis III
290.4x   Multi-infarct dementia, ————
290.00   Senile dementia NOS
            *Specify* etiology on Axis III if known
290.10   Presenile dementia NOS
            *Specify* etiology on Axis III if known
            (e.g., Pick's disease, Jakob-Creutzfeldt disease)

### Psychoactive Substance-Induced Organic Mental Disorders

      Alcohol
303.00   intoxication
291.40   idiosyncratic intoxication
291.80   uncomplicated alcohol withdrawal

291.00   withdrawal delirium
291.30   hallucinosis
291.10   amnestic disorder
291.20   dementia associated with alcoholism

### Amphetamine or similarly acting sympathomimetic
305.70   intoxication
292.00   withdrawal
292.81   delirium
292.11   delusional disorder

### Caffeine
305.90   intoxication

### Cannabis
305.20   intoxication
292.11   delusional disorder

### Cocaine
305.60   intoxication
292.00   withdrawal
292.81   delirium
292.11   delusional disorder

### Hallucinogen
305.30   hallucinosis
292.11   delusional disorder
292.84   mood disorder
292.89   posthallucinogen perception disorder

### Inhalant
305.90   intoxication

### Nicotine
292.00   withdrawal

### Opioid
305.50   intoxication
292.00   withdrawal

### Phencyclidine (PCP) or similarly acting arylcyclohexylamine
305.90   intoxication
292.81   delirium
292.11   delusional disorder

292.84    mood disorder
292.90    organic mental disorder NOS

Sedative, hypnotic, or anxiolytic
305.40    intoxication
292.00    uncomplicated sedative, hypnotic, or anxiolytic withdrawal
292.00    withdrawal delirium
292.83    amnestic disorder

Other or unspecified psychoactive substance
305.90    intoxication
292.00    withdrawal
292.81    delirium
292.82    dementia
292.83    amnestic disorder
292.11    delusional disorder
292.12    hallucinosis
292.84    mood disorder
292.89    anxiety disorder
292.89    personality disorder
292.90    organic mental disorder NOS

*Organic Mental Disorders associated with Axis III physical disorders or conditions, or whose etiology is unknown*

293.00    Delirium
294.10    Dementia
294.00    Amnestic disorder
293.81    Organic delusional disorder
293.82    Organic hallucinosis
293.83    Organic mood disorder
              *Specify*: manic, depressed, mixed
294.80    Organic anxiety disorder
310.10    Organic personality disorder
              *Specify* if explosive type
294.80    Organic mental disorder NOS

PSYCHOACTIVE SUBSTANCE USE DISORDERS

Alcohol
303.90    dependence
305.00    abuse

Amphetamine or similarly acting sympathomimetic
304.40    dependence
305.70    abuse

Cannabis
304.30   dependence
305.20   abuse

Cocaine
304.20   dependence
305.60   abuse

Hallucinogen
304.50   dependence
305.30   abuse

Inhalant
304.60   dependence
305.90   abuse

Nicotine
305.10   dependence

Opioid
304.00   dependence
305.50   abuse

Phencyclidine (PCP) or similarly acting arylcyclohexylamine
304.50   dependence
305.90   abuse

Sedative, hypnotic, or anxiolytic
304.10   dependence
305.40   abuse

304.90   Polysubstance dependence
304.90   Psychoactive substance dependence NOS
305.90   Psychoactive substance abuse NOS

## Schizophrenia

Code in fifth digit: 1 = subchronic, 2 = chronic, 3 = subchronic with acute exacerbation, 4 = chronic with acute exacerbation, 5 = in remission, 0 = unspecified.

Schizophrenia
295.2x   catatonic, _____
295.1x   disorganized, _____

295.3x    paranoid, _____
            *Specify* if stable type
295.9x    undifferentiated, _____
295.6x    residual, _____

    *Specify* if late onset


## DELUSIONAL (PARANOID) DISORDER

297.10    Delusional (Paranoid) disorder

*Specify* type:  erotomanic
                grandiose
                jealous
                persecutory
                somatic
                unspecified


## PSYCHOTIC DISORDERS NOT ELSEWHERE CLASSIFIED

298.80    Brief reactive psychosis
295.40    Schizophreniform disorder
            *Specify*: without good prognostic features or with good prognostic
            features
295.70    Schizoaffective disorder
            *Specify*: bipolar type or depressive type
297.30    Induced psychotic disorder
298.90    Psychotic disorder NOS (Atypical psychosis)


## MOOD DISORDERS

Code current state of Major Depression and Bipolar Disorder in fifth digit:
    1 = mild, 2 = moderate, 3 = severe, without psychotic features, 4 = with
psychotic features (*specify*: mood-congruent or mood-incongruent), 5 = in partial
remission, 6 = in full remission, 0 = unspecified.

For major depressive episodes, *specify* if chronic and *specify* if melancholic type.

For Bipolar Disorder, Bipolar Disorder NOS, Recurrent Major Depression, and
Depressive Disorder NOS, *specify* if seasonal pattern.

*Bipolar Disorders*
            Bipolar disorder
296.6x        mixed, _____

296.4x    manic, _____
296.5x    depressed, _____
301.13   Cyclothymia
296.70   Bipolar disorder NOS

*Depressive Disorders*

          Major Depression
296.2x    single episode, _____
296.3x    recurrent, _____
300.40   Dysthymia (or Depressive neurosis)
          *Specify*: primary or secondary type
          *Specify*: early or late onset
311.00   Depressive disorder NOS

## ANXIETY DISORDERS (OR ANXIETY AND PHOBIC NEUROSES)

296.70   Panic disorder
300.21   with agoraphobia
          *Specify* current severity of agoraphobic avoidance
          *Specify* current severity of panic attacks
300.01   without agoraphobia
          *Specify* current severity of panic attacks
300.22   Agoraphobia without history of panic disorder
          *Specify*: with or without limited symptom attacks
300.23   Social phobia
          *Specify* if generalized type
300.29   Simple phobia
300.30   Obsessive-compulsive disorder (or Obsessive-compulsive neurosis)
309.89   Posttraumatic stress disorder
          *Specify* if delayed onset
300.02   Generalized anxiety disorder
300.00   Anxiety disorder NOS

## SOMATOFORM DISORDERS

300.70   Body dysmorphic disorder
300.11   Conversion disorder (or Hysterical neurosis, conversion type)
          *Specify*: single episode or recurrent
300.70   Hypochondriasis (or Hypochondriacal neurosis)
300.81   Somatization disorder
307.80   Somatoform pain disorder
300.70   Undifferentiated somatoform disorder
300.70   Somatoform disorder NOS

## DISSOCIATIVE DISORDERS (OR HYSTERICAL NEUROSES, DISSOCIATIVE TYPE)

300.14   Multiple personality disorder
300.13   Psychogenic fugue
300.12   Psychogenic amnesia
300.60   Depersonalization disorder (or Depersonalization neurosis)
300.15   Dissociative disorder NOS


## SEXUAL DISORDERS

*Paraphilias*

302.40   Exhibitionism
302.81   Fetishism
302.89   Frotteurism
302.20   Pedophilia
      *Specify*: same sex, opposite sex, same and opposite sex
      *Specify* if limited to incest
      *Specify*: exclusive type or nonexclusive type
302.83   Sexual masochism
302.84   Sexual sadism
302.30   Transvestic fetishism
302.82   Voyeurism
302.90   Paraphilia NOS


*Sexual Dysfunctions*

*Specify*: psychogenic only, or psychogenic and biogenic (*Note*: If biogenic only, code on Axis III.)
*Specify*: lifelong or acquired
*Specify*: generalized or situational

    Sexual desire disorders
302.71   Hypoactive sexual desire disorder
302.79   Sexual aversion disorder

    Sexual arousal disorders
302.72   Female sexual arousal disorder
302.72   Male erectile disorder

    Orgasm disorders
302.73   Inhibited female orgasm
302.74   Inhibited male orgasm
302.75   Premature ejaculation

Sexual pain disorders
302.76   Dyspareunia
306.51   Vaginismus

302.70   Sexual dysfunction NOS

*Other Sexual Disorders*
302.90   Sexual disorder NOS

## SLEEP DISORDERS

*Dyssomnias*

Insomnia disorder
307.42      related to another mental disorder (nonorganic)
780.50      related to known organic factor
307.42   Primary insomnia

Hypersomnia disorder
307.44      related to another mental disorder (nonorganic)
780.50      related to a known organic factor
780.54   Primary hypersomnia
307.45   Sleep-wake schedule disorder
   *Specify*: advanced or delayed phase type, disorganized type, frequently chang-
         ing type

Other dyssomnias
307.40   Dyssomnia NOS

*Parasomnias*

307.47   Dream anxiety disorder (Nightmare disorder)
307.46   Sleep terror disorder
307.46   Sleepwalking disorder
307.40   Parasomnia NOS

## FACTITIOUS DISORDERS

Factitious disorder
301.51      with physical symptoms
300.16      with psychological symptoms
300.19   Factitious disorder NOS

## IMPULSE CONTROL DISORDERS NOT ELSEWHERE CLASSIFIED

312.34   Intermittent explosive disorder
312.32   Kleptomania
312.31   Pathological gambling

312.33   Pyromania
312.39   Trichotillomania
312.39   Impulse control disorder NOS

## ADJUSTMENT DISORDER

Adjustment disorder
309.24      with anxious mood
309.00      with depressed mood
309.30      with disturbance of conduct
309.30      with disturbance of conduct
309.40      with mixed disturbance of emotions and conduct
309.28      with mixed emotional features
309.82      with physical complaints
309.83      with withdrawal
309.23      with work (or academic) inhibition
309.90   Adjustment disorder NOS

## PSYCHOLOGICAL FACTORS AFFECTING PHYSICAL CONDITION

316.00   Psychological factors affecting physical condition
             *Specify* physical condition on Axis III

---

### PERSONALITY DISORDERS
*Note*: These are coded on Axis II.

*Cluster A*

301.00   Paranoid
301.20   Schizoid
301.22   Schizotypal

*Cluster B*

301.70   Antisocial
301.83   Borderline
301.50   Histrionic
301.81   Narcissistic

*Cluster C*

301.82   Avoidant
301.60   Dependent
301.40   Obsessive-compulsive
301.84   Passive-aggressive

301.90   Personality disorder NOS

## V Codes for Conditions Not Attributable to a Mental Disorder That Are a Focus of Attention or Treatment

V62.30    Academic problem
V71.01    Adult antisocial behavior

---

V40.00    Borderline intellectual function
          *Note*: This is coded on Axis II.

---

V71.02    Childhood or adolescent antisocial behavior
V65.20    Malingering
V61.10    Marital problem
V15.81    Noncompliance with medical treatment
V62.20    Occupational problem
V61.20    Parent-child problem
V62.81    Other interpersonal problem
V61.80    Other specified family circumstances
V62.89    Phase of life problem or other life circumstance problem
V62.82    Uncomplicated bereavement

## Additional Codes

300.90    Unspecified mental disorder (nonpsychotic)
V71.09    No diagnosis or condition on Axis I
799.90    Diagnosis or condition deferred on Axis I

---

V71.09    No diagnosis or condition on Axis II
799.90    Diagnosis or condition deferred on Axis II

---

## Severity of Psychosocial Stressors Scale: Adults

| CODE | TERM | EXAMPLES OF STRESSORS | |
| --- | --- | --- | --- |
| | | ACUTE EVENTS | ENDURING CIRCUMSTANCES |
| 1 | None | No acute events that may be relevant to the disorder | No enduring circumstances that may be relevant to the disorder |
| 2 | Mild | Broke up with boyfriend or girlfriend; started or graduated from school; child left home | Family arguments; job dissatisfaction; residence in high-crime neighborhood |
| 3 | Moderate | Marriage; marital separation; loss of job; retirement; miscarriage | Marital discord; serious financial problems; trouble with boss; being a single parent |
| 4 | Severe | Divorce; birth of first child | Unemployment; poverty |
| 5 | Extreme | Death of spouse; serious physical illness diagnosed; victim of rape | Serious chronic illness in self or child; ongoing physical or sexual abuse |
| 6 | Catastrophic | Death of child; suicide of spouse; devastating natural disaster | Captivity as hostage; concentration camp experience |
| 0 | Inadequate information, or no change in condition | | |

## Severity of Psychosocial Stressors Scale: Children and Adolescents

| CODE | TERM | EXAMPLES OF STRESSORS | |
|---|---|---|---|
| | | ACUTE EVENTS | ENDURING CIRCUMSTANCES |
| 1 | None | No acute events that may be relevant to the disorder | No enduring circumstances that may be relevant to the disorder |
| 2 | Mild | Broke up with boyfriend or girlfriend; change of school | Overcrowded living quarters; family arguments |
| 3 | Moderate | Expelled from school; birth of sibling | Chronic disabling illness in parent; chronic parental discord |
| 4 | Severe | Divorce of parents; unwanted pregnancy; arrest | Harsh or rejecting parents; chronic life-threatening illness in parent; multiple foster home placements |
| 5 | Extreme | Sexual or physical abuse; death of a parent | Recurrent sexual or physical abuse |
| 6 | Catastrophic | Death of both parents | Chronic life-threatening illness |
| 0 | Inadequate information, or no change in condition | | |

# Glossary

**A**

**acetylcholine**   One of the chemical neurotransmitters normally present in many parts of the body that enable nerve cells to signal one another.

**addiction**   Dependence on a chemical substance to the extent that a physiologic and/or psychologic need is established. This may be manifested by any combination of the following symptoms: tolerance, preoccupation with obtaining and using the substance, use of the substance despite anticipation of probable adverse consequences, repeated efforts to cut down or control substance use, and withdrawal symptoms when the substance is unavailable or not used.

**adrenergic**   Referring to neural activation by catecholamines such as epinephrine, norepinephrine, and dopamine. *See also* **biogenic amines, neurotransmitters, sympathetic nervous system.**

**adrenergic system**   That system of organs and nerves in which epinephrine (adrenaline) is the neurotransmitter.

**Source:** Stone, E. M., ed. *American Psychiatric Glossary*. Washington, D.C.: American Psychiatric Press, 1989. Used with permission.

**affect**    Subjective experience of emotion accompanying an idea or mental representation. The word *affect* is often used loosely as a generic term for feeling, emotion, or mood. *Affect* and *emotion* are commonly used interchangeably.

**agonist**    In pharmacology, a substance that promotes a receptor-mediated biologic response (contrast with **antagonist**).

**agoraphobia**    Commonly, fear of leaving the familiar setting of one's home. In DSM-III-R, it is almost always a form of panic disorder rather than a phobia.

**akathisia**    Motor restlessness ranging from a feeling of inner disquiet, often localized in the muscles, to inability to sit still or lie quietly; a side effect of some antipsychotic drugs.

**amphetamines**    A group of chemicals that stimulates the cerebral cortex; often misused by adults and adolescents to control normal fatigue and to induce euphoria. Used clinically to treat attention-deficit hyperactivity disorder and narcolepsy.

**anhedonia**    Inability to experience pleasure from activities that usually produce pleasurable feelings.

**antagonist**    A drug that reduces or blocks the action of another drug. For example, naloxone blocks the action of morphine by competing with it for receptor sites in the brain and other tissues. By occupying these sites, naloxone prevents the narcotic from binding to the receptors and exerting its effect.

**anticholinergic effects or properties**    Interference with the action of acetylcholine in the brain and peripheral nervous systems by any drug. In psychiatry, the term generally refers to the side effects of antipsychotic drugs, heterocyclic antidepressants, and antiparkinson drugs. Common symptoms of such effects include dry mouth, blurred vision, and constipation.

**antiparkinson drugs**    Pharmacologic agents that ameliorate Parkinsonlike symptoms. In psychiatry, these agents are used to combat the untoward Parkinsonlike and extrapyramidal effects that may be associated with treatment with phenothiazines and other antipsychotic drugs.

**anxiety**    Apprehension, tension, or uneasiness from anticipation of danger, the source of which is largely unknown or unrecognized. Primarily of intrapsychic origin, in distinction to fear, which is the emotional response to a consciously recognized and usually external threat or danger. May be regarded as pathologic when it interferes with effectiveness in living, achievement of desired goals or satisfaction, or reasonable emotional comfort.

**attention-deficit hyperactivity disorder**    A disorder of childhood or adolescence characterized by overactivity, restlessness, distractibility, short attention span, and difficulties in learning and perceptual motor function. Believed in some cases to be associated with minimal brain dysfunction.

**autonomic nervous system (ANS)**   The part of the nervous system that inner-vates the cardiovascular, digestive, reproductive, and respiratory organs. It oper-ates outside of consciousness and controls basic life-sustaining functions such as heart rate, digestion, and breathing. It includes the sympathetic nervous system and the parasympathetic nervous system.

# B

**barbiturates**   Drugs that depress the activities of the central nervous system; primarily used for sedation or treatment of convulsive disorders.

**benzodiazepines**   The generic name for a group of drugs with potent hypnotic and sedative effects.

**biogenic amines**   Organic substances of interest because of their possible role in brain functioning. Subdivided into catecholamines (e.g., epinephrine, dopamine, norepinephrine) and indoles (e.g., tryptophan, serotonin).

**bipolar disorder**   A mood disorder in which there are episodes of both mania and depression; formerly called manic-depressive psychosis, circular or mixed type. A mild form of bipolar disorder is sometimes labeled *cyclothymic disorder*. Bipolar disorder may be subdivided into manic, depressed, or mixed types on the basis of currently presenting symptoms.

**blood levels**   The concentration of a drug in the plasma, serum, or blood. In psychiatry, the term is most often applied to levels of lithium carbonate, hetero-cyclic antidepressants, and anticonvulsants. Maximum clinical responses to these agents have been correlated with specific ranges of blood levels. *See also* **thera-peutic window**.

**brain metabolism**   The process by which the brain synthesizes, degrades, and alters its cells for repair and function.

# C

**catecholamines**   A group of biogenic amines derived from phenylalanine and containing the catechol nucleus. Certain of these amines, such as epinephrine, norepinephrine, and dopamine, are neurotransmitters and exert an important influ-ence on peripheral and central nervous system activity.

**central nervous system (CNS)**   The brain and the spinal cord.

**cholinergic**   Activated or transmitted by acetylcholine (e.g., parasympathetic nerve fibers). *See also* **parasympathetic nervous system**. Contrast with **ad-renergic**.

**cocaine**   A naturally occurring stimulant drug found in the leaves of the coca plant *Erythroxylon coca*. Its systemic effects include nervous system stimulation, manifested by garrulousness, restlessness, excitement, delusional ideas, and a false feeling of increased strength and mental capacity.

# D

**delirium**   An acute organic mental disorder characterized by confusion and altered, possibly fluctuating, consciousness due to an alteration of cerebral metabolism; it may include delusions, illusions, and/or hallucinations. The condition is reversible if the underlying cause can be identified and treated. It may, however, progress to dementia or death. Often emotional lability, typically appearing as anxiety and agitation, is present.

**delirium tremens**   An acute and sometimes fatal brain disorder (in 10 to 15 percent of untreated cases) caused by total or partial withdrawal from excessive alcohol intake. Usually develops in twenty-four to ninety-six hours after cessation of drinking. Symptoms include fever, tremors, ataxia, and sometimes convulsions, frightening illusions, delusions, and hallucinations. The condition is often accompanied by nutritional deficiencies. It is a medical emergency.

**delusion**   A false belief firmly held despite incontrovertible and obvious proof or evidence to the contrary. Further, the belief is not one ordinarily accepted by other members of the person's culture or subculture.

**dementia**   An organic mental disorder in which there is a deterioration of previously acquired intellectual abilities of sufficient severity to interfere with social or occupational functioning. Memory disturbance is the most prominent symptom. In addition, there is impairment of abstract thinking, judgment, impulse control, and/or personality change. Dementia may be progressive, static, or reversible, depending on the pathology and the availability of effective treatment.

**denial**   A defense mechanism, operating unconsciously, used to resolve emotional conflict and allay anxiety by disavowing thoughts, feelings, wishes, needs, or external reality factors that are consciously intolerable.

**depression**   When used to describe a mood, depression refers to feelings of sadness, despair, and discouragement. As such, depression may be a normal feeling state. The overt manifestations are highly variable and may be culture-specific. Depression may be a symptom seen in a variety of mental or physical disorders, a syndrome of associated symptoms secondary to an underlying disorder, or a specific mental disorder. Slowed thinking, decreased pleasure, decreased purposeful physical activity, guilt and hopelessness, and disorders of eating and sleeping may be commonly seen in the depressive syndrome. DSM-III-R classifies depression by severity, recurrence, and association with hypomania or mania.

**dopamine**   A neurosynaptic transmitter found in the brain, specifically associated with some forms of psychosis and abnormal movement disorders. *See also* **biogenic amines**.

**dopamine hypothesis**    A theory that attempts to explain the pathogenesis of schizophrenia and other psychotic states as due to excesses in dopamine activity in various areas of the brain. This theory is, in part, based on biologic observations that the antipsychotic properties of specific drugs may be related to their ability to block the action of dopamine.

**double bind**    Interaction in which one person demands a response to a message containing mutually contradictory signals, while the other person is unable either to comment on the incongruity or to escape from the situation.

**drug dependence**    Habituation to, abuse of, and/or addiction to a chemical substance. Largely because of psychologic craving, the life of the drug-dependent person revolves around the need for the specific effect of one or more chemical agents on mood or state of consciousness. The term thus includes not only the addiction (which emphasizes the physiologic dependence), but also drug abuse (where the pathologic craving for drugs seems unrelated to physical dependence).

**drug holiday**    Discontinuance of a therapeutic drug for a limited period of time. Sometimes used as a way of evaluating baseline behavior or as a means of controlling or reducing the dosage of psychoactive drugs and side effects.

**drug-induced parkinsonism (pseudoparkinsonism)**    A reversible syndrome resembling the disease parkinsonism, resulting from the dopamine-blocking action of antipsychotic drugs. Pill-rolling movements are less common than in the naturally occurring disorder.

**drug interaction**    The effects of two or more drugs taken simultaneously, producing an alteration in the usual effects of either drug taken alone. The interacting drugs may have a potentiating or additive effect and serious side effects may result. An example of drug interaction is alcohol and sedative drugs taken together, which may cause central nervous system depression.

**drug tolerance**    Repeated use of some substance or drug, often narcotics, so that larger and larger doses are required to produce the same physiologic and/or psychologic effect obtained previously by a smaller dose.


**E**

**electroconvulsive treatment (ECT)**    Use of electric current to induce convulsive seizures. Most effective in the treatment of depression. Introduced by Cerletti and Bini in the mid-1930s. Modifications are electronarcosis, which produces sleeplike states, and electrostimulation, which avoids convulsions. Used with anesthetics and muscle relaxants.

**endorphin**    A naturally produced chemical with morphinelike action; usually found in the brain and associated with the relief of pain. May be the body's own protection against pain.

**enzyme**   An organic compound that interacts with a biologic substrate to form a new chemical, either commonly through the process of synthesis or through degradation. For example, the enzyme monoamine oxidase degrades biogenic amines.

**epinephrine**   One of the catecholamines secreted by the adrenal gland and by fibers of the sympathetic nervous system. It is responsible for many of the physical manifestations of fear and anxiety. Also known as adrenaline.

**extrapyramidal syndrome**   A variety of signs and symptoms, including muscular rigidity, tremors, drooling, shuffling gait (parkinsonism); restlessness (akathisia); peculiar involuntary postures (dystonia); motor inertia (akinesia); and many other neurologic disturbances. Results from dysfunction of the extrapyramidal system. May occur as a reversible side effect of certain psychotropic drugs, particularly phenothiazines.

## G

**gateway drugs**   Term coined by Robert Dupont, M.D., to describe the three drugs that open up the gate to addiction: alcohol, cocaine, and marijuana.

## H

**hallucination**   A sensory perception in the absence of an actual external stimulus. May occur in any of the senses.

**hallucinogen**   A chemical agent that produces hallucinations.

**homovanillic acid (HVA)**   A principal metabolite of dopamine, a catecholamine found in the brain and other organs.

**5HIAA (5-hydroxyindoleacetic acid)**   A major metabolite of serotonin, a biogenic amine found in the brain and other organs. Functional deficits of serotonin in the central nervous system have been implicated in certain types of major mood disorders.

**hypersomnia**   Excessive amount of sleep, sometimes associated with confusion on waking.

## I

**indolamine**   One of a group of biogenic amines, e.g., serotonin, that contains an indole ring and amine group within its chemical structure.

**insomnia**   Inability to fall asleep, difficulty staying asleep, and/or early morning awakening.

# L

**locus coeruleus**    A small area in the brain stem that is considered to be a key brain center for anxiety and fear.

**LSD (lysergic acid diethylamide)**    A potent hallucinogen that produces psychotic symptoms and behavior. Symptoms may include hallucinations, illusions, body and time-space distortions, and, less commonly, intense panic or mystical experiences.

# M

**maintenance drug therapy**    Reducing the dosage of a therapeutic drug after it has reached its maximum efficacy and sustaining it at the minimum level to prevent a relapse.

**major affective disorders**    In DSM-III-R a group of disorders in which there is a prominent and persistent disturbance of mood (depression or mania) and a full syndrome of associated symptoms. The category includes bipolar disorder and major depression. The disorders are usually episodic but could be chronic. In DSM-III-R, the term *major affective disorders* has been changed to *mood disorders* and is divided into *bipolar* and *depressive disorders*.

**mania**    A mood disorder characterized by excessive elation, hyperactivity, agitation, and accelerated thinking and speaking. Sometimes manifested as flight of ideas. Mania is seen in mood disorders and in certain organic mental disorders.

**manic-depressive illness**    A term often used synonymously with bipolar disorder, as defined in DSM-III-R.

**marijuana**    Dried leaves and flowers of *Cannabis sativa* that induce somatic and psychic changes when smoked or ingested in sufficient quantity.

**mental status examination**    The process of estimating psychologic and behavioral function by observing the patient, eliciting his description of self, and formally questioning him. Included in the examination are:

1. evaluation and assessment of any psychiatric condition present, including provisional diagnosis and prognosis, determination of degree of impairment, suitability for treatment, and indications for particular types of therapeutic intervention;

2. formulation of the personality structure of the subject, which may suggest the historical and developmental antecedents of whatever psychiatric condition exists;

3. estimation of the ability and willingness to participate appropriately in treatment. The mental status is reported in a series of narrative statements describing such things as affect, speech, thought content, perception, and cognitive functions. The mental status examination is part of the general examination of all patients, although it may be markedly abbreviated in the absence of psychopathology.

**mescaline**  An alkaloid originally derived from the peyote cactus, resembling amphetamine and adrenaline chemically; used to induce altered perceptions. Also used by Indians of the Southwest in religious rites.

**monoamine oxidase (MAO)**  An enzyme that breaks down biogenic amines (neurotransmitters), rendering them inactive. Found in many body organs, including the brain. Inhibition of this enzyme by certain antidepressant drugs (MAOIs) may result in alleviation of depressed states. *See also* **biogenic amines**.

**monoamine oxidase inhibitor (MAOI)**  A group of antidepressant drugs that inhibit the enzyme monoamine oxidase in the brain and raise the levels of biogenic amines.

**mood**  A pervasive and sustained emotion that, in the extreme, markedly colors one's perception of the world. Common examples of mood include depression, elation, and anger. *See also* **affect**.

# N

**narcotic**  Any opiate derivative drug, natural or synthetic, that relieves pain or alters mood.

**narcotic-blocking drugs (narcotic antagonists)**  Agents structurally similar to the opiates and probably occupying the same receptor sites in the central nervous system. In sufficient doses, they block the effects of opiate drugs by competing for their receptor sites. If given after opiate dependence has developed, they will precipitate an acute abstinence syndrome.

**neuroleptic malignant syndrome**  A rare, idiosyncratic, and sometimes fatal reaction to high-potency neuroleptic drugs; most likely a result of dopamine blockade on the basal ganglia and hypothalamus. Symptoms include muscle rigidity and high fever.

**neuroreceptors**  Binding sites in the central nervous system for psychoactive drugs.

**neurotransmitter**  A chemical found in the nervous system (e.g., dopamine, norepinephrine, and serotonin) that facilitates the transmission of impulses across synapses between neurons. Disorders in the brain physiology of neurotransmitters have been implicated in the pathogenesis of several psychiatric illnesses, particularly major affective disorders and schizophrenia.

**norepinephrine**  A catecholamine neurotransmitter related to epinephrine. It is found in both the peripheral and central nervous systems. Functional excesses in the brain have been implicated in the pathogenesis of manic states; deficits, in certain depressive states. Also called noradrenaline. *See also* **biogenic amines**.

# O

**opiate**   Any chemical derived from opium; relieves pain and produces a sense of well-being.

**orphan drugs**   Drugs that the pharmaceutical companies do not wish to develop either because they cannot be patented (e.g., lithium), because they are used only in rare conditions by very few people, or for a variety of legitimate economic reasons. In such cases, the federal government will work with the companies to make the drugs available to those who need them.

# P

**panic disorder**   Discrete periods of intense fear or discomfort. Listed in DSM-III-R as an anxiety disorder, with or without agoraphobia.

**parasympathetic nervous system**   The part of the autonomic nervous system that controls the life-sustaining organs of the body under normal, danger-free conditions. *See also* **sympathetic nervous system**.

**parkinsonism**   A neurologic disorder characterized by rapid, coarse tremor, pill-rolling movements, masklike facies, cogwheel rigidity, drooling, akinesia, bradykinesia, or gait disturbances. Associated with dopamine depletion in the basal ganglia. *See also* **drug-induced parkinsonism**.

**phobia**   An obsessive, persistent, unrealistic, intense fear of an object or situation. The fear is believed to arise through a process of displacing an internal (unconscious) conflict to an external object symbolically related to the conflict.

**placebo**   A material without pharmacologic activity but identical in appearance to an active drug. Used in pharmacologic research as a method of determining the actual effects of the drug being tested.

**polysomnography**   The all-night recording of a variety of physiologic parameters (e.g., brain waves, eye movements, muscle tonus, respiration, heart rate, penile tumescence) in order to diagnose sleep-related disorders.

**prolactin**   A hormone secreted by the pituitary that promotes lactation in the female and may stimulate testosterone secretion in the male. Prolactin secretion is in part controlled by inhibiting and releasing factors in the brain. Because dopamine is involved in the brain's inhibition of prolactin secretion, the measurement of serum prolactin has been proposed as a way of judging the efficacy of specific antipsychotic drugs that have been thought to act primarily by blocking dopamine's effects.

**psychomotor retardation**   A generalized slowing of physical and emotional reactions. Specifically, the slowing of movements such as eye-blinking; frequently seen in depression.

**psychopharmacology**   The study of the effects of psychoactive drugs on behavior in both animals and people. Clinical psychopharmacology more specifically includes both the study of drug effects in patients and the expert use of drugs in the treatment of psychiatric conditions.

**psychosis**   A major mental disorder of organic or emotional origin in which a person's ability to think, respond emotionally, remember, communicate, interpret reality, and behave appropriately is sufficiently impaired so as to interfere grossly with the capacity to meet the ordinary demands of life. Often characterized by regressive behavior, inappropriate mood, diminished impulse control, and such abnormal mental content as delusions and hallucinations. The term is applicable to conditions having a wide range of severity and duration.

**R**

**receptor**   A specialized area on a nerve membrane, blood vessel, or muscle that receives the chemical stimulation that activates or inhibits the nerve, blood vessel, or muscle.

**S**

**schizophrenia**   A large group of disorders, usually of psychotic proportion, manifested by characteristic disturbances of language and communication, thought, perception, affect, and behavior that last longer than six months. Thought disturbances are marked by alterations of concept formation that may lead to misinterpretation of reality, misperceptions, and sometimes to delusions and hallucinations. Mood changes include ambivalence, blunting, inappropriateness, and loss of empathy with others. Behavior may be withdrawn, regressive, and bizarre.

**serotonin**   A neurotransmitter with an indole structure found both in peripheral ganglia and in the central nervous system. Its transmitter functions in the central nervous system are less clearly demonstrable than in the gastrointestinal tract. It is implicated indirectly in the psychobiology of depression. *See also* **biogenic amines**.

**sympathetic nervous system**   The part of the autonomic nervous system that responds to dangerous or threatening situations by preparing a person physiologically for "fight or flight." *See also* **parasympathetic nervous system**.

**synapse**   The gap between the membrane of one nerve cell and the membrane of another. The synapse is the point at which the transmission of nerve impulses occurs.

**T**

**tardive dyskinesia**   Literally, "late-appearing abnormal movements"; a variable complex of choreiform or athetoid movements developing in patients exposed to antipsychotic drugs. Typical movements include tongue-writhing, -chewing, or -protrusion, lip-puckering, choreiform finger movements, toe and ankle movements, leg-jiggling, or movements of neck, trunk, and pelvis. These movements may be either mild or severe and may occur singly or in many combinations and permutations. These movements may be produced as an adverse effect of antipsychotic medication.

**therapeutic window**    The well-defined range of blood levels associated with optimal clinical response to antidepressant drugs, such as nortriptyline. Levels above or below that range are associated with a poor response.

**toxic psychosis**    An organic mental disorder caused by the poisonous effect of chemicals or drugs.

**tranquilizer**    A drug that decreases anxiety and agitation. Preferred terms are antianxiety and antipsychotic drugs.

**tyramine**    A sympathomimetic amine that acts by displacing stored transmitter from adrenergic axonal terminals; a constituent of many foods such as flat beans, cheese, red wine, etc., which are forbidden when using monoamine oxidase inhibitors because of hypertensive crisis.

# W

**Wernicke-Korsakoff syndrome**    A disease of central nervous system metabolism due to a lack of vitamin $B_1$ (thiamine) seen in chronic alcoholism. Wernicke's disease features irregularities of eye movements, incoordination, impaired thinking, and often sensorimotor deficits. Korsakoff's psychosis is characterized by confabulation and, more important, by a short-term, but not immediate, disturbance that leads to gross impairment in memory and learning. Wernicke's disease and Korsakoff's psychosis begin suddenly and are often found in the same person simultaneously.

**withdrawal symptoms**    Physical and mental effects of withdrawing addictive substances from patients who have become habituated to them. The physical symptoms may include vomiting, tremors, abdominal pain, delirium, and convulsions.

# Index

Page numbers in **bold** type refer to Individual Drug Listings.

# About the Authors

## Stuart C. Yudofsky, M.D.

Stuart C. Yudofsky, M.D. is the D.C. and Irene Ellwood Professor and Chairman of the Department of Psychiatry and Behavioral Sciences of the Baylor College of Medicine in Houston, Texas. He is also the Director of Psychiatry of The Methodist Hospital in Houston. Prior to his current position he was Professor and Chairman of the Department of Psychiatry of the University of Chicago and Director of Psychiatry of the Univesity of Chicago Hospitals. He has held numerous posts at Columbia University College of Physicians and Surgeons including Associate Professor of Clinical Psychiatry, Associate Director of Psychiatric Services at Columbia Presbyterian Medical Center, and Vice Chairman of the Department of Psychiatry. Dr. Yudofsky has also served as Clinical Director and Deputy Director of the New York State Psychiatric Institute, Director of the Department of Psychiatry at Allegheny General Hospital, and Director of Psychiatric Research at the Allegheny Singer Research Institue in Pittsburg. Dr. Yudofsky's area of academic interest is biologic psychiatry, particularly neurospsychiatry, which focuses on psychiatric concomitants of such neurological illnesses as head injury, Alzheimer's disease, stroke, and seizure disorders. His research involves psychopharmacologic treatment of aggressive disorders. He is Chairman of the American Psychiatric Association's Task Force on traumatic brain injury and is Editor in Chief of the *Journal of Neuropshychiatry and Clinical Neurosciences.*

# Robert E. Hales, M.D.

Robert E. Hales, M.D., M.B.A., is the Chairman, Department of Psychiatry, California Pacific Medical Center. He is a Clinical Professor of Psychiatry at the University of California, San Francisco, and at Georgetown University in Washington, D.C. Dr. Hales is President of the Association for Academic Psychiatry. He is the author or editor of over 100 Scientific articles, book chapters, and books, and is co-editor of the *American Psychiatric Press Textbook of Psychiatry* and the *American Psychiatric Press Texbook of Neuropsychiatry, Second Edition*. Dr. Hales is Deputy Editor of the *Journal of Neuropsychiatry and Clinical Neurosciences* and is a member of the editorial boards of *Academic Psychiatry, Hospital and Community Psychiatry*, and the American Psychiatric Press. He is the past chairman of the American Psychiatric Association's (APA) Scientific Program Committee, and is a member of the APA's Task Force on DSM-IV and Task Force on traumatic brain injury. He is also Chair of the American College of Psychiatrists' Committee on the Scientific Program.

# Tom Ferguson, M.D.

Tom Ferguson, M.D. is President of Self-Care Productions in Austin, Texas. He received his M.D. degree from the Yale Universtiy School of Medicine. He is the founding editor of the journal *Medical Self-Care*, and is founder and Editor-in-Chief of the *SelfCare Catalog*. He also served as the medical editor of the *Whole Earth Catalog*.

Dr. Ferguson has received the National Educational Press Association's Distinguished Achievement Award and the Lifetime Extension Award for his writings on the rapidly expanding field of self-help and self-care. His work has been cited by author John Naisbitt in the book *Megatrends* as representing "the essence of the shift from institutional help to self-help." He has appeared on *60 Minutes*, the *Today Show*, and the *Cable News Network* as an expert on self-care and self-help.

Dr. Ferguson's most recent books include *The No-Nag, No-Guilt, Do-It-Your-Own-Way Guide to Quitting Smoking; Hidden Guilt: How to Stop Punishing Yourself and Enjoy the Happiness You Deserve* (with Lewis Engel); *Helping Smokers Get Ready to Quit: A Positive Approach to Smoking Cessation;* and *The Stethoscope Book & Kit* (with Linda Allison).

# Reader Feedback

We have learned a great deal from our patients, and we hope to learn a great deal from our readers as well. We welcome your comments and criticisms.

You can help us improve the next edition by telling us how you used this book. Even more important, please let us know how we can make it more useful.

We will be very grateful for any comments. Please send all responses to:

Stuart Yudofsky, M.D.
Robert Hales, M.D.
Tom Ferguson, M.D.
c/o Grove Weidenfeld
841 Broadway
New York, NY 10003